INTRAOPERATIVE IRRADIATION

CURRENT CLINICAL ONCOLOGY

Maurie Markman, MD, PhD SERIES EDITOR

INTRAOPERATIVE IRRADIATION

Techniques and Results

Edited by

LEONARD L. GUNDERSON, MD, MS
Mayo Foundation and Mayo Medical School, Rochester, MN

CHRISTOPHER G. WILLET, MD
Harvard Medical School and Massachusetts General Hospital, Boston, MA

LOUIS B. HARRISON, MD
Albert Einstein College of Medicine and Beth Israel Cancer Center, New York, NY

FELIPE A. CALVO, MD
University Hospital Gregorio Marañón, Madrid, Spain

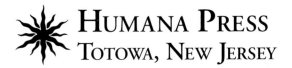

HUMANA PRESS
TOTOWA, NEW JERSEY

Library of Congress Cataloging-in-Publication Data

Intraoperative irradiation : techniques and results / edited by L. Gunderson ... [et al.]
           p.   cm.—(Current clinical oncology ; 1)
      Includes index.
      ISBN 0-89603-523-9 (alk. paper)
      1. Cancer—Intraoperative radiotherapy. I. Gunderson, Leonard L. II. Series: Current clinical oncology (Totowa, N.J.)
      [DNLM: 1. Neoplasms—radiotherapy. 2. Intraoperative Care—methods. 3. Brachytherapy—methods. 4. Radio therapy Dosage. 5. Electrons—therapeutic use. QZ 269 I63 1999]
      RD652.I567 1999
      616.99'40642—dc21
      DNLM/DLC   98-50919
      for Library of Congress   CIP

Dedications

To my wife and eternal partner Katheryn,
  for her love and unfailing support of this project and throughout my career in medicine.

To my secretary Pam Speltz and to the Mayo Central Typing Pool,
  for their Herculean efforts in the preparation of this textbook.

To my colleagues at MGH and Mayo,
  for the opportunity to work as a team to develop and nurture IORT as a component of
  treatment for the past 20 years and in caring for the physical and spiritual needs of our patients.

To the Master Healer,
  for insight into the understanding of and treatment for human malignancy.
                    Leonard L. Gunderson

To my wife (Mary Sunday), children (Elizabeth, Julian, and Andrew), and parents (Alice and Bernanrd)
  for their love and suuport,

To Herman D. Suit, physician, scientist and mentor,
  whose wisdom and insight have improved the care of the cancer patient.
                    Christopher G. Willett

To my wife Ilene and to the rest of my family,
  Robert Tatiner, Lillian and Seymour Harrison, Ellen, and Tammy Harrison,
  thanks for all your love and understanding.

To my children, Barbara and Michelle, to whom I dedicate this book,
  who constantly make me focus on what is truly important in life.

To the administration and my colleagues at Memorial Sloan Kettering Cancer Center,
  Drs. Zvi Fuks, Warren Enker, Lowell Anderson, Murray Brennan, Alfred Cohen, Florence
  Grant, and Bruce Minsky, who provided resources, encouragement, essential input and
  involvement into the development of high dose rate intraoperative irradiation (HDR-IORT) at
  MSKCC.

To Beth Israel Medical Center and St Luke's Roosevelt Hospital Center,
  who have provided enormous resources and encouragement to continue and expand the HDR-
  IORT program in our new department.
                    Louis B. Harrison

To my family: wife Marta and daughters Almudena, Martita, Maria and Covadonga; beloved
  parents Lucia and Felipe, brother Elpidio and sister Tuti,
  my first love, the school of values in which I learned to serve society

To my teachers, especially Drs. José Otero and Luther W. Brady,
  with deep gratitude for the privilege of superb and caring education

To all of my colleagues involved in IORT procedures during the last two decades,
  for their committment to excellence in cancer medicine.
                    Felipe A. Calvo

To the editing staff at Humana Press, especially James Geronimo and Paul Dolgert,
  who have done an excellent job in collating and producing this textbook; it has been a pleasure to interact
  with them in this effort.

PREFACE

Intraoperative Irradiation: Techniques and Results is a comprehensive textbook on intraoperative irradiation (IORT) that covers topics of interest to those working in either intraoperative electrons (IOERT) or high-dose-rate brachytherapy (HDR-IORT), or both. Issues of basic science and physics are covered in addition to techniques, indications, and results by disease-site. This volume is intended for surgeons, radiation oncologists, physicists, anesthesiologists, medical oncologists, and all others involved either in the procedural component of IORT (for instance, radiation therapists and operating room nurses) or in the care of patients with cancer (for instance, internists and nurses). Most disease-site chapters have multinational coauthors and both radiation oncologists and surgeons, which provides a balanced presentation of techniques and results by disease-site and increases the international scope of this book.

Intraoperative Irradiation: Techniques and Results is divided into five major sections. The book begins with chapters on the general rationale for and historical perspectives of IORT and the radiobiology of IORT, and proceeds to a discussion of methods and techniques of treatment, a presentation of normal tissue/organ tolerance to IORT, techniques and results by disease-site, and conclusions and future possibilities.

The rationale for using IORT as a component of treatment is based on the realization that techniques that deliver adequate doses of external beam irradiation (EBRT) often cannot achieve dose levels adequate for local control with reasonable tolerance even with conformal 3-D techniques. As an example, for patients with locally advanced abdominal or pelvic malignancies in whom all disease cannot be surgically removed with negative margins, external beam irradiation (EBRT) by itself or in conjuction with chemotherapy is usually only palliative because EBRT doses greater than 45–50 Gy in 25–28 fractions often cannot be delivered safely owing to the presence of dose-limiting normal structures (stomach, small intestine, liver, kidneys). If doses of 65–70 Gy were attempted to achieve local control, severe treatment-related complications might result that could require hospitalization and operative intervention. A preferred treatment approach is to administer tolerable EBRT doses of 45–50 Gy preoperatively (1.8–2 Gy fractions), often in conjunction with concomitant chemotherapy, and deliver the remaining irradiation as an IORT supplement at the time of surgical exploration and maximal resection. The IORT component of treatment then becomes the optimal conformal irradiation technique, since dose-limiting normal organs such as stomach and small intestine can be surgically displaced while IORT is delivered to the high-risk region of narrow surgical margin or proven residual disease. The high-dose IORT volume is smaller than what could be delivered with any EBRT technique, as is given with appositional IOERT or HDR-IORT applicators.

Methods and techniques of IORT treatment are discussed in Section II in a group of five chapters. Surgical and irradiation philosophies and techniques (EBRT/IORT) are discussed as they apply to IORT in general, and physics aspects of IORT are presented with regard to both IOERT and HDR-IORT. The physics chapters contain practical information concerning issues of dosimetry and applicator design as well as more esoteric factors of facility construction and shielding (for those contemplating a new or retrofitted facility) and specialized equipment (mobile IOERT machine—Mobetron and Novac-7). The technique chapters include discussions of appropriate interactions between surgeon, radiation oncologist, and anesthesiologist; applicator selection for both IOERT and HDR-IORT; energy and dose of IOERT and HDR-IORT dose based on amount of residual disease after maximal resection and other factors of interest to both the surgeon and radiation oncologist. Figures are used amply to discuss some of the above issues. Chapter 7 is a unique, balanced discussion of the comparative advantages and disadvantages of IOERT, HDR-IORT, and perioperative brachytherapy with a senior author whose institution utilizes all three techniques and coauthors being the coeditors of the textbook who have vast experience with IOERT or HDR-IORT (+/- perioperative brachytherapy). The conclusion of the chapter is that large institutions would best serve their patients by having at least two of the three options available in an operating room setting.

Section III contains three chapters that discuss normal tissue tolerance to IORT. Single institution results from NCI and Colorado State University (CSU) present animal tolerance data in a vast array of organs or structures (separate chapters from each institution that also include data from other animal series and some human data as well). The NCI animal data are based totally on the use of single-dose IORT, while the CSU data include invaluable information concerning relative tolerance with EBRT alone (60, 70, or 80 Gy delivered in 30 fractions over 6 wk) vs IORT alone (17.5–55 Gy) vs EBRT plus IORT (EBRT of 50 Gy/ 25 fractions; IORT of 10–47.5 Gy). The remaining chapter contains both animal and human data on the tolerance of peripheral nerve, which is the dose-limiting structure for IORT. These three chapters are essential reading for any individuals who are contemplating a program involving IORT, as the implications of tolerance are far reaching for the patients who will receive IORT as well as for the physicians involved in the delivery of IORT.

The largest section contains the disease-site chapters on every disease-site in which potential merit for IORT has been demonstrated in one or more institutions or countries. Disease-specific treatment factors are presented by the radiation oncology and surgeon coauthors. Results with standard non-IORT treatment are presented for most chapters as a basis for comparing results when IORT is used as a component of treatment. Treatment outcomes data include disease control (local and distant) survival (disease-free and overall) and treatment tolerance. Seven of the 18 disease-site chapters relate to GI cancers (three chapters on colorectal cancer and separate chapters on gastric, pancreatic, biliary tract, and liver); five of the seven chapters contain data with IOERT techniques and four of the seven contain data on either HDR-IORT or perioperative brachytherapy. The remaining 11 disease-site chapters include four on sarcomas (separate chapters on either IOERT or HDR-IORT for retroperitoneal/pelvic sarcoma, IOERT for bone sarcomas, IOERT or perioperative brachytherapy for extremity sarcomas) and single chapters on gynecologic, genitourinary, lung, head/neck, pediatric, CNS, and breast malignancies.

The closing section is a chapter on conclusions and future possibilities written by the four coeditors. The conclusion is that experience has shown that variable combinations of EBRT, IORT (IOERT or HDR-IORT), and maximal surgical resection are feasible and practical in settings where close interdisciplinary cooperation exists. Furthermore, these aggressive approaches that include IORT appear to improve significantly local control, if not survival, in a large number of disease sites when compared to results achieved with standard treatment approaches. However, when gross residual or unresectable disease remains in spite of attempts at a gross total resection or when patients have received prior EBRT in an adjuvant setting, the ability to achieve central or local control is lessened, thus creating the need for prospective trials that address the addition of radiation dose modifiers (sensitizers, hyperthermia, etc.) during both EBRT and IORT. The patients with locally advanced disease who are ideal candidates for the locally aggressive approaches often have moderate to high systemic risks as well. Prospective trials are therefore indicated to address the addition of systemic therapy to optimal locally aggressive combined treatment. Finally, the issue of peripheral nerve tolerance could be addressed by prospective phase II and III studies that evaluate the issue of improving nerve tolerance with the addition of the radioprotector Amifostine. This chapter also includes a discussion on improvements in technology that make IORT more feasible in a larger number of institutions and will facilitate the conduct of the previously mentioned trials (HDR-brachytherapy equipment that can be used in either an outpatient or operating room setting; mobile IOERT equipment including Mobetron and Novac-7).

The editors are indebted to the many international experts who participated in this project as either the primary author or co-authors. As a result of their superb efforts, *Intraoperative Irradiation:* Techniques and Results should be an appropriate resource and reference book for many years to come. The myriad of prospective trials that are indicated to test issues of optimized local control, distant control and tolerance will be best carried out in the setting of a multi-institutional international cooperative group that is reflected in the authorship of this volume.

Leonard L. Gunderson
Christopher G. Willett
Louis B. Harrison
Felipe A. Calvo

CONTENTS

CONTRIBUTORS

SANTIAGO AMILLO, MD, *Department of Orthopedic Surgery, Clínica Universitaria de Navarra, Pamplona, Spain*

LOWELL L. ANDERSON, PhD, *Department of Medical Physics, Memorial Sloan-Kettering Cancer Center, New York, NY*

JAVIER ARISTU, MD, *Department of Oncology, Clínica Universitaria de Navarra, Pamplona, Spain*

IGNACIO AZINOVIC, MD, *Department of Oncology, Clínica Universitaria de Navarra, Pamplona, Spain*

JOYCE A. BATTLE, MD, *Department of Radiation Therapy, Medical College of Ohio, Toledo, OH*

JOSE M. BERIAN, MD, *Department of Urology, Clínica Universitaria de Navarra, Pamplona, Spain*

PETER J. BIGGS, PhD, *Department of Radiation Oncology, Massachusetts General Hospital, Boston, MA*

MURRAY F. BRENNAN, MD, *Department of Surgery, Memorial Sloan Kettering Cancer Center, New York, NY*

PAUL M. BUSSE, MD, PhD, *Joint Center for Radiation Therapy and Harvard Medical School, Boston, MA*

J. C. BUSTOS, MD, *Department of Neurological Surgery, San Francisco de Asís Hospital, Madrid, Spain*

D. CARTER, MD, PhD, *Department of Neurological Surgery, Medical College of Ohio, Toledo, OH*

FELIPE A. CALVO, MD, *Chair of Oncology, University Hospital Gregorio Marañón, Madrid, Spain*

JOSÉ CAÑADELL, MD, *Department of Orthopedic Surgery, Clínica Universitaria de Navarra, Pamplona, Spain*

YUHCHYAW CHEN, MD, PhD, *Department of Radiation Oncology, University of Rochester School of Medicine, Rochester, NY*

JAVIER A. CIENFUEGOS, MD, *General and Digestive Surgery, Clínica Universitaria de Navarra, Pamplona, Spain*

ALFRED M. COHEN, MD, *Colorectal Service, Department of Surgery, Memorial Sloan Kettering Cancer Center, and Department of Surgery, Cornell University Medical College, New York, NY*

RALPH R. DOBELBOWER, MD, PhD, *Department of Radiation Therapy, Medical College of Ohio, Toledo, OH*

JOHN DONOHUE, MD, *Department of General Surgery, Mayo Clinic and Mayo Medical School, Rochester, MN*

ANATOLY DRITSCHILO, MD, *Department of Radiation Medicine, Vincent T. Lombardi Cancer Center, Georgetown University Hospital, Washington, DC*

JEAN-BERNARD DUBOIS, MD, *Department of Radiotherapy, Centre Regional de Lutte Contre le Cancer, Montpellier, France*

MICHAEL EBLE, MD, *Department of Radiation Oncology, University Hospital Heidelberg, Heidelberg, Germany*

WARREN E. ENKER, MD, *Colorectal Service, Department of Surgery, Beth Israel Medical Center, New York, NY and Department of Surgery, Albert Einstein College of Medicine, Bronx, NY*

DOUGLAS B. EVANS, MD, *Department of Surgical Oncology, The University of Texas M. D. Anderson Cancer Center, Houston, TX*

SCOTT FISHER, MD, *Department of Radiation Oncology, Allegheny University Hospitals: Graduate Hospital, Philadelphia, PA*

ROBERT L. FOOTE, MD, *Radiation Oncology, Department of Oncology, Mayo Clinic, Rochester, MN*

PETER GARRETT, MD, *Radiation Oncology, Methodist Hospital, Indianapolis, IN*

JEAN P. GERARD, MD, *Chair of Radiation Oncology, Centre Hospital, Lyon, France*

HOLGER L. GIESCHEN,MD, *Department of Radiation Oncology, Massachusetts General Hospital and Harvard Medical School, Boston, MA*

EDWARD L. GILLETTE, DVM, PhD, *Department of Radiological Health Sciences, Veterinary Teaching Hospital, Colorado State University, Fort Collins, CO*

SHARON M. GILLETTE, DVM, PhD, *Department of Radiological Health Sciences, Veterinary Teaching Hospital, Colorado State University, Fort Collins, CO*

LEONARD L. GUNDERSON, MS, MS, *Professor and Chair of Oncology, Mayo Clinic and Mayo Medical School, Rochester, MN*

F. GUILLEMIN, MD, *Department of General Surgery, Centre A. Vautrin, Nancy, France*

GERALD M. HAASE, MD, *Department of Pediatric Surgery, The Children's Hospital, Denver, CO*

MICHAEL G. HADDOCK, MD, *Radiation Oncology, Department of Oncology, Mayo Clinic and Mayo Medical School, Rochester, MN*

PATRICK J. HARRINGTON, PhD, *Department of Medical Physics, Memorial Sloan-Kettering Cancer Center, New York, NY*

LOUIS B. HARRISON, MD, *Department of Radiation Oncology, Beth Israel Health Care System, and Beth Israel Cancer Center, New York, NY*

HARALD J. HOEKSTRA, MD, PhD, *Department of Surgical Oncology, University Hospital Groningen, The Netherlands*

PETER A. S. JOHNSTONE, MD, *National Cancer Institute, National Institutes of Health, Bethesda, MD*

TIMOTHY J. KINSELLA, MD, MS, *Chair of Radiation Oncology, University Hospitals, Cleveland, OH*

HANS J. KRAMLING, MD, *Department of Surgery, Ludwig Maximilians University, Klinikum Grosshadenn, Munich, Germany*

EDWIN C. MCCULLOUGH, PhD, *Radiation Oncology, Department of Oncology, Mayo Clinic and Mayo Medical School, Rochester, MN*

RAFAEL MARTINEZ-MONGE, MD, PhD, *Department of Oncology, University Clinic of Navarra, Pamplona, Spain*

THOMAS E. MERCHANT, DO, PhD, *Department of Radiation Oncology, St. Jude's Childrens Hospital, Memphis, TN*

HOLLIS W. MERRICK,MD, MS, *Department of Surgery, Medical College of Ohio, Toledo, OH*

THOMAS V. MCCAFFREY, MD, PhD, *Department of Ear, Nose, and Throat Surgery, Mayo Clinic and Mayo Medical School, Rochester, MN*

BRUCE D. MINSKY, MD, *Department of Radiation Oncology, Memorial Sloan Kettering Cancer Center and Department of Radiation Oncology in Medicine, Cornell University Medical College, New York, NY*

SUBIR NAG, MD, *Division of Radiation Oncology, Arthur G. James Cancer Hospital and Research Institute, The Ohio State University, Columbus, OH*

DAVID NAGORNEY, MD, *Department of Surgery, Mayo Clinic and Mayo Medical School, Rochester, MN*

HEIDI NELSON, MD, *Colorectal Surgery, Mayo Clinic and Mayo Medical School, Rochester, MN*

PAUL OKUNIEFF, MD, *Chair of Radiation Oncology, University of Rochester School of Medicine and Dentistry, Rochester, NY*

D. ORTIZ DE URBINA, MD, *Department of Radiation Oncology, San Francisco de Asís Hospital, Madrid, Spain*

S. PALKOVIC, MD, *Klinik und Poliklinik für Stralentherapie, Universität Münster, Germany*

IVY A. PETERSEN, MD, *Radiation Oncology, Department of Oncology, Mayo Clinic and Mayo Medical School, Rochester, MN*

BARBARA E. POWERS, DVM, PhD, *Radiological Health Sciences, Colorado State University, Fort Collins, CO*

DOUGLAS J. PRITCHARD, MD, *Orthopedic Oncology, Department of Orthopedics, Mayo Clinic and Mayo Medical School, Rochester, MN*

WILLIAM RATE, MD, PhD, *Department of Radiation Oncology, Methodist Hospital of Indiana, Indianapolis, IN*

CATHERINE L. SALEM, MD, *Department of Radiation Medicine, Vincent T. Lombardi Cancer Center, Georgetown University Hospital, Washington, DC*

MANUEL SANTOS, MD, *Department of Radiation Oncology, San Francisco de Asís Hospital, Madrid, Spain*

THIERRY SCHMITT, MD, *Service de Radiotherapie, CHU Bellevue, Saint-Etienne, France*

PAULA J. SCHOMBERG, MD, *Chair of Radiation Oncology, Mayo Clinic and Mayo Medical School, Rochester, MN*

PAUL C. SHELLITO, MD, *Department of Surgery, Massachusetts General Hospital, and Harvard Medical School, Boston, MA*

LUIS SIERRASESUMAGA, MD, *Department of Pediatrics, Clínica Universitaria de Navarra, Pamplona, Spain*

WILLIAM F. SINDELAR, MD, PhD, *Department of Surgery, Good Samaritan Hospital of Maryland, Baltimore, MD*

IRA J. SPIRO, MD, PhD, *Department of Radiation Oncology, Massachusetts General Hospital and Harvard Medical School, Boston, MA*

JEAN ST. GERMAIN, MS, *Department of Medical Physics, Memorial Sloan-Kettering Cancer Center, New York, NY*

SRINATH SUNDARARAMAN, MD, *Radiation Oncology Branch, NCI, Bethesda, MD*

JOEL E. TEPPER, MD, *Chair of Radiation Oncology, University of North Carolina School of Medicine, Chapel Hill, NC*

PAULA M. TERMUHLEN, MD, *Department of Surgical Oncology, The University of Texas M. D. Anderson Cancer Center, Houston, TX*

TAKESHI TODOROKI, MD, *Department of Surgery, Institute of Clinical Medicine, University of Tsukuba, Japan*

KJELL M. TVIET, MD, *Department of Medical Oncology and Radiotherapy, Norwegian Radium Hospital, Oslo, Norway*

CAROL WHITE, *Department of Radiation Oncology, Beth Israel Medical Center, New York, NY*

CHRISTOPHER G. WILLETT, MD, *Department of Radiation Oncology, Massachusetts General Hospital and Harvard Medical School, Boston, MA*

NORMAN WILLICH, MD, *Klinik und Poliklinik für Stralentherapie, Westfälische Wilhems Universität Münster, Germany*

TIMOTHY O. WILSON, MD, *Gynecologic Oncology, Department of Gynecology, Mayo Clinic and Mayo Medical School, Rochester, MN*

HORST ZINCKE, MD, *Department of Urology, Mayo Clinic and Mayo Medical School, Rochester, MN*

I

GENERAL RATIONALE AND HISTORICAL PERSPECTIVE

1

General Rationale and Historical Perspective of Intraoperative Irradiation

Leonard L. Gunderson, Felipe A. Calvo, Christopher G. Willett, Louis B. Harrison, and Manuel Santos

CONTENTS

1. INTRODUCTION

Most of the major advances in clinical applications of radiation therapy in the treatment of cancer have been because of differences in dose distribution between tumor and normal tissue. For most tumor types, the likelihood of achieving local tumor control improves if increasing irradiation doses can be delivered to the tumor mass. However, in many clinical situations, the dose that can be delivered safely to the tumor volume is limited by the normal tissues that are in close proximity to the tumor.

Intraoperative irradiation (IORT) in its broadest sense refers to the delivery of irradiation at the time of an operation. This text will discuss the rationale for and results of both intraoperative electrons (IOERT) and intraoperative high-dose-rate brachytherapy (HDR-IORT) when used in conjunction with surgical exploration and resection with or without external-beam irradiation (EBRT) and chemotherapy. Both IORT methods evolved with similar philosophies as an attempt to achieve higher effective doses of irradiation while dose-limiting structures are surgically displaced. After current results and future possibilities are presented for major disease sites, the discussion will center on the future of IORT, including applications and evolution in delivery systems.

From: *Current Clinical Oncology: Intraoperative Irradiation: Techniques and Results*
Edited by: L. L. Gunderson et al. © Humana Press, Inc., Totowa, NJ

2. RATIONALE FOR IORT (IOERT OR IOHDR)

In view of dose limitations of EBRT, IOERT and HDR-IORT have been employed in an attempt to improve the therapeutic ratio of local control complications. In Japanese IOERT trials instituted in the 1960s (1), as well as early United States trials (2), IOERT was usually the sole irradiation modality. Investigators delivered single doses of 20–40 Gy to the site of interest with electron beams and rarely used supplemental EBRT.

Massachusetts General Hospital (MGH) and Mayo Clinic investigators preferred to use IOERT as a "boost" dose in combination with conventional fractionated EBRT with or without chemotherapy and maximal surgical resection as indicated by site (3). This preference was based on several advantages that potentially exist when a combined EBRT–IORT approach is used instead of IORT alone: There is improvement in local/regional control because of a decreased risk of marginal recurrence (areas at risk are included in the EBRT fields) and the radiobiological advantages of fractionated irradiation; and there is less risk of normal tissue damage or necrosis. The excellent long-term results achieved with EBRT plus boost techniques for breast, gynecologic, and head and neck cancers support the concept of this combined approach since good local control is achieved with relatively low morbidity to dose-limiting normal tissues. The only difference is the method of delivering the boost dose. Patients with head and neck and breast lesions require interstitial techniques or fractionated outpatient electrons; gynecologic lesions are treated with an intracavitary technique; IOERT or HDR-IORT are used for intra-abdominal, pelvic, or thoracic lesions.

The combination of IOERT or HDR-IORT with EBRT has the potential to improve the therapeutic ratio of local control vs complications by a multitude of factors. These include a decrease in the volume of the irradiation "boost" field by direct tumor visualization and appositional treatment with IOERT or HDR-IORT; exclusion of all or part of dose-limiting sensitive structures by operative mobilization or shielding and/or the use of appropriate electron-beam energies; and an increase in the "effective" dose by virtue of the prior points. The most ideal setting would be the availability of both IOERT and HDR-IORT in a dedicated IORT suite as exists at Ohio State.

This chapter will discuss the indications for and history of IORT (IOERT, HDR-IORT), patient selection and evaluation, sequencing of EBRT and IORT components of treatment, and guidelines for reporting data from IORT trials. If conventional treatment methods with EBRT, chemotherapy, and surgical resection were providing high local control rates with minimal complications, the addition of IORT as a component of treatment would be unnecessary. Because that is not the situation, there is a need to develop guidelines for determining when the additional treatment is indicated (extent of disease, location, and so on) and what is the best method. General guidelines will be presented in this chapter, and guidelines by disease site will be expanded upon in later chapters.

2.1. EBRT Local Tumor Control or Survival: Selected Disease Sites

The incidence of local relapse with conventional treatment of selected abdominal or pelvic malignancies will be discussed in an attempt to delineate examples in which increased dose may be of benefit or in which there is a need to minimize dose to certain structures. Since the major emphasis with IORT is on gastrointestinal and gynecological carcinomas and retroperitoneal sarcomas, some examples from these tumor sites will be discussed. A more detailed discussion of local control results with standard treatment with or without an IORT supplement will be found in each disease-site chapter.

2.1.1. PANCREAS

For unresectable pancreas cancer, the use of EBRT plus 5-FU-based chemotherapy results in a doubling of median survival (SR) compared with surgical bypass or stents alone (3–6 mo median SR vs 9–13 mo) and an increase in 2-yr SR from 0–5% to 10–20% *(4–6)*. However, 5-yr SR is rare, and local control is low. In a series from Thomas Jefferson University (TJUH) *(6)* with EBRT doses of 60–70 Gy given in 1.8- to 2.0-Gy fractions over 7–8 wk, local failure was still documented in at least two-thirds of the patients. For those treated with EBRT alone, local control was achieved in <20% of patients and with EBRT plus chemotherapy, local control was achieved in approx 30% of patients.

2.1.2. COLORECTAL

EBRT has been combined with resection and chemotherapy for locally advanced colorectal cancers. In separate series from Princess Margaret Hospital (PMH) *(7)* and Mayo Clinic *(8)*, using EBRT alone (PMH, Mayo) or combined with systemic therapy (Mayo), the local relapse rate was >90% in evaluable patients (PMH, primary cancers; Mayo, primary plus locally recurrent). Although a combination of pre- or postoperative EBRT (± 5-FU) with maximal resection for initially unresectable-for-cure cancers produces a local control rate better than no resection, the risk of local relapse remains too high at 30–70% *(9)*. For locally recurrent nonmetastatic rectal cancers, standard treatment with EBRT with or without chemotherapy results in excellent short-term palliation for 6 to 12 mo, but both local control and long-term survival are infrequent (0–5% at 5 yr) *(9)*.

2.1.3. GYNECOLOGIC

A number of centers have treated primary cervical carcinoma patients with metastatic para-aortic nodal disease with EBRT in the hope of producing cures. Although there appears to be definite evidence of the ability to cure a subset of 15–20% of patients if an EBRT dose of 55–60 Gy is employed, the high complication rates in two series *(10,11)* indicate that different radiotherapeutic techniques need to be employed if aggressive treatment to this location is to be done on a large scale.

For patients with relapse in the pelvic sidewalls or para-aortic nodes, salvage therapy results in overall 5-yr SR of 0–5% for endometrial and 2–30% for cervical cancer, according to the size of the relapse. In previously irradiated patients, retreatment with meaningful doses of EBRT is compromised, and utilization of IORT (IOERT or HDR-IORT) as a supplement to low dose EBRT with or without multidrug chemotherapy becomes one of the options available to treat patients with tumor-bed or nodal relapses *(12–16)*.

2.1.4. RETROPERITONEAL SARCOMA

When surgery is the sole treatment modality for retroperitoneal sarcomas, subsequent local relapse rates have been as high as 70–90%. If EBRT is combined with resection, the dose of EBRT that can be delivered safely is much lower than with extremity sarcomas in view of dose-limiting structures (small intestine, stomach, liver, kidney, and spinal cord). In a randomized National Cancer Institute (NCI) trial, patients with primary sarcomas randomized to EBRT alone after marginal resection had a local relapse rate of 80% and excessive acute and chronic small-bowel morbidity *(17)*. The use of IORT supplements with IOERT *(17–20)* or HDR-IORT are therefore reasonable and practical.

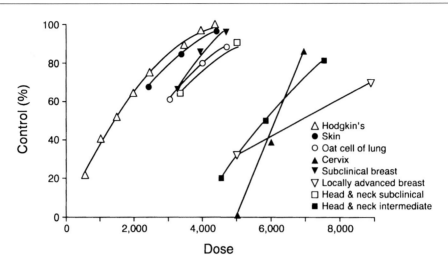

Fig. 1. Local control vs dose of irradiation. ●—skin *(22)*, Δ—Hodgkins *(23)*, O—lung oat cell *(24)*, ▽—breast subclinical *(25,26)*, ▽—breast locally advanced *(25,26)*, ▲—Cervix, ■—head and neck subclinical *(25,26)*, H—head and neck intermediate *(28)*. From ref. *3* with permission.

2.2. Influence of Dose on Local Control

As irradiation dose is increased to a tumor, there is an increased amount of cell killing with an increased likelihood of tumor control. This concept has been validated in many animal experiments in that local tumor control increases sharply with increasing irradiation dose, and the shape of this curve follows closely the theoretical model *(21)*. The animal data also clearly show that the irradiation dose needed to control a certain percentage of tumors will increase as the tumor volume increases and, conversely, that the percentage of tumors that will be controlled at a certain dose level will decrease as the volume of the tumor increases. Thus, although a given irradiation dose may be able to control a small tumor mass with high probability (and with acceptable patient morbidity), that same dose may be quite ineffective against larger volume tumors that contain a larger number of clonogenic cells.

A significant body of information has gradually developed to show that this same concept holds true for human tumors irradiated in vivo. This includes a large spectrum of tumors of various sizes and histologic types as summarized in Fig. 1. One of the earliest series related to tumor control vs dose was reported by Hale and Holmes *(22)* in the treatment of basal- and squamous-cell carcinomas of the skin. They found that the local relapse rate decreased from 33 to 4% as the radiation dose was increased from 24 to 45 Gy, delivered over 1 wk. This analysis is especially valuable since skin cancers are usually well demarcated prior to treatment, are of a fairly uniform size, and can be accurately evaluated for local persistence or relapse, both because of the ease of examination and the small likelihood of metastatic disease and patient death prior to adequate follow-up. Kaplan *(23)* analyzed local control after treatment of Hodgkin's disease with fractionated irradiation alone and demonstrated that the local relapse rate decreased from approx 60% at 10 Gy to 26% at 25 Gy, 11.5% at 35 Gy, and 1.3% at 44 Gy (approx 10 Gy per week, 2 Gy per fraction). The very shallow slope of tumor control vs dose in this clinical situation may be related to the relatively small number of clonogenic cells in even large masses of Hodgkin's disease. Choi and Carey *(24)* analyzed the local control of

Table 1
Tumor Control Probability Correlated With Irradiation Dose and Volume of Cancer

SCC—Upper Aerodigestive Tract

Dose (Gy)	Tumor control probability
50[a]	>90% subclinical
	60% T1 lesions of nasopharynx
	~50% 1-3 cm neck nodes
60[a]	~90% T1 lesions of pharynx and larynx
	~50% T3 and T4 lesions of tonsillar fossa
	~90% 1-3 cm neck nodes
	~70% 3-5 cm neck nodes
70[a]	~90% T2 lesions of tonsillar fossa and supraglottic larynx
	~80% T3 and T4 lesions of tonsillar fossa

ACA of the Breast

Dose (Gy)	Tumor control probability
50[a]	>90% subclinical
60[a]	90% clinically positive axillary nodes 2.5–3 cm
70[a]	65% 2–3 cm primary
70–80 (8–9 wk)	30% >5 cm primary
80–90 (8–10 wk)	56% >5 cm primary
80–100 (10–12 wk)	75% 5–15 cm primary

[a] 10 Gy in 5 fractions each week.
SCC = squamous cell carcinoma; ACA = adenocarcinoma.
Modified from Fletcher, G.H. and Shukovsky, L.J: *J. Radiol. Electrol.* **56;** (1975) 383.

disease in the chests in patients with oat-cell carcinoma of the lung. Control was obtained in 60% of patients who received 30 Gy, 79% at a dose of 40 Gy, and 88% at 48 Gy.

Fletcher and colleagues *(25,26)* performed an extensive evaluation of dose-response curves of human tumors emphasizing adenocarcinoma of the breast and squamous-cell carcinomas of the head and neck (Table 1). Using a retrospective comparison in breast cancer, the probability of controlling subclinical nodal or chest-wall disease was 60–70% with a dose of 30–35 Gy, 85% with 40 Gy, and 95% with 45 to 50 Gy (usual fractionation of 10 Gy per week in 2-Gy fractions). For locally advanced breast cancers, local control can still be obtained, but only when much higher doses are employed. For these large tumors, doses of 50–60 Gy produced local control in 35% of patients in the series of Griscom and Wang *(27)*, compared to 70% local control at doses of 90 Gy (with protracted fraction) obtained by Fletcher *(26)*.

The most extensive information on local control vs dose is available for squamous-cell carcinomas of the head and neck. These data have been summarized by Fletcher and Shukovsky *(25,26)* and Tepper *(28)*. For microscopic disease in lymph nodes, a dose of 30–40 Gy produces local control in 60–70% of patients, compared to greater than 90% control at doses of 50 Gy in 25 fractions over 5 wk. A strong dose-response curve has not been demonstrated for early-stage primary tumors of the head and neck, with good control at virtually all commonly used doses. The lack of a strong correlation is because no centers have had any need to decrease the dose (as morbidity is so low) below that which is commonly used and where high local control rates are obtained. The data

Table 2
Curative Doses of Radiation For Different Solid Cancers

50–60 Gy
  Lymph nodes, metastatic (N_0, N_1)
  Embryonal
  Medulloblastoma
  Retinoblastoma
  Ewing's
  Breast (excised)
60–65 Gy
  Larynx (<1 cm)
  Breast (T_1)
70–75 Gy
  Oral cavity (<2 cm, 2–4 cm)
  Oro-naso-laryngo-pharyngeal
  Breast (T_2)
  Bladder
  Cervix
  Uterine fundal
  Ovarian
  Lymph nodes, metastatic (1–3 cm)
  Lung (<3 cm)
80 Gy or above
  Head and neck (>4 cm)
  Breast (>5 cm)
  Glioblastomas (gliomas)
  Osteogenic sarcomas (bone sarcomas)
  Melanomas
  Soft tissue sarcomas (>5 cm)
  Thyroid
  Lymph nodes, metastatic (>6 cm)

Modified from Rubin, P., *Clinical Oncology: A Multidisciplinary Approach,* 1993.

compiled by Tepper indicate that 20% local control results after a dose of 46 Gy, 50% control with 58.5 Gy, and 80% control only with a very high dose of 75.5 Gy. Thus, a marked improvement in local control results from the ability to increase the tumor dose significantly.

An estimation of curative irradiation dose required for various tumor types on the basis of site, histology, and size was made by Philip Rubin in the text he edits, *Clinical Oncology(29)* (Table 2). As shown, for unresected tumors at most sites, irradiation doses would be ≤ 65 Gy only for early lesions (T_1-larynx, breast) with most lesions requiring 70–80 Gy or higher.

For most abdominal and many pelvic malignancies, the presence of dose-limiting tissues often prevents the use of high radiation doses, and the diagnosis of local relapse can be difficult to define without a reoperation or autopsy. However, as will be discussed in the local failure section for primary locally advanced rectal cancer, a dose-response correlation may exist for patients with only microscopic residual after maximal resection.

That a strong correlation exists between local control and total tumor dose in human tumors seems quite clear, even though a good dose-local control curve cannot be shown

Table 3
Distant Metastasis Rates for Spontaneous Primary
or Locally Recurrent Tumors of the C_3H/Sed Mouse

Tumor size (mm)	Tumor category	Treatment	Distant metastasis	
			F Sa II	SCC VII
6	Primary	Surgery	2.6%	8.0%
		Radiation	3.1%	6.9%
	Recurrent	Surgery	12.5%	43.0%
12	Primary	Surgery	14.3%	41.3%
	Recurrent	Surgery	46.6%	70.3%

FSA = fibrosarcoma; SCC = squamous cell cancer.
From ref. *30* with permission.

for all clinical situations. The fact that this relation exists gives us much optimism that if we can safely increase the total dose given to a tumor mass by using methods such as intraoperative irradiation (IORT) as a supplement to EBRT (with or without concomitant chemo) and maximal resection, increases in local control and total cure rate should result.

2.3. Impact of Local Control on Distant Metastases

In the ASTRO (American Society of Therapeutic Radiology and Oncology) Gold Medal paper of H. Suit *(30)*, the theme of metastases developing from a recurring tumor was discussed as a component of the overall premise that local control benefits survival. Data was presented from several spontaneous tumor systems to suggest that the rate of distant metastases was related to both tumor size and disease presentation as primary vs locally recurrent disease. In both the spontaneous fibrosarcoma FSaII and squamous-cell carcinoma SCC VII lines in the C3H/Sed mouse, Ramsey et al. reported increased rates of distant metastases with 6-mm vs 12-mm tumor size and primary vs recurrent tumors (Table 3) *(31)*. Ramsey's work confirmed an earlier evaluation by Suit et al. *(32)*. In Suit's analysis, 12-mm isotransplants of C3H mouse mammary tumors were treated with single-dose irradiation and evaluated for disease control both locally and distantly. The rate of distant metastases increased with lack of local control with rates of 31% (16 of 52) in mice with local control, 50% (9 of 18) in those with local relapse who were salvaged with further resection, and 80% (12 of 15) of mice with local relapse in whom salvage was not attempted.

Human data were also quoted supporting the thesis of metastases arising from the local relapse. In patients with squamous-cell cervix cancers, the metastatic frequency was higher in patients with local relapse vs those with local control *(33)*. In a Sloan Kettering analysis of prostate-cancer patients treated with I^{125} implants, the rate of distant metastases increased by stage and grade in patients with local relapse vs local control *(34)*. Liebel et al. *(35)* found similar results in disease-outcome analyses of RTOG (Radiation Therapy Oncology Group) patients with head and neck cancers for all sites except nasopharynx.

2.4. Tumor Control vs Complications

For patients with locally advanced abdominal or pelvic malignancies in whom all disease cannot be surgically removed with negative margins, EBRT (with or without chemotherapy) is usually only palliative since doses greater than 45–50 Gy in 25–28

Table 4
GI Radiation Tolerance Doses in Gy[a]

Organ	Injury at 5 yr	1–5% TD$_{5/5}$	25–50% TD$_{50/5}$	Volume or length
Esophagus	ulcer, stricture	60–65	75	75 cm^3
Stomach	ulcer, perforation	45–50	55	100 cm^3
Intestine (small)	ulcer, stricture	45–50	55	100 cm^3
Colon	ulcer, stricture	55–60	75	100 cm^3
Rectum	ulcer, stricture	55–60	75	100 cm^3
Pancreas	secretory functions	—	—	—
Liver	liver failure, ascites	35	45	whole
Biliary ducts	stricture, obstruction	50	70[b]	—

[a]Data based on supervoltage (6–18 MV), 9 Gy/wk (5 × 1.8).
[b]EBRT 50.4 Gy (28 × 1.8 over 5^{1}/$_2$ wk; 20 Gy at 1 cm radius—Ir192).
Modified from ref 36.

fractions often cannot be delivered safely. Gastrointestinal normal-tissue (organ) toler-ance to fractionated EBRT is demonstrated in Table 4 *(36)*. If treated with tolerable doses, patients will usually have local persistence or recurrence of disease with secondary complications that may require hospitalization and/or reoperation for small bowel obstruction, ureteral obstruction, bowel perforation, and so on.

If microscopic residual exists after gross total resection, EBRT doses necessary to accomplish local control are ≥ 60 Gy in 1.8- to 2-Gy fractions. Dose requirements would be even higher if gross residual remains after maximal resection. With doses ≥ 60 Gy, the radiation tolerance of numerous organs and structures in the abdomen and pelvis would be exceeded in both adults and children. Therefore, although an aggressive EBRT phi-losophy may allow better local tumor control, it may also cause severe treatment-related complications that could require hospitalization and operative intervention (*see* solid lines, Fig. 2). If small- or large-bowel problems result from excessive irradiation, com-plications such as fistulae, perforation, and so on can occur that usually require a reoperation.

A preferred treatment alternative for patients with locally advanced malignancies is to give tolerable EBRT doses of 45–50 Gy preoperatively (1.8-Gy fractions) and deliver the remaining irradiation as a supplement at the time of surgical exploration and maximal resection when dose-limiting organs can be excluded as a result of mobilization or shield-ing. This unique approach thereby allows an increase in local control (local control curve shift to the left—dotted line in Fig. 2) with a lower risk of complications than with an EBRT-only approach (complication curve shift to the right—dotted line in Fig. 2).

2.5. Shrinking-Field Techniques

Rationale for the use of shrinking-field irradiation techniques has been in existence for decades using either EBRT alone or EBRT plus brachytherapy. The initial EBRT field is usually designed to include a 3- to 5-cm margin beyond the primary or recurrent tumor plus regional nodal areas that are at risk for metastatic spread. Initial fields are treated to an accepted subclinical dose level of 45–50.4 Gy in 1.8- to 2.0-Gy fractions. Subsequent boost techniques are used to bring gross disease to the level of 65–80 Gy with EBRT or brachytherapy techniques. The excellent long-term results achieved with EBRT plus

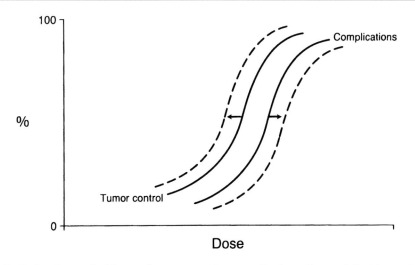

Fig. 2. Radiation dose vs incidence of tumor control or complications. From ref. *3* with permission.

boost techniques for breast, gynecologic, and head and neck cancers support the concept of this combined approach since good local control is achieved with relatively low morbidity to dose-limiting normal tissues.

3. HISTORY OF IORT

3.1. Orthovoltage IORT Era—Europe and United States

The recent discovery in Barcelona (Spain) of an anecdotal, but well documented, case of an IORT-like procedure in early March, 1905, demonstrates the courage and creativity of pioneers in the early medical use of X-rays *(37)*. Comas and Prio *(38)* reported the case of a 33-yr-old patient diagnosed with a squamous-cell carcinoma of the cervix and treated on February 18, 1905, with a total abdominal hysterectomy, pelvic node dissection, and partial cystectomy followed by roentgen therapy. The abdominal wall incision (8 cm in length) was left open, after pelvic tamponage, until May 7. Fractionated intrapelvic irradiation was delivered on March 11 (Fig. 3), 13, 15, 20, and 27, and May 1. Each radiation fraction was administered in three time segments, changing the direction of the tube at each segment in order to encompass the pelvic cavity. The distance from the anticathode to the pelvis ranged from 20 to 28 cm. The surgical incision was protected by lead sheets wrapped in sterilized gauze, and was sutured on May 7 (after monitoring the intrapelvic changes following treatment). Additional external roentgenotherapy was delivered in five abdominal wall sessions, from May 17 to June 10. Endovaginal radiation, 13 applications, was given from July 10 to October 12. In the follow-up period, additional irradiation was delivered at the beginning of 1906 (four fractions of abdominal wall field and one endovaginal application). Ten years after surgery and irradiation, the patient was reported to be alive without evidence of neoplastic disease.

The value of this anecdotal case report is to identify, at the very primitive stages of European radiotherapy practice, a unique association of relevant factors considered key in modern clinical radiotherapy: the indication of adjuvant irradiation after extensive surgery; the design of delivering irradiation through an open surgical incision; the remarkable effort to preserve fractionation in a complex treatment program; and the use

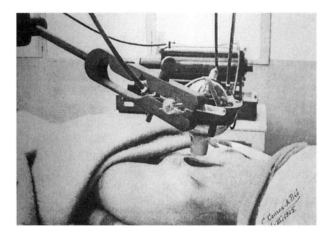

Fig. 3. Photographic document of the case report during intraoperative roentgen treatment. Notice in the lower right-corner of the figure the note with the picture date: 11th March, 1905.

of external and intracavity irradiation to complement treatment to suspected underdosed areas of the target volume. Pioneering work in the field of IORT has been done in Austria *(39)* and Germany *(40)*. However, most of the scientific information generated before the 1980s was of little practical influence in the oncology community *(41–43)*.

The initial use of IORT in the treatment of gastrointestinal cancers was described by Finsterer in 1915 for a patient with advanced gastric carcinoma who received an X-ray treatment with simultaneous jejunostomy *(44)*. The tumor was surgically exposed and irradiated by a technique called "eventration treatment." This approach gained limited popularity for unresectable gastric and colorectal cancer *(45)*.

In the 1930s, surgeons and radiation oncologists readvocated IORT because of the development of shock-proof, 50–100 kvp short-distance X-ray equipment ("contact therapy"). This machine approximated the treatment conditions obtained with radium treatment with regard to dose distribution but offered the advantages of safety, cost, and convenience. The poor tissue penetration of irradiation at this energy prevented extensive use.

Between late 1930 and late 1950, a number of institutions utilized higher-energy orthovoltage units for IORT. In 1937, Eloesser of Stanford reported on the use of intraoperative X-ray therapy with 200 kv energy in six patients with advanced gastric and rectal tumors *(46)*. Sterile lead shields were placed over normal tissues, and doses up to 4500 roentgens were used without the report of acute complications. In 1947, Fairchild and Shorter *(47)* described a technique of "direct" treatment of unresectable gastric carcinoma with 500–1300 roentgens from a 250-kvp unit in the operating room and were the first to propose combining this treatment with postoperative EBRT. Of 32 patients treated in this fashion, two lived beyond 2 yr without any late complications.

A large series of patients with head and neck, thoracic, and abdominal malignancies was reported by Barth in 1959 using intraoperative 90-kvp and 150-kvp X-rays *(48)*. Many patients were treated with "subcutaneous" therapy in which the skin and subcutaneous tissues were temporarily peeled back to allow the delivery of multiple short-distance treatments. By extending this concept to abdominal tumors, Barth was among the first to suggest treatment of malignancy by a combination of preoperative EBRT and a single IORT treatment. Encouraging results, especially with advanced head and neck cancer, were initially reported but long-term follow-up was not published since this was considered mainly palliative therapy. The interest in this technique waned with the introduction of megavoltage X-rays that could deliver high doses to deep structures without the necessity of surgical exposure.

3.2. Megavoltage IORT Era—Japan Experience

The modern approach to IORT began with studies by Abe at the University of Kyoto in the early 1960s (1,48). Their approach to overcoming the limitations of surgery and EBRT in advanced abdominal tumors was to combine surgical excision of the tumor when possible, followed immediately by a single massive dose (25–30 Gy) of radiation during the operation. Higher doses (up to 40 Gy) were used if the tumor was unresectable. The first patients were treated with cobalt-60. In 1965 a betatron was installed in an operating room within the radiotherapy department, and subsequent patients were treated with intraoperative electron irradiation (IOERT). By the early 1980s this technique had spread to 27 hospitals in Japan, and in a 1981 publication, Abe and Takahashi reported the combined Japanese results in 727 patients (48).

3.3. Modern United States Era—IOERT or Orthovoltage

Because of Henschke's earlier interests in intraoperative irradiation (39), in 1970, he and Goldson planned a special IORT facility for the new Howard University Hospital which was under construction. One of the supervoltage suites of the new radiotherapy department was equipped as an operating room. A Varian Clinac 18® MeV linear accelerator was selected as the machine for this undertaking. The first IOERT treatment was given at Howard University in November, 1976, and by December, 1982, 114 patients had been treated with variable electron energies (2,49,50).

Based on the exploratory work performed in Japan and at Howard University, a number of other institutions began investigations into the use of intraoperative electron irradiation (IOERT). The MGH was the second American center to use this technique with the first patient treated in May, 1978 (51). As previously discussed, these investigators made one significant change in that most patients were treated with fractionated conventional EBRT doses of 45–55 Gy in 1.8–2.0 Gy fractions in addition to that delivered intraoperatively. In addition, many patients had surgical resections performed if this was thought to be technically feasible.

The NCI began using IOERT in September, 1979 (52). They also did not use IOERT alone, but rather emphasized the combination of maximal surgical resection with the IOERT and in most clinical situations did not utilize conventional EBRT. As the initial emphasis of the irradiation component of therapy at NCI was on IOERT alone, the field size was often very large, and included abutting as many as three separate electron fields. These large IOERT fields, combined with aggressive surgical resection, were found to be feasible, and no major acute complications were attributed to the IOERT.

In the early 1980s IORT programs also became active at the Mayo Clinic (53) (April, 1981) and the New England Deaconess Hospital (NEDH) division of the Joint Center for Radiation Therapy (54) (January, 1982). At Mayo Clinic, IOERT was incorporated as a component of treatment with the same general approach and philosophy as at MGH. A major difference was the physical plant in that a sterile operating room was developed in the radiotherapy department since patient transfer from normal operating room suites would have been difficult. This facility was used from 1981–1989, when a dedicated facility in the operating room became available. At NEDH, a lower-energy X-ray machine (orthovoltage irradiation) was placed in the operating room with the philosophy that if orthovoltage IORT was shown to be as good as IOERT, this would be advantageous as the low-energy machines were less expensive, required less shielding, and would therefore be more generally available.

3.4. Modern Europe Era—IOERT or Orthovoltage

In the early 1980s several European institutions implemented an IOERT program using either high-energy electron beams or orthovoltage. A literature review of abstracts or publications from International IORT Symposia (55–57) permits identification of some of the very active groups in the mid 1990s that became involved in IORT 7–15 yr earlier. The following list generates a chronogeographical relationship regarding the historical origins of modern European IOERT: Caen (France) 1983, Pamplona (Spain) 1984, Innsbruck (Austria) 1984, Lyon (France) 1985, Milan (Italy) 1985, Munchen (Germany) 1986, Brussels (Belgium) 1987, Groningen (Holland) 1988, Oslo (Norway) 1990, Stockholm (Sweden) 1990, and so on. A modern orthovoltage IORT program was instituted in Montpelier (France) in 1984 with transition to a dedicated IOERT facility in 1996.

There are several remarkable features concerning the expansion of IORT in Europe. First, the number of institutions involved in the modality has increased progressively in every country. Second, IORT has been tested in several tumor sites, histologic types, and disease status (including recurrent and primary cancer) following the initial tendency in Japan to evaluate the technique at the time of a variety of cancer surgical procedures. Third, IORT was adopted very early in the modern clinical experiences as a method of boost-dose irradiation integrated in a treatment program following maximal surgical resection and in which additional fractionated EBRT (pre- or postoperative) was a mandatory treatment component alone or combined with the best established systemic management known.

The European natural evolution of IORT has led to a promising present in which the development of national groups of IORT experts (French, Spanish, and so on) joined efforts including the establishment of a pooled database for outcomes analysis as data matured in terms of patient sample size, treatment homogeneity, and long-term follow-up. These parameters help establish scientific reference points regarding feasibility, treatment tolerance, local control, and survival data to generate the consensus for randomized clinical trials. Generally, active European IORT institutions have been enthusiastic in reporting their results and in supporting transnational ventures to promote improved quality and more influential IORT science, including the recently founded International Society of IORT.

3.5. HDR-IORT—U.S. and Europe

HDR-IORT was developed in the late 1980s in an attempt to combine the technical and dosimetric advantages of brachytherapy with the conceptual and logistic advantages of IOERT (58–67). Although HDR remote afterloaders were initially utilized in 1964 and have become common in modern radiation oncology departments, they have been used primarily in the outpatient setting. HDR-IORT developed as a result of the merging and improvements of this existing technology, applied to the intraoperative setting. It also was developed as a strategy to create new technical possibilities for intraoperative treatment which other IORT approaches could not easily satisfy.

There were several perceived problems preventing the widespread application of IOERT. First, it is expensive to have a dedicated linear accelerator in an operating room. Second, even if the first issue is overcome by transporting anesthetized patients from the OR to the radiation oncology department for their IORT, other medical and logistic issues need to be overcome. Third, by virtue of the infeasibility of electron applicators, it may be difficult if not impossible to treat complex anatomical surfaces such as the deep or anterior pelvis, or lateral or anterior chest with IOERT (*see* Chapter 7). Fourth, the dosimetry of IOERT is akin to EBRT, being quite homogenous (seen as advantageous by those who use IOERT). This does not lend itself to the possibility of dose escalation within a target volume or surface, however, as can be done with the inhomogeneity of brachytherapy dosimetry. HDR-IORT was born out of the desire to deal with some of these issues.

Part of the concept of HDR-IORT is to create a shielded OR in which the entire surgical procedure as well as the radiation can be performed. A complete description of the Memorial Sloan-Kettering Cancer Center facility has already been published elsewhere *(62,63)* as well as in this textbook (Chapters 5, 6, and 16). For institutions building new ORs, or rebuilding existing ORs, introducing proper shielding for HDR-IORT is essential. The development of the Harrison-Anderson-Mick (HAM) applicator *(62,63)* or other superflab applicators *(59,64)* provided a vehicle through which the HDR machine could connect to the desired target surface or volume. Because the HAM applicator is both flexible and transparent, there is literally no surface that cannot be accessed or treated *(66)*. The HDR machine is portable, and can be used either in the outpatient area or the OR. This simple fact makes HDR-IORT a possibility for almost any medical center.

In the late 1980s and early 1990s, HDR-IORT was started in the United States and Europe in an attempt to address some of the above issues and concepts. HDR-IORT using plastic needles in a superflab applicator was first reported from Munich in 1991 by Lukas et al. *(59)*. In 1992, a similar, independently developed protocol was implemented at Memorial Sloan-Kettering Cancer Center (MSKCC) in New York, using superflab HAM applicators in which plastic catheters had been embedded at the time of manufacture *(62,63)*. Prior to these efforts, however, Dritschilo and colleagues at Georgetown University School of Medicine reported HDR-IORT treatments of liver metastases using closed-end needles inserted into the target volume *(58, 60)*. All of the above studies made use of GammaMed (Isolopen-Technik, Haan, Germany) remote HDR afterloaders. A microSelectron (Nucleotron, The Netherlands) HDR machine has been used at Ohio State University Hospital (OSUH) in Columbus for HDR-IORT with assorted applicators, both rigid and flexible *(61,67)*.

In the United States, early clinical experience was developed at MSKCC *(62,63,65,66)*, Georgetown *(58,60)*, and Ohio State University *(61,67)*. The MSKCC experience included colorectal cancers *(62,63,66)* (Chapter 16), pediatric malignancies *(65)* (Chapter 26), retroperitoneal sarcomas (Chapter 19), and selected thoracic and gynecologic cancers (data not yet published). The Georgetown experience was quite different, and concentrated on volume implants for liver metastases (Chapter 17) *(58,60)*. This is a unique experience that needs further exploration. The techniques for the liver IORT program are applicable to pancreas and other sites where gross unresectable disease is often encountered. The early Ohio State clinical experience *(61,67)* was primarily with locally advanced colorectal (Chapter 15) and head and neck cancers (Chapter 25).

Simultaneous with the MSKCC program, investigators in Germany were also evaluating HDR-IORT *(59,64)*. These investigators also concentrated on locally advanced colorectal cancers.

To date, the preliminary data for the clinical studies noted above, including colorectal, sarcoma, pediatrics (multiple sites), and liver reveal promising oncologic outcomes in challenging groups of patients. Most of this early work is presented in the appropriate disease-site-specific chapters of this textbook as stated in prior paragraphs.

New HDR-IORT programs are being developed. A shielded room is being built in a new OR suite at the Beth Israel Medical Center in New York. This is different from the program developed at MSKCC where the shielded OR is in the radiation oncology department. Whereas the MSKCC program works well, the obvious advantages of being in the main OR (resource utilization, professional staffing, accessibility of ancillary staff, sterile supplies, blood products, laboratories, drugs, and so on) will enhance the efficiency of the HDR-IORT program.

Some centers have or plan to acquire both HDR-IORT and IOERT (Ohio State and Mayo Clinic). Whereas it is hard to imagine that one of these techniques will ever be demonstrated to be oncologically preferable, they certainly can be complimentary. We will continue to learn the relative advantages and disadvantages of each. We are also excited that so many new centers will be adding IORT capabilities, which will bring this modality to more patients in desperate need of better local control.

3.6. Summary

Some of the technical problems and nuisance aspects of IORT, encountered in the 1980s and early 1990s, can be overcome with dedicated or semidedicated IOERT or HDR-IORT facilities. This can be built as an operating room (OR) in the radiation oncology department as done for IOERT at NCI, Medical College of Ohio, Thomas Jefferson University, Howard University, and others and as done at MSKCC for HDR-IORT. The most ideal situation is to place a facility within or near the OR suite, which has been done at Mayo Clinic, MGH, MDACC, and some European institutions for IOERT, at Ohio State University for both IOERT and HDR-IORT, and is planned for HDR-IORT at the Beth Israel Medical Center in New York City. Either approach simplifies the treatment of patients, necessitates fewer reoperations (refused by some patients and physicians), and avoids transportation and sterility problems. It also prevents the need to shut down the outpatient treatment machine for a "potential" case. However, the dedicated IORT option in an OR setting is quite expensive if an existing OR has to be retrofitted for proper shielding (for either IOERT or HDR-IORT) and a new linear accelerator is purchased as the electron source for IOERT.

4. PATIENT SELECTION AND EVALUATION

4.1. Patient Selection Criterion

Appropriateness for an IOERT boost should be determined by the surgeon and radiation oncologist in the setting of a joint-preoperative consultation, whenever feasible. This allows input from both specialties with regard to studies that would be helpful for IOERT and EBRT planning as well as whether IOERT is appropriate. An informed consent can be obtained with regard to potential benefits and risks, and optimal sequencing of surgery and EBRT can be discussed and determined.

The following general criterion have guided the selection of appropriate patients for IORT at our institutions:

1. Surgery alone will not achieve acceptable local control (i.e., ≥microscopic residual disease [res(m)] after maximal resection). There must be no contraindications for exploratory surgery and an attempt at gross total resection.
2. EBRT doses needed for adequate local control following subtotal resection or unresectable disease (60–70 Gy in 1.8- to 2.0-Gy fractions for microscopic residual, 70–90 Gy for gross residual or unresected disease) would exceed normal tissue tolerance.
3. IORT will be performed at the time of a planned operative procedure.
4. The IORT plus EBRT technique would theoretically result in a more suitable therapeutic ratio between cure and complications by permitting direct irradiation of unresected or marginally resected tumor with single or abutting fields while surgically displacing or shielding dose-limiting structures or organs.
5. There is no evidence of distant metastases or peritoneal seeding (rare exceptions: resectable single organ metastasis, excellent chemotherapy options, slow progression of systemic disease).

4.2. Patient Evaluation

The pretreatment patient workup should include a detailed evaluation of the extent of the locally advanced primary or recurrent lesion combined with studies to rule out hematogenous or peritoneal spread of disease. In addition to history and physical exam, the routine evaluation includes CBC, liver and renal chemistries, chest film, and tumor-specific serum tests (CEA, CA 19-9, and so on). When palpable pelvic primaries or relapses are immobile or fixed on rectal or bimanual exam or symptoms suggest pelvic recurrence following primary resection, computed tomography (CT) of the pelvis and abdomen can confirm lack of free space between the malignancy and a structure that may be surgically unresectable for cure (i.e., presacrum, pelvic sidewall). In such patients, preoperative EBRT with or without chemotherapy should be given prior to an attempt at resection. Extrapelvic spread to para-aortic nodes or liver can also be determined. If hematuria is present or findings on CT or excretory urogram suggest bladder involvement, cystoscopy is done prior to or on the day of surgical confirmation.

5. SEQUENCING AND DOSES OF EBRT AND IORT

5.1. Sequencing of EBRT, IORT, and Surgery

Whenever feasible, total or gross total resection of disease is performed before or after EBRT. Resection is an almost uniform component of IOERT-containing regimens with both gastric and colorectal cancers but is rarely feasible with biliary and pancreatic cancers. Single-institution pilot studies have evaluated resection plus IOERT following preoperative EBRT and chemotherapy for initially unresectable pancreatic cancers.

Optimal sequencing of surgery and EBRT for locally advanced cancers should be discussed and determined at the time of a joint multispecialty consultation involving a surgeon, radiation oncologist, and medical oncologist. This allows input from all specialists with regard to studies that would be helpful for IORT and EBRT treatment planning as well as whether IORT may be appropriate. For many patients with locally advanced lesions, preoperative EBRT of 45–50 Gy in 1.8- to 2.0-Gy fractions (with or without chemotherapy as indicated by disease site) followed by exploration and resection in

3–5 wk offers the following theoretical advantages over a sequence of resection and IORT followed by EBRT:

1. Deletion of patients with metastases detected at the restaging work-up or laparotomy, thus sparing the potential risks of aggressive surgical resection with or without IORT.
2. Possible tumor shrinkage with an increased possibility of achieving a gross total resection.
3. Potential alteration of implantability of cells that may be disseminated at the time of a marginal or partial surgical resection.
4. Reduction of treatment interval between EBRT and IORT (when resection and IORT are done initially, if postoperative complications ensue, the delay to EBRT with or without chemotherapy may be excessive).

5.2. Irradiation Doses and Technique

The method of EBRT has been fairly consistent in most United States single-institution and group IORT studies. In the Mayo Clinic and MGH trials, doses of 45–54 Gy are delivered in 1.8-Gy fractions, 5 d per week over 5–6 wk in patients who have had no prior irradiation. For pelvic lesions, treatments are given with linear accelerators using ≥ 10 MV photons and four field-shaped external-beam techniques. With extrapelvic lesions, unresected or residual disease plus 3- to 5-cm margins of normal tissues are included to 40–45 Gy, usually with parallel-opposed fields. Reduced fields with 2- to 3-cm margins are treated to 45–54 Gy. With gastrointestinal malignancies, chemotherapy is often given during external irradiation with 5-FU-based regimens (bolus vs infusion 5-FU; alone vs combined with other drugs such as leucovorin, levamisole, cisplatin, mitomycin C).

The technical aspects of both the surgical and irradiation components of IORT procedures will be discussed in detail in Chapters 3 (IOERT) and 5 (HDR-IORT) and will not be reiterated in this chapter. For such procedures, a carefully constructed team needs to exist that includes a surgeon(s), radiation oncologist(s), anesthesiologist(s), operating room nursing, radiation physics and dosimetry, and radiation therapists.

The biologic effectiveness of single-dose IORT is considered equivalent to 2–3 times the same total dose of fractionated EBRT (see Chapter 2 for more complete discussion of this issue). The effective dose in the IORT boost field, when added to the 45–50 Gy given with EBRT, is 65–80 Gy for an IORT dose of 10 Gy, 75–95 Gy with a 15-Gy boost, and 85–110 Gy with a 20-Gy IORT dose.

5.3. Dose-Limiting Structures

In patients with locally advanced malignancies, the issue of morbidity following aggressive treatment is placed into clearer perspective by a comparison with tumor-related morbidity. For instance, when EBRT is used as the main treatment modality for locally advanced rectal cancers, more than 90% of patients have local persistence or relapse of disease and most are dead in 2–3 yr (end result is nearly 100% tumor-related morbidity/mortality). A complete discussion of IORT tolerance of surgically dissected and undissected organs and structures is found in Chapters 8–10.

6. GUIDELINES FOR REPORTING IORT DATA (IOERT, HDR-IORT)

Intraoperative irradiation requires technical sophistication in the local treatment delivery, which implies complexity at the time of data analysis and report. Intraoperative irradiation clinical experiences are established and continued only with remarkable cooperation between surgeons, radiation oncologists, and physicists in the development of a quality IORT component of cancer management. Among the limitations of this technique is the slow patient accrual for the different treatment programs or clinical trials, because of the complexity of professional and institutional coordination (68). Contemporary IORT is usually delivered as a component of therapy (generally integrated in multimodal programs), in an effort to enhance local treatment intensity and promote local tumor control. Since it is a local technique, publications need to include careful analyses of local effects. The impact of possible local benefits in the general outcome of cancer patients have to be evaluated in the context of initial tumor sites and stages, integral treatment intensity and quality of life parameters (69). In addition, the potential impact of improved local control on distant control and survival should also be evaluated and reported.

Analysis and publication of data requires meticulous description of sequential treatment components (local and systemic) with particular emphasis on surgical maneuvers and the IORT parameters. In the last two decades, reports on IORT published in peer-review journals have progressively refined the information presentation, with particular consideration to patient, tumor, and treatment characteristic descriptions, IORT methodology, local effects observations (tolerance of normal tissues and local tumor control rates), patterns of disease relapse, and survival outcomes (Table 5). Institutional experiences have up-dated the results of their pilot studies showing, in consecutive publications, a transition from the description of technical methodology and clinical feasibility towards emphasis on local tissue tolerance and tumor control results (local and distant). Survival (53,70–73) and patterns of disease relapse are generally reported, but phase I–II-oriented studies (or comparison with existing historical control data from conventional treatment programs in comparable tumor sites, histology, and stage) should be interpreted with caution (74).

6.1. Local Normal Tissue Tolerance Analyses

Local normal tissue tolerance in clinical IORT trials in Western institutions have been prospectively analyzed. Patients entered in controlled studies and their long-term events were monitorized periodically. Unquestionable data is available identifying peripheral nerves as dose limiting and ureters as dose-sensitive in IORT experiences (72,73,75). Anecdotal reports have described severe toxicity in IORT patients in bone (vertebral collapse) (76), vessels (fatal bleeding) (77), and brain (demyelinization) (78). Local toxicity in IORT trials is, by definition, a multifactorial event in which the biological conditions of the tissues at risk for complications is modulated by multiple possible causes of tissue damage. Although the predominant factor for a biological lesion might be the IORT component of treatment, the clinical observation needs to be interpreted in the context of other risk factors (i.e., other components of treatment including the magnitude of current surgery, EBRT, chemotherapy, and prior treatment with surgery or EBRT; disease factors including extent of disease and normal tissue toxicity produced by the malignancy such as peripheral neuropathy, and so on). Table 6 describes a systematic and integral analysis scheme for evaluation of local toxicity.

6.2. Local Tumor Control Analyses

Intraoperative irradiation is generally used after a surgical alteration of the normal anatomy, either by tumor resection or normal tissue manipulation (for instance biliary-digestive bypass in unresected pancreatic cancer). Postsurgical changes (presacral hematoma) ought to be well documented by pre- and postoperative image techniques in an effort to establish a base-line condition for comparison in the follow-up period.

Table 5
Guidelines of Relevant Data Base Information
for Reporting Intraoperative Irradiation Trials or Experiences

General Information
Patient's name
Institution
Chart number
Surgeon
Radiation oncologist
Medical oncologist
Physicist
Anesthesiologist
Date of IORT
Time of IORT

Patient characteristics
Age
Sex
Karnofsky
Symptoms
Previous illnesses
Previous treatments
Tumor markers
Disease status
   Primary
   Recurrent

Tumor characteristics
Site/size/location
Stage
   T description
   N description
Histology
Cellular differentiation
Molecular findings

Treatment characteristics
General factors
   Integral program description
   Modality segments sequence
   Place of IORT component
Surgery
Type of procedure (name)
Distant disease
Margins
   involved
   close
Residual disease (area/size)
   no resection
   resection
      macroscopic
      microscopic
      high risk (negative, narrow)
Adjacent organ manipulation
Reconstruction of surgical defect
Maneuvers for IORT exposure

External beam irradiation
Preoperative
Postoperative
Chemoradiation
Volume
Fractionation
Total dose
Dates

Chemotherapy
Neoadjuvant
Adjuvant
Concurrent
Drugs
Courses
Dates

Treatment for recurrent disease

IORT Characteristics
Target volume definition
Normal tissues included
Normal tissues excluded
Number of IORT fields
Applicator size/shape/beveled end
Electron Energy
Total dose

Toxicity and complications
IORT related
   Date of observations
   Type of damage
   Severity scale
   Evolution
IORT unrelated
   Responsible modality
   Date of observation
   Type of damage
   Severity scale
   Evolution

Patterns of tumor relapse
Date of observation
Central
   Infield IORT
   Marginal IORT
Local
   External beam field
Distant
   Site(s)
Mixed (local plus distant)

Patient follow-up
Date of last follow-up
Status
   Disease related
      NED
      AWD
      DWD
      DFD (cause)
   Toxicity related
      improving
      worsening
      stable
   Treatment related
      Responding
      Progressing
      Stable

Table 6
Valuable Information for Normal Tissue Toxicity Interpretation in IORT Trials

1. Pre-IORT identification of biological compromised tolerance:
   Symptomatic or imaging evidence of tissue deterioration.
   Symptoms suggesting direct tumor involvement.
   Surgical manipulation.
   Previous treatments: radiotherapy, chemoradiation, chemotherapy.

2. IORT *per se* contribution to tissue damage:
   Type of tissues at risk in the IORT volume.
   Tissue structure and dimensions at IORT risk.
   Estimated dose received (location in the IORT dosimetric treatment volume).

3. Post-IORT parameters of additional damage:
   Local infections, abscesses, and so on.
   Surgical reinterventions with further tissue manipulation.
   Macro and microvascularization status.
   Complementary treatments: external beam irradiation, chemoradiation, chemotherapy,
      and so on.
   Tumor relapse and involvement of toxic tissues.

The determination of the IORT treatment volume is not homogeneous among institutions. The use of surgical clips, or other means, to identify the IORT boost region is a valuable system to be able to distinguish central recurrences (in the IORT field), from local/marginal relapse (in the EBRT field). This information is not generally available in the literature except for highly expert institutions (72,73). There are anatomical limitations for such a precise evaluation. For instance, in the pelvic cavity, the technical difficulties for applicator positioning implies uncertainty of the dosimetric behavior of the electron beam (lateral pelvic wall region).

In contemporary radiation oncology, the principle that tumor control probability is a function of the total dose of irradiation is still valid. Local recurrences, when suspected, need to be histologically proven when feasible. The documentation of this event requires a retrospective reconstruction of the integral dosimetric plan designed for that particular case, and its relationship with the present anatomical findings of the recurrence. Through the meticulous analysis of local recurrences, expert scientists will establish the limitations and indications of precision radiation boost techniques (with IOERT or HDR-IORT brachytherapy) and their role as a loco-regional treatment intensification modality (79) (Fig. 4).

6.3. Institutional IORT Methodology Description

Active IORT institutions are recommended to publish their program description, with particular emphasis in technical methodology adopted, the dosimetric characteristics of their IORT devices (applicators, flaps, and so on), the criteria for radiation-dose prescription and the intramural protocols developed for quality-control parameters. This report has been generally published by expert institutions at the time of IORT program initiation (80–82), and does not need to be up-dated unless new technology is incorporated with time (83). The methodology description report is frequently coded in the "Methods and Materials" portions of clinical results publications and offers the opportunity to interpret the data in terms of technical methodological similarity among institutions (situation in

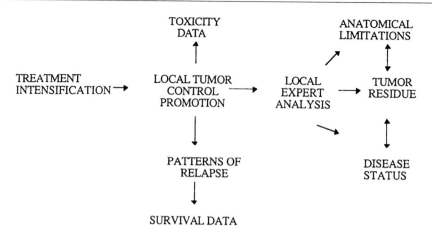

Fig. 4. Process of disease control and tolerance analyses in IORT clinical experiences and trials.

Table 7
Description of Relevant Parameters for an IORT Institutional Methodology Report

1. Materials:
   Radiation source(s).
   IORT applicators
      sizes
      shapes
   Image documentation system.
   Check list protocols for professionals involved.
   Multidisciplinary protocol for individual IORT procedure description.

2. Methods:
   Dosimetric properties of applicators.
   Dosimetric treatment planning.
   Dose-specification criterion.
   Surgical-radiation oncology interaction: case discussion, technical cooperation for applicator
      positioning, consensus in target volume selection.
   Anesthesiology-radiation oncology interaction: transportation and/or patient monitoring
      during IORT.
   Prospective follow-up protocols: selective analysis of local effects and disease outcome.

3. Institution:
   Hospital description.
   Clinical oncology coordination characteristics.
   Surgical oncology characteristics activity.
   IORT program implementation:
      Dedicated unit
      Semi-dedicated unit
      Prolonged transportation required

which homogeneous clinical results are expected unless patient selection varies) or the opposite situation wherein technology and clinical decisions involved in IORT treatment are markedly different (different radiation quality, applicators sizes and shapes, dosimetric properties, and dose-specification criterion) *(84)*. In Table 7, relevant parameters of IORT institutional methodology are listed for the elaboration of a program-descriptive report.

REFERENCES

1. Abe M, Fukada M, Yamano K, et al. Intraoperative irradiation in abdominal and cerebral tumours, *Acta Radiol.,* **10** (1971) 408–416.
2. Goldson A. Preliminary clinical experience with intraoperative radiotherapy, *J. Nat. Med. Assoc.,* **70** (1978) 493–495.
3. Gunderson LL, Tepper JE, Biggs PJ, et al. Intraoperative ± external beam irradiation, *Curr. Probl. Cancer,* **7** (1983) 1–69.
4. Gunderson LL, Nagorney DM, Martenson JA, et al. External beam plus intraoperative irradiation for gastrointestinal cancers, *World J. Surg.,* **19** (1995) 191–197.
5. Gunderson LL and Willett C. Pancreas and hepatobiliary tract cancer, In Perez CA, Brady LW (eds.), *Principles and Practice of Radiation Oncology,* 3rd ed. Lippincott, Philadelphia, 1997, pp. 1467–1488.
6. Whittington R, Solin L, and Mohiuddin M. Multimodality therapy of localized unresectable pancreatic adenocarcinoma, *Cancer,* **54** (1984) 1991–1998.
7. Brierly JD, Cummings BJ, Wong CS, et al. Adenocarcinoma of the rectum treated by radical external radiation therapy, *Int. J. Radiat. Oncol. Biol. Phys.,* **31** (1995) 255–259.
8. O'Connell MJ, Childs DS, Moertel CG, et al. A prospective controlled evaluation of combined pelvic radiotherapy and methanol extraction residue of BCG (MER) for locally unresectable or recurrent rectal carcinoma, *Int. J. Radiat. Oncol. Biol. Phys.,* **8** (1982) 1115–1119.
9. Gunderson LL, Cohen AM, Dosoretz DE, et al. Residual, unresectable or recurrent colorectal cancer: external beam irradiation and intraoperative electron beam boost ± resection, *Int. J. Radiat. Oncol. Biol. Phys.,* **9** (1983) 1597–1606.
10. Tewfik HH, Buchsbaum HJ, Latourette HB, et al. Para-aortic lymph node irradiation in carcinoma of the cervix after exploratory laparotomy and biopsy proven aortic nodes, *Int. J. Radiat. Oncol. Biol. Phys.,* **8** (1982) 13–18.
11. Piver MS and Barlow JJ. High dose irradiation in biopsy confirmed aortic node metastases from carcinoma of the uterine cervix, *Cancer,* **39** (1977) 1243–1246.
12. Delgado G, Goldson AL, Ashayeri E, et al. Intraoperative radiation in the treatment of advanced cervical cancer, *Obstet. Gynecol.,* **63** (1984) 246–252.
13. Garton GR, Gunderson LL, Webb MJ, et al. Intraoperative irradiation in gynecologic cancer: the Mayo Clinic experience, *Gyn. Oncol.,* **48** (1993) 328–332.
14. Haddock M, Petersen I, Webb MJ, et al. Intraoperative irradiation therapy for locally advanced gynecologic malignancies, In Vaeth J, Meyer J (eds) *The Role of Intraoperative Radiation Therapy in the Treatment of Cancer.* S. Karger, Basel, *Front. Radiat. Ther. Oncol.,* **31** (1997) 256–259.
15. Stelzer K, Koh W, Greer B, et al. Intraoperative electron beam therapy (IOEBT) as an adjunct to radical surgery for recurrent cancer of the cervix, In Schildberg FW, Willich N, Kramling H (eds), *Intraoperative Radiation Therapy,* Verlag Die Blaue Eule, Verlag, 1993, pp. 411–414.
16. Mahe M, Dargent D, Chabert P, et al. Intraoperative radiation therapy (IORT) in recurrent carcinoma of the uterine cervix: report of the French IORT group about 70 patients, *Lyon Int'l. IORT Abst. Hepatogastroenterol.,* **41** (1994) 6.
17. Sindelar WF, Kinsella TJ, Chen PW, et al. Intraoperative radiotherapy in retroperitoneal sarcomas: final results of a prospective, randomized trial, *Arch. Surg.,* **128** (1993) 402–410.
18. Gunderson LL, Nagorney DM, McIlrath DC, et al. External beam and intraoperative electron irradiation for locally advanced soft tissue sarcomas. *Int. J. Radiat. Oncol. Biol. Phys.,* **25** (1993) 647–656.
19. Petersen I, Haddock M, Donohue J, et al. Use of intraoperative electron beam radiation therapy (IOERT) in the management of retroperitoneal and pelvic soft tissue sarcomas, ASTRO Abst. *Int. J. Radiat. Oncol. Biol. Phys.,* **36(1)** (1996) 184.
20. Willett CG, Suit HD, Tepper JE, et al. Intraoperative electron beam radiation therapy for retroperitoneal soft tissue sarcoma, *Cancer,* **68** (1991) 278–283.
21. Suit HD. Radiation biology: a basis for radiotherapy, In Fletcher GH. (ed.), *Textbook of Radiotherapy,* 2nd ed. Lea and Fabiger, Philadelphia, 1973, pp. 75–121.
22. Hale CH and Holmes GW. Carcinoma of skin: influence of dosage on the success of treatment, *Radiology,* **48** (1947) 563–569.
23. Kaplan HS. Evidence for a tumoricidal dose level in the radiotherapy of Hodgkin's disease, *Cancer Res.,* **26** (1966) 1221–1224.
24. Choi CH and Carey R. Small cell anaplastic carcinoma of lung: reappraisal of current management, *Cancer,* **37** (1976) 2651–2657.

25. Fletcher GH. Clinical dose response curves of human malignant epithelial tumors, *Brit. J. Radiol.,* **46** (1973) 1–12.

26. Fletcher GH and Shukovsky LJ. The interplay of radiocurability and tolerance in the irradiation of human cancers, *J. Radiol. Electrol.,* **56** (1975) 383–400.

27. Griscom NT and Wang CC. Radiation therapy of inoperable breast carcinoma, *Radiology,* **79** (1962) 18–23.

28. Tepper J. Clonogenic potential of human tumors: a hypothesis, *Acta Radiol. Oncol.,* **20** (1981) 283–288.

29. Rubin P and Siemann DW. Principles of radiation oncology and cancer radiotherapy, In Rubin P, McDonald S, Qazi R, (eds.), *Clinical Oncology: A Multidisciplinary Approach,* 7th ed. Saunders, Philadelphia, 1993, pp. 71–90.

30. Suit HD. Local control and patient survival *Int. J. Radiat. Oncol. Biol. Phys.,* **23** (1992) 653–660.

31. Ramsay J, Suit HD, and Sedlacek R. Experimental studies on the incidence of metastases after failure of radiation treatment and the effect of salvage surgery, *Int. J. Radiat. Oncol. Biol. Phys.,* **14** (1988) 1165–1168.

32. Suit HD, Sedlacek RS, and Gillette EL. Examination for a correlation between probabilities of development of distant metastasis and of local recurrence, *Radiology,* **95** (1970) 189–194.

33. Suit HD. Potential for improving survival rates for the cancer patient by increasing the efficacy of treatment of the primary lesion, *Cancer,* **50** (1982) 1227–1234.

34. Fuks Z, Leibel SA, Wallner KE, et al. The effect of local control on metastatic dissemination in carcinoma of the prostate: long-term results in patients treatment with 125-I implantation, *Int. J. Radiat. Oncol. Biol. Phys.,* **21** (1991) 537–547.

35. Leibel SA, Scott CB, Mohiuddin M, et al. The effect of local-regional control on distant metastatic dissemination in carcinoma of the head and neck: results of an analysis for RTOG head and neck database, *Int. J. Radiat. Oncol. Biol. Phys.,* **21** (1991) 549–556.

36. Gunderson LL and Martenson JA. Gastrointestinal tract radiation tolerance. In Vaeth JM and Meyer JE (eds.), radiation tolerance of normal tissues, Karger, Basel, *Front. Radiat. Ther. Oncol.,* **23** (1989) 277–298.

37. Medina R, Casas F, and Calvo FA. Radiation oncology in Spain: historical notes for the radiology centennial, *Int. J. Radiat. Oncol. Biol. Phys.,* **35** (1996) 1075–1097.

38. Comas C and Prió A. Irradiation röetgen préventive intra-abdominale, aprés l'intervention chirurgicable dans un cas de cancer de l'uterus. Communication an III an. Congres International d'Electrólogie 1906. Barcelona: Imprenta Francisco Badia, 1907, pp. 5–14.

39. Finsterer H. Zur Therapie inoperabler Magen-und Darmkarzinome mit Freileung und nachfolgender Rontgenbenstrahlung, *Strahlentherapie,* **6** (1915) 205.

40. Henschke G and Henschke V. Zur technik der operations-strahlung, *Strahlentherapie,* **74** (1944) 223–239.

41. Barth G. Erfahrungen und Ergebnisse mit der Nahbestrahlung operativ freigelegten tumorem, *Strahlentherapie,* **109** (1953) 386.

42. Fuchs G and Uberall R. Die intraoperative Roentgentherapie des Blasenkarzinoms, *Strahlentherapie,* **135** (1968) 280.

43. Sabitzer H, Manfreda D, Millonig H, Primik F, Redtenbacher M, and Schneider F. Chirurgischradiologisch kombinierters therapieverfahren beim Pankreaskarzonoma-Falldemonstration-Zukunftsasperte, *Wien. Klin. Wochenschr.,* **95** (1983) 523.

44. Beck C. On external roentgen treatment of internal structures (eventration treatment), *NY Med. J.,* **89** (1919) 621–622.

45. Eloesser L. The treatment of some abdominal cancers by irradiation through the open abdomen combined with cautery excision, *Ann. Surg.,* **106** (1937) 645–652.

46. Fairchild GC and Shorter A. Irradiation of gastric cancer, *Br. J. Radiol.,* **20** (1947) 511–522.

47. Barth G. Erfahrungen und ergebnisse mit der nahbestrahlung operative freigelegter tumoren, *Strahlentherapie,* **91** (1959) 481–527.

48. Abe M and Takahashi M. Intraoperative radiotherapy: the Japanese experience, *Int. J. Radiation Oncol. Biol. Phys.,* **7** (1981) 863–868.

49. Goldson AL. Past, present and future prospects of intraoperative radiotherapy (IOR), *Sem. Oncol.,* **8** (1981) 59–65.

50. Goldson AL. Update on 5 years of pioneering experience with intraoperative electron irradiation. In *Session II—intraoperative electron therapy*, Varian Users Proceedings, (1982) 21–27.

51. Gunderson LL, Shipley WU, Suit HD, et al. Intraoperative irradiation: a pilot study combining external beam photons with "boost" dose intraoperative electrons, *Cancer,* **49** (1982) 2259–2266.

52. Tepper J and Sindelar W. Summary on intraoperative radiation therapy, *Cancer Treat. Rep.,* **65** (1981) 911–918.
53. Gunderson LL, Martin JK, Earle JD, Voss M, Kelly K, and Rorie D. Intraoperative and external beam irradiation ± resection: Mayo Pilot experience, *Mayo Clin. Proc.,* **59** (1984) 691–699.
54. Rich TA, Cady B, McDermott W, Kase K, Chaffey JT, and Hellman S. Orthovoltage intraoperative radiotherapy: a new look at an old idea, *Int. J. Radiat. Oncol.,* **10** (1984) 1951–1965.
55. Dobelbower RR and Abe M. (eds). *Intraoperative Radiation Therapy.* CRC Press, Boca Raton, FL, 1989.
56. Abe M and Takahashi M. (eds). *Intraoperative Radiation Therapy. Proceedings of the Third International Symposium on Intraoperative Radiation Therapy.* Pergamon Press, Philadelphia, 1991
57. Schildberg FW, Willich N, and Krämling HJ (eds). *Intraoperative Radiation Therapy. Proceedings 4th International Symposium.* Die Blane Eule, Essen, 1993.
58. Dritschilo A, Harter KW, Thomas D, et al. Intraoperative radiation therapy of hepatic metastases: technical aspects and report of a pilot study, *Int. J. Radiat. Oncol. Biol. Phys.,* **14** (1988) 1007–1011.
59. Lukas P, Stepan R, Ries G, et al. A new modality for intraoperative radiation therapy with a high dose-rate-afterloading unit, *Radiology,* **181** (1991) 251.
60. Thomas DS, Nanta RJ, Rodgers JE, et al. Intraoperative high dose rate interstitial irradiation of hepatic metastases from colorectal carcinoma, *Cancer,* **71** (1993) 1977–1981.
61. Nag S and Orton C. Development of intraoperative high dose rate brachytherapy for treatment of resected tumor beds in anesthetized patients, *Endcurieth Hyperth. Oncol.,* **9** (1993) 187–193.
62. Harrison LB, Enker WE, and Anderson L. High dose rate intraoperative radiation therapy for colorectal cancer - part 1, *Oncology,* **9** (1995) 679–683.
63. Harrison LB, Enker WE, and Anderson L. High dose rate intraoperative radiation therapy for colorectal cancer - part 2, *Oncology,* **9** (1995) 737–741.
64. Huber FT, Stepan R, Zimmerman F, Fink V, Molls M, and Siewart JR. Locally advanced rectal cancer: resection and intraoperative radiotherapy using the flab method combined with preoperative or postoperative radiochemotherapy, *Dis. Colon Rectum,* **39** (1996) 774–779.
65. Zelefsky MJ, LaQuaglia MP, Ghavimi F, Bass J, and Harrison LB. Preliminary results of phase I/II study of high dose rate intraoperative radiation therapy for pediatric tumors, *J. Surg. Oncol.,* **62** (1996) 267–272.
66. Harrison LB, Minsky BD, Enker WE, et al. High dose rate intraoperative radiation therapy (HDR-IORT) for locally advanced unresectable primary and recurrent rectal cancer, 1997 ASTRO Abstracts *Int. J. Radiat. Oncol. Biol. Phys.,* **39S** (1997) 168.
67. Nag S, Martinez-Monge R, and Gupta N. Intraoperative radiation therapy using electron-beam and high-dose-rate brachytherapy, *Cancer J.,* **10** (1997) 94–101.
68. Calvo FA, Brady LW, and Micaily B. Intraoperative radiotherapy: a positive view, *Am. J. Clin. Oncol.,* **16** (1993) 418–423.
69. Calvo FA, Santos M, and Brady LW (eds). *Intraoperative Radiotherapy. Clinical Experiences and Results.* Springer Verlag, Heidelberg, Germany, 1992.
70. Willett CG, Shellito PC, Tepper JE, et al. Intraoperative electron beam radiation therapy for primary locally advanced rectal and rectosigmoid carcinoma, *J. Clin. Oncol.,* **9** (1991) 843–849.
71. Tepper JE, Gunderson LL, Orlow E, et al. Complications of intraoperative radiation therapy, *Int. J. Radiat. Oncol. Biol. Phys.,* **10** (1984) 1831–1839.
72. Gunderson LL, Nelson H, Martenson JA, et al. Intraoperative electron and external beam irradiation with or without 5-fluorouracil and maximum surgical resection for previously unirradiated, locally recurrent colorectal cancer, *Dis. Colon Rectum,* **39** (1996) 1379–1395.
73. Gunderson LL, Nelson H, Martenson JA, et al. Locally advanced primary colorectal cancer: intraoperative electron and external beam irradiation +/– 5-FU, *Int. J. Radiat. Oncol. Biol. Phys.,* **37** (1997) 601–614.
74. Gunderson LL. Past, present and future of intraoperative irradiation for colorectal cancer, *Int. J. Radiat. Oncol. Biol. Phys.,* **34** (1996) 741–744.
75. Shaw EG, Gunderson LL, Martin JK, et al. Peripheral nerve and ureteral tolerance of intraoperative radiation therapy: clinical and dose response analysis, *Radiother. Oncol.,* **18** (1990) 247–255.
76. Calvo FA, Henriquez I, Santos M, et al. Intraoperative and external beam radiotherapy in advanced resectable gastric cancer: technical description and preliminary results, *Int. J. Radiat. Oncol. Biol. Phys.,* **17** (1989) 183–189.
77. Villa VV, Calvo FA, Bilbao JI, et al. Arteriodigestive fistula: a complication associated with intraoperative and external beam radiotherapy following surgery for gastric cancer, *J. Surg. Oncol.,* **49** (1992) 52–57.

78. Goldson AL, Streeter OE, Ashayeri E, et al. Intraoperative radiotherapy for intracranial malignancies, *Cancer,* **54** (1984) 2807–2813.

79. Hoekstra HJ, Restrepo C, Kinsella TJ, and Sindelar WF. Histopathological effects of intraoperative radiotherapy on pancreas and adjacent tissues: a postmortem analysis, *J. Surg. Oncol.,* **37** (1988) 104–108.

80. Fraass BA, Miller RW, Kinsella TJ, et al. Intraoperative radiation therapy at the National Cancer Institute: technical innovations and dosimetry, *Int. J. Radiat. Oncol. Biol. Phys.,* **11** (1985) 1299–1311.

81. Archambeau JO, Aitken D, Potts TM, and Slater JM. Cost-effective, available-on-demand intraoperative radiation therapy, *Int. J. Radiat. Oncol. Biol. Phys.,* **15** (1988) 775–778.

82. Wolkow BB, Chenery SG, Asche DR, et al. Practical and technical considerations in establishing an intraoperative radiation therapy program in the community practice, *Radiology,* **168** (1988) 255–258.

83. Merrick HW, Milligan AJ, Woldenberg LS, et al. Intraoperative interstitial hyperthermia in conjunction with intraoperative radiation therapy in a radiation-resistant carcinoma of the abdomen: report on feasibility of a new technique, *J. Surg. Oncol.,* **36** (1987) 48–51.

84. Tepper JE, Gunderson LL, Goldson AL, et al. Quality control parameters in intraoperative radiation therapy, *Int. J. Radiat. Oncol. Biol. Phys.,* **12** (1986) 1687–1695.

2 Biology of Large Dose per Fraction Radiation Therapy

Paul Okunieff, Srinath Sundararaman,
and Yuhchyaw Chen

CONTENTS

1. INTRODUCTION

Experimental radiobiology has inadvertently studied the implications of intraoperative and high-dose-per-fraction radiotherapy in more detail than it has standard fractionated radiotherapy. This is because the majority of radiobiological literature of tumor and normal tissue features in vivo and in vitro studies in which the radiation was given in a single fraction. Similarly, when fractionation is used experimentally, the experiment rarely features fraction sizes near the clinical 1.8- to 2-Gy size used for most external beam irradiation (EBRT). As a result much of our understanding of tumor and normal tissue response should and does relate well to that observed clinically for intraoperative irradiation (IORT).

The first and most important implication of single, large-fraction irradiation is the clear advantage it gives to tumor compared to normal tissue. The majority of radiosensitive organs, including the lung, kidney, small bowel, and brain have substantial ability to recover between daily radiation treatments *(1)*, whereas the ability of the tumor is typically much less pronounced *(2)*. Thus, on first principles, intraoperative radiation puts normal tissues at a disadvantage if they remain in the IORT field (Fig. 1). Add to that the other classical advantages of fractionation, including reoxygenation and redistribution of the cell cycle, and it is hard to justify single-fraction intraoperative radiation as the sole method of irradiation on radiobiological grounds. In particular, the dose required to control 50% of tumors is on average only minimally changed with fractionation because of reoxygenation, redistribution, and repopulation (Fig. 2).

From: *Current Clinical Oncology: Intraoperative Irradiation: Techniques and Results*
Edited by: L. L. Gunderson et al. © Humana Press, Inc., Totowa, NJ

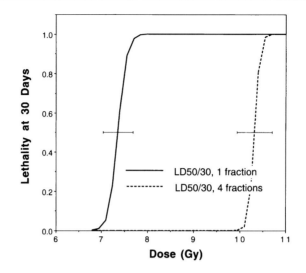

Fig. 1. Normal tissues benefit greatly from fractionation. The greatest benefit to fractionation is found in late-reacting tissues like the lung, but even acutely reacting normal tissues benefit from fractionation. Bone marrow for example is an acutely reacting tissue. If whole-body irradiation is given to C3H mice in a single fraction the $LD_{50/30}$ is 7.4 ± 0.2 Gy vs 10.3 ± 0.3 Gy if the treatment is given in four fractions over 2 d. The calculated dose-modifying factor of 1.4 is significant (95% CI 1.29· · ·1.51) *(99)*. The error bars represent the 95% CI of $LD_{50/30}$. Late-reacting tissues have larger dose-modifying factors with fractionation compared to single fraction, usually greater than 2.

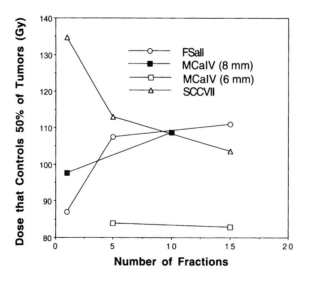

Fig. 2. On average, tumor benefits little from fractionation because of competing effects of reoxygenation and cell-cycle redistribution between fractions. Data from three different C3H-tumor models and the dose that controls 50% of tumors (TCD_{50}) are shown. Tumors are the FSaII fibrosarcoma, the MCaIV mammary carcinoma, and the SCCVII squamous-cell carcinoma. The therapeutic-gain factors with fractionation were not significantly different from 1, and ranged from 0.77 to 1.28, with an average of 1.05 ± 0.23 *(64,65,100)*. The absence of a clear increase in TCD_{50} is remarkable considering that there can be substantial tumor growth between fractions, if the interfraction interval is long *(101)*.

The entire advantage of IORT is the ability to exclude nontarget normal tissues from the radiation field. The success of IORT therefore, requires a full knowledge of the partial organ tolerances of normal tissues, and the accurate delineation of the tumor so that normal tissues can be maximally excluded. The radiobiologic literature falls short in one aspect of single-fraction radiation effects, and that is the toxicity modification caused by partial organ radiation.

In this chapter we will review the classical radiobiological principles and some of the experimental and clinical data to help better understand the tolerances of normal tissues and tumor to large radiation doses.

1.1. Model Used to Predict Radiation Effects

Several models have been used over the years to understand and quantify the radiation tolerances of tumor and normal tissues (3). Perhaps the most successful and useful models are the clonogenic-cell survival models. Based on these models, successful treatment results if all tumor clonogenic cells are killed by the treatment. By the same model, normal organ damage results if a regenerative unit is not preserved. The tumor model has withstood extensive experimental scrutiny and has generally performed well. Use of the clongenic model has been less successful in predicting normal tissue tolerance. The normal tissue model predicts tolerance best when the whole organ is treated. In addition, the normal tissue model requires the invention of a regenerative unit of tissue (1,4). This tissue unit is hard to define based on known organ physiologic and proliferative function.

Two clonogenic survival models are commonly used: the linear-quadratic model, and the multitarget model. The former predicts that survival of clonogenic units follows the shape of a parabola on log-linear coordinates. The second model predicts that low doses of radiation kill few clonogenic units, whereas at higher doses, the survival curve becomes linear on log-linear coordinates. The formulas for each of these survival curves are

$$\text{Linear-Quadratic Surviving Fraction} = S/S_0 = [e^{(-\alpha d - \beta d^2)}]^n$$

$$\text{Multitarget Surviving Fraction} = S/S_0 = [1 - (1 - e^{-d/d_o})^N]^n$$

where d is the fraction dose, n is the number of fractions, and the remaining variables (N, d_o, α, β) are fit parameters for the two models. In general, the linear-quadratic formula fits experimental data better at low doses (e.g., under 3 Gy), whereas the multitarget model better explains results at survivals under approx 10^{-3} (e.g., above 10–15 Gy). In the dose range typically used for IORT (10–20 Gy) both models work comparably well.

Using the linear-quadratic model, the shape of the survival curve is determined by the α/β ratio. This ratio has units of radiation dose. A low α/β ratio is typical of late-reacting normal tissues. Most late reacting tissues have α/β ratios less than 5 Gy, whereas acute reacting tissues and tumor often have α/β ratios of over 7. The simple exponential mathematics make estimations of equivalent doses using the linear-quadratic model convenient. Equivalent doses to compare IORT to standard 2-Gy fractionation can be estimated using the equation:

$$D_{IORT} = (1/2) \{[(\alpha/\beta)^2 + 4 D_{2Gy} (\alpha/\beta + 2)]^{0.5} - \alpha/\beta\}$$

A graphical comparison of estimated equivalent doses, based on the above equation, is given in Fig. 3. For example, if one estimates the EBRT dose required to control a squamous-cell carcinoma at 60 Gy delivered at 2-Gy per daily dose ($D_{2\,Gy} = 60$) and the

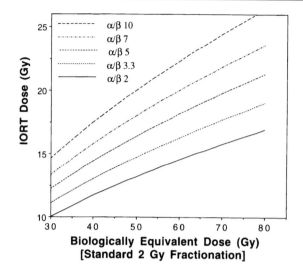

Fig. 3. The estimated biological effect of a given IORT dose is compared to that of radiation given in standard 2 Gy daily fractionation. α/β are chosen for conservative late-reacting normal tissue 2 Gy, brain 3.3 Gy *(102)*, acute reacting normal tissue 7 Gy *(103)*, and tumor 10 Gy *(104,105)*.

α/β of a squamous-cell tumor at 10 Gy, then the equivalent single fraction needed to control the tumor would be D_{IORT} = 22.3 Gy. This dose is in good agreement with the approx 20 Gy estimated by classical Strandqvist plots *(5,6)*.

Using the same equation, but instead calculating the tolerance of peripheral nerve, using a conservative α/β of 2 Gy and a generous tolerance dose of 70 Gy at 2 Gy per fraction, yields an equivalent IORT tolerance dose of only 15.8 Gy. This number is similar to those obtained in canine and human studies. For the sacral plexus, the canine 5-yr ED_{50} was 16.1–17.2 Gy, though the safe dose to nerve was 10 Gy and 25% of animals had sacropathy at 15 Gy *(7)*. Sacral plexopathy in humans occurs at a slightly lower dose with an estimated ED_{50} of 15 Gy at 2 yr. The lower dose is probably related to the associated external beam, concurrent disease such as atherosclerosis, and chemotherapy *(8)*.

With fractionation, the tolerance of peripheral nerve was initially higher than the tumor control dose. When radiation is given in a single fraction, the tumor-control dose becomes greater than the tolerance of the peripheral nerve. Thus, the normal tissue had a greater loss of tolerance because of the absence of fractionation. This phenomenon underscores the potential disadvantage inherent in any large-dose-per-fraction radiation treatment approach. To be advantageous therefore, IORT must take advantage of the surgical procedure to either exclude the nerve or other dose-limiting structure from the radiated volume, or to accomplish a gross total resection of tumor so that lower IORT doses can be used. Since nerve can rarely be excluded from IORT fields, IORT should be used as a boost dose to supplement adjuvant EBRT (typically 45–50 Gy at 1.8- to 2.0-Gy fractions) and maximal resection as discussed in Chapter 10 of this text.

2. RADIOBIOLOGY OF NORMAL TISSUES

2.1. Dose Response of Normal Tissues

Over the years, the tolerance doses of normal tissues have been estimated and tabulated by several authors, based primarily on clinical studies with laboratory confirmation *(9)*.

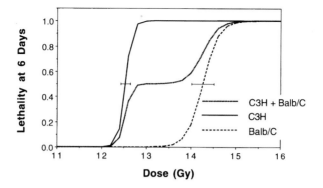

Fig. 4. Radiation toxicity to normal tissues typically occurs with a steep dose response. Figure 1 shows the steep dose response of bone marrow. In this figure gastrointestinal toxicity is measured using the lethal dose at 6 d (LD$_{50/6}$) following radiation. For C3H mice, gastrointestinal death is rare below 11 Gy, and survival is rare above 14 Gy. A steep increase in lethality occurs between 11 and 14 Gy, with half the animals dying at a dose of 12.5 ± 0.1 Gy. Gastrointestinal death occurs with a similarly steep dose response in Balb/C mice, but at a much higher dose. The effect of gastrointestinal irradiation of human subjects is likely to be just as steep for any individual. When populations of patients, each with individual genetic predispositions to gastrointestinal complications are treated, the dose-response curve will appear to be less steep. In the example, this is illustrated by the dose-response curve that might have been obtained had half the animals been C3H and half Balb/C. Also, note that if the C3H + Balb/C combination models human population studies, one might conclude that mortality was 50% at 13 Gy, a dose at which no gastrointestinal deaths are expected in the Balb/C component of the population.

The dose-response curve of normal tissue is very steep. That is, small changes in dose near tolerance can result in large changes in the rate of complication *(3).* For example, in estimating the whole-body dose of radiation that causes half of C3H mice to die of gastrointestinal (GI) lethality (e.g., LD$_{50/6}$) none will die at doses under 11 Gy, and none will survive doses over 14 Gy (Fig. 4); at 12.5 ± 0.1 Gy half will survive the GI endpoint.

Clinically the steepness of the response curve and the impact of fraction size can be easily seen. Two patients treated a few months apart with mantle irradiation fields are shown in Fig. 5. The first (left) was treated using single daily fields, anterior or posterior, using ^{60}Co at 80 cm. The second (right) was treated with opposed fields. Both had a fraction size at midplane near 2 Gy, however, the latter patient also had Mustargen hydrochloride (mechlorethamine hydrochloride), Oncovin (vincristine), procarbazine, and prednisone (MOPP) chemotherapy. The prescribed dose to the first patient was 40 Gy, but the effective fractionation at maximum, because of the inhomogeneous technique, was 3.5 Gy × 10 fractions (anterior field) + 1 Gy × 10 fractions (posterior field) = 45 Gy. The second had 1.8 Gy × 25 fractions = 45 Gy. Despite the added chemotherapy, the late effects including muscle wasting and permanent hair loss are evident in the patient treated with large fraction size. Hence, the dose response was steep enough, that the change in fraction size impacted severely on late effects even though the total dose was similar. Rib fragility, pulmonary fibrosis, pericardial constriction, and myocardial ischemia are other risks of altered fractionation schemes.

The steepness of the dose response curve aids in the choice of dose and of targets in IORT. If the radiation oncologist can maintain the IORT dose below the threshold dose for complication, then risk of complication is expected to be minimal. Alternatively, if the radiation dose is above the tolerance range, then the oncologist can expect that the

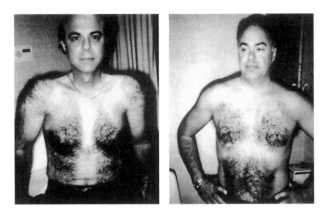

Fig. 5. Clinically the steepness of the response curve and the impact of fraction size can be easily seen. Two patients treated a few months apart are shown. The first (on left) was treated using single daily fields, anterior or posterior, using ^{60}Co at 80 cm. The second (on right) was treated with opposed fields using 4 MV X-rays at 100 SAD. Both had a fraction size at midplane near 2 Gy. The prescribed dose to the first patient was 40 Gy, but the effective fractionation at maximum, because of the inhomogeneous technique, was 3.5 Gy × 10 fractions (anterior field) + 1 Gy × 10 fractions (posterior field) = 45 Gy. The second had 1.8 Gy × 25 fractions = 45 Gy. The late effects, including muscle wasting and permanent hair loss, are dramatically evident with the larger fraction size.

organ will be damaged and can determine how important loss of that function will be to a patient. When organ function is critical, the oncologist must either choose to omit the IORT or lower the dose delivered.

2.2. Vascular Effects of Single-Fraction Irradiation

Radiation has a number of effects on vascular healing and angiogenesis. Vascular damage caused by radiation is greatest for the smallest vessels, and is more pronounced in arteries compared to veins *(10,11)*. Capillaries are probably the most severely effected by radiation, in part because of their natural fragility, and in part because antiangiogenic effects of radiation can prevent their regeneration *(11)*. As with other late-responding tissues, damage to blood vessels is dependent on both total dose and on the dose of each fraction. It is already possible to detect differences in angiogenesis in skin after 6 Gy in mice, and after 11–16 Gy given in a single fraction there is a vast decrease in the capacity of mouse skin to generate microvasculature (Fig. 6). Likewise, in response to radiation-induced antiangiogenesis, angiogenic factors are among the early genes activated in irradiated connective tissue. These cytokines are, however, unable to completely correct the antiangiogenic deficit induced by radiation. Interestingly, large vessels have a complex response to irradiation that is incompletely understood. In the case of angioplasty damage to pig coronary arteries, low doses of radiation appear to increase intimal proliferation compared to angioplasty alone, whereas intermediate doses of radiation reduce the natural intimal proliferation seen 1–6 mo after angioplasty *(12)*. In contrast to the beneficial prevention of endothelial proliferation at lower doses, fractionated radiation taken to a total dose over 40 Gy is associated with a detectable increase in ischemic heart disease in pediatric lymphoma patients followed for over 5 yr *(13)*. Hence, radiation can both increase (Fig. 7) and decrease hyperplasia of larger arteries, each with a different time course and dose response.

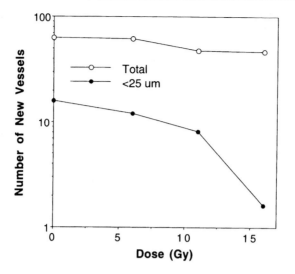

Fig. 6. Radiation doses of 0, 6, 11, or 16 Gy were given to the skin of C3H mice immediately prior to the injection of intradermal FSaII tumor cells. The tumor cells supply an angiogenic stimulus. Three days later the angiogenesis is measured by a photographic technique *(11)*. Preirradiation of the skin results in a reduction of neovascular formation that is most severe as the dose exceeds 11 Gy in a single fraction. Large vessel number is well preserved at the full range of doses. Microvessels, however, were severely reduced, indicating that capillaries and nutritive vasculature are the most severely effected by radiation of normal tissues. Conduit flow, which occurs in larger vessels, is better preserved.

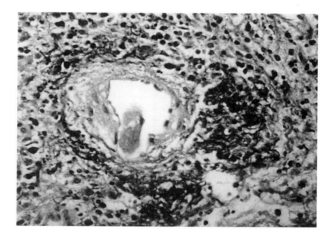

Fig. 7. The pulmonary arteries are normally thin-walled vessels. Four months after radiation to a dose of 62 Gy at 2 Gy per fraction, there is substantial perivascular connective-tissue proliferation, intimal proliferation, exposure of vascular basement membrane, and associated platelet thrombus. Vascular effects of large-dose-per-fraction radiation are complex and can be hard to predict, however, in most cases the damage is more severe than with fractionated radiation.

Studies of vascular tolerance in IORT of canine and human subjects appear to reproduce this complex dose and time response. Most vascular complications, like many of the neurological complications are associated with fibrovascular proliferation and stenosis. In contrast, some data suggest that at the highest IORT doses (e.g., ≥25 Gy) radiation may actually decrease the natural intimal proliferation after vascular anastomosis *(14)*. Vas-

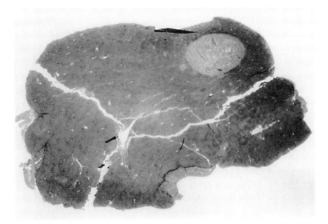

Fig. 8. Canine liver was irradiated using a point source. At 1 mo following radiation, the liver shows a region of necrosis 3 cm in diameter, corresponding to the 15-Gy isodose volume. The animal had no detectable increase in liver function tests and no detectable hepatic dysfunction. Necrosis-inducing doses of radiation are well tolerated with no detectable metabolic abnormalities if only a small portion of the liver is irradiated *(99)*.

cular rupture and aneurysm have also been described when large arteries must be taken to full dose. In this case, it appears that the vasa vasorum that feed the arterial wall have been damaged, and the small-vessel disease then precipitates the large-vessel complication *(15)*.

The lack of a clear understanding of the dose-time effects of radiation on arteries limits our ability to fully understand the toxicity to any perfused tissue. Canine and clinical studies of radiation tolerance of large arteries, however, suggest that clinically significant complications are rare under 15–17 Gy and become common if circumferential radiation over approx 20 Gy is given. In contrast, fractionated radiation is usually safe even to coronary arteries at doses up to 40 Gy. Other large arteries are commonly taken over 60 Gy safely when fractionation is employed. When fractionated and single-fraction IORT radiation are both given, the frequency of complication is similar to that expected from the IORT treatment alone. In either case, vascular ischemic complications increase with time, are dose dependent, and can take over a decade to occur.

2.3. Partial Organ Tolerance

The radiation dose safely tolerated by many critical organs is determined by the volume of tissue irradiated. For the central nervous system, the dose-volume relationship is well understood and can be easily quantified using several models *(16–18)*. The volume-response curve, like the dose-response curve is steep. Namely, at a given radiation dose, the frequency of toxicity is rare at small volume, and above a threshold-like volume, complication frequency rises quickly to near certainty. As an example, the frequency of complication with single-dose treatment of brain is minimal for targets under 3 mL (frequency under 3%) and rises to 40% for volumes over 10 mL *(19)*. Likewise, lung tolerance is generally quoted as under 20 Gy with standard fractionation of the whole lung and under 16 Gy for total-body irradiation *(9)*. Nevertheless, pulmonary dysfunction is rarely symptomatic even when doses of over 70 Gy are given to small lung volumes *(20)*. Similar observations have been made in partial organ treatment of the liver (Fig. 8) *(21)*.

Unfortunately, exact rules for estimating partial-organ tolerance are not available; however, certain rules apply. Circumferential treatment to high dose is unwise for any hollow viscus or large vessel *(14,22)*. Transmural treatment is tolerated less well than glancing treatment of hollow organs. Organs involved by tumor are at higher risk for fibrovascular complication. For example ureteral and peripheral nerve tolerance appear to be lowered by tumor involvement *(23)*. Care should be made to limit irradiation of vascular grafts and bowel anastomoses, and all sutures should be placed securely and with some redundancy. Likewise, if there are multiple arterial supplies to an organ, it is advantageous to avoid irradiation of as much of the vascular supply as possible. Finally, portions of organs that can be sacrificed surgically can also often be safely treated to high radiation dose (i.e., lung, liver). Exceptions include the small bowel, which might perforate or obstruct if overdosed compared to resection of the same region of bowel, and major arteries for which aneurysm can result from damage to vasa vasorum *(14,22)*.

2.4. Dose-Rate Effects

Dose-rate effects rarely enter into IORT. This is because the surgical procedure must be completed in a timely manner. Dose-rate effects do not become important clinically until rates under 5–10 cGy/min are achieved *(24,25)*. Experimental models suggest that even lower dose rates are required to take full advantage of dose-rate effect *(26)*. In clinical practice, it is rarely, if ever, possible to slow dose rate to these levels when IORT is employed, since the procedure duration would be lengthened by a minimum of 2–5 h.

2.5. Clinical Modifiers of Normal Tissue Radiosensitivity

Patients undergoing IORT have commonly already undergone several surgical procedures, previous EBRT, and multiple cycles of chemotherapy. Patients may also have other conditions including cardiovascular disease, diabetes, collagen-vascular disease, autoimmune disease, or undetected genetic instability syndromes (e.g., heterozygosity of ataxia telangiectasia, heterozygosity of Fanconi's anemia) *(27–29)*.

The interaction between standard radiation or surgery on the IORT site is usually limited to the specific anatomy or its physiology. Delayed treatment-induced fibrosis is known to be more pronounced in patients who undergo irradiation before, after, or with a surgical manipulation. Delayed fibrosis can worsen with time. Acute toxicities are also sometimes worsened by irradiation. Toxicities include impaired granulation of irradiated tissue, and wound strength can be reduced. In performance of IORT it is usually possible to avoid treatment of skin, making the frequency of wound closure complications low. The interaction of radiation and surgery, however, in the tumor bed cannot be avoided.

Radiation and surgery can sometimes interact in more complex ways. For example, in animal models, if the left kidney is removed, and the entire right kidney is irradiated 1 mo later, the radiation tolerance of the right kidney increases substantially *(30,31)*. The hypertrophic response apparently led to radiation protection in this animal model. In contrast, if the entire left kidney is irradiated, and the right kidney is immediately nephrectomized, the left kidney develops nephritis at a reduced dose *(30,31)*. Here, the induction of a proliferative response seems to result in a stress that is poorly handled by an irradiated kidney. We have been in a related situation clinically. A right nephrectomy and IORT were performed for treatment of a retronephric sarcoma several years after bilateral renal irradiation. (The patient had a distant history of a right-sided Wilms tumor, the treatment of which included 10-Gy EBRT to the whole abdomen delivered at 1.5 Gy per fraction.) Perhaps because of the long time lapse between therapies, this patient has done well for

4 yr with no recurrent disease and stable renal function. In most cases of combined radiation and surgery, however, the interaction can be predicted based on the physiology and local anatomy.

2.6. Chemical Modifiers of Normal Tissue Radiosensitivity

The impact of chemotherapy on radiosensitization of tumor and normal tissues is difficult to predict. The enhancement ratio is a measure of radiosensitization induced by combinations of drug and radiation. The enhancement ratio is the differential cell kill obtained by the combination of radiation and drug after correction for the independent cytotoxicity of the drug itself. The enhancement ratio may increase either because of a steeper slope and/or reduction in the shoulder of the radiation dose-response curve.

In general, a therapeutic gain is only obtained if the normal tissues irradiated are not also sensitized by the combination of radiation and drug. If the enhancement ratio seen by the tumor is also experienced by the normal tissue, and the normal tissues must be irradiated, radiosensitizing drugs are of no theoretical advantage. IORT can be advantageous from this perspective, since it is frequently possible to exclude sensitized organs from the IORT port.

Enhancement ratios for chemical sensitizers are almost always greater when given with large radiation doses, such as IORT. This is because the enhancement ratio is diluted in a fractionated course of radiotherapy. An enhancement ratio of 2 indicates that cell kills normally seen at a given dose will be seen at one-half that dose. If such effects were seen clinically, responses would be dramatic. However, fractionation severely dilutes the enhancement ratios that are seen when radiation is given in a single fraction. It is common for large enhancement ratios of 2 or 3 to decrease to 1.1 or less with fractionation. This dilution is probably because of redistribution of tumor cells in the cell cycle, repopulation of tumor between fractions, reoxygenation, and other modifiers of the radiation dose-response curve. Since IORT emulates the experimental model in which radiation is given in a single fraction, the utility of combinations of radiation and radiosensitizing drugs is expected to be significant. Thus, radiosensitizing drugs with enhancement ratios of 1.1 to 1.5 might still be expected to be important biologically when radiation is given in large single fractions.

The interaction between drugs and radiation is most pronounced when both are used simultaneously (32). Some drugs interact with radiation even if separated substantially in time, a phenomenon termed recall (Table 1). The most well known drug in this category is doxorubicin, and related intercalating drugs include bleomycin (33,34). For other chemotherapeutic drugs, the interaction seems to be more pronounced if the chemotherapy is given following radiation. The possibility of deleterious interaction is much less if the drug is completed well before radiation. An example of a drug in this category is high-dose methotrexate (35). This is probably because of the chronic subclinical radiation effects interacting with a drug toxicity that would have also otherwise been subclinical and temporary.

In animal models and probably humans, alkylating agents can worsen pulmonary toxicity if given in close proximity to irradiation (36,37). Cis-platinum, a bifunctional alkylating agent, is a powerful radiosensitizer of both tumor and normal tissues (38–45). The effects are most pronounced at low doses (46–49). At higher doses, cisplatinum kills tumor cells and thus cannot sensitize those cells (cells cannot die twice). At low drug doses however, radiation appears to enhance the sublethal drug toxicity. Both oxic and

Table 1
Radiosensitizing Drugs with Potential Application to IORT

Drug	Proposed Mechanism	Mode of Radiosensitization
Adriamycin, bleomycin, actinomycin D and mitomycin C	Antibiotics: Intercalation into DNA where it can remain for long periods of time.	Greatest radiosensitizing effect if given concurrent with radiation. Radiosensitization sometimes seen when given months or years before or after irradiation. Commonly associated with pulmonary fibrosis or cardiac toxicity.
Cisplatinum	Alkylating agent.	Sensitizer of hypoxic cells even at very low concentration.
Cyclophosphamide	Alkylating agent.	Primarily interacts in lung and heart. Toxicity greatest when given in close proximity to radiation.
5-FU and gemcytabine	Antimetabolite: Primarily S-phase cytotoxin. Complex mechanism of action.	Sensitizer of cells in the most radioresistant portion of the cell cycle. Particularly useful for gastrointestinal malignances.
Methotrexate	Antimetabolite.	Primarily interacts in CNS. Worse if given with or after irradiation.
Paclitaxel	Tubulin binder. Synchronizes cells in G_2/M.	Places cycling cells in the most radiation-sensitive portion of the cell cycle. Sensitization requires appropriate schedule of drug before irradiation.
Topotecan and camptothecin	Topoisomerase inhibition.	Greatest effect when given concurrently or in close proximity. Believed to sensitize by unraveling DNA and contributing to double strand breaks.
Misonidazole, SR2508	Nitromidazole. Radiosensitizers. Oxygen mimetic, hypoxic cell radiosensitization.	Typically neurotoxic at radiosensitizer dose levels.
IUDR and BUDR	Halogenated pyrimidines. Thymidine replacement in DNA.	Sensitizes only actively replicating cells.

hypoxic tumor cells are prone to cisplatinum-induced radiosensitization *(50,51);* hypoxic cells might, however, be more sensitized *(46–49).*

Other chemotherapy drugs with independent cytotoxicity have also been studied with clinical success. Perhaps the most important of these being fluorouracil (5-FU) *(52,53).* This drug has a complex mechanism of action, and is particularly cytotoxic to S-phase cells. The S-phase is the least sensitive portion of the cell cycle and killing of these cells undoubtedly is a component of the 5-FU-mediated synergistic effects. Another cycle-active drug, paclitaxel, sensitizes cells by synchronizing them in G_2/M, the most radiosensitive portion of the cell cycle *(54–56).*

A final category of radiosensitizing drugs worth discussing are the topoisomerase inhibitors *(57–60).* Topoisomerases uncoil supercoiled DNA by nicking one strand and serving as a swivel to allow uncoiling without tearing of the remaining single strand of DNA. By inhibiting the swiveling of the DNA, topoisomerase inhibitors preserve the single-strand break. The uncoiled DNA provides a better target for radiation. Also, the effective single-strand break may allow for easier breakage of the remaining DNA strand, leading to a lethal double-strand break. The effects of topoisomerase inhibitors are primarily observed in cycling cells, but topoisomerase activity occurs in all cells.

3. RADIOBIOLOGY OF TUMOR

3.1. Tumor Oxygenation and Hypoxic Radiation Sensitization

When experimental tumors are treated with a single fraction, tumor response is usually determined by the hypoxic fraction of cells. This is because well-oxygenated cells are far more sensitive to radiation than those with poor oxygenation. The differential sensitivity is exponential with dose. Hence, even if oxygenated cells outnumber the hypoxic cells by one or two orders of magnitude, the hypoxic cells can still dominate as the cause of treatment failure. When fractionation of the radiation dose is employed, the impact of hypoxia is harder to detect because of a reassortment of the oxygenation between treatments, a process termed reoxygenation *(61).* Whereas in experimental animals the hypoxic fraction of tumor consistently increases with tumor size, in humans the relation is less consistent. Thus, even small tumors can be hypoxic in human subjects. Hypoxic fractions for human tumors are often similar to that of small murine tumors, and like small murine tumors, oxygenation is quite variable even among tumors of the same size and histologic type. Thus, many human tumors have no significant hypoxia, and in others, hypoxic cells can comprise more than half the tumor. The impact of vascular ligation, clamps, and anesthesia during surgery add to the potential of increased tumor hypoxia during IORT.

Several clinical approaches have been taken to reduce hypoxia. First, patients are anesthestized and blood pressure is maintained by appropriate hydration and transfusion. Anesthesia can cause vasodilation, which in the absence of concomitant hypotension can actually improve tumor blood flow. During the irradiation, patients can be ventilated with near pure oxygen. In this case, increasing the oxygen partial pressure can improve the oxygen-carrying capacity modestly, and does appear to at least temporarily increase tumor oxygenation *(62).* Interestingly, tumor metabolism is often oxygen limited, and when oxygen breathing is allowed to continue for over approx 30 min, some tumors will augment their metabolic rate and consume the added oxygen. Hence, the inspired oxygen should not be unnecessarily increased until just before the radiation is to be delivered.

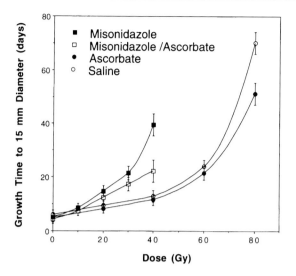

Fig. 9. In single-fraction irradiation treatment, the response of tumor is primarily determined by the fraction of tumor cells that are radiobiologically hypoxic. For example, using the hypoxic sensitizer misonidazole at a dose of 0.3 mg/g body weight, dose modifying factors of 1.5–2.5 are typically observed (64,65). Likewise, drugs that only radioprotect well-oxygenated cells, like ascorbate, do not protect tumor in single-fraction studies. Ascorbate can reduce some of the sensitizing effects of oxygen-mimetic drugs like misonidazole. The data shown were measured using FSaII fibrosarcoma tumors growing in C3H mice. Tumors were irradiated at 8-mm diameters and time to reach 15 mm was tabulated. Values are means ± 1 SE. At 40 Gy, some misonidazole-treated tumors had permanent control. Likewise, at 80 Gy some ascorbate or control animals were permanently controlled.

Hypoxic radiosensitizing drugs, and in particular the nitroimidazole drugs, have been used in combination with IORT. Whereas the data is still inconclusive, this approach has much theoretical merit. The major toxicity of the nitroimidazole radiosensitizers is neurologic. The effect is cumulative with total drug dose. Because humans appear to tolerate these drugs less well than rodents, the concentrations of drug that are required to significantly sensitize tumor are often prohibitive in fractionated studies. As a result, many studies of fractionated radiation have given the drug at doses that do not even sensitize animal tumors treated in a single fraction. Successful use of these drugs with fractionated radiation, a condition in which hypoxia is less important than single-fraction irradiation, has thus been difficult to achieve. Single-fraction therapies, like IORT, allow for a therapeutic dose of nitroimidazole radiosensitizer to be delivered. Only hypoxic cells would be sensitized by this therapy, and dose-modifying factors over 2 are typically achieved with these drugs (Fig. 9) (63–65). If a doubling of dose effect were to be observed in the clinic, it should have an important benefit to patients.

Whereas most normal tissues are well oxygenated and are thus not expected to be sensitized by increased inspired oxygen or nitroimidazole drug, it is known that brain involved by tumor can be quite hypoxic (66,67). Skin and liver are two other organs that commonly have high natural hypoxia and would be sensitized by procedures aimed at hypoxic cells (68). Normal tissue radiation tolerance, therefore, can sometimes occur when tissue oxygenation is increased. For example, augmenting the inspired oxygen in the case of IORT for brain tumors might be expected to increase the oxygenation of the normal brain and thus increase the risk of necrosis. Hence, an understanding of the actual physiology of the tissues being treated should be taken into consideration when any radiosensitizer is employed.

Oxygen diffusion distances change depending upon the metabolic rate of tumor, on the cell density of tumor, and on the availability of carbon substrate (e.g., sugars and protein). Over the years, several drugs have been developed for improving tissue hypoxic cell sensitivity. These drugs include the oxygen-mimetic sensitizers, oxygen-unloading drugs, vasodilatory drugs, hyperbaric and hyperoxic breathing, blood doping, hypo- and hyper-thermia, drugs that alter the oxygen-consumption rate, and therapies that alter tumor angiogenesis. The diffusion of oxygen is primarily limited by metabolism, and since the latter is rarely known, the oxygen status is rarely known. Hence, the ability to evaluate toxic drug therapies, aimed only at hypoxic cells, is plagued by the problem of delivery of these toxic drugs to patients with tumors that have no substantial hypoxia *(69)*. Progress is being made in imaging hypoxia using positron emission tomography (PET) and elec-trode technology and this should ultimately impact on the successful routine use of hypoxic radiosensitizers *(70)*.

Many drugs with independent tumor cytotoxicity are known to function as radiosen-sitizers, and some are routinely used clinically. These drugs are of obvious interest as an adjunct to IORT. Some chemotherapy, interestingly, are very effective at killing hypoxic cells and thus might synergize with radiation given during IORT *(71–74)*.

3.2. Dose Response of Human Tumors and Implications for IORT Dose

There is little discussion of dose response for tumor control in the IORT literature despite the large range of doses used in various studies. In contrast, there is great discus-sion of the dose response for production of complications. Thus, it appears that the heterogeneity of tumor response to IORT may be more determined by the ability to safely include the tumor and less by the dose chosen. Radiobiologically this can be explained if even the lowest IORT doses are already sufficient for infield control of most tumors.

The dose response of human tumors have been published in multiple clinical series and organized by several authors *(75–78)*. The median dose range that locally controls 50% of adult solid tumors (TCD_{50}) is approx 45–65 Gy in standard fractionation (Fig. 10). The TCD_{50} for microscopic residual disease is closer to 25–50 Gy for typical adult solid tumors *(75)*. As previously discussed, the dose response curve is steep. The $gamma_{50}$ factor was defined to estimate the steepness of the dose-response curve *(4,75)*. It has units of percentage change in local control divided by percentage change in dose measured at the TCD_{50}. Thus, a $gamma_{50}$ of 1 to 2, which is typical of most tumors, suggests that a 1% increase in dose near the TCD_{50} level will increase controls by 1–2%. As an example, if the TCD_{50} is 50 Gy, then 55 Gy (10% increase in dose) would increase local control to 60–70%.

No detailed analyses are possible for IORT because of the complexity of cases treated, and the routine combination of EBRT and IORT. As an estimate, however, an IORT boost of 10, 15, or 20 Gy, using data in Fig. 3, preceded or followed by 45 Gy of fractionated EBRT, would have a theoretical biological effect equivalent to 61, 76, or 95 Gy assuming an α/β of 10. Since these doses safely exceed the expected TCD_{50} for most solid tumors, there is little radiobiological justification to ever exceed total IORT doses of 15–20 Gy, if EBRT is also delivered. Perhaps the only exception to this rule would be in the case of a known severely hypoxic tumor. The experience with stereotactic radiosurgery of brain metastases supports the conclusion that tumor can be locally controlled with radiation

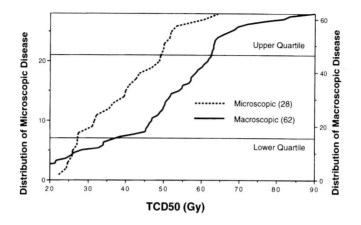

Fig. 10. The distribution of 100 dose-response curves for human malignancies were collected based on single and multi-insitutional studies *(75)*. Sixty-two calculations of TCD_{50} were made for unresectable tumor, and 28 calculations for patients at high risk of recurrance or with positive margins. The calculated TCD_{50}s are displayed as a cumulative histogram. Typical tumors, based on the middle quartiles, had TCD_{50}s of 45–65 Gy for gross tumor, and 25–50 Gy for resected tumor. In most studies the radiation was given with standard fractionation using external beam. The lowest TCD_{50}s occurred in hematopoietic and pediatric malignancies, the highest TCD_{50}s were for unresectable esophageal cancer. In the context of steep dose-response curves, these data suggest that total effective doses over 70 Gy are rarely indicated for control of macroscopic disease and that doses over 60 Gy should obtain infield control for microscopic disease.

doses ≤15 Gy when combined with external beam. Fractionated whole-brain radiation doses of 30–40 Gy, combined with 10- to 15-Gy stereotactic boosts, yields local control of approx 90% of patients *(79)*. Though the success of stereotactic radiation is compelling evidence that doses of IORT over 15 Gy may not be necessary, competing causes of mortality make determination of local control difficult. Late failures, therefore, may have been missed.

3.3. Radiobiologic Benefits of Low-Dose IORT When Full-Dose Cannot be Safely Delivered: Rationale for Field within a Field

Having discussed the steepness of the radiation dose-response curve, one might predict that if doses of radiation near the tumor-control dose cannot be safely given or are not delivered for other reasons, the utility of IORT is in question. This concept however is true only when IORT is the only therapy being delivered. If the patient has received preoperative EBRT, is expected to be given postoperative EBRT, or has had a gross total resection, then IORT could yield tumor control even if total dose must be limited. The rationale for this comes from the expectation that the largest number of potentially surviving clonogenic tumor cells are in the primary mass or surgical bed, and that disease outside the field can be controlled by EBRT, chemotherapy, or surgical excision. Under these circumstances, even a low boost dose of radiation given by IORT may improve control rates *(77,80)*. Theoretical estimations of improved control rates have been made by several authors. The concept of partial tumor boost is still controversial, but the conditions of IORT make its consideration particularly important. Some estimates suggest that for many tumors as much as 10% of the tumor can be excluded from the IORT boost field and still yield 10–20% improvements in local control *(4,81)*. Theoretically, therefore, if the entire tumor cannot be safely taken to full dose, it is still worth considering giving the safe dose to the entire tumor and a further intraoperative dose (field within a field) to the volume excluding the sensitive tissue.

4. FUTURE OF RADIOBIOLOGY AND RELEVANCE TO IORT

4.1. New Biological Parameters of Consideration

It has long been known that patients with certain inherited abnormalities are substantially more radiation sensitive than "normal" patients (28,82). It has also been hypothesized that many apparently normal people are more radiosensitive than true "normals" because of undetected heterozygosity for an inheritable disorder (27). With recent advances in molecular technique, it is becoming possible to test for disorders of DNA repair. In primitive eukaryotes, yeast, there are over a dozen DNA repair pathways, each of which has multiple genes acting in concert, and mutants have been isolated for each repair pathway. Interestingly, each repair mutant has increased radiation sensitivity. Radiation may be unique in this ubiquitous affect; cytotoxic drugs typically effect only one or two DNA repair pathways. The results suggest that there could be a large number of individuals with abnormalities of complex pathways that must be intact for fully normal DNA repair following radiation. As the enzymes and genes are sequenced and mutant patterns identified, it might ultimately be possible to identify patients with increased risk for complications from IORT. An example of a genetically unspecified difference that alters gastrointestinal radiosensitivity is shown in Fig. 4. Interestingly, IORT may still be safe and effective for these patients if the radiation dose is appropriately adjusted. For example, patients with ataxia telangiectasia or heterozygosity for that disorder, might benefit from a reduction in the radiation dose. There is already substantial experience to suggest that the tumors and leukemias that occur in many of these subjects are comparably sensitized by the DNA-repair disorder (28,29,83,84) and thus tumor response should not suffer when dose is adjusted.

Recent studies of cytokine expression also suggest that toxicities to normal tissues resulting from IORT may be predicted in the future. Rubin et al. showed that TGFβ (transforming growth factor β) was elevated preceding the development of radiation pneumonitis (85). TGFβ is one of many fibrogenic and proinflammatory cytokines induced to different degrees in animal and human following radiation. Experimentally, the levels of expression of these cytokines appear to depend on animal species and strain, the type of tumor growing in the animal, and type of therapy delivered. As with different mouse strains, the levels of expression in different human subjects is highly variable (86,87). Correlative studies in man confirm that many tumors produce TGFβ and that individuals who have chronically elevated levels of these cytokines, whether endogenous, disease-induced, or therapy-induced, are at increased risk for late radiation complications. TGFβ and tumor necrosis factor (TNF) for example have been associated with pulmonary and/or hepatic fibrosis following radiation or chemotherapy (86,87). These cytokines can already be easily measured by ELISA, paving the way for predictive assays. It is interesting to speculate that medications to alter the chronic expression of these cytokines will prevent some complications of IORT.

4.2. Oncogenesis

The oncogenic potential of radiation is well known. In general, as with other complications of radiation, the frequency of late radiation-induced cancers are related to fraction size, total dose, and field size. Oncogenesis in the IORT field is common in canines (88), though not yet reported in human subjects. Malignancies attributed to IORT, however, must originate in the IORT field, must be of a different histology than the original primary, and must occur after a significant time lag (usually over 6 mo and often years or decades). Radiation-induced oncogenesis can include leukemias, carcinomas, and sarcomas *(89)*. IORT-induced malignancies in canines, however, are most commonly sarcomas of bone or soft tissue. The type of cancer generated by treatment is related to the type of radiation used, the target tissue irradiated and the size of the radiation dose used for the treatment. For example, orthovoltage techniques have the disadvantage of severe dose inhomogeneity and thus high-dose regions can occur in nonmalignant tissues included in the IORT field. Likewise, electrons have significant dose heterogeneity when traversing bone, leading to inadvertent overdose of this organ. Murine models suggest that single doses of ≥35 Gy are associated with near certain sarcomatous degeneration *(90)*. Estimates of carcinogenesis in canine models are typically not actuarially corrected and, thus underestimate long-term risk of malignancy. In two canine studies from the National Institutes of Health, one found that animals that received over 20 Gy have a crude long-term malignancy rate of 1/8 (12%), and in a shorter analysis 10/46 (22%) developed sarcomas, all but one of which received over 20 Gy *(88)*. None of the sham-irradiated animals in either study developed cancers.

The frequency of malignancy caused by IORT is difficult to discern in patients. Unlike the animal models, most patients treated with IORT already have aggressive tumors and a high rate of death from other causes, follow-up is often short because of high mortality, and the IORT dose is usually 10–20 Gy. Perhaps for these reasons, oncogenesis is and will remain rare in patients treated with IORT.

The mechanism of radiation-induced oncogenesis is unknown in most cases because few cancers occur within the first years after irradiation. However, it is unlikely that direct DNA damage from the irradiation is the primary cause of most cancers. In some cases the mechanism of radiation-induced oncogenesis is known. For example, patients with hereditary retinoblastoma are at high risk of developing multiple malignancies including sarcomas of bone and soft tissue. Cancers in these patients develop because of radiation-induced mutation of the remaining normal Rb gene *(91–93)*. Recently it was discovered that cycles of hypoxia and reoxygenation can select for cells with p53 mutations *(94)*. As previously discussed, radiation causes a prolonged antiangiogenic effect that includes intimal proliferation, thrombosis, and intermittent vascular occlusion *(11)*. An important action of p53 is the promotion of apoptosis of cells with genetic damage *(95)*. p53-mutant cells selected by the years of impaired blood flow would fail to naturally undergo apoptosis and could, therefore, accumulate genetic damage *(96,97)*. If this proves to be an important mechanism of oncogenesis, strategies aimed at preventing the vascular effects of radiation might also reduce the incidence of radiation-induced malignancy.

The authors would like to suggest a final mechanism that could predispose to oncogenesis. As previously discussed, the normal tissues in the IORT bed can in some subjects develop chronically elevated proliferative and fibrogenic cytokine levels. It is now known that high levels of many cytokines inhibit apoptosis by mechanisms that, can but often do not include, the p53 pathway *(98)*. As with p53, this process could predispose to oncogenesis, and might be preventable using anticytokine therapies.

With long-term survivals becoming common, the frequency of oncogenesis is likely to increase. For most patients it is a very late effect, occurring many years after successful therapy of the primary. The effect is associated with fraction dose, the organ irradiated, previous surgery or chemotherapy, and the patient's underlying genetics. As we better understand the mechanisms of radiation-induced cancers, it is reasonable to expect that therapies to alter those mechanisms can be developed to reduce the long-term risk.

5. CONCLUSIONS

Classical radiobiology teaches that fractionation benefits normal tissue over tumor, and is probably the most effective method we have of improving tumor response and preventing late normal-tissue toxicity. The current requirement that IORT be given in a single dose results in the potential disadvantages for IORT that have been previously discussed. The most important advantage of IORT is the potential for radiation of the tumor, while minimizing radiation to nontarget tissues. Another advantage of IORT is the potential of delivering concurrent radiosensitizing drugs under circumstances in which the minimum of normal tissue will experience the sensitization affects. Because tumor response to single fraction is predominantly determined by the hypoxic fraction, drugs and other strategies aimed at this population of tumor cells should be studied. However, it must also be recognized that hypoxia does exist in some normal tissues, and the effects of these drugs may not be selective in some circumstances. Normal-tissue complications are the main limitation of IORT, and they can be minimized by avoidance of full-organ irradiation and by procedures designed to reduce dose to nontarget organs. Reducing dose is reasonable in many cases since there is experimental and theoretical evidence that even low-dose IORT can improve local control when employed in conjunction with other therapies. Late side effects of radiation are currently difficult to predict, and occur with a steep dose and volume response. Ongoing research into the mechanisms and genetics of fibrosis, angiogenesis, and oncogenesis suggest that some of these effects will eventually be alleviated by appropriate therapeutic interventions.

REFERENCES

1. Thames HD, Withers HR, Peters LJ, and Fletcher GH. Changes in early and late radiation responses with altered dose fractionation: implications for dose-survival relationships, *Int. J. Radiat. Oncol. Biol. Phys.,* **8** (1982) 219–226.
2. Thames HD and Suit HD. Tumor radioresponsiveness versus fractionation sensitivity, *Int. J. Radiat. Oncol. Biol. Phys.,* **12** (1986) 687–691.
3. Tucker SS, Thames HD, and Taylor JM. How well is the probability of tumor cure after fractionated irradiation described by Poisson statistics?, *Radiat. Res.,* **124** (1990) 273–282.
4. Niemierko A and Goitein M. Implementation of a model for estimating tumor control probability for an inhomogeneously irradiated tumor, *Radiother. Oncol.,* **29** (1993) 140–147.
5. Strandqvist M. Time-dose relationship, *Acta Radiologica,* **55** (1944) 1–300.
6. Andrews JR and Coppedge TO. The dose-time relationship for the cure of squamous cell carcinoma, *Am. J. Roentgenol.,* **65** (1951) 934–939.
7. Johnstone PAS, DeLuca AM, Bacher JD, et al. Clinical toxicity of peripheral nerve to intraoperative radiotherapy in a canine model, *Int. J. Radiat. Oncol. Biol. Phys.,* **32** 1995) 1031–1034.
8. Vujaskovic Z, Gillette SM, Powers BE, et al. Intraoperative radiation (IORT) injury to sciatic nerve in a large animal model, *Radiother. Oncol.,* **30** (1994) 133–139.
9. Emami B, Lyman J, Brown A, et al. Tolerance of normal tissue to therapeutic irradiation, *Int. J. Radiat. Oncol. Biol. Phys.,* **21** (1991) 109–122.
10. Fajardo LF. *Pathology of Radiation Injury.* Masson Publishing, New York, 1982.
11. Okunieff P, Dols S, Lee J, et al. Angiogenesis determines blood flow, metabolism, growth rate, and ATPase kinetics of tumors growing in an irradiated bed: 31P and 2H nuclear magnetic resonance studies, *Cancer Res.,* **51** (1991) 3289–3295.
12. Mazur W, Ali MN, Khan MM, et al. High dose rate intracoronary radiation for inhibition of neointimal formation in the stented and balloon-injured porcine models of restenosis: angiographic, morphometric, and histopathologic analyses, *Int. J. Radiat. Oncol. Biol. Phys.,* **36** (1996) 777–788.

13. Hancock SL, Donaldson SS, and Hoppe RT. Cardiac disease following treatment of Hodgkin's disease in children and adolescents, *J. Clin. Oncol.,* **11** (1993) 1208–1215.

14. Johnstone PAS, Sprague M, DeLuca AM, et al. Effects of intraoperative radiotherapy on vascular grafts in a canine model, *Int. J. Radiat. Oncol. Biol. Phys.,* **29** (1994) 1015–1025.

15. Rubin P and Cassarett GW. *Clinical Radiation Pathology.* Saunders, Philadelphia, 1968.

16. Flickinger JC, Lunsford LD, and Kondziolka D. Dose prescription and dose-volume effects in radio-surgery, *Stereotactic Radiosurgery,* **3** (1992) 51–59.

17. Flickinger JC, Lunsford LD, Wu A, and Kalend A. Predicted dose-volume isoeffect curves for stereo-tactic radiosurgery with the ^{60}Co gamma unit, *Acta Oncologica,* **30** (1991) 363–367.

18. Flickinger JC. An integrated logistic formula for prediction of complications from radiosurgery, *Int. J. Radiat. Oncol. Biol. Phys.,* **17** (1989) 879–885.

19. Kapp DS, Fischer D, Gutierrez E, Kohorn EI, and Schwartz PE. Pretreatment prognostic factors in carcinoma of the uterine cervix: a multivariable analysis of the effect of age, stage, histology and blood counts on survival, *Int. J. Radiat. Oncol. Biol. Phys.,* **9** (1983) 445–455.

20. Roberston JM, Ten Haken RK, Hazuka MB, et al. Dose escalation for non-small cell lung cancer using conformal radiation therapy, *Int. J. Radiat. Oncol. Biol. Phys.,* **37** (1997) 1079–1085.

21. Cromheecke M, Vermeij J, Grond AJK, Konings AWT, Oldhoff J, and Hoekstra HJ. Tissue tolerance of normal and surgically manipulated canine liver to intraoperative radiation therapy (IORT), *Int. J. Radiat. Oncol. Biol. Phys.,* **27** (1993) 1141–1146.

22. Sindelar WF, Tepper JE, Kinsella, TJ, et al. Late effects of intraoperative radiation therapy on retro-peritoneal tissues, intestine, and bile duct in a large animal model, *Int. J. Radiat. Oncol. Biol. Phys.,* **29** (1994) 781–788.

23. Shaw EG, Gunderson LL, Martin JK, Beart RW, Nagorney DM, and Podratz KC. Peripheral nerve and ureteral tolerance to intraoperative radiation therapy: clinical and dose-response analysis, *Radiother. Oncol.,* **18** (1990) 247–255.

24. Down JD, Tarbell NJ, Thames HD, and Mauch PM. Syngeneic and allogeneic bone marrow engraft-ment after total body irradiation: dependence on dose, dose rate, and fractionation, *Blood,* **77** (1991) 661–669.

25. Tarbell NJ, Amato DA, Down JD, Mauch P, and Hellman S. Fractionation and dose rate effects in mice: a model for bone marrow transplantation in man, *Int. J. Radiat. Oncol. Biol. Phys.,* **13** (1987) 1065–1069.

26. Hall EJ. Radiation dose-rate: a factor of importance in radiobiology and radiotherapy, *Br. J. Radiol.,* **45** (1972) 81–85.

27. Helzlsouer KJ, Harris EL, Parshad R, Perry HR, Price FM, and Sanford KK. DNA repair proficiency: potential susceptibility factor for breast cancer, *J. Natl. Cancer Inst.,* **88** (1986) 754–755.

28. Hart RM, Kimler BF, Evans RG, and Park CH. Radiotherapeutic management of medulloblastoma in a pediatric patient with ataxia telangiectasia, *Int. J. Radiat. Oncol. Biol. Phys.,* **13** (1987) 1237–1240.

29. Deeg HJ, Socie' G, Schoch G, et al. Malignancies after marrow transplantation for aplastic anemia and Fanconi anemia: a joint Seattle and Paris analysis of results in 700 patients, *Blood,* **87** (1996) 386–392.

30. Soranson J and Denekamp J. Precipitation of latent renal radiation injury by unilateral nephrectomy, *Br. J. Cancer,* **53 (Suppl VII)** (1986) 268–272.

31. Otsuka M and Meistrich ML. Acceleration of late radiation damage of the kidney by unilateral nephre-ctomy, *Int. J. Radiat. Oncol. Biol. Phys.,* **22** (1992) 71–78.

32. Brock WA, Baker FL, and Tofilon PJ. Tumor cell sensitivities to drugs and radiation, In Chapman JD, Peters LJ, Withers HR (eds.), *Prediction of Tumor Treatment Response.* Pergamon, New York, 1989, pp. 139–156.

33. Donaldson SC, Click JM, and Wilbur JR. Adriamycin activating a recall phenomenon after radiation therapy, *Ann. Intern. Med.,* **81** (1974) 407–408.

34. Belli JA and Piro AJ. The interaction between radiation and adriamycin damage in mammalian cells, *Cancer Res.,* **37** (1977) 1624–1630.

35. DeAngelis LM and Shapiro WR. Drug/radiation interactions and central nervous system injury. In Gutin PH, Leibel SA, Sheline GE (eds.), *Radiation Injury to the Nervous System.* Raven, New York, 1991, pp. 361–382.

36. Dorie MJ, Bedarida G, and Kallman RF. Protection by interleukin 1 against lung toxicity caused by cyclophosphamide and irradiation, *Radiat. Res.,* **128** (1991) 316–319.

37. Jagannath S, Dicke KA, Armitage JO, et al. High-dose cyclophosphamide, carmustine, and etoposide, and autologous bone marrow transplantation for relapsed Hodgkin's disease, *Ann. Intern. Med.,* **104** (1986) 163–168.

38. Kyriazis AP, Yagoda A, Kereiakes JG, Kyriazis AA, and Whitmore WF. Experimental studies on the radiation-modifying effect of Cis-diamminedichloroplatinum II (DDP) in human bladder transitional cell carcinomas grown in nude mice, *Cancer,* **52** (1983) 452–457.

39. Stewart FA, Luts A, and Begg AC. Tolerance of previously irradiated mouse kidneys to *cis*-Diamminedichloroplatinum(II), *Cancer Res.,* **47** (1987) 1016–1021.

40. Shipley WU, Coombs, LJ, Einstein AB, Soloway MS, Wajsman Z, Prout GR, and National Bladder Cancer Collaborative Group. Cisplatin and full dose irradiation for patients with invasive bladder carcinoma: a preliminary report of tolerance and local response, *J. Urol.,* **132** (1984) 899–903.

41. Stewart F, Bohlken S, Begg A, and Bartelink H. Renal damage in mice after treatment with cisplatinum alone or in combination with x-irradiation, *Int. J. Radiat. Oncol. Biol. Phys.,* **12(6)** (1986) 927–933.

42. Stewart FA, Oussoren Y, and Barelink H. The influence of cisplatin on the response of mouse kidneys to multifraction irradiation, *Radiother. Oncol.,* **15** (1989) 93–102.

43. Coughlin CT and Richmond RC. Biologic and clinical developments of cisplatin combined with radiation: concepts, utility, projections for new trials, and the emergence of carboplatin, *Sem. Oncol.,* **16** (1989) 31–43.

44. Dewit L, Oussoren Y, and Bartelink H. Early and late damage in the mouse rectum after irradiation and cis-diamminedichloroplatinum(II), *Radiother. Oncol.,* **8** (1987) 57–69.

45. Dritschilo A, Piro AJ, and Kelman AD. The effect of cis-platinum on the repair of radiation damage in plateau phase Chinese hamster (V-79) cells, *Int. J. Radiat. Oncol. Biol. Phys.,* **5** (1979) 1345–1349.

46. Sun JR and Brown JM. Lack of differential radiosensitization of hypoxic cells in a mouse tumor at low radiation doses per fraction by cisplatin, *Radiat. Res.,* **133(2)** (1993) 252–256.

47. Walther MM, DeLaney TF, Smith PD, et al. A phase I trial of photodynamic therapy in the treatment of recurrent superficial transitional carcinoma of the bladder, *Urology,* **50 (2)** (1997) 199–206.

48. Melvik JE and Pettersen EO. Oxygen- and temperature-dependent cytotoxic and radiosensitizing effects of cis-dichlorodiammineplatimum (II) on human NHIK 3025 cells in vitro, *Radiat. Res.,* **114(3)** (1988) 489–499.

49. Skov KA, Farrell NP, and Adomat H. Platinum complexes with one radiosensitizing ligand [PtC12(NH3) (sensitizer)]: radiosensitization and toxicity studies in vitro, *Radiat. Res.,* **112(2)** (1987) 273–282.

50. Pfeffer MR, Teicher BA, Holden S, Al-Achi A, and Herman TS. The interaction of cisplatin plus etoposide with radiation ± hyperthermia, *Int. J. Radiat. Oncol. Biol. Phys.,* **19** (1990) 1439–1447.

51. Teicher BA, Holden SA, Al-Achi A, and Herman TS. Classification of antineoplasic treatments by their differential toxicity toward putative oxygenated and hypoxic tumor subpopulations in vivo in the FSaIIC murine fibrosarcoma, *Cancer Res.,* **50** (1990) 3339–3344.

52. McGinn CJ, Shewach DS, and Lawrence TS. Radiosensitizing nucleosides, *J. Natl. Cancer Inst.,* **88** (1996) 1193–1203.

53. Gunderson LL, Nelson H, Martenson JA, et al. Locally advanced primary colorectal cancer: intraoperative electron and external beam irradiation ± 5-FU, *Int. J. Radiat. Oncol. Biol. Phys.,* **37** (1997) 601–614.

54. Milas L, Hunter NR, Mason KA, Kurdoglu B, and Peters LJ. Enhancement of tumor radioresponse of a murine mammary carcinoma by paclitaxel, *Cancer Res.,* **54** (1994) 3506–3510.

55. Milross CG, Mason KA, Hunter NR, Chung WK, Peters LJ, and Milas L. Relationship of mitotic arrest and apoptosis to antitumor effect of paclitaxel, *J. Natl. Cancer Inst.,* **88** (1996) 1308–1314.

56. Liebmann J, Cook JA, Fisher J, Teague D, and Mitchell JB. Changes in radiation survival curve parameter in human tumor and rodent cells exposed to paclitaxel (Taxol), *Int. J. Radiat. Oncol. Biol. Phys.,* **29** (1994) 559–564.

57. Kaufmann SH, Peereboom D, Buckwalter CA, et al. Cytotoxic effects of topotecan combined with various anticancer agents in human cancer cell lines, *J. Natl. Cancer Inst.,* **88** (1996) 734–741.

58. Kim JH, Kim SH, Kolozsvary A, and Khyil MS. Potentiation of radiation response in human carcinoma cells in vitro and murine fibrosarcoma in vivo by topotecan, an inhibitor of DNA topoisomerase I, *Int. J. Radiat. Oncol. Biol. Phys.,* **22** (1992) 515–518.

59. Takimoto CH and Arbuck SG. Clinical status and optimal use of topotecan, *Oncology,* **11** (11) (1997) 1635–1646.

60. Chen AY, Okunieff P, Pommier Y, and Mitchell JB. Mammalian DNA topoisomerase I mediates the enhancement of radiation cytotoxicity by camptothecin derivatives, *Cancer Res.,* **57** (1997) 1529–1536.

61. Hendry JH and Thames HD. Fractionation sensitivity and the oxygen effect, *Br. J. Radiol.,* **63** (1992) 79–80.

62. Grau C, Nordsmark M, Khalil AA, Horsman MR, and Overgaard J. Effect of carbon monoxide breathing on hypoxia and radiation response in the SCCVII tumor in vivo, *Int. J. Radiat. Oncol. Biol. Phys.,* **29** (1994) 449–454.

63. Overgaard J. Sensitization of hypoxic tumour cells—clinical experience, *Int. J. Radiat. Biol.,* **56** (1989) 801–811.

64. Okunieff PG and Suit HD. Toxicity, radiation sensitivity modification, and combined drug effects of ascorbic acid with misonidazole in vivo on FSaII murine fibrosarcomas, *J. Natl. Cancer Inst.,* **79** (1987) 377–381.

65. Suit HD, Maimonis P, Michaels HB, and Sedlacek R. Comparison of hyperbaric oxygen and misonidazole in fractionated irradiation of murine tumors, *Radiat. Res.,* **87** (1981) 360–367.

66. Rampling R, Cruickshank G, Lewis A, Fitzsimmons SA, and Workman P. Direct measurement of pO_2 distribution and bioreductive enzymes in human malignant brain tumors, *Int. J. Radiat. Oncol. Biol. Phys.,* **29** (1994) 427–431.

67. Oberhaensli RD, Bore PJ, Rampling RP, Hilton-Jones D, Hands LJ, and Radda GK. Biochemical investigation of human tumours in vivo with phosphorus-31 magnetic resonance spectroscopy, *Lancet,* **5** (1986) 8–11.

68. Vaupel P, Kallinowski F, and Okunieff P. Blood flow, oxygen and nutrient supply, and metabolic microenvironment of human tumors: a review, *Cancer Res.,* **49** (1989) 6449–6465.

69. Okunieff P, Dunphy EP, Höckel M, Terris DJ, and Vaupel P. The role of oxygen tension distribution on the radiation response of human breast carcinoma, *Adv. Exp. Med. Biol.,* **345** (1984) 485–492.

70. Koh WJ, Rasey JS, Evans ML, et al. Imaging of hypoxia in human tumors with [F-18]Fluoro-misonidazole, *Int. J. Radiat. Oncol. Biol. Phys.,* **22** (1992) 199–212.

71. Teicher BA, Lazo JS, and Satorelli AC. Classification of antineoplastic agents by their selective toxicities toward oxygenated and hypoxic tumor cells, *Cancer Res.,* **41** (1981) 73–81.

72. Tannock IF. Response of aerobic and hypoxic cells in a solid tumor to adriamycin and cyclophosphamide and interaction of the drugs with radiation, *Cancer Res.,* **35** (1975) 1147–1153.

73. Sindelar WF, Kinsella TJ, and Chen PW, et al. Intraoperative radiotherapy in retroperitoneal sarcomas: final results of a prospective, randomized, clinical trial, *Arch. Surg.,* **128** (1993) 402–410.

74. Weinstein GD, Rich TA, and Shumate CR, et al. Preoperative infusional chemoradiation and surgery with or without an electron beam intraoperative boost for advance primary rectal cancer, *Int. J. Radiation Oncol. Biol. Phys.,* **32** (1995) 197–204.

75. Okunieff P, Morgan D, Niemierko A, and Suit HD. Radiation dose response of human tumors, *Int. J. Radiation Oncol. Biol. Phys.,* **32** (1994) 1227–1238.

76. Brahme A. Dosimetric precision requirements in radiation therapy, *Acta Radiat. Oncol.,* **23** (1984) 379–391.

77. Thames HD, Schultheiss TE, Hendry JH, Tucker SL, Dubray BM, and Brock WA. Can modest escalations of dose be detected as increased tumor control?, *Int. J. Radiat. Oncol. Biol. Phys.,* **22** (1992) 241–246.

78. Williams MV, Denekamp J, and Fowler JF. Dose-response relationships for human tumors: implications for clinical trials of dose modifying agents, *Int. J. Radiat. Oncol. Biol. Phys.,* **10** (1984):1703–1707.

79. Coia LR, Aaronson N, Liggood R, Loeffler J, and Priestman TJ. A report of the consensus workshop panel on the treatment of brain metastases, *Int. J. Radiat. Oncol. Biol. Phys.,* **23** (1992) 223–227.

80. Withers HR. From bedside to bench and back. In Dewey WC, Edington M, Fry RJM, Hall EJ, and Whitmore GF (eds.), *Radiation Research: A Twentieth-Century Perspective.* vol. II, Academic, San Diego, 1992, pp. 30–70.

81. Goitein M and Niemierko A. Intensity modulated therapy and inhomogeneous dose to the tumor: a note of caution, *Int. J. Radiat. Oncol. Biol. Phys.,* **36** (1996) 519–522.

82. Suit HD, Skates S, Taghian A, Okunieff P, and Convery K. Clinical implications of heterogeneity of tumor response to radiation therapy, *Radiother. Oncol.,* **25** (1992) 251–260.

83. Kohli-Kumar M, Morris C, DeLaat C, et al. Bone marrow transplantation in Fanconi anemia using matched sibling donors, *Blood,* **84** (1994) 2050–2054.

84. Gluckman E, Auerbach AD, Horowitz MM, et al. Bone marrow transplantation for Fanconi Anemia, *Blood,* **86** (1995) 2856–2862.

85. Rubin P, Finkelstein J, and Shapiro D. Molecular biology mechanisms in the radiation induction of pulmonary injury syndromes: interrelationship between the alveolar macrophage and the septal fibroblast, *Int. J. Radiat. Oncol. Biol. Phys.,* **24** (1992) 93–101.

86. Anscher MS, Peters WP, Reisenbichler H, Petros WP, and Jirtle RL. Transforming growth factor b as a predictor of liver and lung fibrosis after autologous bone marrow transplantation for advanced breast cancer, *N. Engl. J. Med.,* **328** (1993) 1592–1598.

87. Anscher MS, Murase T, and Prescott DM, et al. Changes in plasma TGFb levels during pulmonary radiotherapy as a predictor of the risk of developing radiation pneumonitis, *Int. J. Radiat. Oncol. Biol. Phys.,* **30** (1994) 671–676.

88. Barnes M, Duray P, DeLuca A, Anderson W, Sindelar W, and Kinsella T. Tumor induction following intraoperative radiotherapy: late results of the National Cancer Institute canine trials, *Int. J. Radiat. Oncol. Phys.,* **19** (1992) 651–660.

89. Mauch P. Second malignancies after curative radiation therapy for good prognosis cancers, *Int. J. Radiat. Oncol. Biol. Phys.,* **33** (1995) 959–960.

90. Zietman AL, Suit HD, Okunieff PG, Donnelly SM, Dieman S, and Webster S. The life shortening effects of treatment with doxorubicin and/or local irradiation on a cohort of young C3Hf/Sed mice, *Eur. J. Cancer,* **27(6)** (1991) 778–781.

91. Cance WG, Brennan MF, Dudas ME, Huang CM, and Cordon-Cardo C. Altered expression of the retinoblastoma gene product in human sarcomas, *N. Engl. J. Med.,* **323** (1990) 1457–1462.

92. Helton KJ, Fletcher BD, Kun LE, Jenkins J 3rd, and Pratt CB. Bone tumors other than osteosarcoma after retinoblastoma, *Cancer,* **71** (1993) 2847–2853.

93. Fung YK and T'Ang A. The Role of the retinoblastoma gene in breast cancer development, *Cancer Treat. Res.,* **61** (1992) 59–68.

94. Graeber TG, Osmanian C, Jacks T, et al. Hypoxia-mediated selection of cells with diminished apoptotic potential in solid tumours, *Nature,* **379** (1996) 88–91.

95. Norimura T, Nomoto S, Katsuki M, Gondo Y, and Kondo S. p53-dependent apoptosis suppresses radiation-induced taratogenesis, *Nature Med.,* **2** (1996) 577–580.

96. Harvey M, McArthur CA, Montgomery CAJr, Butel JS, Bradley A, and Donehower LA. Spontaneous and carcinogen-induced tumorigenesis in p53-deficient mice, *Nat. Genet.,* **5** (1993) 225–229.

97. Donehower LA, Godley LA, Aldaz CM, et al. Deficiency of p53 accelerates mammary tumorigenesis in wnt-1 transgenic mice and promotes chromosomal instability, *Genes Devel.,* **9** (7) (1995) 882–895.

98. Fuks Z, Persaud RS, Alfieri A, et al. Basic fibroblast growth factor protects endothelial cells against radiation-induced programmed cell death *in vitro* and *in vivo, Cancer Res.,* **54** (1994) 2582–2590.

99. Ding I, Huang KD, Wang X, Greig JR, Miller RW, and Okunieff P. Radioprotection of hematopoietic tissue by fibroblast growth factors in fractionated radiation experiments, *Acta Oncologica,* **36** (1997) 337–340.

100. Suit HD, Sedlacek R, Silver G, et al. Therapeutic gain factors to fractionated radiation treatment of spontaneous murine tumors using fast neutrons, photons plus O_2 at 1 or 3 ATA, or photons plus misonidazole, *Radiat. Res.,* **116** (1988) 482–502.

101. Suit HD and Brown JM. Relative efficacy of high-pressure oxygen and misonidazole to reduce TCD50 of a mouse mammary carcinoma, *Br. J. Radiol.,* **52** (1979) 159–160.

102. Flickinger JC and Kalend A. Use of normalized total dose to represent the biological effect of fractionated radiotherapy, *Radiother. Oncol.,* **17** (1990) 339–347.

103. Brenner DJ and Hall EJ. Conditions for the equivalence of continuous to pulsed low dose rate brachytherapy, *Int. J. Radiat. Oncol. Biol. Phys.,* **20** (1991) 181–190.

104. Hall EJ, Marchese M, Hei TK, and Zaider M. Radiation response characteristics of human cells grown in vitro. *Radiat. Res.,* **114** (1988) 415–424.

105. Brenner DJ, Martel MK, Hall EJ. Fractionated regimens for stereotactic radiotherapy of recurrent tumors in the brain, *Int. J. Radiat. Oncol, Biol. Phys.,* **21** (1991) 819–824.

II METHODS AND TECHNIQUES OF TREATMENT

3 Physical Aspects of Intraoperative Electron-Beam Irradiation

Edwin C. McCullough and Peter J. Biggs

CONTENTS

1. INTRODUCTION

In intraoperative electron-beam irradiation (IOERT), a single dose of radiation (e.g., 10–20 Gy) is delivered to a selectively defined volume of tissue. Usually, the IOERT treatment is a boost therapy added to another course of treatment using standard external-beam techniques to irradiate a volume much larger than, but always including, the volume treated intraoperatively. IOERT places certain technical demands on equipment and documentation. There are several technical aspects unique to IOERT in addition to those items one normally associates with conventional external-beam irradiation (EBRT) treatments.

The most common radiation modality used to date for IOERT is the stationary megavoltage electron beam. Although at least one institution has reported on the use of orthovoltage X-rays *(1)*, this report will only be concerned with the use of electron beams in IORT. Existing linear accelerators are easily adapted for IOERT *(2–8)*, but there also appears to be some interest in dedicated units *(9)* that are particularly attractive for use in IOERT because they are easy to install in existing operating suites, are magnetron driven to reduce cost, have electron-only operation, have specific safety and monitoring features, and possibly have multidirectional head motion.

There are a number of physical aspects relating to IOERT that need to be appreciated and discussed. These include: treatment equipment and apparatus; facility design and shielding; beam dosimetry and characterization; and quality assurance.

From: *Current Clinical Oncology: Intraoperative Irradiation: Techniques and Results*
Edited by: L. L. Gunderson et al. © Humana Press, Inc., Totowa, NJ

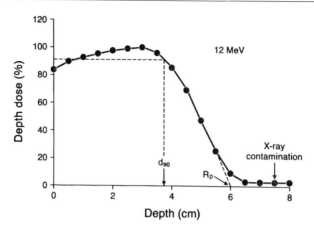

Fig. 1. Central axis dose vs depth for a 12-MeV electron beam from a 15 × 15-cm square applicator. Data are for a VARIAN Clinac 2100C linear accelerator with phantom surface at isocenter.

2. TREATMENT EQUIPMENT AND APPARATUS

Equipment needed for electron-beam IORT includes: a treatment machine for providing electron beams of sufficient penetration, a means of collimating the electron beam while at the same time providing a mechanism for keeping normal tissues out of the treatment area, and access to dosimetric equipment to characterize the physical properties of electron beams such as applicator ratios or given dose/monitor unit (GD/MU), relative surface and buildup doses, central axis percent depth doses, isodose curves, and beam profiles.

2.1. Accelerator

2.1.1. THE ELECTRON BEAM

Currently available clinical linear accelerators can produce electron beams with energies between 4 and 23 MeV. The maximal or practical range of these electron beams, R_p, is given in millimeters by the formula E_0 (in MeV)/0.2, in which E_0 is the energy of the electron beam at the surface. For example, 15 × 15-cm square-field electron beams with nominal energies of 6, 12, and 18 MeV, would have R_ps of approx 30, 60 (Fig. 1), and 90 mm, respectively. The depth at which the dose is normally prescribed in IOERT is that for 90% of the given dose, usually designated as D_{90} (Fig. 1). This value is chosen as a way of having the surface dose be similar to the prescription dose, yet limiting the maximum dose received to less than 10% over prescription dose. Table 1 lists values of d_{90} for some IOERT beams from a VARIAN Clinac 2100 (Varian Oncology Systems, Palo Alto, CA) linear accelerator.

To allow for coverage of both resectable and unresectable lesions over a reasonable depth it is desirable to have equipment with a maximum D_{90} of 45–50 mm. IOERT treatments commonly require applicators that have beveled ends, with angles between 15 and 45° to the perpendicular to the surface of the treated area. When beveled applicators are used, the depth of D_{90} measured perpendicular to the surface is reduced relative to applicators with flat ends (Fig. 2), as documented by Biggs (10). This fact combined with the data for flat-end applicators as shown in Table 1 would indicate optimal IOERT requires electron beams up to a maximum energy of 18–20 MeV, an observation borne

Table 1
Depth at Which Electron Percent Depth
Dose Falls to 90% of its D_{max} Value

Energy	Diameter	D_{90}
6 MeV	50 mm	16 mm
	70	17
	90	17
12 MeV	50 mm	33 mm
	70	36
	90	36
18 MeV	50 mm	48 mm
	70	52
	90	53

VARIAN 2100C; circular applicator; no bevel; phantom surface at isocenter

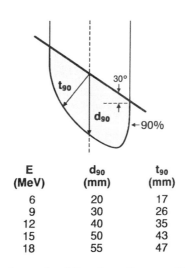

E (MeV)	d_{90} (mm)	t_{90} (mm)
6	20	17
9	30	26
12	40	35
15	50	43
18	55	47

Fig. 2. Isodose line (90% of maximum dose) for a 9 cm diameter, 30° beveled methyl methacrylate intraoperative applicator. The thickness of tissue treated to 90% of given dose, t_{90}, is listed along with the central axis D_{90} values for electron beams from a VARIAN Clinac 18.

out by an analysis by McCullough and Gunderson *(11)*. It is interesting to note that a subsequent analysis in 1996 showed that only approx 30% of 827 IOERT fields were treated with electron energies in excess of 12 MeV, whereas the 1988 analysis *(11)* showed this to be close to 60%. The difference is that since April of 1989, there has been a marked decrease in the number of unresectable pancreas cases and IOERT has been administered at Mayo Clinic in a dedicated OR, which allowed delivery of IOERT after resection of locally advanced and locally recurrent lesions at any site instead of for selected sites.

Electron beams are characterized by a widening of the isodose curves at depth (Fig. 3), which will be very important information to have available if abutting-field treatments are contemplated. In addition, having isodose curves for beveled-applicator treatments

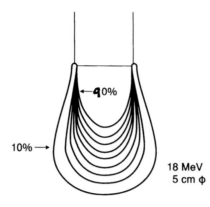

Fig. 3. Isodose distribution for a 5-cm circular-diameter applicator irradiated with an 18-MeV electron beam.

lets one choose a field size to compensate for isodose asymmetry about central axis (Fig. 2) and to ensure adequate depth of d_{90}.

Electron-beam fields generated by high Z-scattering foils will generate a bremsstrahlung tail (Fig. 1). Most modern linear accelerators have a bremsstrahlung tail less than 4–5% of the electron dose at the highest energy and 1–2% at the lowest energies. Even though this bremsstrahlung is low in terms of patient dose, it is an important consideration for the shielding design of a dedicated IOERT facility located above the ground floor.

2.1.2. DEDICATED UNITS

Dedicated treatment accelerators for IOERT have been a subject of much discussion, and at least one commercial machine, the Siemens Mevatron ME (Siemens Oncology Systems, Concord, CA) has been manufactured, though it is no longer available. An interesting new technical development is that of the Mobetron, which was developed by Intraop (Santa Clara, CA), and is being manufactured in partnership with Siemens (Fig. 4). This machine is a magnetron-driven X-band linac with energies between 4 and 12 MeV. However, unlike a conventional linac, it is not mounted on a fixed gantry but on one that can be moved within and between operating rooms because of its low overall weight and self shielding. The choice of 12 MeV as the maximum energy was dictated by the need to reduce neutron photoproduction as much as possible.

Generally, such dedicated linear accelerators might have the following, cost-reducing features:

1. Accelerate only electrons so that a lower power, and hence cheaper, microwave source can be used.
2. Fixed circular secondary collimator eliminating the need for adjustable photon collimation and monitoring.
3. Use of magnetron-driven power unit vs the much more expensive klystron.
4. Substitution of a suitably adapted, completely motorized operating table for the usual manufacturer-supplied standard patient support assembly. The table should allow for fine adjustments in not only x, y, and z directions but also pivoting side-to-side and head-to-toe.
5. Provision for motion of the treatment head in more than one plane (realized in Mobetron).

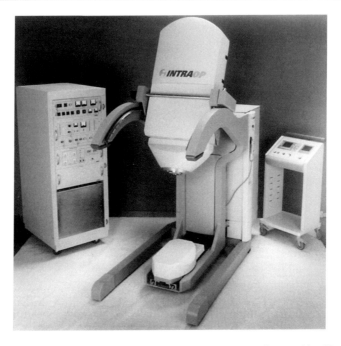

Fig. 4. The Mobetron IOERT machine designed by Intrap and manufactured by Siemens Oncology Systems. Unit is self shielding so can be used in existing operating rooms. Electron energies up to 12 MeV are provided. (Photograph courtesy of Intraop, Santa Clara, CA).

6. A reduction in gantry size and weight which, combined with a different mounting mechanism, would permit retrofitting into an existing operating room suite or moving between operating rooms

Dedicated IOERT machines (Siemen Mevatron-ME) were installed in operating room (OR) confines at M.D. Anderson (Houston, TX; MDA) in a retrofitted OR *(9)*, and at the Massachusetts General Hospital (Boston, MA) in new OR construction in 1996. Mayo Clinic (Rochester, MN) refurbished a VARIAN Clinac 18 that was installed in a large newly constructed operating room on the second floor of Rochester Methodist Hospital in early 1989 (Fig. 5). Dedicated IOERT machines have also been installed in several European centers. The initial Mobetron (Fig. 4) was placed at the University of California in San Francisco (UCSF) in Spring 1997.

2.1.3. BEAM COLLIMATION

The technical area within IOERT with the most activity since 1987 has been in beam collimation. The initial collimation systems followed the lead of the Japanese and Howard University in using a single aluminum tube rigidly attached to the face of the linear accelerator collimator assembly. Into this tube were placed polymethylmethacrylate (Lucite, Plexiglas) circular tubes of various inner diameters utilizing spacing annuli *(2,4)*. This type of collimator is commercially available (Radiation Products Design, Albertville, MN; Bionix Corporation, Toledo, OH). In addition to circular applicators, rectangular and elliptical (originally built at MGH) geometries have been constructed. McCullough and Gunderson reported on the relative use of various applicator sizes and shapes used in over 200 IOERT procedures at Mayo Clinic *(11)*. IOERT applicators have also been

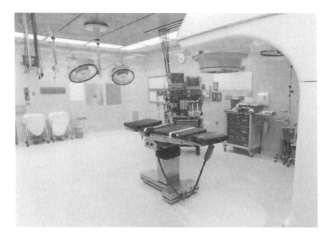

Fig. 5. Clinac 18 (VARIAN Associates, Palo Alto, CA) linear accelerator (electrons only) in a dedicated operating room on second floor of Methodist Hospital, Rochester, MN.

equipped for TV-assisted viewing *(3)*. However, the original two-tube hard-docking system presented some problems including:

1. Machine motions had to be disengaged during the treatment to ensure patient safety.
2. The hard-docking system provides a direct electrical connection between the patient's inner tissues and the accelerator (perspiration-coated plastic is a good conductor).
3. Visualization is not easily accomplished.

For these and other reasons, two major IOERT centers (Thomas Jefferson University Hospital [TJUH] and MDA) have developed and reported on so-called soft- or nondocking systems *(12–14)*. In such systems, the applicator inserted into the patient is not directly connected to the linear accelerator and is aligned using either four pairs of laser lines and dots (Siemens) *(12,14)* or a mechanical jig plus cross-wire light-field projections (Philips Medical Systems [now Elekta Oncology Systems], Stamford, CT; *13)*.

The TJUH and MDA groups have reported on leakage values for their nonhard-docking applicator systems *(12–14)*. In particular, the MDA group reported on leakage values for both brass- and lucite-walled applicators. For 18-MeV electrons, the maximum leakage dose (as a percent of given dose) was 18% for 5-mm Lucite walls, whereas it was approx 8% for a 1-mm brass wall. An additional 1 g/cm^2 is needed for a further 50% reduction. As this is 10 mm of Lucite vs 1 mm of brass, brass is indicated as the material of choice for the applicator walls. The TJUH applicators are made of 6 mm thick Lucite and it is reported that at 22 MeV there is leakage as high as 22% of given dose at the top of the applicator. Bagne and colleagues at Toledo *(15)* reported on leakage for Lucite applicators used in a hard-docking system. Specifically, they emphasize that penumbra is directly related to the size of the photon collimator jaw setting and electron energy. At D_{max} in a phantom located at the end of the applicator, their reported values of 5–15% (of given dose) are consistent with those of McCullough and Anderson *(4)*. However, neither of these groups *(4,15)* report on doses along the outside of the applicator walls themselves.

Electrons scattering off the inside walls of the applicators can introduce a significant lack of field flatness in IOERT treatments. Furthermore, the field flatness value is a sensitive function of electron energy, photon collimator jaw setting, applicator dimension and shape, as well as the depth in tissue. In general, "horns" are developed at the edge of the field if the photon collimator jaw setting is much greater than the applicator dimension. Simple solutions to produce flatter beam profiles such as internal annuli *(12,13)* are not without problems, causing either isodose line contraction *(12)* or being useful for only two or three of the energies. It is a question of clinical judgment whether to develop beams with flat profiles and a rounded 90% isodose line or beams with horns and a 90% isodose line that is less constricted.

3. FACILITY DESIGN AND SHIELDING

IOERT requires a surgical suite and a high-energy electron accelerator. Accelerators for IOERT have been provided in three major locales:

1. Use of an existing machine in a radiation oncology department room that doubles as an operating room (OR).
2. Use of an existing machine in a radiation oncology department room that is located next to an operating suite in the radiation oncology department.
3. Use of an existing machine in radiation oncology with transport from a hospital OR.
4. An electron-only accelerator placed in an existing or new operating room within a complex of ORs in a hospital (generally above basement level).

The ideal situation is to have the IOERT machine and OR combined (choices 1 and 4). This does not interrupt the surgical process and minimizes the problem of maintaining a sterile field. Choice 1 causes major disruptions in radiation oncology treatments, which are somewhat avoided by choice 2. Choices 1–3 introduce problem of anesthesia and surgical support at a remote site. A drawback to having the OR remote from the IOERT machine (choice 3), other than inconvenience, is the potential for infection during transport. However, this risk has been reported to be very low *(16)*. The disadvantages of an IOERT machine in a hospital-based OR (choice 4) are the high construction cost, the low use factor, and the intrusion of non-IOERT cases. These and several other aspects are discussed in the AAPM Task Group Report *(7)*. In particular, it is pointed out in the work of Nyerick et al. *(14)* that a dedicated IOERT machine might have a 1–2% lower X-ray bremsstrahlung tail, which would reduce the floor and wall shielding needed for a dedicated unit.

In an existing room already shielded for megavoltage photons in a radiation oncology department, no additional wall or door shielding is needed. Of course, there is still bremsstrahling X-ray background, which precludes personnel staying in the room during treatment.

3.1. Dedicated Facilities

In responding to a perceived need, manufacturers and hospitals are considering plans for placing dedicated IORT machines in operative suites. Most of the machines being considered are electron-only linear accelerators. Even though one might initially assume that little or no shielding might be needed, there is sufficient X-ray and neutron leakage from a conventional linear accelerator operated up to 18 MeV to warrant significant wall, floor, ceiling, and door shielding. In addition, the shielding needed for the in-beam X-ray contamination turns out to be surprisingly high.

As a general guideline, at 1 m one can expect 0.002% contamination for both X-ray and neutron leakage components with 15–20 MeV electrons *(17)*. Assuming an IOERT workload of 200 electron Gy/wk (including warm-up time), one quickly calculates that for a design level of 20 mSv/wk, 100% occupancy, and a source-to-location distance of

Table 2
Thicknesses to Shield
Against "Leakage" Radiations
from an 18-MeV Electron Accelerator

Material	X-Rays	Neutrons
Concrete	74 cm	33 cm
Steel	16.5 cm	—
Lead	10 cm	—
Polyethylene	—	15.5 cm

20,000 MU/wk; 3 meters from machine; 100% occupancy.

Design limit = 10 mSv/wk for X-ray and neutron components.

3 m, approximately 1.6 TVLs (tenth value layers) are required for both the X-ray and neutron components, assuming the contribution from each is 10 mSv/wk. Table 2 shows some typical material thicknesses to provide 1.6 TVLs.

In general, 38–46 cm of concrete with an 8-cm thick steel door with 6–8 cm of borated polyethylene (for neutrons) on the machine side will suffice for leakage-radiation shielding about an electron-only IOERT accelerator. These values are less than those listed in Table 2 as the IOERT machine will not always be run at 15–18 MeV (10), the distance to the area of protection will usually exceed 3 m and, for noncontrolled areas, occupancy most likely will be less than 100%. Furthermore, the shielding for other acceptable design limits are a factor of 5 and 50 higher; for example, design limits of 50 mSv per week (uncontrolled, "occasional occupancy") needs approx 0.4–0.7 TVL (depending on the exact occupancy assumption), whereas for 500 mSv per week (controlled, 100% occupancy) requires little or no shielding.

No maze is needed unless it is desirable to sacrifice space for a simplified and lighter door design. However, care must be taken to ensure adequate overlap at the door. Another significant problem is the shielding of the air conditioning ducts which are usually larger in the OR than in radiation oncology treatment rooms because a higher turnover rate of air is required. If the shielding consists of lead and borated polyethylene, the overall thickness will be 15–22 cm so the ducts have to be carefully placed in the room and designed so that they can be adequately shielded.

Because of neutron production in the accelerator, capture gammas of approx 2.2 MeV are produced from hydrogen in the concrete wall at the rate of 1 gamma per capture. Utilizing the approach of Schmidt (18) as discussed in National Council on Radiation Protection (NCRP) Report 38 (19), we have calculated that through a 30-cm concrete wall, the dose equivalents for X-rays : neutrons : capture gammas exist in the ratio 5:1:2. Therefore, with 0.3 mSv of 10 MV leakage X-rays (energy expected from 18–20 MeV electron operation) incident upon 46 cm concrete, one calculates an expected total dose equivalent of 20 mSv.

The X-ray contamination in the electron beam is an interesting problem. Assuming a workload of 200 Gy/wk at isocenter, a distance of 2 m to the floor and 5% in-beam X-ray contamination, one calculates a weekly X-ray exposure of 2.5 Gy at the floor. Reduction to 20 mSv/wk requires approx 5.1 TVLs which, assuming a TVL of 18 in concrete for 20 MV X-rays, yields a total concrete thickness of in excess of 92 in. Lead and/or steel is an efficient substitute for concrete and will reduce the floor thickness to acceptable levels. Photoproduction of neutrons by the bremsstrahlung X-rays in the primary beam has also been observed *(17)*. Hence, installing a dedicated electron-beam-only machine into an existing room presents some challenging shielding problems. This thickness of shielding will probably require the use of in-room shields, a raised floor under which 25–30 cm of lead is located or a level floor in which the lead is built into a submerged floor.

The above calculations are representative, conservative (i.e., in-beam contamination are usually 2–3%), and really are presented to alert the reader to the need to consider X-ray and neutron shielding for dedicated electron-beam IOERT machines. Furthermore, vendors should guarantee, in writing, the head leakage levels of a machine, so that radiation-protection design limits can be met.

Upon installation of the refurbished VARIAN Clinac 18 in new construction at Rochester Methodist Hospital, the environs of the dedicated machine (18 MeV maximum) were surveyed as well as badged for a 400 Gy exposure (projected maximum 2-wk workload). Results of this are shown in Fig. 6. These data show measurable values of neutrons (approx 0.2 Sv/wk) at the door for 200 Gy/wk, half of which was run at 18 MeV. The door next to the scrub sink has 3 mm (1/8 in) lead, whereas the door to the vestibule has 75 mm (3 in) of borated polyethylene (BPE) plus 38 mm (1.5 in) of lead on its vestibule side (to attenuate the BPE-produced capture gammas). Boyer et al. have written up the MDA experience for the shielding of their dedicated IOERT machine in the setting of a retrofitted OR *(9)*.

4. DOSIMETRY AND CHARACTERISTICS OF IOERT BEAMS

4.1. Dosimetric Equipment

With the exception of the Siemens ME and Intraop Mobetron machine, the electron beams produced from standard linear accelerators are not suitably optimized for IOERT collimation systems. The shapes of the isodose curves therefore depend very heavily on both the geometry and the setting of the photon collimator jaws. Isodose curves therefore do not resemble the isodose curves obtained with the manufacturer's standard applicators and should be measured for most if not all IOERT applicators (beveled as well as all small diameter (e.g., ≤6 cm) flat-ended applicators).

In IOERT it is important to ensure that the dose delivered at the surface of the treated volume is within an acceptable amount of the prescribed dose. In addition, if thermoluminescent dosimetry (TLD) is to be used as an in-vivo dosimeter, knowledge of percent surface dose is needed to relate surface dose to given dose. As a result, one must document the surface dose delivered using each IOERT applicator and electron energy.

4.2. Dosimetric Measurements

At the time of the IOERT procedure, the physicist staff must have available the following information in a rapidly accessible form:

1. Surface dose, depths of the 80 and 90% doses and applicator ratios for all applicators and beam energies.
2. Central axis depth-dose curves for all applicators and beam energies.
3. Isodose curves of beveled cones for a range of diameters plus smaller-diameter flat-end applicators for all electron-beam energies.
4. Bolus thickness to achieve 90% surface dose.

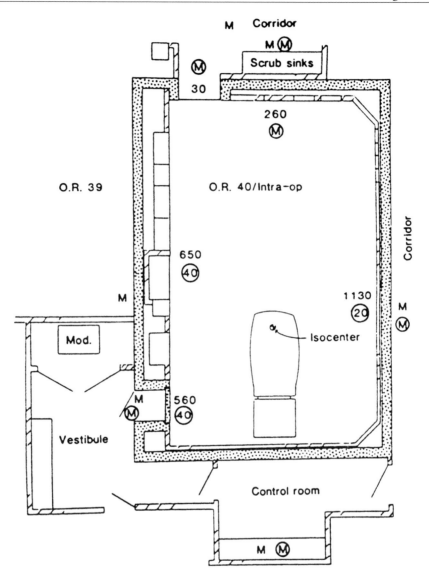

Fig. 6. Photon and neutron (results circled) TLD readings (in mrems) for a 40,000 MU exposure (2-wk workload). Monitor units of 20,000 MU at 18 MeV; 10,000 MU at 15 MeV; and 10,000 MU at 12 MeV were run with a 7 cm diameter applicator and the electron beam striking a phantom. Data (From Robert A. Dahl, MSc) is for a VARIAN Clinac 18 at Methodist Hospital, Rochester, MN. The designation M means a reading of less than 0.1 mSv.

5. Lead thickness (in number of lead sheets of the available thickness) needed to achieve a given transmission level (e.g., 10%) for each electron energy.
6. Field width, if significantly different from inner physical dimensions of the applicator.
7. Factors for nonstandard source-to-skin distances (SSDs) for those situations in which a simple inverse-square law correction is inappropriate.

Dosimetric parameters and techniques that need to be documented prior to instituting IOERT treatments are summarized in Table 3.

Table 3
Dosimetric Parameters of Interest
in Intraoperative Electron Beam-Therapy

Applicator Ratios
  Applicator ratio
  SSD corrections
Central Axis Percent Depth Doses
  Surface dose
  D_{max}, D_{90}, or D_{80}
  X-ray contamination
Beam Profiles
  Flatness/symmetry
  Field width (e.g., W_{90})
  Penumbra
  Isodose curves
Verification
  Thermoluminescent dosimetry system calibration and precision
Shielding (internal)
  Transmission values

A number of papers have discussed measurement of these parameters for both polymethylmethocrylate (PMMA) *(2,4)* and metallic applicators *(12–14,20)*.

4.2.1. APPLICATOR RATIOS

Applicator ratios, or given-dose-per-monitor unit, must be determined for each combination of applicator and electron energy. The applicator ratio is usually defined as the ratio of the dose at the depth of maximum dose, D_{max}, for the intraoperative applicator, to the dose at D_{max} for the calibration applicator, generally 15×15 cm^2 *(21)*, at the usual SSD, both measurements being taken along the central axis and for the same electron energy. Although the depth of D_{max} is not necessarily the same in each case, the difference is sufficiently small to have little effect on the ionization-to-dose conversion factor, so the ratio of ionization readings is used for this ratio. Applicator ratios are usually near 1.00 for circular applicator sizes > 6 cm in diameter and for energies > 9 MeV at the nominal SSD of the accelerator *(4)*.

For hard-docking systems, it is not always possible to dock the plastic applicator completely within the aluminum tube, so the given dose must be corrected to account for this difference in SSD. The validity of a simple inverse-square-law factor correction using the virtual SSD should be verified over the range of energies and applicator sizes and shapes. If this correction does not follow the inverse-square law within an acceptable tolerance (e.g., 2%), a table of values needs to be generated for those applicators and electron energies that exceed the discrepancy tolerance.

4.2.2. CENTRAL AXIS DOSE VS DEPTHS

There is a need to document central-axis depth-dose values because there could be a significant change in these values with both applicator size and shape as well as beam energy. Obviously, D_{max} needs to be documented for all applicator/beam energy combinations, so applicator ratios can be measured at the actual, D_{max} values for each applicator as recommended by the American Association of Physicists in Medicine (AAPM) TG-25 *(21)*.

Values of D_{max} for beveled applicators are usually specified along the applicator central axis and isodose curves used to find t_{90} (Fig. 2). If a sophisticated water-phantom-scanning system is not available, central-axis percent-depth-dose values along the applicator axis can be measured using a tiltable water phantom *(22)*.

It is important to measure central-axis percent-dose-depth values for all applicators and electron energies since, as noted previously, the depth of 90% of maximum dose (D_{90}) can change very dramatically for small field sizes, particularly at high energies (i.e., $\geq$ 12 MeV). Percent-depth-dose curves for beveled applicators must also be measured since it has been shown *(4,10)* that even when the dose is measured along the central axis of the beam, the depth-dose curves are a function of the angle of incidence of the beam with respect to the surface. Depth-dose curves should be measured for all electron energies. These are usually measured as a function of the distance along the beam axis, but, as noted above, are more usefully presented as a function of distance perpendicular to the surface.

In intraoperative, just as in conventional electron-beam therapy, one will need to know D_{90} or D_{80} for each applicator size and shape to assist in the selection of an electron-beam energy. For beveled applicators, one has the additional consideration (as shown in Fig. 2) that the 90% depth perpendicular to the treated surface (t_{90}) is less than the central axis distance (D_{90}) by a factor close to the cosine of the bevel angle. For a 30° bevel, this factor is 0.87. The physicist should ensure that the physicians understand this.

Unlike conventional electron-beam treatments in which the target volume usually does not extend to the surface of the treated area, in intraoperative electron-beam therapy the surface of the treatment area usually contains tumor and, thus, it is important to ensure an adequate surface dose. A particularly interesting problem has arisen as vendors have striven to improve percent-dose-depth values by reducing the mass of their ionization monitoring chambers (e.g., through the use of plastic foil rather than metallic or mica monitor chamber walls). This produces a substantially lower surface dose value than with nonfoil-walled chambers, which usually gave surface doses >88% for E $\geq$ 9 MeV and 90% for E $\geq$ 15 MeV *(2,23)*. Increasing the surface dose of beams using these new chambers can be achieved in practice by placing a thin plastic, honey-combed disc not far from the surface. This effectively increases the surface dose by scatter but does not significantly reduce the percent-depth doses. The exact change depends on the relative hole to total area and the distance of the disc from the surface. The important point is that it is necessary to document the adequacy of surface-dose values for all applicators and electron energies.

The X-ray contamination of an electron beam may be defined as the dose 100 mm beyond the practical range as a percentage of the dose at D_{max}. X-ray contamination for intraoperative fields has been reported to be below 4% for all electron-beam energies on the Clinac 18 accelerator *(4)*. For a dedicated machine such as the Siemens ME, it is approx 2.5–3% at 18 MeV. For the Mobetron, the X-ray contamination is specified to be < 1% at the depth 100 mm beyond the depth of the 10% isodose line. Since the X-ray contamination is independent of field size, if the applicator ratio decreases with field size, then the percent bremsstrahlung will increase. It is important, therefore, that it be measured over the range of applicator sizes to be used. The X-ray contamination is also related to the choice of photon collimator jaw settings *(2)*. For settings close to the applicator size, the percent background will be large. However, it decreases rapidly with increasing field size and changes less rapidly for large settings of the photon collimator jaws.

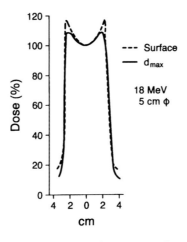

Fig. 7. Electron relative-dose profile as measured at D_{max} and surface for 18 MeV for a 5 cm diameter circular applicator. Data is expressed as a percentage of the central-axis value.

4.2.3. BEAM PROFILES

Isodose curves and beam profiles at D_{max} are required to document the off-central-axis behavior of IOERT beams. Width of the 90% isodose line, W_{90}, beam flatness, and symmetry can be determined from a beam profile at D_{max}. These data are particularly important for beveled or small-diameter circular applicators, in which the isodose distributions tend to be bullet-shaped (Fig. 3). Profiles taken at the surface may also be useful, but these can only be taken with film.

In present collimator systems, one generally does not see perfectly flat beams because of the effect of scatter from the walls of the applicator. This gives rise to a significant lack of flatness at the surface which, however, is reduced at D_{max} (Fig. 7). This lack of flatness, even though it is of concern, translates to much smaller inhomogeneity values since these IOERT treatments are generally given as a boost in combination with 45–50 Gy of fractionated EBRT (generally 1.8–2.0 Gy per fraction in the United States). Also, any misalignment of the applicator will lead to an asymmetry in the region where this scatter component is important. If there is one major problem remaining in the dosimetry of intraoperative electron beams, it is the modification of the collimator/applicator design to improve surface flatness. It is to be anticipated that dedicated intraoperative equipment might have as one of its features an integrated system of scattering devices and applicators that might permit customization of the isodose contours.

Field width may be defined in terms of the distance between the 90% isodose lines at a certain depth below the surface (e.g., D_{max}, D_{90}, or D_{80}). The radiation-defined field width should be close to that defined geometrically by the end of the applicator, and, if this is not the case, these discrepancies must be documented. McCullough and Anderson *(4)* showed that for flat-ended applicators, the radiation width (W_{90}) and geometrically defined field size were within a few millimeters of each other. This discrepancy is probably not of much importance unless margins less than 5 mm are being used (usual recommendation is 1-cm margin around target volume—i.e., 5 cm target results in 7-cm applicator). For beveled applicators one has a more complicated situation, and adequate coverage is best assessed by having isodose-curve information (Fig. 2) available at the time of the IOERT procedure.

Penumbra is generally defined as the distance required for the dose to fall from 80–20% of its central axis value at the depth of D_{max}. For circular applicators, the penumbra should be measured both for planes parallel to the photon collimator jaws and along the diagonal direction of the jaws because of the mismatch between the square shape of the photon collimator jaw-defined field and the circular-shaped applicator. If the dose outside the applicator is in excess of 10% more than 10 mm from the outside edge of the cone, a brass attenuator may need to be added to the top of the applicator. This does not apply to a machine line the Siemens ME which has a single circular precollimator in the head of the treatment machine.

4.3. Verification Dosimetry

Because of the single-dose nature of the IOERT procedure, it is advisable to have an independent check on the overall accuracy of dose delivery. This can be done by monitoring surface dose using TLD. For example, one can hermetically seal several TLDs in a small plastic pouch or in tubes to which a long piece of surgical thread has been attached. These are then placed on top of the tumor bed usually through a hole at the upper end of the applicator. Use of at least three high precision (that is, ±5%) TLD chips per measurement appears satisfactory. When calculating the expected dose from the number of monitor units delivered, a correction factor may have to be applied for the thickness of the encapsulation material if it is of significant thickness. Experience at Mayo with TLD monitoring has been disappointing. Dose variations of up to 35% were noted even though values obtained on top of plastic phantoms were within 5% of expected values. Much of the lack of agreement for patient measurements can be attributed to the poor flatness of the IOERT beam, the fact that the body tissues tend to push up into the open end of the applicator, and in some cases, the accumulation of fluid on the treatment surface.

4.4. Field Shaping

During IOERT it may sometimes be necessary to shield a portion of the field and/or those tissues behind the volume to be treated because of normal-tissue tolerance issues. To accomplish this, pieces of lead of adequate size (e.g., $10 \times 10\,cm^2$, $20 \times 20\,cm^2$) should be available in sterilized packages. Sterilized scissors should also be available. Measurement of the transmission curve of lead for the various energies and for a few applicator sizes needs to be measured since there is an initial build-up effect. As a general rule of thumb, it requires approx 0.5 mm Pb per MeV to completely stop the electron beam. Thus, a 16-MeV electron beam requires approx 8 mm Pb. One should use relatively thin pieces of lead (≤1 mm) so they can be easily cut and shaped. These are usually placed within saline-soaked gauze. As a general rule, since the lead is on the surface, the applicator ratios do not change much if the shielding is small and peripheral. For area reductions greater than 33%, measurements should be made after the procedure. Unfortunately, in practice, one has no way of determining the exact effect of lead shielding on applicator ratios during the IOERT procedure.

5. QUALITY ASSURANCE (QA)

5.1. Treatment Machine QA

The single-treatment nature of IOERT indicates that it is highly desirable to have a comprehensive and frequent quantity assurance (QA) program. Certain parameters that are routinely monitored in conventional external therapy (e.g., accuracy of gantry angle

Table 4
Representative Quality Assurance Program for Dedicated IOERT Machine
(Mayo Clinic)

1. Biweekly
   A. Output constancy/calibration
   B. Collimator-jaw size
   C. Audiovisual, door lights
   D. Door interlocks
   E. Deadman switch

2. Monthly
   A. Safety checks
      1. Beam-direction interlocks (if so equipped)
      2. Emergency offs
   B. Energy (% DD)
   C. Flatness/symmetry (GA = 0° IEC)

NOTE: Tests II.B and II.C. are performed with a standard electron applicator.

3. Annual
   A. Monitor system
      1. Short-term (hours)
      2. Long-term (days) stability
      3. Linearity
      4. Dose-rate independence
      5. Independence with gantry angle
   B. Symmetry
      1. Interlocks
      2. Stability with gantry angle
   C. Radiation isocenter
      1. Collimator Rotation
   D. Applicator output factors (spot check)
   E. D_{90} (spot check)

indicators) may not be particularly relevant for IOERT machinery. On the other hand, there are some parameters that are not routinely checked on a daily basis on conventional equipment (e.g., photon-jaw setting accuracy when utilizing electron applicators) whose value may be critical for the next IOERT treatment.

A representative physics QA program for a dedicated IOERT machine is seen in Table 4. Note that this is only one possible QA program. Radiation-safety requirements of various states may differ from each other. For example, the Commonwealth of Massachusetts requires that the door interlocks be checked only monthly. Different aspects of quality assurance related to IOERT treatments are covered in several papers (7–8,24–27).

5.2. Treatment Documentation

It is desirable to have a prepared sheet on which one can list all the various physical details for each intraoperative treatment. Table 5 presents a minimal listing of physics data to be included on a sheet documenting a patient's treatment. Additional bookkeeping items might include spaces to check off and initial that photon-collimator-jaw size was checked and power to gantry and table were removed just prior to treatment.

Table 5
Minimum Physics Data Required for Documentation of Intraoperative Treatments

1. Nominal-beam energy
2. Applicator size and angle
3. Photon-collimator-jaw setting
4. A. Target depth
   B. Target dose
   C. Given dose (GD)
   D. Applicator ratio (GD/MU^a)
   E. SSD corrections (if any)
   F. Total MU^a delivered
5. Depth of 90% dose, D_{90}, etc.
6. Dose specifications to other sites of interest (e.g., spinal cord or kidneys)
7. Surface dose (if desired)
   A. Calculated
   B. By thermoluminescent dosimetry
8. Field blocking and any additional dosimetric calculations (use diagram if necessary)

^{a} MU = monitor units.

6. CONCLUSION

IOERT involves the use of an electron-treatment beam collimated by an applicator placed within the patient and adjacent to normal tissues. A single treatment of 10–20 Gy is usually given as an adjunct to a course of external photon-beam irradiation (with or without chemotherapy) and maximal surgical resection. Equipment selection (or adaptation) as well as facility location and design are important precursors to mounting a successful IOERT program. The unique geometry of IOERT requires scrupulous and careful documentation of all relevant dosimetric and treatment data.

REFERENCES

1. Rich TA, Cady B, and McDermott WV. Orthovoltage intraoperative radiotherapy: a new look at an old idea, *Int. J. Radiat. Oncol. Biol. Phys.,* **10** (1984) 1957–1965.
2. Biggs PJ, Epp ER, and Ling CC. Dosimetry, field shaping and other considerations for intraoperative electron therapy, *Int. J. Radiat. Oncol. Biol. Phys.,* **7** (1981) 875–884.
3. Fraass BA, Harrington FS, Kinsella TJ, and Sindelar WF. Television system for verification and documentation of treatment fields during intraoperative radiation therapy, *Int. J. Radiat. Oncol. Biol. Phys.,* **9** (1983) 1409–1411.
4. McCullough EC and Anderson JA. The dosimetric properties of an applicator system for intraoperative electron beam therapy utilizing a Clinac-18 accelerator, *Med. Phys.,* **9** (1982) 261–268.
5. Abe M and Dobelbower RR, eds. *Intraoperative Radiation Therapy.* CRC Press, Boca Raton, FL, 1989.
6. Jones D. Apparatus, techniques and dosimetry of intraoperative electron beam therapy. In, Vaeth JM and Meyer JL (eds). *The Role of High Energy Electrons in the Treatment of Cancer. Front. Radiation Ther. Oncology,* **25** (1991) 233–245.
7. AAPM Radiation Therapy Task Group 48. Intraoperative electron beam radiation therapy: technique, dosimetry and dose specification, *Int. J. Radiat. Oncol. Biol. Phys.,* **33** (1995) 725–746.
8. McCullough EC and Biggs PG. Intraoperative electron beam radiation therapy, In Kereiakes J, Barn C, and Elson H, (eds.). *Radiation Oncology Physics,* American Association of Physicists in Medicine, College Park, MD, 1987.
9. Mills MD, Almond PR, and Boyer AL. Shielding considerations for an operating room based intraoperative electron radiotherapy unit, *Int. J. Radiat. Oncol. Biol. Phys.,* **18** (1990) 1215–1221.
10. Biggs PJ. The effect of beam angulation on central axis percent depth dose for 4-29 MeV electrons, *Phys. Med. Biol.,* **29** (1984) 1089–1096.

11. McCullough EC and Gunderson LL. Energy as well as applicator size and shape utilized in over 200 intraoperative electron beam procedures, *Int. J. Radiat. Oncol. Biol. Phys.*, **15** (1988) 1041–1042.

12. Hogstrom KR, Boyer AL, and Shiu AS. Design of metallic electron beam cones for an intraoperative therapy linear accelerator, *Int. J. Radiat. Oncol. Biol. Phys.*, **18** (1990) 1223–1232.

13. Palta JR and Suntharalingham N. A non-docking intraoperative electron beam applicator system, *Int. J. Radiat. Oncol. Biol. Phys.*, **17** (1989) 411–417.

14. Nyerick CE, Ochran TG, Boyer AL, and Hogstrom KR. Dosimetry characteristics of metallic cones for intraoperative radiotherapy, *Int. J. Radiat. Oncol. Biol. Phys.*, **21** (1991) 501–510.

15. Bagne FR, Samsani N, and Dobelbower RR. Radiation contamination and leakage assessment of intraoperative electron applicators, *Med. Phys.*, **15** (1988) 530–537.

16. Noyes RD, Weiss SM, Krall JM, et al. Surgical complications of intraoperative radiation therapy: the Radiation Therapy Oncology Group experience, *J. Surg. Oncol.*, **50** (1992) 209–215.

17. Biggs PJ. Evidence for photoneutron production in the lead shielding of a dedicated intra-operative electron-only facility, *Health Physics,* submitted.

18. Schmidt FAR. The attenuation properties of concrete for shielding of neutrons of energy less than 15 MeV. Oak Ridge National Laboratory, Oak Ridge, TN, 1970.

19. NCRP Report No. 38. Protection against neutron radiation. National Council on Radiation Protection, Washington, DC, 1971.

20. Nelson CE, Cock R, and Rakfal S. The dosimetric properties of an intraoperative radiation therapy applicator system for a Mevatron-80, *Med. Phys.*, **16** (1989) 794–799.

21. AAPM Radiation Therapy Committee Task Group 25. Clinical electron-beam dosimetry, *Med. Phys.*, **18** (1991) 73–109.

22. Dahl RA and McCullough EC. Determination of accurate dosimetric parameters for beveled intraoperative electron beam applicators, *Med. Phys.*, **16** (1989) 130–131.

23. Biggs PJ and McCullough EC. Physical aspects of intraoperative electron beam energy. In Gunderson LL and Tepper, JE (eds.), *Intraoperative +/– External Beam Irradiation,* Yearbook Medical, Chicago, 1983.

24. Tepper JE, Gunderson LL, Goldson AL, et al. Quality control parameters of intraoperative radiation therapy, *Int. J. Radiat. Oncol. Biol. Phys.*, **12** (1986) 1687–1695.

25. Davis MG and Ochran TG. A quality assurance program for intraoperative linear accelerator. In Physics Starkschall, G. and Horton, J (eds.), *Quality Assurance In Radiotherapy,* American College of Medical Physics, Reston, VA, 1991.

26. Hazle JD, Chu JCH, and Kennedy P. Quality assurance for intraoperative electron radiotherapy clinical trials: ionization chamber and mailable thermoluminescent dosimeter results, *Int. J. Radiat. Oncol. Biol. Phys.*, **24** (1992) 559–563.

27. McCullough EC. Intraoperative electron beam radiation therapy (IORT). In Purdy JA (ed.), *Advances in Radiation Oncology Physics,* American Association of Physicists in Medicine, College Park, MD, 1991.

4 IOERT Treatment Factors

Technique, Equipment

Christopher G. Willett, Leonard L. Gunderson, Paul M. Busse, David Nagorney, Joel E. Tepper, and Felipe A. Calvo

CONTENTS

1. INTRODUCTION

Intraoperative electron-beam irradiation (IOERT) is a treatment modality designed to combine the efforts of surgery and radiation therapy to increase local-tumor-control rates in cancer therapy. In the past 20 yr, there have been impressive gains in understanding the optimal interaction of IOERT with surgery as well as technical advances in the administration of IOERT. This knowledge has translated into improved local control with low rates of treatment-related toxicity. This chapter summarizes issues involved in treatment factors of IOERT.

2. FACILITY LOCATION, EQUIPMENT

2.1. Dedicated IOERT Suites

In the United States, there are four dedicated IOERT suites within operating rooms—the Massachusetts General Hospital, Mayo Clinic, M.D. Anderson Hospital, and Ohio State University (Fig. 1). These facility designs involved a multispecialty effort including anesthesia, surgery, radiation oncology, operating room (OR) nursing, and hospital

From: *Current Clinical Oncology: Intraoperative Irradiation: Techniques and Results*
Edited by: L. L. Gunderson et al. © Humana Press, Inc., Totowa, NJ

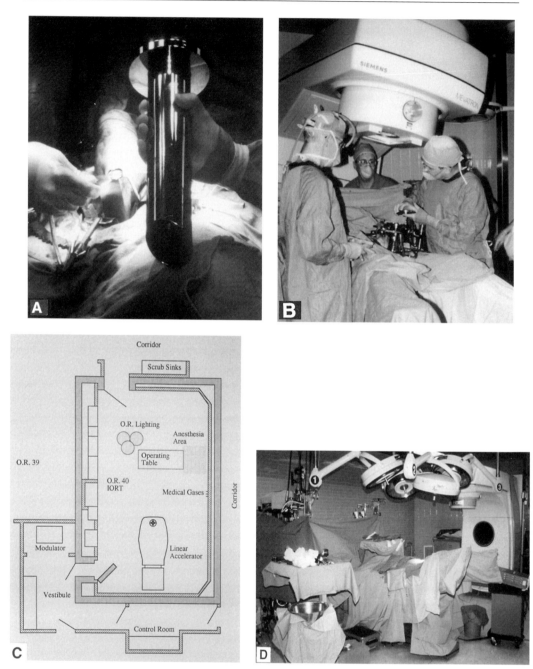

Fig. 1. Dedicated IOERT suite within an operating room: (**A,B**) Massachusetts General Hospital (MGH). Applicator is selected with 30° bevel (**A**) and immobilized in pelvis with Buckwalter system (**B**). (**C,D**) Mayo Clinic—Artist's depiction (**C**) (reprinted with permission from ref. 7); Actual (**D**).

administration. These rooms permit complete operating-room capability as well as delivery of IOERT. Three of the facilities (Massachusetts General Hospital, M.D. Anderson Hospital, and Ohio State University) use the Siemen's ME accelerator (Siemans, Concorde, CA), which provides electron energies ranging from 6 to 18 MeV, whereas the

Mayo Clinic utilizes a refurbished Varian Clinac 18 accelerator (VARIAN Associates, Palo Alto, CA) that provides electrons from 6 to 18 MeV.

Dedicated IOERT suites within an operating room represent the ideal as these facilities simplify the integration of IOERT with surgery. There is no requirement of a transport process from the operating room to a radiation-therapy suite and operating-room personnel (anesthesiogists, OR nursing, and surgeons) remain in a familiar working environment.

An alternative approach is to have a dedicated IOERT suite with full OR capability within the radiation oncology department as currently exists at Medical College of Ohio in Toledo and Thomas Jefferson University. This is a lower-cost alternative as it utilizes an existing radiation oncology treatment room (with shielding) and equipment. All surgical components of the procedure are performed in the OR suite, and patients are transported to the adjacent linear accelerator room only for the IOERT delivery. A potential disadvantage of such a facility is its potential distance from anesthesia and routine OR support should a surgical emergency occur. Surgeons may therefore be less willing to do extensive cases in such a setting.

2.2. Transport from Operating Room to Radiation Therapy Suite

In many institutions using IOERT, the patient must be transported from the regular operating room to the radiation oncology department for treatment and back to the operating room if necessary *(1)*. From 1978 to 1996 at the Massachusetts General Hospital (MGH), initial explorations were done in the regular operating rooms, with resection performed as appropriate. If there were no metastases beyond the regional lymph nodes and if a site at high risk for local failure could be defined by the surgeon and the radiation oncologist, the patient was considered an appropriate candidate for IOERT. After decisions were made regarding optimal placement and applicator selection, the patient was then prepared for transport to the radiation oncology department. After adequate hemostasis had been obtained, the abdominal wound was closed with a few stay sutures and then covered with a plastic adhesive sterile drape (Fig. 2A,B). A few additional layers of drapes were placed over the patient. The patient was transferred to a Surgi-Lift stretcher and switched to portable anesthesia equipment (Fig. 2C). Operating-room personnel wore an additional layer of gowns and gloves, and the patient was then transported to the radiation oncology department through corridors and elevators (Fig. 2D,E).

The room in the radiation oncology department was prepared so that it could be used effectively as an operating room. Full surgical supplies were available and portable operating-room lights were supplied. The patient was transferred onto the radiation-therapy treatment couch and returned to standard anesthesia equipment (Fig. 2F). After the operating room team was regowned and regloved, the patient was reprepped and redraped and the wound was re-exposed. The previously selected applicator was then placed over the treatment area in the patient (Fig. 2G,H). Docking followed and the patient was treated with IOERT. If no additional major surgery was required, the incisions of the patient were closed in the radiation oncology department and the patient then transferred to the recovery room. If additional surgery was required, the patient was transported back to the operating room.

In the past, there has been concern regarding the safety of a room that does not have standard operating-room air-exchange rates and about the possibility of infectious complications in patients who are transported through the corridors to the radiation oncology department. However, in a large experience of over 330 patients at the MGH transported

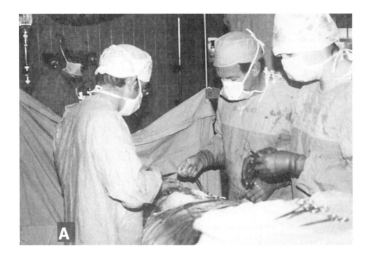

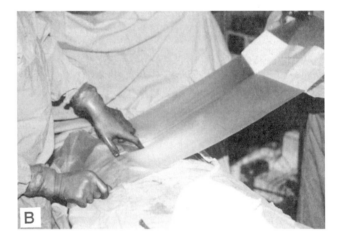

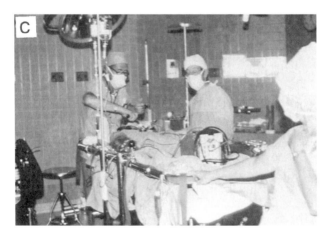

Fig. 2. Patient transfer from the operating room to radiation oncology department for IOERT at Massachusetts General Hospital (MGH). (**A,B**) Abdominal wound temporary closure; covered with sterile drape. (**C**) Transfer of patient to Surgi-Lift stretcher for transfer. (**D,E**) Transportation through corridors and elevators. (**F**) Transfer of patient to linear accelerator treatment couch in Radiation Oncology Department. (**G,H**) Placement of applicator prior to treatment with IOERT.

D

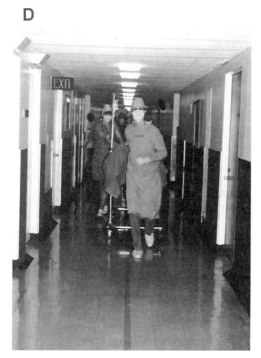

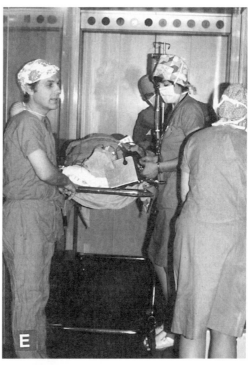

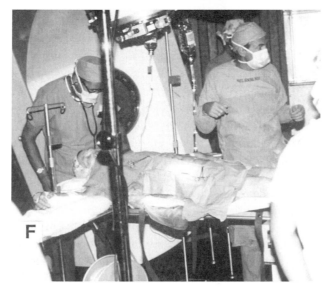

Fig. 2. (*continued*)

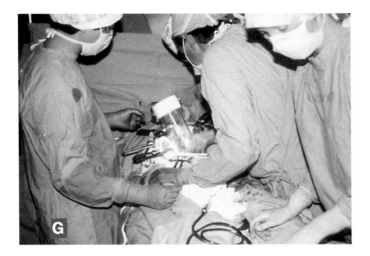

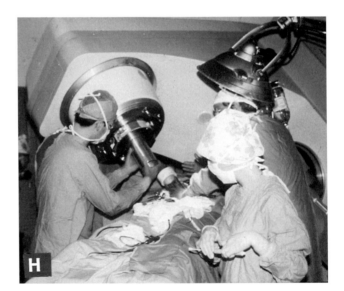

Fig. 2. (*continued*)

from the operating room through a number of corridors as well as two sets of elevators from 1978 to 1996, neither of these factors seem to be a major problem. In the first 105 patients who were treated at the MGH with transportation from the OR to the radiation oncology department, the wound-infection rate was 7%, with other miscellaneous infections in 14 of the 105 patients (2). These infection rates are comparable to a series of surgical patients at the MGH without IOERT.

The transportation procedure and surgery performed outside of the operating room has not been a clinical problem, although the logistics are substantial. Most IOERT patients have been treated with intravenous antibiotics at the time of the surgical procedure, which minimizes the potential adverse affects of taking a patient out of the standard OR environment. Furthermore, we have observed no anesthesia, cardiac, or respiratory problems from transporting patients. Nonetheless, the use of transportation from the OR to the radiation therapy department is not ideal, and should be avoided if possible.

3. INTERACTIONS WITH
SURGEONS IN OR AND SURGICAL FACTORS

It is essential that all realize that IOERT is truly a combined modality approach in which the knowledge and expertise of both the surgeon and the radiation oncologist are essential in making treatment decisions throughout the operative procedure (1–4). In performing the surgery itself, good operative exposure is essential so that the tumor is treated completely with proper sparing of the adjacent normal tissue. In many situations this may require modifying the surgical incision. A small midline incision, adequate for a pancreatic carcinoma biopsy, may not be sufficient for a thorough abdominal evaluation and optimal treatment with IOERT. The surgeon and radiation oncologist must discuss the potential approaches so that proper exposure can be obtained. Decisions regarding surgical resections and the extent of the radiation must be made by the surgeon and the radiation oncologist combined. Thus, if a resection is to be performed, the radiation oncologist must be in the operating room at the time of resection to evaluate the location of the tumor, mode of spread, and to define where the IOERT port will be located. Often, details of the surgical procedure are affected by the abilities and limitations of the IOERT. This applies as much to normal tissue, which may be adversely affected by the IOERT, as it does to the optimal treatment for eradicating the tumor. An adequate dissection to determine the extent of the tumor is necessary. This often involves more dissection than just determining a tumor's unresectability.

The importance of identifying and excluding patients with metastatic disease cannot be overemphasized. It is critical for most abdominal tumors that the liver, bowel mesentery, abdominal cavity, and pelvis be carefully palpated for metastatic disease and whenever possible that biopsies (including frozen sections) be obtained of areas suspicious for tumor.

The actual surgical procedure must of course vary for each individual patient and disease site. The definition of the extent of an appropriate surgical resection is not constant between institutions or even surgeons. A regional pancreatectomy for pancreatic carcinoma had been thought to be a proper combination with IOERT at the National Cancer Institute (NCI), but was not accepted at other institutions. All agree, however, that when the operative risks are acceptable, such as in a patient who can have an abdominoperineal resection for a rectal carcinoma or a gastrectomy for a gastric carcinoma, this is appropriate.

In patients with potentially unresectable tumors, high dose (45–55 Gy) preoperative irradiation, with or without concomitant chemotherapy as indicated by site, should be considered to reduce tumor mass, which will then facilitate the surgical resection. In addition, areas in which either gross or microscopic tumor is transsected may be at a lower risk for surgical seeding of tumor cells either into the peritoneal cavity or the systemic circulation. In situations in which resection is not to be performed, it may still be helpful to give a component of the radiation preoperatively to prevent seeding as a result of surgical manipulation.

Once the evaluation and resection (if possible) have been performed, the patient is fully evaluated for the delivery of the intraoperative irradiation. It is helpful to mark areas of residual tumor or the tumor bed with either sutures or surgical clips (Fig. 3A,B). These help define the extent of the IOERT field for placement of the treatment cylinder. In patients who are receiving some of their EBRT postoperatively, clips help define the fields for the postoperative treatment (Fig. 3C–E).

It is important that all standard surgical procedures are followed. Dead spaces should be minimized by appropriate drainage. After an abdominoperineal resection, unless the

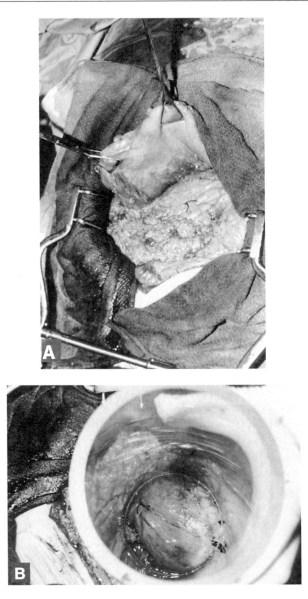

Fig. 3. Surgical placement of suture(s) or clips can help define IOERT and EBRT fields: (**A,B**) Silk sutures mark extent of unresectable pancreas cancer with overlying stomach mobilized superiorly (**A**). View down applicator (**B**). (**C–E**) Clip placement assists in definition of EBRT fields in conjunction with CT abdomen in Mayo Clinic patient with unresectable body of pancreas cancer (reprinted with permission from ref. 8).

area is properly drained, there can be a large perineal dead space that may lead to poor healing with abscess and fistula formation. These tissues may be heavily traumatized by extensive tumor, high-dose preoperative EBRT with or without chemotherapy, surgical resection, and IOERT such that infection and fluid accumulation may be more likely than after a standard resection.

In planning the IOERT, the radiation oncologist and surgeon must define precisely all normal tissues that will be in the radiation-therapy field. Clinical experience and animal

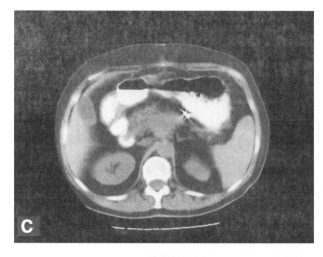

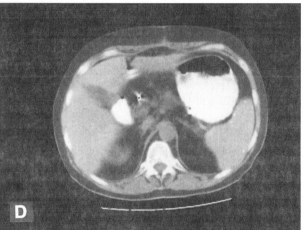

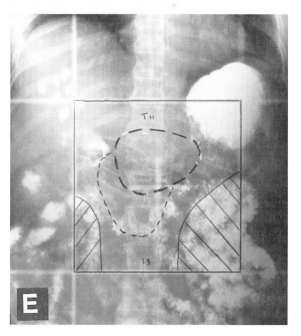

Fig. 3. (*continued*)

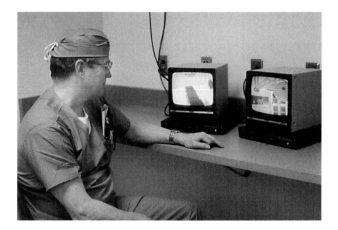

Fig. 4. Anesthesia monitoring of IOERT procedure at Mayo Clinic with closed circuit television.

research indicate normal tissues that may not tolerate high-dose IOERT. Portions of the intestine that have not been defunctionalized by surgical bypass may develop strictures, and the stomach may be prone to ulceration. Surgical anastomoses should, if possible, be excluded from the radiation field, although healing can probably take place even with the IOERT. Ureters, which are relatively resistant to EBRT, are relatively sensitive to the high single doses delivered with IOERT and should be moved from the radiation field unless ureteral obstruction is acceptable or the ureter is involved with tumor. Likewise, a functional bile duct will likely develop obstruction secondary to IOERT although recanalization may occur after high-dose treatment. Catheterization of the biliary system may be needed for a year or more after IOERT to the bile duct. Large blood vessels and nerves in the radiation field should be defined as well as possible so that one can interpret meaningfully the significance of any late complications. Similarly, bone which is in the IOERT field should be defined because late bone necrosis is possible. Certain important structures may be in the low-dose portion (deep) of the IOERT field and precise dose to these structures should also be determined, if feasible, and as indicated. Specifically, in the treatment of pancreatic carcinoma or other intra-abdominal malignancies, the IOERT field will often be directly overlying the spinal cord. Depending upon the exact beam energy and quality, a moderate dose of radiation may still be delivered to the cord. This dose should be determined because IOERT is usually combined with high-dose EBRT.

4. ANESTHETIC FACTORS

The anesthesiology team is critically and intimately involved with the entire surgical and IOERT process. For patients requiring transport from the operating room to the radiation therapy suite to receive IOERT, anesthesiology oversees the transfer and monitoring of the patient from standard anesthesia equipment in the operating room to portable anesthesia equipment during transport to the radiation oncology department and to resumption of standard anesthesia equipment in the radiation therapy suite. During the IOERT treatment, all personnel leave the room for the 3–5 min of irradiation. The patient and the anesthesia equipment are monitored by closed-circuit television from outside the treatment room (Fig. 4). Access to the patient is available within seconds if malfunction of anesthesia equipment or other difficulties arise.

Table 1
IOERT Applicator Size Availability at MGH, Mayo, Madrid, and Ohio State University

IOERT Applicators (size in cm)	MGH	Mayo	Madrid	OSU
Circular flat and 22° bevel				
(4–12 cm diameter)	—	—	—	Y
Circular flat, 15° and 30° bevel				
(0.5 cm increments, 4.5–9.5 cm)	Y	Y	Y[a]	—
Circular 45° bevel	Y	N	Y	N
Elliptical (flat and 20° bevel)	Y	Y	N	N
6 × 11, 7 × 12, 9 × 12				
8 × 15, 8 × 20 cm				
Rectangular (20° bevel)	Y	Y	N	N
7 × 9, 8 × 12, 8 × 15 cm				

[a]Circular applicators in 1 cm increments include 12 and 15 cm size for large field cases such as retroperitoneal sarcomas

5. APPLICATOR SELECTION

When an institution is going to embark on the use of IOERT, a full set of treatment applicators must be made available with full physics calibration (1–4). The exact applicators to be used will depend on the tumors to be treated at that institution. It is essential that a large variety are available, because even one tumor type will require many different sizes for adequate treatment. For treatment of the tumors that are commonly irradiated (rectal cancer with pelvic sidewall or sacral involvement, pancreas, bile duct, gastric bed, and abdominal or pelvic lymph-node diseases), we recommend the assortment of applicators (shown in Table 1). As a minimum, round applicators should be available at 6, 7, 8, and 9 cm both with no bevel on the edge of the applicator and with a 15° and a 30° for each of the nominal applicator diameters (Fig. 5A). Small diameter applicators of 3 and 4 cm are sometimes useful, but have a more limited application. For treatment of some pancreatic tumors and for intra-abdominal tumors such as gastric carcinoma, retroperitoneal sarcomas, and colonic tumors, either rectangular or elliptical applicators should be available. Elliptical applicators of 9 × 7, 12 × 7, 12 × 9, 15 × 8, and 20 × 8 have been very helpful for both abdominal and extremity cases, and are easier to position than rectangular ones (Fig. 5A–D). The NCI has an applicator called the "squircle" which has one end circular and the other end rectangular. This simplifies the problem of field abutment in patients who require more than one IOERT field.

At the time of surgery, the tumor volume (tumor bed after resection or unresectable tumor) to be irradiated is defined by the surgeon and radiation oncologist and marking sutures are placed around the perimeter of the lesion. An applicator is then selected that encompasses the tumor bed, usually with a 1-cm margin. A margin of at least 1 cm is optimal to allow for both dose and tumor variabilities. When visualizing the tumor or tumor bed through the applicator, the marking sutures should be readily identified well within the perimeter of the applicator, thus ensuring adequate coverage of the tumor volume.

If an applicator with a bevel is used, it is easy to overestimate the beam coverage towards the heel of the bevel (depth of penetration is less at heel vs toe end of beveled applicator) (Fig. 6). Because tissues directly below the heel may be underdosed, the

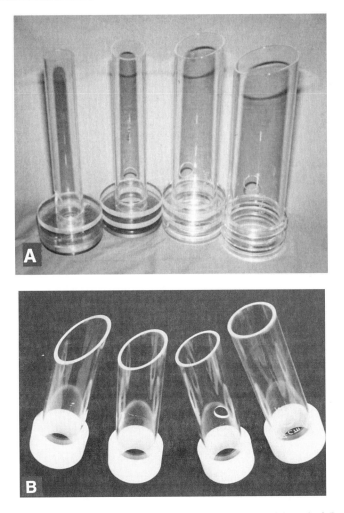

Fig. 5. Applicator options: (**A**) Circular (Mayo) 4.5 cm–flat and 15° bevel; 6.5 and 8.5 cm with 15° bevel. (**B**) Circular (MGH)—flat, 15°, 30°, and 45° bevel. (**C,D**) Rectangular (MGH).

treatment cylinder must be carefully placed. In addition, the bevel decreases the total beam penetration from what would be obtained without a bevel.

Although the IOERT applicator can often function adequately as a normal tissue retractor to hold sensitive normal structures out of the IOERT field, patient respiration or spontaneous movement of the bowel can allow normal tissues to move under the applicator and insinuate themselves inside the IOERT field. The applicator must be observed to confirm that this is not occurring. If there is evidence that bowel or other normal tissues slip into the IOERT field, surgical packing must be used to hold them out of the way. It is important that the packing itself does not enter into the field as this will decrease the electron-beam penetration, resulting in underdosage of a portion of the tumor volume.

There are certain situations in which normal tissues cannot be physically moved out of the radiation field. Thus, it is essential that a technique be available for secondary shielding. Standard lead sheets, which can be cut to the appropriate shape, should be available and an appropriate number used to attenuate 90% of the radiation beam. The

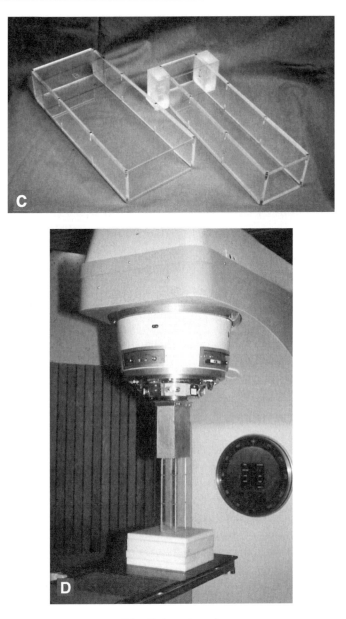

Fig. 5. (*continued*)

lead is covered with saline-soaked gauze and placed over the normal tissues. Lead shielding is often essential if abutting IOERT fields are to be used. Other methods for secondary collimation may be employed, but this method has been found to be effective.

6. METHOD OF DOCKING

There are two types of docking systems: "hard" and "soft." The hard-dock system is the most commonly employed, and in this system the treatment applicator is physically attached to the radiation therapy machine (Fig. 7A–H). In a soft-dock system, there is no physical contact between the applicator and linear accelerator (Fig. 1A,B, Fig. 7I).

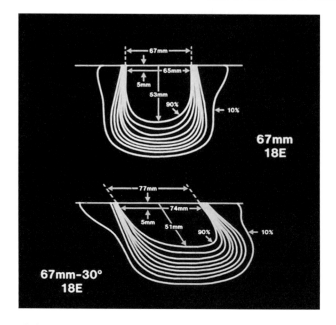

Fig. 6. Dosimetry of circular applicator with 30° bevel angle at end of applicator compared with flat end applicator (reprinted with permission from ref. *9*).

In a hard-dock system, this attachment process of applicator to machine is quite easy for most abdominal tumors (Fig. 7A–D), but for a tumor involving the pelvic sidewall (Fig. 2G,H, Fig. 7E,F) or located under the rib cage, the angulation of the treatment applicator can be quite difficult and requires a well-coordinated three-dimensional movement of the treatment table. The applicator is immobilized by hand (Fig. 7A,C) or with a Bookwalter stabilizer (Fig. 7E,F) (Codman Co., Raynham, MA) during this attachment procedure. After the applicator has been attached to the therapy machine, a periscope is inserted above the treatment applicator to confirm the proper positioning of the treatment field.

In the soft-dock system, the applicator is also secured in the patient by a modified Bookwalter retraction system (Fig. 1B). There is no further movement of the applicator in the patient after it has been immobilized. Once the patient is under the radiation-therapy machine, geometric alignment of the treatment applicator with the gantry head is achieved by a laser-alignment system with appropriate couch movement and gantry rotation (Fig. 7I).

7. ENERGY AND DOSE VS AMOUNT OF RESIDUAL DISEASE OR FLUID ACCUMULATION

IOERT is currently utilized as a component of a comprehensive treatment program of pre- or postoperative EBRT (45–54 Gy in 25–28 fractions) frequently with concurrent chemotherapy and surgery (maximal resection) for a locally advanced malignancy. Because most patients have received a course of full-dose preoperative EBRT, IOERT doses are usually in the range of 7.5–20 Gy.

The selection of dose as well as electron energy are dependent on the amount of residual tumor remaining after maximal resection. Doses in our institutions are quoted

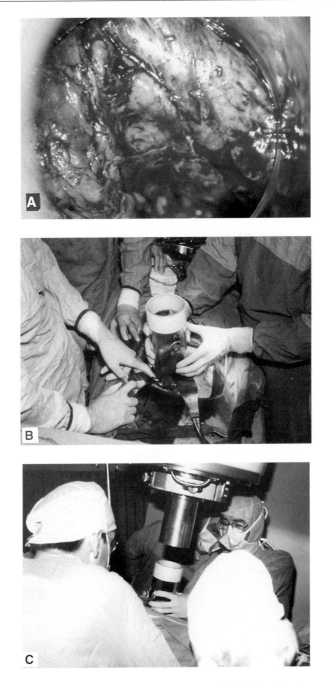

Fig. 7. Method of applicator docking and immobilization. (**A–F**) Hard dock system. Placement of applicator in upper presacrum (**A,B**) with applicator stabilized by hand (**C**) and docking accomplished (**D**). Pelvic sidewall tumor with applicator immobilized by Buckwalter device (**E**) and ready for treatment (**F**) (reprinted with permission from ref. 4). (**G**) Modification of treatment head to improve safety of hard docking system, Mayo Clinic. (**H**) IOERT at Univ. Hospital Gregorio Maranon (Madrid) with a conventional linear accelerator. Simulation of IOERT with a 7 cm applicator with 30° bevel to left pelvic sidewall with gantry angle rotation of 26° and patient on surgical table in oblique position (accelerator table removed). (**I**) Soft dock system with laser lights in dedicated IOERT facility at MGH. Geometric alignment of the applicator and gantry has been achieved, and patient is ready to treat.

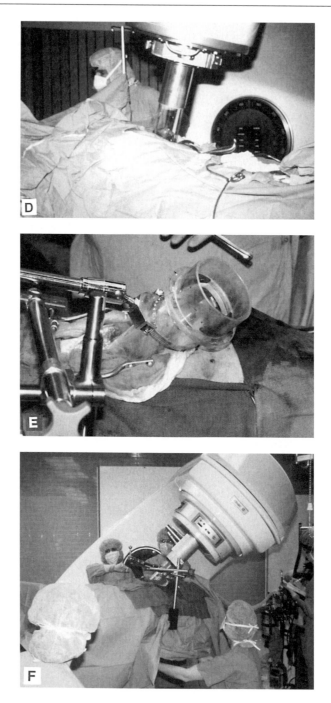

Fig. 7. (*continued*)

at the 90% isodose line and D_{max} as recommended by the NCI IORT working group guidelines (*1*). Electron energies are chosen so that the 90% depth dose encompasses the maximum thickness of any residual or unresectable tumor. After gross total resection, energies of 6 and 9 MeV are commonly used with or without surface bolus (with bolus to improve surface dose, if necessary).

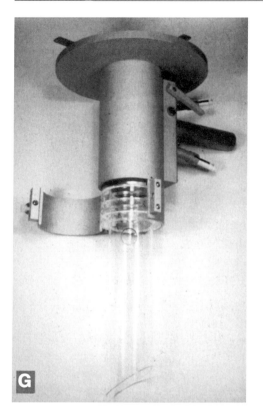

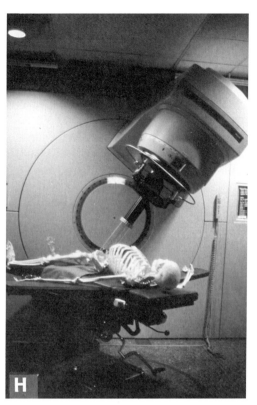

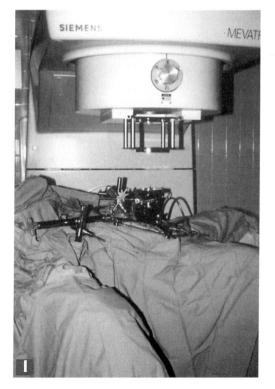

Fig. 7. (*continued*)

Guidelines used at MGH and Mayo Clinic are as follows for doses at the 90% isodose line: resection margin negative but narrow—7.5–10 Gy, margin microscopically positive or res(m)—10–12.5 Gy, gross residual-res(g) 2 cm or less in largest diameter—15 Gy, unresected or res(g) of 2 cm or greater—17.5–20 Gy. Doses of 20 Gy or higher are not utilized unless there have been limitations of delivery of EBRT.

One of the major problems that can occur during the actual delivery of the IORT is a build-up of fluid in the field. This is especially a problem in dependent areas, such as the posterior portion of the pelvis, when relatively low electron energies are employed. Accumulation of 1.0–1.5 cm of fluid will decrease the beam penetration by an equivalent amount and may result in underdosing of tissues at risk for tumor involvement. Therefore, suction always needs to be available at the time of the IORT procedure. It is usually adequate to place the suction on the outside of the base of the treatment applicator (Fig. 8). However, if the most dependent area is in the center of the applicator, an alternative suction device such as the Micromat may have to be considered.

8. SPECIALIZED EQUIPMENT—MOBETRON AND ORTHOVOLTAGE

Many considerations must be taken into account when embarking upon an operating room-based IOERT program. These include the frequency of utilization of IOERT, the type of cases that will be irradiated, architectural constraints of the building, and finally but not insignificantly, the cost of the project. Two alternative solutions are the Mobetron *(5)* and orthovoltage photon irradiation.

Conventional linear accelerators, even those modified for electron beam IOERT use, produce a significant amount of stray X-ray irradiation from the accelerator itself because of the design of these linacs. In order to provide multiple energies for clinical use, conventional linacs use a bending magnet to achieve energy selection. To assure a narrow energy spectrum and beam stability, tungsten slits are located in the magnet to restrict the energy of the emerging electron beam to within 5% of the nominal energy selected. Unfortunately, these electron slits also result in the generation of a substantial amount of energetic X-rays for which provisions for protection of operating personnel must be made. In practice, this requires about a foot of concrete equivalent shielding material to be placed in the walls, ceiling, and floor of the room. Together with the weight of conventional linacs (about 8 tons), the shielding required for a conventional IOERT unit installed in the OR adds another 20 or more tons of weight. The cost of the construction is substantial and has limited the widespread use of conventional linacs in ORs for IOERT.

8.1. Mobetron

A new and different approach is used in the Mobetron, a mobile and self-shielded electron beam linear accelerator designed specifically for IOERT use (*see* Chapter 3, Fig. 4). In the Mobetron, energy control is achieved without resorting to a bending magnet, thereby avoiding the high levels of radiation leakage produced by that type of system. The accelerator system consists of two collinear accelerator guides. By adjusting the power phase of the rf waves in the second accelerator guide, multiple electron energies with very tight energy control are achieved. The injector design, together with a prebuncher and beam alignment system, assures a narrow energy spectrum and low radiation leakage. The only significant stray radiation emanating from this approach comes from the patient-generated bremsstrahlung. A beamstopper is used to absorb the more energetically directed X-rays in the forward direction. At 3 m from the patient, with

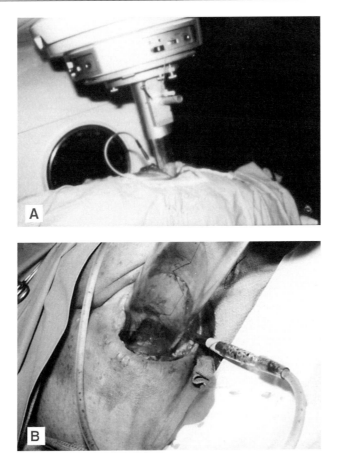

Fig. 8. Use of suction to prevent fluid build-up within surgical/IOERT field. (**A**) Unresectable pancreas. (**B**) Pelvic sidewall with patient in decubitus position.

no additional shielding required in the OR, this design leads to a maximum exposure to personnel of less than 2 mrem for a delivered dose of 20 Gy to the tumor.

The Mobetron is also substantially lighter than conventional linacs. Because it uses higher-frequency microwaves to generate the electron energies required, there is a substantial reduction in both size and weight of the linac system. The Mobetron weighs about 2750 lb, about 1/6 the weight of conventional linacs. The mobility of the Mobetron allows the unit to be shared between ORs, permitting greater utilization of IOERT. Because it can fit on most elevators, the Mobetron can also be removed to another location when maintenance or annual physics quality assurance tests are required, thereby not tying up an OR for these purposes.

8.2. Orthovoltage IORT

Orthovoltage IORT has been the approach taken for IORT at the New England Deaconess Hospital since 1982. The original IORT equipment was a heavily filtered Philips 305 kVp therapy unit permanently installed in the corner of a retrofitted and shielded operating room. A series of lead-lined brass treatment applicators were available that ranged in internal diameter from 6.1 to 9.9 cm. The length of the applicator could be varied, either 25 or 30 cm, and the end could be beveled at 0, 15, and 30°. Once the

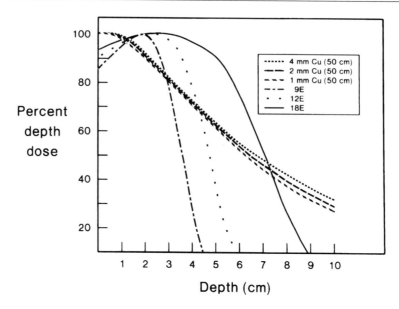

Fig. 9. Dosimetry of orthovoltage IORT compared with IOERT dosimetry.

position was determined, the applicator was fixed into position through a modified Bookwalter retractor that prevented movement and patient injury during the docking and treatment procedures. The output at the surface of the applicator ranged from 0.98 to 1.5 Gy, the time required to deliver a prescribed dose of 20 Gy at depth was in the order of 20 min.

In 1995, a new Deaconess Hospital was constructed and an entirely new IORT suite was designed. Since the experience thus far with orthovoltage was favorable, it was decided to continue with this form of radiation. Several modifications were made from the original IORT suite, the most important was the installation of ceiling tracks that allowed the treatment head to move from the side of the room to directly over the operative field. This obviated the cumbersome move of an anesthesized patient. The entire room was lead-lined and appropriate changes in the supporting structure were made to accommodate the additional weight of the shielding. The control module for the therapy unit was placed in an adjacent room as well as a separate anesthesia cart and television monitors.

The new IORT unit is a modified Oldelft (The Netherlands) Therapax DXT 300 which is microprocessor controlled. The peak voltage ranges from 30 to 300 kVp although only 300 and 100 kVp are used for IORT. A series of stainless-steel applicators were specially designed according to specifications and the internal diameter ranges from 4 to 10 cm. The focus to surface distance (FSD) is either 40 or 50 cm and applicators can be bevelled at 0, 15, and 30°. As before, a modified Bookwalter retractor system keeps the applicators rigidly in place during the procedure. The dose rate at the surface is approx 250 cGy/min.

The percentage depth dose curve for 300 kVp is 85% at 2 cm and 60% at 5 cm. At 100 kVp, the corresponding values are 47 and 20%. Because of the limited penetration at treatment depths over several centimeters, orthovoltage IORT is utilized almost exclusively in the setting of minimal residual disease. The dose heterogeneity is acceptable through 2 cm and compares favorably to electron-beam IORT (Fig. 9). The disadvantage of orthovoltage IORT is the unavoidable tail of the percent depth-dose curve. Because of this, more normal tissue is irradiated than with electron-beam IORT. Fortunately, this is without adverse clinical effect as has been the experience at the New England Deaconess Hospital where over 230 patients have been treated with this modality.

REFERENCES

1. Tepper JE, Gunderson LL, Goldson AL, et al. Quality control parameters of intraoperative radiation therapy, *Int. J. Radiation Oncol. Biol. Phys.*, **12** (1986) 1687–1695.
2. Tepper JE, Gunderson LL, Orlow E, et al. Complications of intraoperative radiation therapy, *Int. J. Radiation Oncol. Phys.*, **10** (1984) 1831–1839.
3. Gunderson LL, Tepper JE, and Biggs PJ. Intraoperative ± external beam irradiation, *Curr. Problems Cancer,* **7** (1983) 1–69.
4. Gunderson LL, Willett CG, Harrison LE, Petersen I, and Haddock MG. Intraoperative irradiation— current status, *Semin. Oncol.,* **24** (1997) 715–731.
5. Meurk M, Goer D, Schonberg R, et al. The Mobetron: a new concept for intraoperative irradiation. In JM Vaeth (ed.) *Intraoperative Radiation Therapy in the Treatment of Cancer,* 6th International IORT Symposium, 1996, San Francisco, CA. Basal, Karger, *Front. Radiation Oncol. Biol. Phys.,* **31** (1997) 65–70.
6. Kim HK, Jessup JM, Beard CJ, et al. Locally advanced rectal carcinoma: pelvic control and morbidity following radiation therapy, resection, and intraoperative radiation therapy, *Int. J. Radiation Oncol. Biol. Phys.,* **38** (1977) 777–783.
7. Gunderson LL, Dozios RR. Intraoperative irradiation for locally advanced colorectal carcinomas. *Persp. Colon Rectal Surg.* **5** (1992) 1–23.
8. Gunderson LL, Meyer JE, Sheedy P, and Munzenrider JE. Radiation oncology. In AR Margolis and AJ Burhenne (eds.) *Alimentary Tract Radiology, 3rd ed.* Mosby, St. Louis, MO (1983), pp. 2409–2446.
9. McCullough EC and Anderson JA. The dosimetric properties of an applicator system for intraoperative electron beam therapy using a Clinac-8 accelerator. *Med. Phys.* **9** (1982) 261–268.

5 Physics of Intraoperative High-Dose-Rate Brachytherapy

Lowell L. Anderson, Patrick J. Harrington, and Jean St. Germain

Contents

1. INTRODUCTION

Intraoperative irradiation by high-dose-rate remote-afterloading brachytherapy (HDR-IORT) requires, in addition to capabilities in surgery and radiation oncology, specialized physical equipment and facilities, appropriate computer software for treatment planning and, as an integral part of the interdisciplinary team, physicists trained in dose planning, dose delivery, and quality-assurance procedures. The rationale for HDR-IORT is related, in large part, to the physical advantages it affords of confining the therapeutic dose to a highly localized target and sparing normal structures either by moving them away or shielding them. These advantages may substantially offset the radiobiological disadvantage associated with a single-fraction treatment (*see* Chapter 2). Although only a few institutions are currently performing HDR-IORT, sufficient experience has been acquired to establish its feasibility with respect to such physical factors as available source strength, suitable applicators, and acceptable treatment durations.

2. CHARACTERISTICS OF HDR REMOTE AFTERLOADERS

Since its introduction more than 20 yrs ago, high-dose-rate remote afterloading with a single ^{192}Ir source under stepping-motor control has become a prominent brachytherapy modality. Because it virtually eliminates radiation exposure to staff and because it facilitates treatment planning by permitting a variable dwell time at each source location, its role is still expanding, most recently to include intraoperative brachytherapy. At the same time, the potential for harm to both patients and staff from an uncontrolled source is such

From: *Current Clinical Oncology: Intraoperative Irradiation: Techniques and Results*
Edited by: L. L. Gunderson et al. © Humana Press, Inc., Totowa, NJ

Table 1
Characteristics of Currently Used High-Dose-Rate Remote Afterloaders

	μ-Selectron HDR	Gamma Med 12i	VariSource
Number of channels	18	24	20
Number of steps/channel	48	40	20
Step increment	2.5 mm, 5.0 mm	1.0–10.0 mm	2.0–99.0 mm
Minimum dwell time	0.1 s	1 s	0.1 s
Maximum dwell time	999.9 s	999 s	360 s
Direction of treatment	forward	backward	backward
Source travel	1500 mm	1300 mm	1500 mm
Storage safe	tungsten	uranium	tungsten
Active length	3.5 mm	3.5 mm	10.0 mm
Active diameter	0.6 mm	0.6 mm	0.34 mm
Capsule diameter	1.1 mm	1.2 mm	0.59 mm

that a high level of caution is necessary in all aspects of facility and machine maintenance on the one hand and treatment planning and delivery on the other.

2.1. Operational Capabilities

The concept of afterloading in brachytherapy, introduced in 1960 (1), heralded a significant reduction in radiation exposure to staff. The subsequent introduction of HDR remote afterloading only a few years later essentially eliminated staff exposure, as the patient is alone in a shielded room during treatment. Moreover, the short treatment times associated with HDR remote afterloading permitted enhanced accuracy of dose delivery, because of less patient motion during treatment; lower doses to normal tissue by greater retraction of adjacent structures; and treatment on an outpatient basis. Independent development efforts led, in 1964, to the introduction of high-dose-rate remote afterloaders at four widely dispersed centers (2–5). Three of the four were for intracavitary treatment of uterine cervix cancer. The fourth, the Gamma Med unit, was used interstitially to treat brain tumors.

The most significant event in the subsequent commercial development of remote afterloading was the incorporation of stepping-motor control of source position in the design of the Gamma Med II unit (6). In this unit, dwell time for a single ^{192}Ir source (nominally 10 Ci) could be programmed to the nearest second at up to 20 uniformly spaced positions, 0.5 or 1.0 cm apart, along the treatment catheter. Automatic correction for source decay was performed by an internal microprocessor. This design was soon recognized to facilitate greatly the optimization of treatment plans, and other manufacturers of HDR machines were not long in adopting that feature. Later models of the Gamma Med and of other machines were designed primarily for interstitial treatments, each with a narrow, elongated source for use with small diameter catheters, and an indexer to allow the source to be projected into multiple channels.

The ^{192}Ir stepping-source HDR remote afterloaders currently marketed in the United States are the micro-Selectron HDR (Nucletron, Veenendaal, The Netherlands), the GammaMed 12i (Isotopen-Technik Dr. Sauerwein, Haan, Germany), and the VariSource (Varian-Crowley, Crowley, England). A detailed description of their characteristics has been published (the VariSource is a new version of the Omnitron afterloader described in this work) (2). Machine specifications are summarized in Table 1.

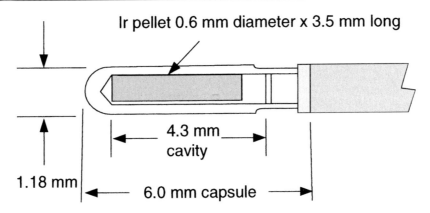

Fig. 1. [192]Ir source in stainless-steel capsule, which is welded to a stainless-steel cable.

2.2. Sources—Design and Dosimetry

[192]Ir is currently the only radionuclide suitable for HDR remote afterloading. Other radionuclides that might be considered would produce, for the same source dimensions, a much lower dose rate as a result of too long a half life (and, therefore, too low a specific activity) and/or too low an air-kerma-rate constant. The air-kerma-rate constant for ^{192}Ir is 4.08 cGy cm^2 mCi^{-1} h^{-1}, corresponding to an exposure-rate constant of 4.65 R cm^2 mCi^{-1} h^{-1}, the value calculated by Glasgow and Dillman *(8)* as adjusted to the currently accepted value (0.877 cGy R^{-1}) of exposure-to-dose correction factor (they were using 0.869 cGy R^{-1}). Thus, a 10-Ci point source of ^{192}Ir would deliver dose to air 1 cm away at a rate of 680 cGy min^{-1} (or 755 cGy min^{-1} to water).

Whereas the Gamma Med II afterloader used a cylindrical ^{192}Ir source of active dimensions 1×1 mm and was intended primarily for intracavitary applications, the interstitial afterloaders introduced later required sources of smaller diameter that were, of necessity, longer. A longitudinal cross section of the source used with the GammaMed 12i afterloader is shown in Fig. 1. The dimensions of the micro-Selectron/HDR source are similar to those of the GammaMed 12i, whereas the VariSource source is still longer and thinner, but with roughly the same active volume.

Accuracy in dose delivery depends on accuracy in both source calibration and in single-source reference data. For routine source calibrations, options such as a well chamber or a phantom jig may be used. In the United States, well-chamber calibrations for HDR sources are available at two Accredited Brachytherapy Calibration Laboratories (ABCLs; accredited by the American Association of Physicists in Medicine, these laboratories are operated by K & S Associates in Nashville, TN, and the University of Wisconsin Medical Physics Department in Madison, WI).

In-air calibration remains the standard for HDR sources whether performed at an ABCL or at the local institution. A generally recommended approach to in-air calibration is that of Goetsch et al. *(9)*. Source calibration calls for some measure of redundancy when considered as part of the quality-assurance program. At Memorial Sloan-Kettering Cancer Center, for example, the practice has been to perform an in-air measurement of the strength of each new source and to compare the value obtained with the value predicted from the in-air measurement at the previous source-change by applying the new source/old source ratio of well-chamber measurements; agreement within 2% is considered acceptable.

With respect to dose-reference data, the experimentally validated Monte Carlo calculated results of Kirov et al. are applicable to the 3.5×0.6-mm sources used in both the micro-Selectron/HDR and GammaMed 12i afterloaders (10). The dose-rate constant was found to be 1.115 cGy h^{-1} U^{-1} and the value of the anisotropy function at 1 cm on the longitudinal axis was 64%. Good agreement with these data were seen in a similar study by Watanabe et al., who also performed experimental and Monte Carlo evaluations of dose distribution around the partially shielded ovoid source position of a Henschke applicator (11). Recently presented Monte Carlo calculations and validating film measurements of dose distribution around the VariSource source show the dose-rate constant to be 1.04 cGy h^{-1} U^{-1} and the axial anisotropy function at 1 cm to be approx 45% (12). In treatment configurations for which lines of target points are parallel to lines of closely spaced (0.5–1.0 cm) dwell positions, such as planar tumor-bed implants, inexact anisotropy data may make little contribution to error in the treatment dose. In volume-implant configurations, on the other hand, anisotropy-related error will be more significant.

2.3. Safety Features

The three afterloading machines mentioned above share certain capabilities that relate to safe and accurate treatment delivery. Of prime importance is the automatic retraction of the source when all dwell positions in a given channel have been treated or when potentially dangerous situations arise. Abnormal circumstances that should cause automatic retraction of an extended source include a distorted or obstructed source-guide tube that creates unacceptable resistance to source motion, opening of the treatment room door, operation of the interrupt switch on the console, operation of one of the emergency switches (mounted on the console, on the wall near the door, and on the afterloader itself). Similarly, extension of the source from its shield will be prevented if no source-guide tube is connected to the selected channel or a treatment-room door is open. System operation from rechargeable batteries assures source retractability in the event of power failure. Radiation detectors in the afterloader and/or elsewhere in the treatment room activate visual or audible signals when the source is extended, allowing staff to check that a given treatment is proceeding as expected and, in an emergency, to determine if measures to reshield the source have been successful. Each source extension for treatment is preceded by extension of a "dummy" cable to check that the planned travel path is unobstructed and of appropriate length. Duplicate timers allow detection of an error in either during treatments. A manual source-retraction system is available in the event all other retraction methods fail. Finally, key locks at both the console and the afterloader limit access to authorized personnel.

3. CONSTRUCTION OF THE HDR-IORT FACILITY

Many HDR facilities are currently housed within a treatment room designed for use with a higher-energy modality, e.g., a linear accelerator or a ^{60}Co teletherapy unit. The shielding of the higher energy unit is more than adequate to shield the HDR source. Because of the special surgical and anesthesia requirements for HDR-IORT, these facilities are not usually adaptable to HDR-IORT. Relatively few institutions have OR facilities designed to house accelerators with capability for intraoperative electron irradiation (IOERT). In most IOERT institutions, the patient is transported to the IOERT treatment room from an operating room in a nearby space. Although the shielding in electron-accelerator facilities may be adequate for HDR-IORT, the other medical requirements usually cannot be met. It may be possible in a given set of circumstances to convert an operating room for HDR-IORT, but the most satisfactory solution is the construction of a dedicated facility (13).

3.1. Shielding Design

The shielding design follows the general principles outlined for primary barriers in Report No. 49 of the National Council on Radiation Protection and Measurements (NCRP) (14). This report is currently under revision. The report's methodology involves calculating the barrier transmission factor required to achieve a specified weekly exposure limit to a point of interest outside the room from a radiation source inside the room, taking into account the point-to-source distance, the strength of the source, and the fraction of the time it will be "on" (exposed), as well as the fraction of the on-time the point of interest may be occupied by a given person. Graphs are included from which one may read the thickness of a lead or a concrete barrier corresponding to the calculated transmission factor.

The permissible doses in surrounding areas and the occupancy of such areas need to be examined by the physicist. Based on the recommendations of the NCRP Report No. 116, a dose limit of 1 mSv/yr (100 mrem/yr) would apply in unrestricted areas (15). For restricted areas, a dose limit of 50 mSv/yr (5000 mrem/yr) would apply. For unrestricted areas, the corresponding weekly design limit is 0.02 mSv/wk (2 mrem/wk). For restricted areas, a design limit of 0.1 mSv/wk (10 mrem/wk) is recommended as it is to be anticipated that occupational dose limits may continue to decrease and the personnel will wish to work in as low an irradiation field as possible.

For shielding purposes, the source may be considered to approximate a point source. Its position may be taken as the point of closest approach of the operating couch to the shielding barrier. Although each barrier needs to be calculated individually, shielding barriers for restricted areas will usually contain approx 30–45 cm (12–18 in) of concrete (147 lb ft^{-3}) or concrete equivalent. The larger thickness corresponds to the 0.1 mSv/wk design limit recommended here, whereas the smaller thickness corresponds to the 1 mSv/wk design limit that would be allowed by NCRP Report No. 116.

The use of a maze wall will reduce the shielding of the door, but a maze requires additional space. A shielded door for a "no maze" design will typically contain a thickness of Pb that provides the same transmission factor as does the concrete wall. For ^{192}Ir, the "equivalent thickness" of Pb is very close to a factor of 10 smaller than that of concrete, leading to a range for Pb of 3.0–4.5 cm (1.2–1.8 in). Note that one cannot obtain the equivalent thickness from the ratio of tabulated tenth-value layers, since the latter are derived from the heavily shielded portion of the transmission curve and our focus here is on a barrier for an unshielded source. In a no-maze design, the weight of the shielding door will mandate an electric operator. In the event of an emergency, such as a power failure, the door design should allow for mechanical operation.

Finally, provision should be made for an instrument port for calibration purposes in addition to the necessary penetration(s) for mechanical and electrical services.

3.2. Operational and Safety Design

As in most radiation-treatment rooms, the shielded operating room must be equipped with two video cameras, patient communication systems, door interlocks, and a room-radiation monitor (see Fig. 2). A shielded receptacle large enough to contain the entire applicator should be positioned near the afterloader during treatment, for emergency use in the event of a nonretracting or dislodged source. In addition, anesthesia and surgical

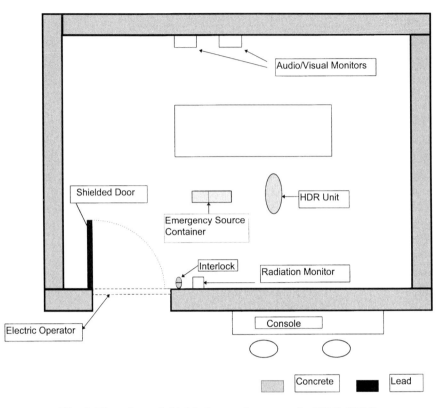

Fig. 2. Plan view of shielded operating room for HDR-IORT.

monitors will be within the room and duplicated at a remote location, either near the treatment console or in an adjacent room or corridor. Provision for placement of equipment on the hospital emergency generator should be part of the planning process. An emergency "crash cart" should be within the immediate area. The console area should be large enough to accommodate not only all the monitors required but also the operating-room personnel, who must wait outside the room during treatment. One should consider providing a special anteroom for people who must remain sterile during treatment in case emergency reentry is required; this area should have its own video monitor to observe the operative field and the progress of the treatment. A portable survey meter should be available at the console for use in emergencies and in monitoring.

4. TREATMENT PLANNING AND DOSE DELIVERY

As recounted in Chapter 1, HDR-IORT of tumor beds using plastic needles in a superflab applicator was first reported in 1991 by Lukas et al. of the Klinikum rechts der Isar in Munich *(16)*. Treatment planning and delivery methods were described in a subsequent publication *(17)*. The following year a similar, independently developed protocol was implemented at Memorial Sloan-Kettering Cancer Center (MSKCC) in New York, using superflab HAM (Harrison-Anderson-Mick) applicators in which plastic catheters had been embedded at the time of manufacture *(18,19)*. Prior to these efforts, however, Pirkowski and colleagues at Georgetown University School of Medicine (GUSM) in Washington, D.C. had employed curved needles in a segmented acrylic

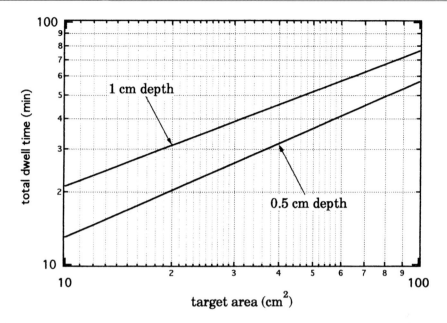

Fig. 3. Time to deliver a uniform dose of 10 Gy to a rectangular target plane for a 3.78 cGy cm^2 sec^{-1} (or 3.33 Ci) ^{192}Ir source at two depths from the applicator surface, which itself is 0.5 cm from the source plane.

applicator to treat diaphragmatic cancer by HDR-IORT *(20),* pursuant to still earlier HDR-IORT treatments of liver metastases using closed-end needles inserted into the target volume *(21).* All of the above studies made use of Gamma Med remote afterloaders. A microSelectron HDR machine has been used at Ohio State University Hospital (OSUH) in Columbus for HDR-IORT with assorted applicators, both rigid and flexible *(22).* The HDR-IORT experience at all four of these centers has been summarized as of early 1993 *(13).*

4.1. Applicators

It is clear from the early experience of the Munich group that some separation is required between the HDR-source catheters and the tissue surface being treated, in order to avoid necrosis and other complications *(13).* Too large a distance, however, can result in an inconveniently long treatment time, and the most commonly employed distance between source plane and applicator surface is 0.5 cm. In connection with initial feasibility estimates, the MSKCC group made use of Paterson-Parker planar-mold data *(23)* to generate approximate relationships between treatment area and total treatment dwell time at given distances, for a source at the end of its useful life (just before a source change). The Paterson-Parker data give the cumulated source strength (mg hr) to deliver 1000 R uniformly over a rectangular target as a function of target area **a** (cm^2) for various distances between source and target planes. When multiplied by appropriate correction factors to account for updated values of exposure-rate constant and f-factor for water, the data for 1 and 1.5 cm distances are well approximated by 93.6 $a^{0.642}$ and 185 $a^{0.557}$, respectively. Translated from milligram-hours of radium into curie-minutes (Ci-min) of ^{192}Ir and divided by 3.33 Ci, these formulas become 2.96 $a^{0.642}$ and 5.85 $a^{0.557}$ and give the total dwell time required for treatment with a source that has been allowed to decay to one-third of its nominal starting strength. Plotted in Fig. 3, they indicate treatment

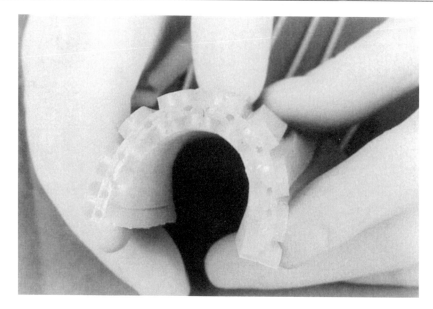

Fig. 4. Silicone mold "ALPA-SIL 10:1" applicator with grooves on either side, alternating midway between catheters to enhance flexibility (courtesy of Isotopen-Technik Dr. Sauerwein GMBH, Haan, Germany).

times that are already becoming problematic with larger treatment areas for a 1 cm distance (0.5 cm from the applicator surface), suggesting that source-surface distances greater than 0.5 cm would be logistically difficult.

Both of the groups that began treating tumor beds with mold applicators made of superflab are now using similar applicators made of a silicone rubber material. Although not as flexible as the superflab, the silicone material is more easily sterilized and, because it is stable even with repeated steam sterilization, is reusable *(24)*. For the silicone applicators supplied by Sauerwein Isotopen Technik, enhanced flexibility has been achieved in the transverse direction by surface grooves parallel to the catheters (*see* Fig. 4) and in the longitudinal direction by using catheters of softer material. Applicator length, as well as width, may be adjusted in the operating room prior to insertion of sterile catheters. For the silicone HAM applicators supplied by Mick Radio-Nuclear Instruments (Bronx, NY), improved flexibility has been accomplished by reducing the applicator thickness to 0.8 cm, yet retaining the 0.5 cm distance between source plane and treatment surface (*see* Fig. 5). Clear labeling of the "thin" side is required to make sure it is not used as the treatment surface. Embedded catheters in the HAM applicators may themselves preclude steam sterilization and discourage reuse, although these limitations do not apply to applicators furnished without catheters.

HDR-IORT at OSUH has involved several applicator types, including rigid applicators of "delrin" (a DuPont trademark), flexible foam-based applicators, and semiflexible applicators of "silastic" (the Dow Corning trademark for a particular silicone material) *(22,13)*. Selection is based on topographic features of the anatomical surface to be treated. A unique applicator design, flexible in the catheter direction, was developed for HDR-IORT at GUSM in subdiaphragmatic treatments (*see* Fig. 6). The design was based on anatomic molds of the diaphragmatic surface in cadavers and provided for longitudinal curvatures from planar to a full right angle *(20)*.

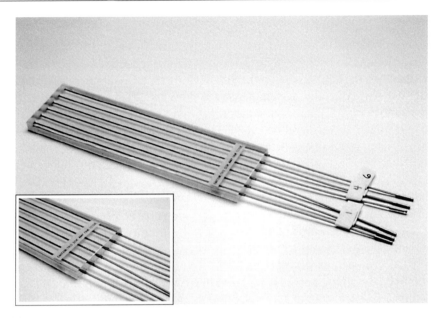

Fig. 5. Silicone mold HAM applicator with embedded catheters (manufactured by Mick Radio-Nuclear Instruments, Bronx, NY).

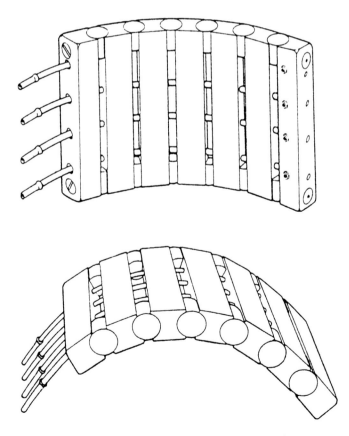

Fig. 6. Segmented 7-cm-width acrylic IOHDR applicator conforming to curved steel needles (Reprinted with permission from *Int. J. Radiation Oncol. Biol. Phys.*, **22** (1992) 1105–1108.)

4.2. Dose Specification

Although dose specification in brachytherapy usually refers to the evaluated dose reported as having been delivered, in the case of tumor-bed HDR-IORT treatments with mold applicators, the methodology is usually lacking for an evaluation separate from the planning and one generally assumes that the dose specified is the same as the dose prescribed and planned. There are two aspects of dose specification. First, at what depth from the applicator surface will the dose be prescribed and second, will the dose at that depth be constant or variable over the target surface? From the literature available to date, it appears that there are interinstitutional differences (and, perhaps, intra-institutional differences, as well) in the approach to these questions.

In the standard protocol described by Kneschaurek et al., a reference dose was specified at a reference point on the surface of the applicator in the center of the target region, and all source positions were assigned the same dwell time (17). This approach assures a significant variation in dose within the target plane, a greater variation for smaller areas. The MSKCC protocol, on the other hand, is different both in that the dose is prescribed at 0.5 cm from the applicator surface and in that dwell times are optimized to achieve a closely uniform dose throughout the target plane at 0.5 cm depth (19). A uniform target dose is the usual goal in external-beam treatments and in the Manchester system of brachytherapy. The treatment policy reported by Nag at OSUH is intermediate between those just mentioned in that, whereas dose is prescribed at 0.5 cm depth, equal dwell times are used at all source positions for reasons of lower chance of error in data entry, probable higher tumor burden near the target center, and simplified interinstitutional comparison of results (25). Dose specification at various depths, depending on disease assessment, is implied by Pirkowski et al. for the subdiaphragmatic treatments at GUSM (20).

4.3. Planning

Since uniform dwell time characterized the standard HDR-IORT method in Kneschaurek et al., the total time selected was that which would deliver the reference dose to the surface reference point (17). For a rectangular grid of source positions spaced at 1 cm in both directions, tables were prepared, for various applicator thicknesses, to give the dwell time required for a 10-Gy reference dose as a function of grid dimensions. Other doses were obtained by appropriate scaling of the dwell time. Source positions were always in the central plane of the applicator, whatever its thickness. For a 1-cm-thick applicator, total dwell time ranged from 82 s for a 3×3 array of source positions to 990 s for a 15×15 array. These are nominal dwell times, of course, for a nominal source strength of 11.3 Gy cm^2 sec^{-1} (10 Ci); actual dwell times are usually longer, reflecting automatic decay corrections implemented by the afterloading machine. In the case of a 1.5-cm applicator, the total dwell time is 52% longer for the 3×3 array and 23% longer for the 15×15 array. For a 9×9 array of sources, corresponding to a 7×7 cm target size, depth doses for these two thicknesses along a perpendicular to the applicator at the reference point are shown in Fig. 7. Although the 1.5-cm thickness affords significantly better penetration, it would probably result in unacceptable rigidity in the silicone applicators now in use. The dose on the applicator surface at the corner of the target area in this case, for the 1.5-cm thickness, is only 76% of the reference dose.

Departures from the standard protocol were effectuated when called for (17). For a nonrectangular target, dwell positions outside a 1-cm extension of the target boundary were not loaded. Also not loaded, or with dwell times reduced by about a factor of two,

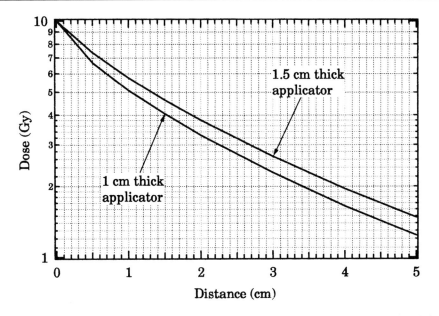

Fig. 7. Dose along an axis perpendicular to the applicator at its center for applicator thicknesses of 1.0 cm and 1.5 cm.

were positions in the immediate neighborhood of critical structures adjacent to the target area. Finally, in selected cases it was desirable to achieve a constant dose over the target area. In such cases, dwell times were optimized to achieve the reference dose at nine reference points (ends and midpoints of target boundary lines as well as target center), producing a practically homogeneous dose to the target area. The requisite increase in dwell times near the target border, for a 9×9 source array, resulted in a 50% increase in total dwell time compared to the standard method.

Planning for a given HDR-IORT tumor-bed treatment at MSKCC, once the dimensions of the target area have been specified by the radiation oncologist, consists of retrieving the correct plan from a computer atlas of plans *(19)* and verifying it by plotting isodose lines in the central transverse plane and by printing out dwell-time data for the specified number of channels. The current version of the atlas contains over 5000 plans, for all combinations of source-array dimensions from 3×3 to 24×40, for two dose levels (10 and 15 Gy), and for cylindrically curved applicators (10 cm radius) in both catheter and transverse directions as well as flat applicators *(26)*. Both catheters and source position are spaced at 1 cm. In addition to a uniform dose in the target plane 0.5 cm from the applicator, planning goals included a comparable degree of uniformity at the applicator surface.

Least-squares optimization of dwell times was employed in atlas construction, with a two-term objective function in which the first term was the sum of squares of differences between achieved and desired doses at target points, and the second term was the sum of squares of differences between doses at applicator-surface points and the average dose among all surface points *(26)*. An analytic (rather than iterative) least-squares method was used because it is made possible by the fact that dwell times are essentially continuous variables in HDR treatments and it involves a global (rather than local) minimization of the objective function, thereby assuring the best possible solution for a given set of parameters. In addition to the targeted dose, the parameters included a weighting factor applied to the second term, a factor that was generally adjusted to bring about the same percent standard deviation among doses at "uniformity" (surface) points as among target points. The initial approach to identifying nonnegative solutions to the least-squares problem was to derive a set of n linear equations in n unknowns (dwell times) by differentiating the objective function with respect to each unknown, in turn, setting equal to zero and then solving the system by determinants. If the solution contained negative dwell times, further solutions were found for the n sets of $n-1$ equations in $n-1$ unknowns formed by setting each of the unknowns separately equal to zero. If still no nonnegative solutions emerged, each of the n sets was reduced in size again to get solutions for $n-1$ sets of $n-2$ equations in $n-2$ unknowns. This reduction process proceeded one level beyond the level at which the first nonnegative solution appeared and, if more than one nonnegative solution was found, the one accepted was the one with the lowest standard deviation. Although this approach is straightforward, it is obviously inefficient, because reduction of large matrices by several levels could involve solving thousands of sets of equations. A much faster analytic method used currently to get the same answers is the *nnls* (nonnegative least squares) algorithm described by Lawson and Hanson *(27)*. In this method, the objective function is formulated as the difference between the product of an $m \times n$ matrix of doses per unit dwell time and a solution vector of n dwell times, and a vector of which the m components are the desired doses at target and uniformity points. The solution is obtained by matrix methods, subject to the constraint that dwell times must be greater than zero.

The procedure for atlas formulation involves first running a *spec* program that reads user specifications concerning target and uniformity point locations as well as source positions (number of lines and number per line) and then generates an input file for *brachy,* the standard brachytherapy dose computation program at MSKCC, setting a keyword in the file to direct *brachy* to produce an "individual contributions" (.ics) output file containing the dose per unit dwell time at each target and uniformity point. The *brachy* program is then run, followed by an auxiliary program, *rals* (remote afterloading least squares), which reads the .ics file and calls the *nnls* subroutine to perform the actual optimization. Before calling *nnls,* the *rals* program subtracts from each uniformity-matrix element the average of all uniformity-matrix elements, thereby targeting zero dose difference among them. Automation of the above steps, using a command-language program, facilitated timely production of the atlas.

An evaluation of the "goodness of fit" achieved by least-squares optimization was performed for the atlas as configured initially for the Gamma Med IIi afterloader, with source-array dimensions ranging from 3×3 to 12×20. Mean dose among target points for each atlas plan was at worst 1.1% different from the desired dose, whether for flat or curved applicators; averaged over the full range, the difference was only 0.1%. The worst-case and average standard deviations for flat applicators were 2.5% and 1.4%, respectively, for target points and 4.8% and 1.9%, respectively, for uniformity (surface) points. For curved applicators, these figures did not exceed 4.0% and 2.3%, respectively, for target points and 6.8% and 4.2%, respectively, for uniformity points. Also evaluated was the effect of planning for one curvature and treating with another. These results, given in Table 2, indicate worst-cast dose differences of 6–7%.

The computer window for HDR-IORT atlas implementation is shown in Fig. 8. Labeled edit boxes are provided for entry of the patient's name, medical record number, and prescribed dose. Longitudinal and transverse target area dimensions (cm) are chosen

Table 2
For Various Array Sizes and a Planned Dose of 10 Gy, Target-Point
Doses Calculated if Curvature Is Different from that Assumed in Planning

Curvature Direction	Number of Lines × Number of Positions	Planned Radius (cm)	Actual Radius (cm)	Average Dose (cGy)	Extreme Dose (cGy)
Transverse	4 × 6	flat	15	982	942
		10	7	987	932
	11 × 11	flat	15	979	957
		10	7	990	938
Longitudinal	4 × 6	flat	15	969	935
		10	7	984	915
	11 × 11	flat	15	972	941
		10	7	986	941
Transverse	10 × 10	flat	3	964	935
		10	3	992	955

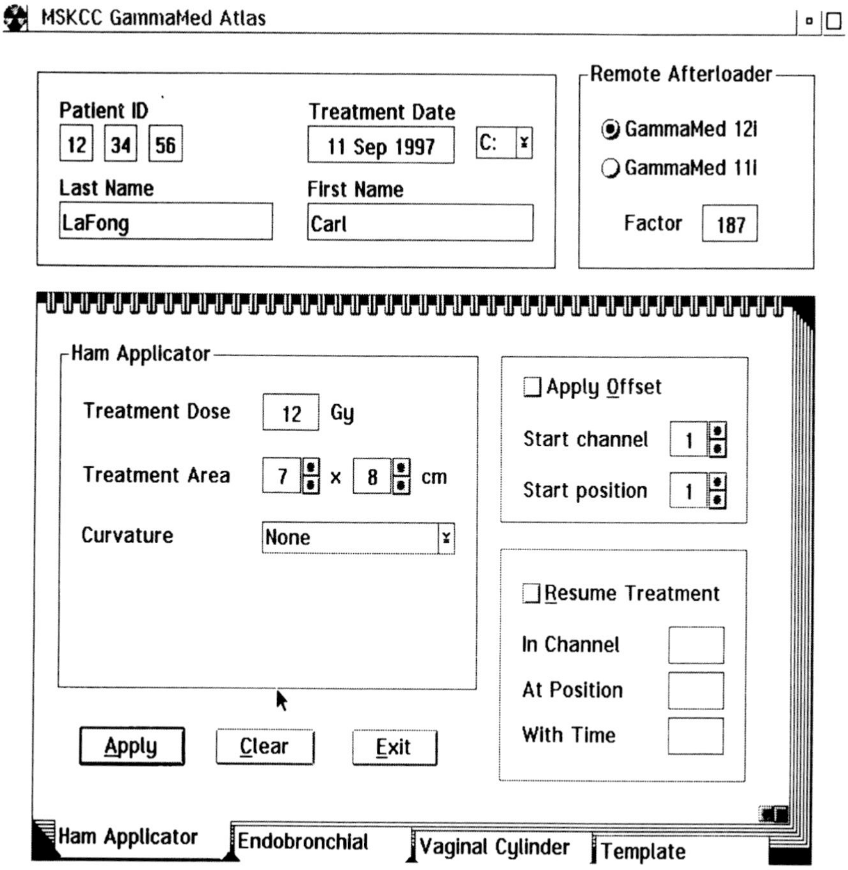

Fig. 8. Atlas window for HDR brachytherapy at MSKCC.

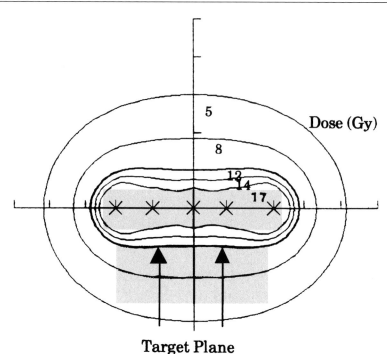

Target Plane

Fig. 9. Isodose plot in central transverse plane of IOHDR application to treat a rectangular area 4 cm wide and 8 cm long. Together with dwell-time data printout, serves to verify retrieval of correct plan from computer atlas. Overlay of applicator cross-section and target surface has been added.

from pop-up menus, as well as applicator curvature (flat, longitudinal, or transverse) and prescribed dose. Each dimension is increased by one by the computer program to get the source array size. On the basis of these responses, the program locates the corresponding plan and, if the dose specified is not 10 or 15 Gy, scales the dwell times appropriately from whichever stored plan has the closest dose. A *brachy* input file is generated automatically and *brachy* is run to obtain the verification isodose plot and printout of dwell-time data.

Treatment planning calculations for HDR-IORT at OSUH and at GUSM made use of commercially available planning systems *(22,20)*. Although no detailed description has been found in the literature, it is inferred that the planning methodology was similar to that of Kneschaurek et al. *(17)*. At OSUH, plans were precalculated for applicators of various sizes to avoid the delay of treatment planning following applicator selection *(13)*.

4.4. Quality Assurance in Dose Delivery

Whether the treatment plan is retrieved from an atlas or computed just prior to treatment, it is important that its correctness be verified by a second physicist. An example of the central-plane isodose plot generated for plan verification at MSKCC is shown in Fig. 9. The names and signatures of both the planning and the checking physicist should appear prominently on the hard copy version of the plan. Planning data entered at the afterloader console keyboard or transferred to the console electronically should also be checked by a second person before the dose is delivered.

It is exceedingly important to proper dose delivery that the applicator be in contact with the tissue surface throughout the entire target area and for the entire treatment time. From Fig. 7 it is seen that, for a 1-cm-thick applicator, even a 0.5 cm separation can result in a reduction of more than 30% in dose to tissue along the central perpendicular to the applicator. The effect is only slightly less severe for a 1.5 cm applicator or for dwell times optimized to produce uniform dose over the target area *(17)*.

Quality assurance (QA) procedures specific to HDR-IORT include checks of the applicators to be used. At MSKCC, each HAM applicator is inspected and tested when received from the manufacturer (Mick Radio-Nuclear Instruments). It is first physically inspected to assure that there are no loose connectors or visible defects. Then the length of each channel of the applicator-source guide tube assembly is measured for ± 1 mm conformity with specification. Finally, the applicator is autoradiographed to ascertain that all channels will accept the source and that interchannel tube alignment is acceptable.

As is the case for all applications of HDR brachytherapy, extensive QA checks of the afterloading machine and treatment facility must be performed prior to HDR-IORT. For most other applications it is feasible to perform these checks on the same day as treatment. For HDR-IORT, however, where preparations for surgery typically start at approx 7:00 AM, same-day QA requires a physicist to arrive at 6:00 AM for uninterrupted access to the operating room. Because of the scheduling difficulties presented by this circumstance at MSKCC, for example, QA procedures are carried out on the day preceding any scheduled HDR-IORT, and early morning QA occurs only for clinical procedures on Monday. The MSKCC radioactive materials license to operate the afterloader requires complete QA following any move from one room to another, thereby ruling out the possibility of performing same-day QA in an adjacent shielded room. At OSUH, a license modification was obtained to permit moving the remote afterloader from the radiation oncology department to the shielded operating room for a treatment *(22)*.

HDR QA checks in general have been thoroughly described elsewhere *(28)*. Broad categories as well as specific procedures are represented in the QA checklist (Fig. 10) used at MSKCC, where two shielded rooms are in use, each with a different remote afterloader. At the operator's console, after the functionality of indicator lights, intercom, and video monitors has been established, the source decay correction factor displayed on the screen is compared with that on a computer-generated calendar prepared at the time of the last source change. The treatment room radiation monitor is unplugged to be sure its backup batteries are good, and its alarm-light response to a ^{137}Cs source held near its ceiling location is verified. Checks are made of the operational safety features of the machine and facility to determine that the backlighted sign near the treatment room door is on when the source is extended; the source will not project unless a guide tube is connected; Gamma Med 12i errors are reported if the guide tube/applicator connected is either too long or too short; the source will not project if the treatment room door is open and, if extended, will retract if the door is open; and an extended source will retract if either the interrupt button or the emergency button is actuated. Treatment functionality of the indexer is addressed by projecting the source, on a rotating basis, in 4 of the 24 channels for the 12i machine and 3 of the 12 channels for the IIi machine, recording which channels were tested on a given occasion. By video monitor observation of the source-step viewer, the source's entry-exit time is measured at a dwell position programmed for 60 s, dividing the stopwatch reading by the decay correction factor should produce a number within 0.5 s of the programmed time. Finally, position accuracy is checked via an autoradiograph of incremental source positions in a QA phantom with a built-in tungsten-wire scale that is also imaged on the film *(29)*.

Emergency procedures should be prominently posted in the console area and should be familiar to all HDR brachytherapy staff. These procedures detail a hierarchy of

GammaMed Quality Assurance Report

☐ Operating Room   ☐ GammaMed 12i   *Date* [   ]
☐ Procedure Room   ☐ GammaMed IIi

Operator's Console

☐ Video Monitors   ☐ Intercom   ☐ Indicator Lights

☐ Source Decay Factor [   ]

Treatment Room Radiation Monitor

☐ Battery Backup   ☐ Check Source Response

GammaMed Operational Safety

☐ GAMMAMED ON Light
☐ Source Guide Tube Interlock
☐ Source Guide Tube Too Long (GammaMed 12i only)
☐ Source Guide Tube Too Short (GammaMed 12i only)
☐ Treatment Room Door Interlock
☐ Treatment Interrupt
☐ Emergency Source Retraction

GammaMed Treatment Functionality

☐ Source Indexer
  Channels Exercised [ ] [ ] [ ] [ ]
☐ Timer Accuracy
  Stopwatch Reading (secs) [   ]

☐ Source Positioning Autoradiograph
☐ Printer (Ribbon, Paper)   *Physicist* [   ]

Fig. 10. Quality assurance checklist/report used at MSKCC for HDR brachytherapy.

increasingly severe measures that must be taken in the event the source has failed to retract. In the case of HDR-IORT, the most extreme measure prescribed, involving emergency entry of the room, must be formulated in a way that would prevent a dislodged source from falling into the operative field. For this reason, it would generally call for removal and shielding of the applicator without disconnecting any guide or transfer tubes from the machine. During each treatment, in order to assure rapid response to a source emergency, the physicist in attendance should be alert to any failure of the radiation level in the room to drop when either the treatment program or the operator has called for a source retraction. Also, awareness of which channel the source was in just prior to such an event will allow emergency removal of the applicator to be performed with reduced radiation exposure, should it become necessary.

5. CONCLUSIONS

The stepping-source HDR remote afterloader and its interstitial extensions, the small diameter source, and the indexer, have made possible the HDR-IORT brachytherapy that has now been implemented at several medical centers in the United States and Europe. Its confinement to date to a few centers is no doubt related to the fact that it requires a shielded operating room. Although some volume treatments have been performed, most HDR-IORT has involved treating the tumor bed using a mold applicator. Various silicone applicators are currently available, usually providing for a source plane 0.5 cm from the treatment surface. Because dwell positions of the HDR ^{192}Ir source in the applicator are well defined relative to the target surface, custom planning is generally not necessary and reference instead to a planning atlas is readily feasible. For the same reason, applicator curvature within broad limits can often be ignored. However, good contact with the tissue surface is essential to accurate dose delivery. No consensus yet exists regarding the depth at which dose is specified or whether dose uniformity over the target surface is desirable. Least-squares optimization of dwell times is a practical method of achieving good uniformity over a target surface at depth, with comparable uniformity over the applicator surface at the same time. All of the safety precautions and quality-assurance measures required for other types of HDR brachytherapy must be taken for HDR-IORT, including those directed specifically at the applicators used.

REFERENCES

1. Henschke UK. Afterloading applicator for radiation therapy of carcinoma of the uterus, *Radiol.,* **74** (1960) 834.
2. Henschke UK, Hilaris BS, and Mahan GD. Remote afterloading with intracavitary applicators, *Radiol.,* **83** (1964) 344–45.
3. O'Connell D, Joslin CAF, Howard N, Ramsey NW, and Liversage WE. A remotely-controlled unit for the treatment of uterine carcinoma, *Lancet, 2* (1965) 570.
4. Wakabayashi, Masuru, Ohsawa T, Mitsuhashi H, Kikuchi Y, Mita M, Watanabe T, Saito K, Suda Y, Yushii M, Dato S, Koshibu R, Furuse W, and Wakabayashi M. High dose rate intracavitary radiotherapy using the RALSTRON. Introduction and Part I (Treatment of carcinoma of the uterine cervix), *Nippon Acta Radiologica, 31* (1971) 340–378.
5. Mundinger F and Sauerwein K. Gamma med, ein Gerat zur Bestrahlung von Hirngeschwulsten mit Radioisotopen, *Acta Radiologica, 5* (1966) 48–51.
6. Busch M, Makosi B, Schulz U, and Sauerwein K. Das Essener Nachlade-Verfahren für die intrakavitare Strahlentherapie, *Strahlentherapie,* **153** (1977) 581–88.
7. Glasgow GP and Anderson LL. High dose rate remote afterloading equipment, In Nag S, (ed.), *High Dose Rate Brachytherapy: A Textbook,* Futura Publishing, Armonk, NY, 1994, pp. 41–57.
8. Glasgow GP and Dillman LT. Specific γ-ray constant and exposure rate constant of ^{192}Ir, *Med. Phys.,* **6** (1979) 49–52.
9. Goetsch SJ, Attix FH, Pearson DW, and Thomadsen BR. Calibration of ^{192}Ir high-dose-rate afterloading systems, *Med. Phys.,* **18** (1991) 462–467.
10. Kirov AS, Williamson JF, Meigooni AS, and Zhu Y. TLD, diode and Monte Carlo dosimetry of an ^{192}Ir source for high dose-rate brachytherapy, *Phys. Med. Biol.,* **40** (1995) 2015–2036.
11. Watanabe Y, Roy J, Harrinton PJ, and Anderson LL. Experimental and Monte Carlo dosimetry of Henschke applicator for HDR ^{192}Ir remote afterloading, *Med. Phys.,* **25** (1998) 736–745.
12. Fessenden KK, DeMarco JJ, Solberg TD, Smathers JB, Wright AE, and Kleck JH. Measured and calculated dosimetry for the VariSource HDR source, *Med. Phys., 23* (1996) 1149.
13. Nag D, Lukas P, Thomas DS, and Harrison L. Intraoperative high dose rate remote brachytherapy, In Nag S, (ed.), *High Dose Rate Brachytherapy: A Textbook,* Futura Publishing, Armonk, NY, 1994, pp. 427–445.
14. National Council on Radiation Protection and Measurements. NCRP Report No. 49, Structural Shielding Design and Evaluation for Medical Use of X-rays and Gamma Rays of Energies Up to 10 MeV. National Council on Radiation Protection and Measurements, Washington, DC, 1976.

15. National Council on Radiation Protection and Measurements. NCRP Report No. 116, Limitation of Exposure to Ionizing Radiation. National Council on Radiation Protection and Measurements, Washington, DC, 1993.

16. Lukas P, Stepan R, Ries G, Kneschaurek P, Fink U, Siewert R, et al. New modality for intraoperative radiation therapy with a high-dose-rate afterloading unit, *Radiology,* **181S** (1991) 251. Abstract.

17. Kneschaurek P, Wehrmann R, Hugo C, Stepan P, and Molls M. Die Flabmethode zur intraoperative Bestrahlung, *Strahlenther. Onkol.,* **171** (1995) 61–69.

18. Harrison LB, Enker WE, and Anderson LL. High dose-rate intraoperative radiation therapy for colorectal cancer - part 1, *Oncology,* **9** (1995) 679–683.

19. Harrison LB, Enker WE, and Anderson LL. High dose-rate intraoperative radiation therapy for colorectal cancer - part 2: Technical aspects of brachytherapy/remote afterloader, *Oncology,* **9** (1995) 737–741.

20. Pirkowski M, Holloway R, Delgado G, Barnes W, Thomas D, Torrisi J, Popescu G, Rodgers J, and Dritschilo A. Radiotherapy of malignant subdiaphragmatic implants in advanced ovarian carcinoma: a new technique, *Int. J. Radiat. Oncol. Biol. Phys.,* **22** (1992) 1105–1108.

21. Dritschilo A, Harter KW, Thomas D, Nauta R, Holt R, Lee TC, Rustgi S, and Rodgers J. Intraoperative radiation therapy of hepatic metastases: technical aspects and report of a pilot study, *Int. J. Radiat. Oncol. Biol. Phys.,* **14** (1988) 1007–1011.

22. Nag S and Orton C. Development of intraoperative high dose rate brachytherapy for treatment of resected tumor beds in anesthetized patients, *Endocurietherapy/Hyperthermia Oncol.,* **9** (1993) 187–193.

23. Meredith WJ (ed.). *Radium Dosage, The Manchester System.* E. & S. Livingstone Ltd., Edinburgh, 1967.

24. Ries G, Lukas P, and Seelentag W. A new flab-technique for IORT with HDR-afterloading units, *Sauerwein Isotopen Technik GammaNews,* **4** (1997) 4–7.

25. Nag S. The Harrison/Enker/Anderson article reviewed, *Oncology,* **9** (1995) 742–748.

26. Anderson LL, Hoffman MR, Harrington PJ, and Starkschall G. Atlas generation for intraoperative high dose-rate brachytherapy, *J. Brachytherapy Int.,* **13** (1997) 333–340.

27. Lawson CL and Hanson RJ. *Solving Least Squares Problems.* Society for Industrial and Applied Mathematics, Philadelphia, PA (an unabridged, revised republication of the work first published in 1974 by Prentice-Hall, Inc., Englewood Cliffs, NJ) 1995.

28. Williamson JF, Ezzell GA, Olch A, and Thomadsen BR. Quality assurance for high dose rate brachytherapy, in Nag S (ed.), *High Dose Rate Brachytherapy: A Textbook,* Futura Publishers, Armonk, NY, 1994, pp. 147–212.

29. Anderson LL, Mick FW, Zabrouski K, and Watanabe Y. Photoelectrons facilitate autoradiography for ^{192}Ir remote afterloaders, *Med. Phys.,* **22** (1995) 1759–1761.

6

High-Dose-Rate Intraoperative Irradiation (HDR-IORT)

Technical Factors

Louis B. Harrison, Alfred M. Cohen, and Warren E. Enker

CONTENTS

1. FACILITY LOCATION AND EQUIPMENT

At Memorial Sloan-Kettering Cancer Center (MSKCC), a new program was developed in 1992 for intraoperative radiation therapy. This program attempts to combine the technical and dosimetric advantages of brachytherapy with the conceptual and logistic advantages of intraoperative electron-beam irradiation. The entire procedure takes place in a full service and shielded operating room in a Brachytherapy Suite in the Department of Radiation Oncology which became available in November 1992 (*see* Chapter 5, text and figures). No intraoperative patient transportation is required. For the radiation-therapy delivery, a high-dose-rate remote afterloader *(1,2)* is used instead of a linear accelerator-based electron beam *(3–5)*. Because the remote afterloader is a portable unit, it can also be utilized for other procedures in the outpatient facility when it is not needed for intraoperative cases. The use of a remote afterloader enhances the cost effectiveness of the program, potentially making it possible for a larger number of world centers to consider an IORT program that is economically feasible.

2. APPLICATOR SYSTEM

At MSKCC an applicator system was developed for high-dose-rate intraoperative irradiation (HDR-IORT), known as the Harrison-Anderson-Mick (HAM) applicator, which has been previously described (Fig. 1) *(1,2)*. It is composed of transparent, flexible material that is precut to specific sizes and thickness. Source-guide tubes are incorporated

From: *Current Clinical Oncology: Intraoperative Irradiation: Techniques and Results*
Edited by: L. L. Gunderson et al. © Humana Press, Inc., Totowa, NJ

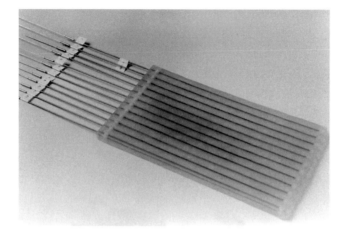

Fig. 1. Harrison-Anderson-Mick (HAM) applicator.

into the applicator pad, and are 5 mm from the surface of the applicator. The applicator bends and contours to any surface within the pelvis, abdomen or chest, thus becoming an intraoperative surface mold. Treatment is customized as any size applicator can be used, and any portion of an applicator can be included in or excluded from the treated region.

3. SURGICAL AND IRRADIATION FACTORS

It must be emphasized that this entire program is a coordinated effort between the surgery and radiation oncology teams. The goal of the HDR-IORT procedure is to deliver a large single fraction of irradiation to the target area, with minimal doses to the surrounding normal tissues. This procedure takes advantage of the intraoperative exposure of the cancerous region, and the ability to move normal structures out of the way of the radiation therapy. The therapeutic ratio is significantly enhanced because the normal tissue dose is minimized, whereas the tumor dose is quite high.

The IORT technique is feasible only when total or near gross total resection can be accomplished. The maximum thickness of residual disease after maximal resection should be ≤1 cm on the basis of depth-dose factors. Therefore, the use of HDR-IORT is best suited for institutions with aggressive surgeons by whom gross total resection is routinely attempted.

3.1. Treatment Field Delineation

After the surgeon completes the resection, the area to be treated with HDR-IORT is delineated jointly by the surgeon and the radiation oncologist. Adequate margins are placed around the surface to allow for proper anatomic coverage and to include the periphery where microscopic disease may surround the dimensions of the tumor bed. The HAM applicator is then placed onto the appropriate surface, and is fixed in place with proper packing and/or sutures (Fig. 2). Dummy sources are placed in the channels of the applicator, and intraoperative X-rays are taken to document the position of the applicator and of the sources. Because of anatomical constraints, it is not always possible to take these X-rays (Fig. 3).

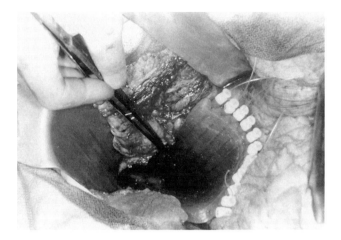

Fig. 2. HAM applicator on a pelvic surface. On the left is a large retractor displacing the bladder anteriorly. The applicator is sitting on the presacral space, and curving to cover the left (inferior of figure) and right (superior of figure) pelvic sidewalls.

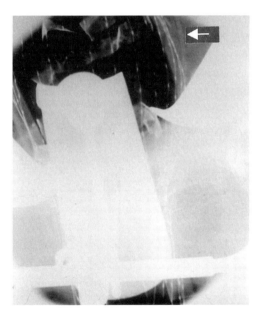

Fig. 3. This is an anterior–posterior (AP) view of the pelvis with dummy wire in the HAM applicator. A large retractor is seen. On the lateral aspects of the pelvis, as the applicator curves anteriorly, the channels appear superimposed. The arrow shows the stent in the ureter, which is displaced from the applicator as much as possible.

3.2. HDR-IORT Dosimetry

The intraoperative setting does not allow the luxury of time to prepare the dosimetry for the brachytherapy application. For this reason, an atlas of dosimetry has been prospectively developed that it utilized for this purpose. The rationale as well as the details of this atlas are described in Chapter 5. With the aid of this atlas, a plan for the high-dose-rate

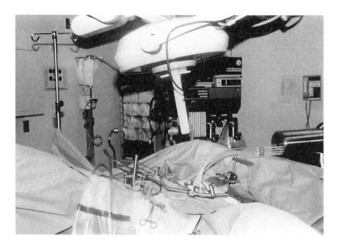

Fig. 4. View of the operating room with the staff out of the room and treatment to begin. The source guide tubes are seen as they exit the applicator and are connected to the HDR remote afterloader. A video camera is incorporated into the OR light so that the team can monitor the procedure from outside the room.

treatment is rapidly determined, and the computer-operated afterloader can be programmed. This process is completed within 10 min. The atlas allows for consideration of a large variety of field sizes, contours, and depth doses. Several thousand plans are stored, and are ready for use *(1,2)*.

3.3. HAM Applicator Attachment to HDR Machine

The HAM applicator is then connected to the high-dose-rate remote afterloader using dedicated source-guide cables that have been manufactured for this project. The cables attach to the applicator on one end and insert into the appropriate channel of the remote afterloader on the other end. In order to stabilize the source-guide tubes properly, a special securing bar attached to a Martin arm is attached to the operating table (Fig. 4). By clamping the source-guide tubes securely, vibration and other unwanted motion of the cables is eliminated allowing for a smooth passage of the source from the machine into the applicator.

3.4. HDR-IORT Treatment Factors

After the appropriate connections have been made, the radiation oncologist reviews the treatment plan and dose distribution. Once this is approved, the dwell times of the source are programmed by the physics staff.

During HDR-IORT delivery, all personnel must leave the room. To assure patient safety, a remotely controlled video system is activated. Monitors for this system are placed outside the operating room, in a region where the radiation oncologist, surgeon, and operating nurse can remain gowned and gloved. A separate monitoring area for the anesthesiology team allows them to monitor the patient's vital signs, EKG, arterial line, and to regulate iv fluids. A video camera that is installed in the handle of the operating room light, allows the operative field, the packing, and the irradiated area to be monitored. The applicator and its connection to the source-guide tube is observed. The radiation oncologist and the surgeon can monitor the source travelling in and out of each tube. Any inappropriate connection, disruption of the applicator, or movement of the

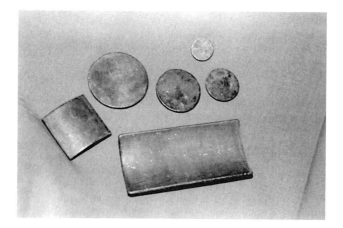

Fig. 5. Lead discs of various shapes, sizes, and curvatures can be used to protect normal tissue.

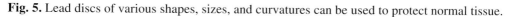

brachytherapy system would be observed, and can be rapidly corrected. In such an event, the source would be retracted and the door to the operating room opened. The room can be entered within seconds, any type of problem corrected, and the treatment immediately resumed. The same process would be followed if there were any bleeding or other problems in the surgical field, or for any urgent problem that requires the attention of the anesthesiologist. In practice, it has been uncommon for the room to be entered during the treatment.

Depending on the total HDR-IORT dose to be delivered, and the activity of the source, the treatment time will vary as discussed in Chapters 7, 16, 18, and 24. The usual single dose of HDR-IORT delivered at MSKCC following gross total resection is 12 or 15 Gy. The dose is calculated at a 0.5–1.0 cm depth in most patients in the MSKCC pilot studies.

Once the HDR-IORT treatment is completed, the guide tubes are disconnected from the remote afterloader, and the applicator itself is removed. At this point, the surgical team can complete the operative procedure and close the patient.

3.5. Normal-Tissue Shielding

To aid in the protection of normal tissue, intraoperative lead disks have been prepared. They come in a variety of shapes, sizes, and curvatures. These disks can be placed adjacent to normal tissues, to augment radiation protection. These disks have proven particularly useful to protect the distal rectum in order to allow for a primary anastomosis and to protect the perineal skin from the distal applicator in cases in which low-lying lesions must be treated. Other uses include protecting the ureter, or an extraneous loop of bowel that cannot be moved far enough away from the treatment field for the inverse-square law to provide protection (Fig. 5).

4. CONCLUSIONS AND FUTURE POSSIBILITIES

In conclusion, the MSKCC HDR-IORT approach has shown itself to be feasible and versatile. Early treatment results with colorectal cancer *(1,2,6)* are consistent with other data using electron beam IORT *(3–5,7–10)*. This approach may have certain technical, dosimetric, and logistic advantages, and may offer a cost-effective approach to the majority of world centers that cannot afford IORT with a linear accelerator-based electron program.

Whereas the MSKCC physical facility arrangement has worked well, it would have been wiser to have this dedicated OR as part of the main OR facility. This would have allowed more efficient utilization of staff, instruments, and a proximity to the recovery room and the surgical ICU. Groups looking to develop such a facility may wish to weigh the relative merits of the location of the OR, and make the decision based upon the logistics that will work best for their particular program. In conjunction with a professional transition of two of the authors from MSKCC to Beth Israel Medical Center (LBH, WEE), a dedicated shielded facility for HDR-IORT is accordingly being developed in a new OR suite at Beth Israel.

REFERENCES

1. Harrison LB, Enker WE, and Anderson L. High dose rate intraoperative radiation therapy for colorectal cancer—Part 1, *Oncology,* **9** (1995) 679–683.
2. Harrison LB, Enker WE, and Anderson L. High dose rate intraoperative radiation therapy for colorectal cancer—Part 2, *Oncology,* **9** (1995) 737–741.
3. Gunderson LL, Cohen AC, Dosoretz DD, et al. Residual, unresectable, or recurrent colorectal cancer. External beam irradiation and intraoperative electron beam boost ± resection, *Int. J. Radiat. Oncol. Biol. Phys.,* **9** (1983) 1597–1606.
4. Tepper JE, Cohen AM, Wood WC, Hedberg SE, and Orlow E. Intraoperative electron beam radiotherapy in the treatment of unresectable rectal cancer, *Arch. Surg.,* **121** (1986) 421–423.
5. Gunderson LL and Dozois RR. Intraoperative irradiation for locally advanced colorectal carcinomas, *Perspect. Colon Rectal Surg.,* **5** (1992) 1–24.
6. Harrison LB, Minsky B, Enker W, et al. High dose rate intraoperative radiation therapy (HDR-IORT) as part of the management strategy for locally advanced primary and recurrent rectal cancer, *1997 ASTRO Abstracts Int. J. Radiation Oncol. Biol. Phys.,* in press.
7. Willett C, Shellito PC, Tepper JE, et al. Intraoperative electron beam radiation therapy for primary advanced rectal and rectosigmoid carcinoma, *J. Clin. Oncol.,* **9** (1991) 843–849.
8. Wallace HJ, Willett CG, Shellito PC, et al. Intraoperative radiation therapy for locally advanced recurrent rectal or rectosigmoid cancer, *J. Surg. Oncol.,* **60** (1995) 122–127.
9. Gunderson LL, Nelson H, Martenson J, et al. Locally advanced primary colorectal cancer—intraoperative electron and external beam irradiation ± 5-FU, *Int. J. Radiat. Oncol. Biol. Phys.,* **37** (1997) 601–614.
10. Gunderson LL, Nelson H, Martenson J, et al. Intraoperative electron and external beam irradiation ± 5-FU and maximal surgical resection for previously unirradiated locally recurrent colorectal cancer, *Dis. Colon Rectum,* **39** (1996) 1379–1395.

7

Intraoperative Irradiation with Electron-Beam or High-Dose-Rate Brachytherapy

Methodological Comparisons

Subir Nag, Leonard L. Gunderson, Christopher G. Willett, Louis B. Harrison, and Felipe A. Calvo

CONTENTS

INTRODUCTION
TREATMENT FACTORS
INTRAOPERATIVE IRRADIATION: METHODOLOGICAL ALTERNATIVES
REFERENCES

1. INTRODUCTION

Intraoperative irradiation (IORT) refers to delivery of a single dose of irradiation to a surgically exposed tumor or tumor bed while the normal tissues are protected from the irradiation either by retracting the mobilized tissue or by shielding the anatomically fixed tissues. IORT has traditionally been performed by using an electron beam as the source of irradiation.

A limitation of intraoperative electron-beam irradiation (IOERT) is that it can only be used in areas accessible to the nonflexible IOERT applicator. Narrow cavities, steeply sloping surfaces, or areas where treatment delivery requires turning a corner may not be accessible to the applicator. Therefore, IOERT may be less feasible in sites such as the skull base, paranasal sinuses, diaphragm, deep pelvis, and retropubic areas which are frequent sites of residual disease after maximal surgical resection of cancers in those locations. Intraoperative high-dose rate brachytherapy (HDR-IORT) may be technically more feasible in locations that are potentially inaccessible for IOERT, if the surgeon can accomplish a gross total or near gross total resection, thus extending the usefulness and applicability of IORT *(1)*.

The terminology and abbreviations used in IORT literature can be confusing. In this chapter, IORT will be used to define any radiation treatments delivered in a single dose

From: *Current Clinical Oncology: Intraoperative Irradiation: Techniques and Results*
Edited by: L. L. Gunderson et al. © Humana Press, Inc., Totowa, NJ

while the patient is still under anesthesia. IOERT will be used to refer to intraoperative irradiation delivered with electron beams, and HDR-IORT will refer to intraoperative HDR brachytherapy.

2. TREATMENT FACTORS (*see* expanded discussion in Chapters 3–6)

2.1. Shielded Facility in OR vs Radiation Oncology

A shielded operating room is required for a dedicated IORT facility, either in the radiation oncology department or in the hospital operating suite. The shielding can be accomplished by lining an existing operating room with lead, using an existing shielded treatment room, or constructing a room with appropriately thick concrete walls.

The shielding requirements for HDR-IORT are slightly greater than those for IOERT. At OSU, therefore, a mobile lead shield is positioned between the HDR-IORT treatment site and the scrub room (where the surgical personnel wait), and personnel entry to the adjacent passageway is restricted during IORT treatments. Another possibility being considered for HDR-IORT by some institutions, where completely shielded ORs are unavailable, is to treat the patient within a lead-lined box permanently placed in the OR (room within a room) after resection has been accomplished and the applicator for HDR-IORT has been positioned.

Institutions not having a dedicated shielded OR can perform IORT by moving the anesthetized patient from the operating room to the radiation oncology department for either IOERT or HDR-IORT. A special transportation cart and strict procedural policy are required to facilitate the transfer of the patient. Another alternative is to build an operating room (unshielded) adjacent to the shielded radiation treatment room. Hence, the patient will have to be moved only for a short distance for IORT treatment. The latter situation exists and has functioned well at Medical College of Ohio in Toledo and at Thomas Jefferson University and some other centers. However, it requires the institution to provide or at least consider the availability of OR services such as specimen transport, blood bank support, sterilization, pharmacy, and so on in a location remote from the routine ORs.

2.2. Operative Techniques

The radiation oncologist and surgeon should interact before and during the operative procedure with regard to issues such as selective organ preservation and optimum exposure for both resection and IORT. When IORT procedures are being initiated in an institution, it is useful for the radiation oncologist to join the surgeon in the operating room before tumor resection to allow visualization of the relationship of the tumor to the surrounding tissues for correlation with preoperative imaging studies. The radiation oncologist and the surgeon can then jointly discuss the volume of the tissue that optimally would be removed and which tissues may be able to be preserved. In general, a gross total resection with negative or only microscopically positive margins is preferable, if this can be accomplished without substantial destruction of functional tissues and if anatomic and/or functional reconstruction appears feasible.

In addition to accomplishing the tumor resection, the surgeon may need to optimize exposure for IORT treatment or shielding. This may include modification of the skin incision, resect/mobilize surrounding tissues to better expose the tumor bed, retract radiosensitive structures (e.g., small or large bowel, stomach, heart, ureter, kidney) out of the irradiation field. It is possible to resect bone (e.g., maxilla) and regraft it after IORT, if this is required to gain access to the tumor bed.

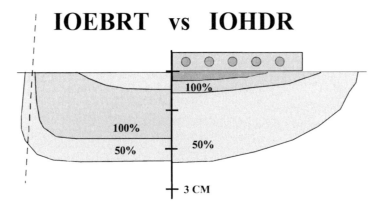

Fig. 1. Dose distribution characteristics of IOERT and HDR-IORT at OSU. IOERT with 6 MeV electrons using a 9 cm diameter applicator; HDR-IORT with a 9-cm-wide, 1-cm-thick surface applicator, with dose prescribed at 0.5 cm depth (i.e., 1 cm from the catheter plane).

The target area to be treated by IORT is the tumor bed, including microscopically positive margins, areas of close margins, and any gross residual disease as determined jointly by the surgeon and the radiation oncologist. The tumor bed or residual disease should be marked with radio-opaque surgical hemoclips (to define the tumor margins on radiographs for future EBRT planning).

2.3. IOERT Technique

IOERT is usually delivered by a linear accelerator electron beam in the 6–20 MeV energy range (see electron isodose characteristics Chapters 3 and 4 and Fig. 1). The linear accelerator (linac) could be an electron-beam-only unit in a dedicated operating room or an existing linac, with photon and electron capability, in the radiation oncology department.

If a dedicated linac in the OR is used, the unit can be "warmed up," and the output checked before the patient is brought to the OR. If this cannot be accomplished because the patient is already in the room, the linac should be able to produce a very stable output under "cold start" conditions. Linacs should be calibrated and checked under cold start conditions to ensure their performance. If beam cannot be produced to check the linac, certain key operational parameters of the machine can be checked to get an indication whether the machine is operating normally.

The following is a description of the laser-guided soft-docking technique in a dedicated operating room as used at the Ohio State University Hospital (OSUH). When the tumor bed is accessible to the IOERT applicator, an appropriate-sized electron-beam applicator is selected to cover the target area (Fig. 2). Applicator sizes at OSUH range from 5 to 12 cm diameter with a choice of flat or 22.5° beveled ends. A majority of OSUH patients are treated with 5–8 cm diameter applicators.

To maximize the possibility of being able to treat with IOERT, a wide assortment of applicator sizes and shapes are recommended. Applicator options available at Mayo and Massachusetts General Hospital (MGH) include circular applicators from 4.5 to 9.5 cm in 0.5-cm increments (flat, 15°, and 30° bevel), and a variety of elliptical and rectangular applicators (flat and 20° bevel for elliptical, 20° bevel for rectangular). Madrid has an even wider range of circular applicators, in 1-cm increments, that include 12 and 15 cm diameters for large fields such as abdominal and extremity sarcomas.

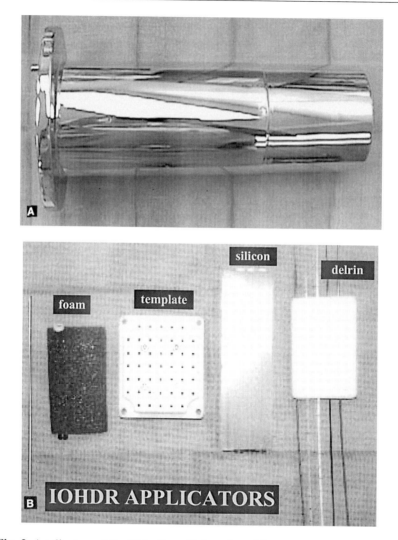

Fig. 2. Applicators at the Ohio State University: (**A**) IOERT. (**B**) HDR-IORT.

The applicator is manually positioned over the area of high risk and attached to the table using a Buckwalter clamp assembly. Gauze packing or retractors are used whenever possible to displace normal tissues from the treatment field and, occasionally, to pull suspected tumor tissues (e.g., resected margin in base of tongue) into the treatment field. Custom pliable-lead shields 1–2 mm thick can be used within the treatment field to protect critical normal structures. The patient is then positioned beneath the dedicated linac in the operating room.

The gantry of the dedicated linac at OSUH can be rotated by only +/– 25° from the vertical axis because of shielding issues. At Mayo, MGH, and Madrid, the gantry angle can exceed +/– 90°, which may be necessary for treatment of anterior pelvic structures such as the base of the prostate after an abdominal-perineal resection (APR) (Fig. 3A–F) or the retropubic region after pelvic exenteration (Fig. 3G–I). For pelvic sidewall (Fig. 3J—M), abdominal or chest sidewall fields or distal presacrum (Fig. 3N) the gantry angle necessary to treat a patient can also exceed 25°. The availability of both

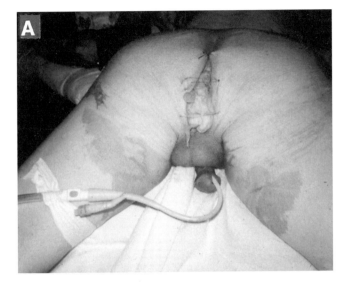

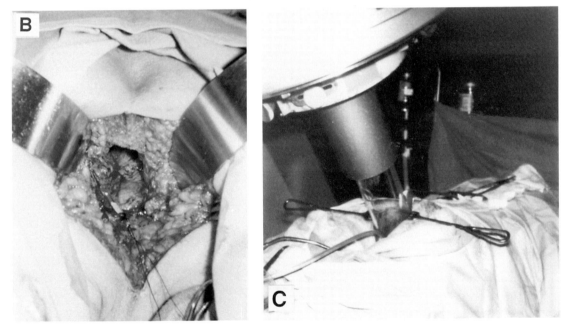

Fig. 3. Examples of abdominal or pelvic IOERT cases requiring gantry angle rotation of 30° to >90°. **(A–F) Treatment of Prostate ± Base of Bladder After Abdominoperineal Resection. (A–C)** *Patient Prone*—Sandbags under hips to produce flexion (**A**); exposure of prostate via perineal incision with TLD in place (**B**); applicator in patient and "docked" with accelerator (**C**). **(D–F)** *Patient Supine*—Applicator immobilized in position with Buckwalter retractor; patient is in trendelenberg position with legs in stirrups and retracted (**D**); Prostate visualized within IOERT applicator (**E**); linear accelerator in position for treatment with gantry rotation > 90° (**F**). **(G–I)** Treatment of Retropubic Region after Pelvic Exenteration. Applicator (8.0 cm with 30° bevel) in position with visualization of retropubic region including prostatic fossa (**G**); immobilization with Buckwalter retractor (**H**); linear accelerator in position with gantry rotation > 45° (**I**). **(J–M) Treatment of Lateral Pelvic Sidewall. (J,K)** Via abdominal incision. **(L,M)** Treatment of sidewall via perineal approach after abdominal perineal resection with patient in decubitus position with permission from ref. *14*. **(N)** Treatment of distal presacrum via perineal incision with patient in supine lithotomy position. (Figs. 3B, C, J, K, and N from ref. *14* with permission from ref. *15*.)

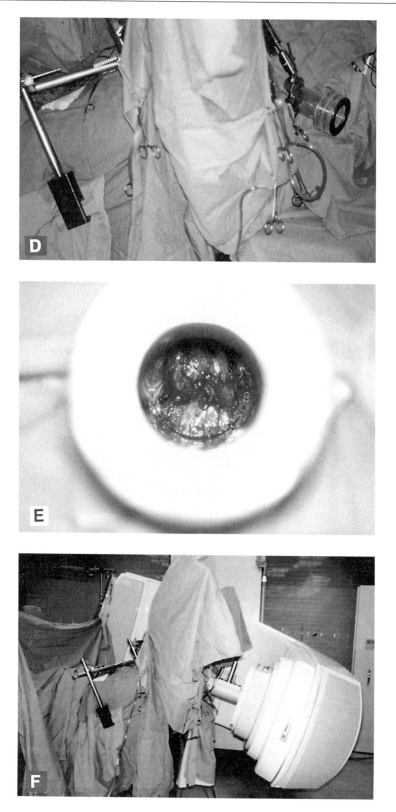

Fig. 3. (*continued*)

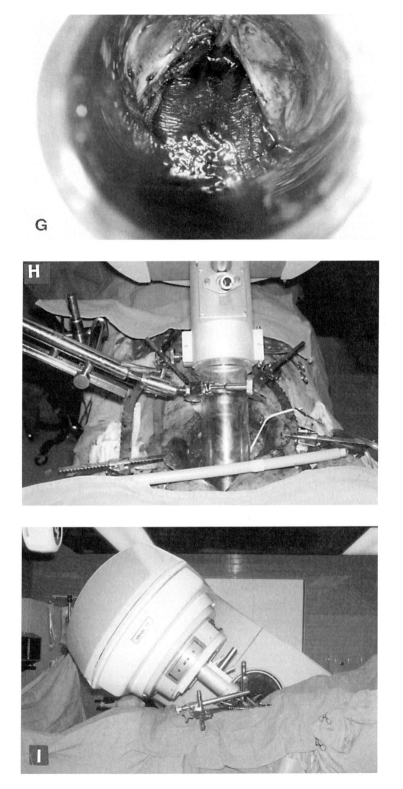

Fig. 3. (*continued*)

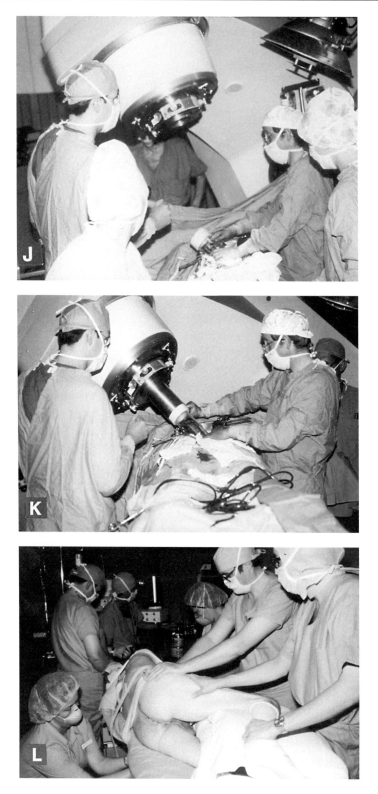

Fig. 3. (*continued*)

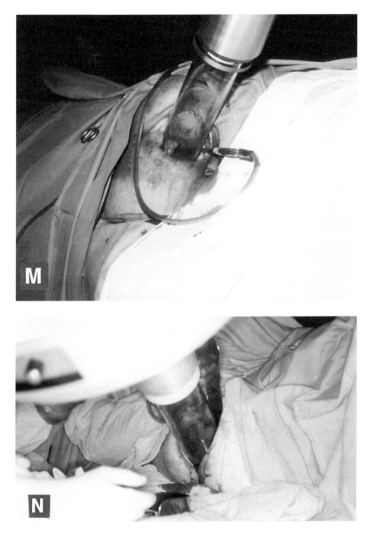

Fig. 3. (*continued*)

flat and beveled applicators, combined with gantry rotation and table angulation, provides some degree of freedom in treating accessible curved surfaces. For pelvic IOERT treatment, applicators with 30° bevel are used almost exclusively at Mayo. In Madrid, applicators with 45° bevel are commonly selected to encompass the presacral region in the adjuvant IOERT treatment of resected high-risk rectal cancers.

The applicator is aligned to the linac at both OSUH and MGH by moving the table under the guidance of a laser-docking system. There is no physical contact between the linac and the applicator, hence the term "soft-docking" (*see* Chapter 4). Finally, the treatment field is suctioned to prevent any accumulated fluids from acting as a bolus. The staff then exits the operating room, and the patient is observed with remote monitors while the IOERT is delivered. Other institutions, including Mayo and Madrid, use a "hard-docking" technique whereby the applicator is similarly positioned over the target volume with a Buckwalter retractor but is then physically attached to the gantry of the linac by adjusting the treatment couch height and location (*see* Chapter 4). For hard-docking systems, the procedure is facilitated by the availability of a Macquet table that has 5 cm of movement both in a superior/inferior and left/right mode. In addition, the aluminum adapter on the linac gantry has been modified from a fixed circular opening to a hinged system that opens to a half circle during the hard-docking procedure.

2.4. HDR-IORT Technique

HDR-IORT treatment is given with a HDR remote afterloader that has a nominal 10-Ci ^{192}Ir source encapsulated in a small (4×1 mm) capsule attached to the end of a metal wire. This single source is moved by mechanically pushing the wire under remote control through transfer tubes into the hollow catheters that are placed in the tumor or tumor bed. In most departments, if an HDR afterloader is available, it is used and kept in the radiation oncology department. Since it is mobile, it can be transferred, as needed, to the operating room. Such movement of the HDR unit requires modification of the user's license with the Nuclear Regulatory Commission. At OSUH, the HDR afterloader is transferred from the radiation oncology department to the OR for treatment; whereas at Memorial Sloan Kettering Cancer Center (MSKCC) a dedicated intraoperative suite is available in the radiation oncology department. The MSKCC suite has several rooms; the afterloader is moved from the procedure room to the OR, depending on the OR findings in a particular case.

In conventional brachytherapy, catheters are sutured onto the tumor bed, and then treatment-planning dosimetry is performed after obtaining orthogonal radiographs and digitizing the data (Fig. 1B). For HDR-IORT brachytherapy, since the patient is under anesthesia, the entire treatment must be performed rapidly, but accurately. To accomplish this, HDR-IORT surface-template applicators and corresponding precalculated dosimetry tables have been developed at OSUH *(1,2,4)*. Several types of HDR-IORT applicators (with catheters embedded parallel and 1 cm apart), are available in sizes suitable for various sites (Fig. 2B). For flat tumor beds, a rigid delrin applicator is used. For curved surfaces, flexible applicators made of silastic, silicone, supermold, or foam are used. After the tumor resection, an appropriate applicator is placed on the tumor bed, and localization radiographs are obtained using dummy sources. These radiographs are obtained for documentation and are not used for dosimetry calculations. The foam or silicone applicators can be easily cut or trimmed in the operating room, if required, to fit into irregular or tapered tumor beds. In these circumstances, the preplanned dosimetry is modified by turning off the appropriate dwell positions and repeating the treatment plan before proceeding with the treatment. Hence, treating with modified, custom-made applicators requires an extra 10–20 min. At MSKCC, Harrison-Anderson-Mick (HAM) surface applicators are used *(3)*, and applicators made of superflab are used in München *(5)*.

At MSKCC, a dosimetry atlas with several thousand plans is used to determine the plan and source loading for each case. The radiation oncologist determines the field size, total dose, prescription depth, and severity of curvature of the target surface. The physicist then can use the plan from the atlas that corresponds to the intraoperative situation. A similar atlas exists for volume implants and flexiguide needles. Many times, localization films are not taken because it is not possible to obtain accurate films with a C-arm unit. However, this has not limited the capability of delivering treatment. The remote-control system has a video hook-up, allowing the treatment site and delivery to be recorded for documentation purposes, if this is felt to be necessary.

Surface applicators are most suitable for treatment of tumor beds less than 0.5 cm thick. Tumors greater than 0.5 cm thick can be treated by placing needles interstitially through a template into the gross tumor. The latter technique has been used to treat metastatic liver tumors at Georgetown University *(8,9)*. At OSUH, although a template is available for interstitial HDR-IORT, metastatic liver tumors are treated with permanent ^{125}I brachytherapy, which involves a far easier technique *(10,11)*.

If HDR-IORT is found to be more suitable than IOERT at OSUH, the remote afterloading machine is transported by the physicist and brachytherapy technologist and cleaned with an antiseptic before entering the operating room. The preplanned treatment program is retrieved from the computer and transferred on a disk to the treatment control panel. After the applicator has been secured on the tumor bed (packing with gauze, or suturing as indicated), radiosensitive structures are carefully displaced using retractors or are shielded with sterilized lead foils. Sterilized transfer cables are attached to the ends of the catheters. The catheters are checked for patency, and the proper length is confirmed by using a dummy source cable. A quality-assurance check, which is mandated by the Nuclear Regulatory Commission, is performed with all personnel out of the room. The treatment plan is checked for accuracy. The transfer cables from the applicator are then attached to the treatment machine, and the treatment is performed with the patient still anesthetized. After the treatment, the applicator is removed from the treatment site, and the surgeon closes the incision.

3. INTRAOPERATIVE IRRADIATION: METHODOLOGICAL ALTERNATIVES

3.1. IORT vs No IORT

The numerous potential advantages of IORT make it a useful addition to the radiation therapy armamentarium. The target volume can be visually defined with accuracy and directly irradiated, thus minimizing the risk of a geographical miss. Dose-limiting radiosensitive normal tissue can usually be retracted away from the volume to be irradiated. Tissues that cannot be retracted can often be shielded to reduce normal tissue toxicities, unless they are part of the target volume or are anatomically immobile or deep to the treatment field (peripheral nerve). Irradiation can be given during surgery, hence eliminating delay in treatment. IORT can be delivered as a supplement to tolerable moderate doses of EBRT (45–55 Gy in 1.8- to 2.0-Gy fractions), thus allowing delivery of a higher total radiation dose to marginally resected or unresected tumor. In an adjuvant setting, the use of IORT may allow a decrease in the dose of the EBRT-treatment component thereby improving the integral tolerance of the irradiation program. Finally, the procedure is relatively brief (IOERT requiring an additional 45–60 min after maximal resection; HDR-IORT, 1–2 h).

However, IORT does have its potential disadvantages. First is the radiobiology of a large single dose, which does not allow repair of sublethal damage. This disadvantage can be minimized, however, if a small dose of IORT is given as a boost to the immediate tumor bed to supplement modest doses of EBRT delivered to a larger target volume (Table 1). A practical disadvantage of IORT is that it requires a shielded operating room or transportation of an anesthetized patient, as previously discussed, hence limiting the widespread use of IORT.

3.2. IORT vs Conventional Perioperative Brachytherapy

IORT has some similarities to conventional (permanent or removable perioperative) brachytherapy. Both techniques allow delivery of high-dose irradiation to the tumor or

Table 1
IORT Equivalent of Fractionated EBRT Doses[a]

IORT Dose	Tumor Effect[b]	Late Tissue Effect[c]	Late Tissue Effect[d]
10 Gy	17 Gy	26 Gy	8 Gy
15 Gy	31 Gy	54 Gy	16 Gy
20 Gy	50 Gy	92 Gy	26 Gy
25 Gy	73 Gy	140 Gy	39 Gy

[a]Assume EBRT dose of 2 Gy per fraction in calculating equivalent doses.
[b]Assume α/β ratio of 10, EBRT dose of 2 Gy per fraction.
[c]Assuming no dose reduction to normal tissues, α/β ratio of 3.
[d]Assuming a 50% dose reduction to normal tissues, α/β ratio of 3.

tumor bed while minimizing dose to the normal tissues. Both techniques require a surgical procedure, although in some cases perioperative brachytherapy can be given without exposing and/or resecting the tumor. In both cases, additional irradiation can be given to supplement EBRT to an initially unresectable tumor at the time of subsequent planned resection without giving the tumor a chance to proliferate as may occur if further irradiation were to be accomplished with a postoperative EBRT supplement.

IORT differs from perioperative brachytherapy in the following respects. IORT (IOERT or HDR-IORT) is given in a short interval that does not allow for repair of sublethal damage or reoxygenation of hypoxic tissues. In contrast, conventional brachytherapy is typically given over a few days, thus allowing for repair of sublethal damage or reoxygenation of hypoxic tissues during the irradiation. Hence, IORT is preferably given in moderate doses of 10–20 Gy as a supplement to adjuvant doses of EBRT and not as the sole modality; whereas brachytherapy can be used either as a boost treatment with EBRT or as the sole modality. IORT has been used as the sole irradiation modality in previously irradiated patients, but has its best potential value in that capacity if a gross total resection has been achieved, and a dose of 25–30 Gy is tolerable to normal structures.

Most clinical trials have shown greater benefit of IORT in the treatment of microscopic residual disease after maximal resection rather than for the treatment of gross residual disease, perhaps because of the radioresistance of hypoxic cells. Although perioperative brachytherapy does not suffer from this handicap, its efficacy in this regard is unclear. It can be used in the treatment of both gross and microscopic residual disease provided the implant is technically feasible and dose-limiting structures can be displaced away from the implant volume over the protracted time required for conventional brachytherapy.

The dose distribution of each technique is different. Electron-beam irradiation gives a more homogeneous dose distribution both to a large surface and at depth; whereas in perioperative brachytherapy, the dose is highest at the center of the implant volume. This difference in dose distribution and the location of the normal and tumor tissue with the target volume must be remembered when selecting the technique. A potential (uncertain) advantage of the brachytherapy dosimetry is that of dose escalation within the target volume.

3.3. IORT with Electrons or HDR Brachytherapy

The potential differences (advantages, disadvantage) between IOERT and HDR-IORT are summarized in Tables 2 to 7. Factors including accessibility, depth of tissue at risk, field size, treatment time, and rationale for having both modalities, if feasible, will be discussed.

Table 2
Potential Differences Between IOERT and HDR-IORT

	IOERT	HDR-IORT
Actual treatment time	2–4 min	5–30 min
Total procedure time	30–45 min	45–120 min
Treatment sites	Accessible locations	All areas where depth at risk is ≤ 0.5 cm from surface of applicator[a]
Surface dose	Lower (75%–93%)[b]	Higher (150–200%)
Dose at depth (2 cm)	Higher (70%–100%)[b]	Lower (30%)
Dosimetric homogeneity (surface to depth)	$\leq$10% variation	$\geq$100% variation

[a] Precludes aortocaval region, mediastinum, and any unresected disease >0.5 cm. Gross tumors >0.5 cm thick in the liver have been treated by HDR-IORT using interstitially placed needles (8,9).

[b] Based on electron energy of 6 MeV at OSUH and energies of 6–18 MeV with 7-cm flat-end lucite applicator at Mayo Clinic (see Table 3).

3.3.1. ACCESSIBILITY

Although HDR-IORT can be used to treat both easily accessible and poorly accessible sites, at OSUH, IOERT is used for sites that are accessible to the electron-beam applicator because the treatment time and the setup time are both shorter, and a greater depth dose can be achieved, if required, when compared with the usual HDR-IORT surface-applicator system. However, since the electron beam only travels in a straight line, and the electron-beam applicator has a finite diameter, IOERT may be unsuitable for treatment of sites deep in the inferior pelvis, subpubic locations, some lateral pelvic sidewalls, anterior abdominal walls, subdiaphragmatic areas, anterior and/or lateral interior chest wall, and narrow cavities like the paranasal sinuses. HDR-IORT, if available, usually becomes the modality of choice at OSUH for these difficult locations. Both of the HDR-IORT coauthors of this chapter (SN, LH) agree that there is literally no site or surface for which HDR-IORT cannot be used (Table 5).

If IOERT is the only available option for intraoperative irradiation and an adequate assortment of applicators exist, an innovative radiation oncologist and surgeon can find a way to treat most sites. Modification of surgical incisions and gantry angle rotation of +/– 90° or greater may be necessary to accomplish such (Figs. 3, 4).

3.3.2. DEPTH OF TISSUE AT RISK

The dose-distribution characteristics for HDR-IORT and IOERT differ (Fig. 1 and Tables 2 and 3). The percentage depth-dose characteristics at OSUH for HDR-IORT and IOERT with 6-MeV electrons are seen in Table 3. The dose is prescribed at 1 cm from the plane of catheters (0.5 cm from the applicator surface) for HDR-IORT, and at D_{max} for 6-MeV electrons for IOERT. The dose at the surface is higher for HDR-IORT than for IOERT. However, the dose at depth (for example, at 2 cm) is greater for IOERT than for HDR-IORT (usual single-plane surface applicator). Since HDR-IORT gives a far greater surface dose, investigators at OSUH prefer to use HDR-IORT for treating small microscopic tumor beds (see subsequent section on field size). However, HDR-IORT (using surface applicators) is not suitable for treating residual tumors more than 0.5 cm

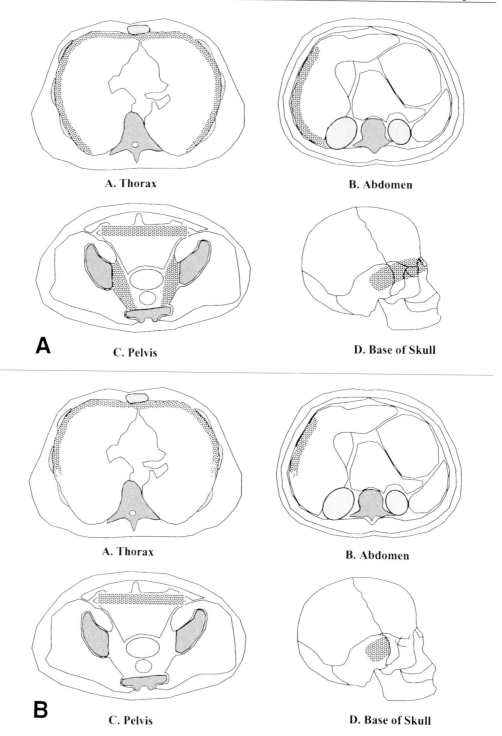

Fig. 4. (A) Shaded areas represent locations where HDR-IORT may be easier to use than IOERT if gantry angle rotation of linear accelerator is limited to ± 25–30°. **(B)** If gantry rotation of linear accelerator is unlimited except for patient anatomy, shaded areas represent locations where IOERT may be difficult or impossible to use unless surgical incision is altered to yield different exposure (i.e., can treat posterior to sternum with a lateral thoracotomy approach). (The assistance of Dr. Rafael Martinez-Monge in creating this diagram is acknowledged.)

Table 3

Percentage Depth Dose for HDR-IORT Brachytherapy and IOERT (6 MeV) at OSUH; Variable Energy IOERT and Variable Applicator Bevel Angle at Mayo Clinic

Tissue Depth (cm)	OSU % Depth Dose[a]		Mayo IOERT % DD, Variable Electron Energy, and Applicator Bevel[b]									
	HDR-IORT	6 MeV IOERT	6 MeV Flat	6 MeV Bevel	9 MeV Flat	9 MeV Bevel	12 MeV Flat	12 MeV Bevel	15 MeV Flat	15 MeV Bevel	18 MeV Flat	18 MeV Bevel
0	200	75	82	82	87	87	90	90	93	93	93	93
0.5	100	85	—	—	—	—	—	—	—	—	—	—
1.0	60	95	D_{max}^{c} 1.2	90 (1.2)	—	—	—	—	—	—	—	—
1.5	40	100	90 (1.7)	75	D_{max}^{c} 1.5	—	—	—	—	—	—	—
2.0	30	90	70	50	—	90 (2.1)	D_{max}^{c} 2.0	—	D_{max}^{c} 2.0	—	D_{max}^{c} 2.0	—
2.5	20	50	30	20	90 (2.6)	80	—	—	—	—	—	—
3.0	15	20	10	10 (2.9)	70	60	—	90	—	—	—	—
3.5	—	—	—	—	45	40	90	77	—	—	—	—
4.0	—	—	—	—	20	20	77	62	—	—	—	—
4.5	—	—	—	—	10 (4.4)	10	60	48	90 (4.3)	90 (3.8)	—	—
5.0	—	—	—	—	—	—	40	30	82	75	90 (5.2)	90 (4.9)
6.0	—	—	—	—	—	—	10	10 (6.1)	68	62	74	68
7.0	—	—	—	—	—	—	—	—	37	38	50	48
8.0	—	—	—	—	—	—	—	—	10	10 (7.4)	23	28
9.0	—	—	—	—	—	—	—	—	—	—	10 (8.7)	10 (9.4)

[a] For OSUH figures, dose of HDR-IORT is prescribed at 1 cm from catheter plane or 0.5 cm from applicator surface and for IOERT at 90% isodose for 6-MeV electrons.
[b] At Mayo, IOERT doses are prescribed at D_{90} and the surface dose for most applicator sizes and beam energies is within 5% of D_{90}. Figures listed are for 7 cm lucite applicator with flat and 30° bevel ends using a collimator jaw setting of 10 × 10 cm (see ref. 7 and Chapter 3).
[c] D_{max} in cm.

Table 4
Applicator Size Availability of IOERT and HDR-IORT

IOHDR Applicators

OSUH	Memorial
Various sized from 2 × 2 cm to 15 × 12 cm Custom-made sizes and shapes can be made in OR	Any size or shape feasible

IOERT Applicators (size in cm)	Mayo	MGH	Madrid	OSU
Circular flat and 22° bevel (4 to 12 cm diameter)	—	—	—	Y
Circular flat, 15°and 30° bevel (0.5-cm increments, 4.5–9.5 cm)	Y	Y	Y*	—
Circular 45° bevel	N	Y	Y	N
Elliptical (flat and 20° bevel) 6 × 11, 7 × 12, 9 × 12, 8 ×15, 8 × 20 cm	Y	Y	N	N
Rectangular (20° bevel) 7 × 9, 8 × 12, 8 × 15 cm	Y	Y	N	N

*Circular applicators in 1-cm increments include 12- and 15-cm size for large field cases such as retroperitoneal and extremity sarcomas

thick. Gross tumors, thicker than 0.5 cm, have been treated by HDR-IORT at Georgetown University using interstitially placed needles *(4,8)*.

For purpose of comparison, Table 3 also contains data on depth-dose characteristics of various energy electrons with the applicator system used at Mayo. The depth-dose advantages of IOERT over HDR-IORT are demonstrated for tumor residual ≥0.5 cm depth.

For both IORT treatment approaches, the radiation oncologist and surgeon must address the issue of fluid build-up after resection which could alter depth-dose characteristics unless dealt with in appropriate fashion. It is necessary to maintain suction during the delivery of treatment when such risks exist.

3.3.3. Field Size (Table 4) and Treatment Time

For HDR-IORT, the treatment time depends on the total area to be treated and the activity of the source, because a single source is used to treat the entire tumor bed. The actual HDR-IORT treatment time at OSUH generally varies from 5–30 min because generally only small areas are treated with HDR-IORT. Larger tumor beds (up to 12 cm in diameter) are generally treated with IOERT at OSUH. Extremely large tumor beds are less suitable for IORT treatments except in cases in which gross total resection can be accomplished, as for large retroperitoneal and extremity sarcomas. In such instances, IOERT institutions (Mayo, MGH, National Cancer Institute [NCI], Pamplona, Madrid) have used abutting fields to cover the area at risk, and MSKCC uses large HAM applicators for HDR-IORT, which may result in treatment times up to 145 min (median 44 min, range 17–145).

A comparison of applicator sizes available for IOERT and HDR-IORT at the authors' institutions is seen in Table 4. For HDR-IORT there is basically no applicator size limitation, and custom-made applicators can be constructed in the OR. IOERT applica-

Table 5
Potential Applicability of IOERT, HDR-IORT,
and Perioperative Brachytherapy by Treatment Site

Treatment Site	(LLG, CW, FC)[a] IOERT	(LLG, CW, FC)[a] Brachy Periop	(SN)[b] IOERT	Brachy[b] (SN) HDR IORT	Brachy[b] (SN) Periop	Brachy (LH)[c] HDR IORT	Brachy (LH)[c] Periop
Pelvis							
Posterior	Y	+	Y	Y	Y	Y	Y
Lateral	Y	+	±	Y	Y	Y	Y
Anterior	+, ±	N	Y	Y	Y	Y	±
Abdomen							
Aortocaval	Y	N	Y	Y	Y	Y	±
Abdominal wall							
Posterior	Y	N	Y	Y	Y	Y	+
Lateral	±	N	±	Y	Y	Y	Y
Anterior	±, N	N	Y	Y	Y	Y	Y
Chest							
Mediastinum	Y	N	Y	Y	Y	Y	Y
Inner chest wall							
Posterior	Y	±	Y	Y	Y	Y	Y
Lateral	+, ±	±	N	Y	Y	Y	Y
Anterior	±, N	±	N	Y	Y	Y	Y
Head/Neck							
Neck	Y	Y	Y	Y	Y	Y	Y
Oral Cavity	Y	Y	Y	Y	Y	Y	Y
Base of skull	±	N	N	Y	Y	Y	+
Extremity (sarcoma)	Y	Y	Y	Y	Y	Y	Y
Brain	+, ±	+	±	+	Y	Y	±

Y = yes; N = no; + = possible; ± = may be possible (technically challenging situation); Periop = perioperative; brachy = brachytherapy.

[a]Response of chapter coauthors, LG, CW and FC, who have availability of IOERT and perioperative brachytherapy but not HDR-IORT.

[b]Response of chapter primary author, SN, who has availability of IOERT, HDR-IORT and perioperative brachytherapy.

[c]Response of chapter coauthor, LH, who has both HDR-IORT and perioperative brachytherapy.

Note: The authors are aware that author's choices are to some degree operator dependent and reflect a combination of bias and other available treatment options in a given institution.

tors by definition cannot be custom made, although lead sheets can be custom made for purpose of field shaping and protection of dose-limiting tissue or organs that cannot be surgically mobilized.

3.4. Rationale for Having IOERT, HDR-IORT, and Perioperative Brachytherapy Available in the OR (Tables 5–7)

A comprehensive intraoperative program should have combinations of IOERT, HDR-IORT, or perioperative brachytherapy facilities available to treat all disease sites and situations. For some institutions, this will mean having or obtaining both IOERT and HDR-IORT, at others it may be having expertise in both HDR-IORT and perioperative brachytherapy, and a few institutions may have expertise in all three options. These modalities are not competitive but rather complement each other. Tables 5–7 discuss the

Table 6
Relative Advantage or Disadvantage of IOERT vs HDR-IORT Brachytherapy
after Gross Total or Near Total Resection (Maximum Thickness ≤ 0.5 cm)

IOERT Potential Advantage if Technically Feasible

Better dose homogeneity[a]
Faster treatment time
Less shielding required in OR
Can treat full thickness of organ or structure at risk with relative homogeneity[a]
    (i.e., aorta or vena cava, bladder sidewall)

Potential Disadvantages of IOERT	*Potential Solution*
Surface dose <90% with 6 ± 9 MeV	Add bolus over tumor bed to improve surface dose; use HDR-IORT
Unable to include area at risk in single field within either abdomen or pelvis	Use abutting IOERT fields (difficult in pelvis); use HDR-IORT
Area at risk is technically inaccessible due to location	Use HDR-IORT; surgically displace small bowel or stomach with vascularized flap (omentum, muscle) and give postoperative EBRT boost or perioperative brachytherapy

[a] The chapter authors have differing opinions with regard to the relative advantage or disadvantage of dose homogeneity with IOERT or inhomogeneity with HDR-IORT (i.e., authors SN and LH feel dose escalation within a target may be advantageous rather than disadvantageous)

potential applicability of each method by both site and amount of residual disease after maximal resection.

IORT is preferred for the treatment of microscopic tumor beds (Table 6). At OSUH, IOERT is preferred in accessible sites and HDR-IORT for poorly accessible sites for the reasons previously discussed. The choice of IORT modality at other centers may differ as they may have either IOERT or HDR-IORT, but the overall concept and treatment outcome are the same.

Interstitial brachytherapy may be preferable for the treatment of gross residual tumor if the residual disease can be uniformly implanted, and dose-limiting structures can be displaced for 3–7 d (Table 7). IOERT combined with EBRT and concomitant chemotherapy has been used quite successfully in the treatment of limited gross residual or unresectable disease, however, provided the volume can be encompassed within a single applicator. Results could potentially be improved with the addition of a dose modifier during IORT such as sensitizers or hyperthermia.

Fractionated EBRT (with or without concomitant chemotherapy) should be used in adjuvant level doses of 45–54 Gy in 1.8- to 2.0-Gy fractions, whenever feasible, to irradiate the entire area of potential microscopic disease. For locally advanced primary or recurrent lesions where marginal resection would exist, preoperative EBRT with or without chemotherapy is generally preferable over postoperative EBRT with or without chemotherapy for reasons previously discussed. Depending on the volume and location of the tumor and the available expertise and equipment, IOERT or HDR-IORT and/or perioperative brachytherapy could be used along with EBRT and surgery for the optimal management of malignancies. The best IORT results are obtained when used as a con-

Table 7
Potential Advantage or Disadvantage of IOERT, HDR-IORT and Perioperative Brachytherapy for Unresected Tumor or Gross Residual Disease > 0.5 cm thickness

Perioperative Brachytherapy, Potential Advantages

Hypoxia and sublethal damage repair less of an issue because of longer treatment time (reoxygenation, repair of sublethal damage)
Higher central dose
Less risk to normal tissues

Perioperative Brachytherapy, Potential Disadvantages

Unable to do homogeneous implant[a] (adjacent to vessels, curved pelvic surface)
Unable to displace dose-limiting organs for prolonged interval
Inhomogeneous dose distribution with potential issues regarding both tumor and normal structures
Increased whole-body irradiation exposure
Radiation exposure to personnel

IOERT - Potential Advantages	*over*	*HDR IORT*	*or*	*Perioperative Brachytherapy*
More homogeneous dose distribution[a]		Y		Y
Better displacement of dose-limiting structures		N		Y

IOERT Disadvantages Relative to Perioperative Brachytherapy	*Potential Solutions*
Hypoxia within unresectable tumors	Add dose modifiers (hypoxic cell sensitizers, hyperthermia)
Peripheral nerve risks	Evaluate radioprotectors

[a]See footnote in Table 6 regarding dose homogeneity (IOERT) and inhomogeneity with target dose escalation (HDR-IORT).

formal boost to the tumor bed after maximal resection and incorporation with other modalities including EBRT and chemotherapy (concomitant with EBRT with or without maintenance) or other systemic therapies (future may include gene or immunotherapy).

REFERENCES

1. Nag S and Orton C. Development of intraoperative high dose rate brachytherapy for treatment of resected tumor beds in anesthetized patients, *Endcurieth Hyperth. Oncol.,* **9** (1993) 187–193.
2. Nag S, Martinez-Monge R, and Gupta N. Intraoperative radiation therapy using electron-beam and high-dose-rate brachytherapy, *Cancer J.,* **10** (1997) 94–101.
3. Harrison LB, Enker WE, and Anderson LL. High dose rate intraoperative radiation therapy for colorectal cancer. Part I, *Oncology,* **9** (1995) 679–684.
4. Nag S, Lukas P, Thomas DS, and Harrison L. Intraoperative high dose rate remote brachytherapy, In Nag S (ed.), *High Dose Rate Brachytherapy: A Textbook,* Futura Publishing, Armonk, NY, 1994, p. 427–445.
5. Lukas P, Stepan R, Ries G, et al. A new modality for intraoperative radiation therapy with a high-dose-rate-afterloading unit, *Radiology,* **181** (1991) 251.

6. McCullough E and Anderson JA. The dosimetric properties of an applicator system for intraoperative electron beam therapy utilizing a Clinic-8 accelerator, *Med. Phys.,* **9** (1982) 261–268.

7. Gunderson LL, Nelson H, Martenson JA, et al. Locally advanced primary colorectal cancer. Intraoperative electron and external beam irradiation ± 5FU, *Int. J. Radiat. Oncol. Biol. Phys.,* **37** (1997) 601–614.

8. Dritschilo A, Harter KW, Thomas D, et al. Intraoperative radiation therapy of hepatic metastases: technical aspects and report of a pilot study, *Int. J. Radiat. Oncol. Biol. Phys.,* **14** (1988) 1007–1011.

9. Thomas DS, Nauta RJ, Rodgers JE, et al. Intraoperative high-dose rate interstitial irradiation of hepatic metastases from colorectal carcinoma. Results of a phase I-II trial, *Cancer,* **71** (1993) 1977–1981.

10. Nag S. Radiotherapy and brachytherapy for recurrent colorectal cancer. *Sem. Surg. Oncol.,* **7** (1991) 177–180.

11. Erickson B and Nag S. Bile duct and liver. In Nag S (ed.), *Principles and Practice of Brachytherapy,* Futura Publishing, Armonk, NY, 1997, pp. 367–391.

12. Calvo FA, Azinovic J, and Escude LL. Intraoperative radiotherapy in cancer management. *Appl. Radiol.,* **27** (1992) 19–23.

13. Calvo FA, Santos JA, and Lozano MA. Intraoperative radiotherapy: methodological development and early clinical experience, *Oncologia,* **20** (1997) 435–443.

14. Gunderson LL, Tepper JE, Biggs PJ, et al. Intraoperative ± external beam irradiation. *Curr. Probe Cancer,* **7** (1983) 1–69.

15. Gunderson LL, Cohen AM, Dosoretz DE, et al. Residual, unresectable or recurrent colorectal cancer: external beam irradiation and intraoperative electron beam boost ± resection. *Int. Radiat. Oncol. Biol. Phys.* **9** (1983) 1597-1606.

III | NORMAL TISSUE TOLERANCE—IORT

8 Normal Tissue Tolerance to Intraoperative Irradiation

The National Cancer Institute Experimental Studies

William F. Sindelar, Peter A.S. Johnstone, Harald J. Hoekstra, and Timothy J. Kinsella

CONTENTS

1. INTRODUCTION

In early clinical applications of intraoperative electron irradiation (IOERT), reliable radiobiologic information was unavailable on the tolerance of normal tissues to single, large (>10 Gy) radiation doses. In concert with the development of IOERT clinical protocols at the National Cancer Institute (NCI), an extensive experimental program was instituted examining the tolerance of both intact and surgically manipulated tissues exposed to varying doses of IOERT in a large animal (canine) model *(1)*. Early evidence suggested that the radiosensitivities of normal tissues were similar in both humans and dogs to these large, single radiation doses *(2)*. Consequently, a comprehensive examination of canine normal-tissue responses to IOERT was undertaken at the NCI. Findings in the canine experiments were applied in the design of clinical applications of IOERT to patients with various malignant diseases. Dogs were subjected to surgical procedures and the application of IOERT to various anatomic sites (Fig. 1). All studies were conducted under the supervision of the NCI Institutional Review Board for large animal research.

The goals of the experimental IOERT studies at the NCI were to assess both the acute and late (up to 5 yr of follow-up) normal-tissue toxicities following a range of single doses of IOERT using a large animal model. The overall design of these studies was to mimic

From: *Current Clinical Oncology: Intraoperative Irradiation: Techniques and Results*
Edited by: L. L. Gunderson et al. © Humana Press, Inc., Totowa, NJ

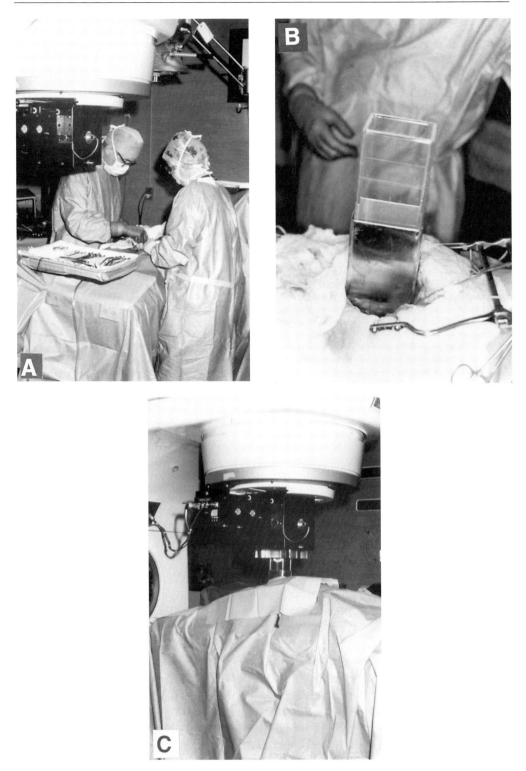

Fig. 1. Procedure performed in intraoperative irradiation facility. (**A**) Surgical procedures in combined radiation-therapy-surgical suite. (**B**) Placement of radiation treatment application defining intraoperative field to be irradiated. (**C**) Irradiation procedure.

procedures used in human cancer surgery in the thoracic and abdominal cavities and to accrue normal-tissue toxicity data following a limited range of single IOERT doses delivered to a variety of anatomic locations in healthy adult American foxhounds (wt 20–25 kg). This larger dog species was used principally in the NCI studies instead of the more commonly used beagle model (as used by Colorado State investigators; *see* Chapter 9) because many of the more technically demanding surgeries such as biliary-jejunal anastomosis and aortic transection with anastomosis would be more easily accomplished with fewer surgical complications in the larger animal. Additionally, the foxhound is without a predilection for spontaneous tumor development, a serious problem with many dog breeds. Whereas radiation (IOERT) carcinogenesis was not a primary endpoint at the formulation of the NCI experimental studies, the absence of known spontaneous tumor rates in this dog breed was fortuitous in later analysis of IOERT-related tumors. An overall listing of the experimental normal-tissue studies performed at the NCI is shown in Table 1. The IOERT radiation parameters for the various studies are outlined in Table 2. An overall summary of the tolerance of IOERT doses derived from these normal-tissue toxicity studies in intact canine tissues is found in Table 3, whereas a summary for surgically manipulated canine tissues is found in Table 4. A more detailed discussion of the design of these normal tissue studies as well as the conclusions (or recommendations) for the maximum IOERT doses tolerated by a specific normal tissue is presented as follows:

2. GASTROINTESTINAL TRACT

The gastrointestinal tract includes some of the most radiosensitive tissues. Consequently, several NCI experimental protocols examined the acute and late normal-tissue toxicities to varying portions of the gastrointestinal tract to IOERT doses as high as 50 Gy.

2.1. Esophagus, Full-Thickness

Thirty-seven dogs underwent right thoracotomy with mobilization of the esophagus and IOERT on two protocols *(3,4)*. Segments of esophagus received full-thickness electron-beam IOERT of 0, 20, or 30 Gy. Clinical examinations, barium swallows, and esophagoscopy were performed to assess toxicity for up to a 2-yr follow-up period. No toxicities were noted in the first week postoperatively. No clinical toxicities were noted over the entire follow-up period in the sham-irradiated controls and in the 20-Gy animals. Endoscopic examinations were normal in all control and 20-Gy animals through 12 mo of follow-up.

All 30-Gy animals suffered signs of dysphagia and weight loss that was relieved by dietary modifications. These symptoms resolved within 3 mo in all animals. One animal was noted to have circumferential esophageal ulcers 3 mo after receiving 30 Gy. This animal subsequently succumbed to exsanguination caused by an esophagoaortic fistula, presumably IOERT-related. All 30-Gy animals exhibited severe inflammatory changes that progressed between 6 wk and 3 mo postoperatively. Mucosal ulceration and strictures developed in all 30-Gy dogs by 12 mo. These abnormalities also appeared on barium swallows and were confirmed at necropsy.

Five-year follow-up was obtained in 5 of 37 animals treated *(5)*. One control animal had an uncomplicated course. Two of the three animals treated with 20 Gy had no abnormalities, whereas the third developed achalasia without stricture that necessitated a liquid diet. A single 30-Gy animal survived without clinical stigmata but did have an

Table 1
NCI Experimental Normal Tissue Studies

Study Name	Surgical Procedure	IOERT Field	No. Dogs Total	No. IOERT	No. Sham
1. Retroperitoneum	Laparotomy with exposure of unilateral retroperitoneum	Retroperitoneum, including portions of kidney and ureter	20	16	4
2. Aortic anastomosis and small intestinal suture line	Laparotomy, transection aorta and reanastomosis, Roux-en-Y with formation of blind loop of small bowel	Aorta segment, blind bowel loop (separate field)	4	3	1
3. Aortic anastomosis	Laparotomy, transection of aorta and reanastomosis	Aorta segment	11	10	1
4. Small intestinal suture line	Laparotomy, Roux-en-Y with formation of blind loop of small bowel	Blind bowel loop	18	15	3
5. Intact bile duct	Laparotomy, mobilization of biliary tree	Bile duct and lateral duodenum	7	6	1
6. Biliary-jejunal anastomosis	Laparotomy, Roux-en-Y biliary-jejunal anastomosis	Biliary anastomosis	9	7	2
7. Bladder	Laparotomy and cystotomy	Bladder trigone	18	15	3
8. Lung and mediastinum	Right thoracotomy	Lung segment, atrium (separate field)	24	21	3
9. Bronchial stump	Left pneumonectomy	Bronchial stump	15	12	3
10. Esophagus	Right thoracotomy, mobilization of esophagus	Esophagus segment	13	12	1
11. Peripheral Nerve (high dose)	Laparotomy, exposure of unilateral lumbosacral plexus	Lumbosacral plexus	27	21	6
12. Peripheral Nerve (low dose)	Laparotomy, exposure of unilateral lumbosacral plexus	Lumbosacral plexus	12	12	0
13. Arterial vascular grafts	Laparotomy, segmental resection of infrarenal aorta and immediate grafting	Aorta segment including graft	30	24	6
14. Spinal cord	Laparotomy, exposure of midline retroperitoneum	Lumbar vertebrae	25	22	3
Total Dogs			227	196	31

NCI = National Cancer Institute; IOERT = intraoperative electron irradiation.

Table 2
IOERT Radiation Parameters Used in NCI Studies

Study No.	Target Tissues Irradiated	IOERT Field Size/Shape/Electron Energy	Dose Delivered, Gy (No. Treated)
1.	Paravertebral soft tissues, aorta, vena cava, one ureter, lower pole one kidney	4 × 15 cm/Rectangle/11 MeV	0 (4), 20 (4), 30 (4), 40 (4), 50 (4)
2.	Paravertebral soft tissues, aorta, vena cava, blind end loop of jejunum	3.5 × 15 cm/Rectangle/11 MeV	0 (1), 20 (1), 30 (1), 45 (1)
3.	Abdominal aorta, vena cava, one ureter	3.5 × 15 cm/Rectangle 11 MeV	0 (1), 20 (4), 30 (3), 45 (3)
4.	Retroperitoneal soft tissues, blind end loop of jejunum	3.5 × 15 cm/Rectangle/11 MeV	0 (3), 20 (5), 30 (5), 45 (5)
5.	Extrahepatic bile duct	5 cm dia./Circle/11 MeV	0 (1), 20 (3), 30 (2), 45 (2)
6.	Extrahepatic bile duct with anastomosis to jejunum	5 cm dia./Circle/11 MeV	0 (2), 20 (3), 30 (2), 45 (2)
7.	Trigone of bladder (through cystotomy)	5 cm dia./Circle/12 MeV	0 (3), 20 (3), 25 (3), 30 (3), 35 (3), 40 (7)
8.	A. Upper lobe of right lung	5 cm dia./Circle/9 MeV	0 (3), 20 (7), 30 (7), 40 (7)
	B. Mediastinal soft tissues (right atrium large vessels, phrenic nerve, bronchi)		
9.	Left bronchial stump, pulm. artery and vein esophagus, aorta, pericardium, segment of left atrium and ventricle	5 cm dia./Circle/13 MeV	0 (3), 20 (4), 30 (4), 40 (4)
10.	Esophagus	6 cm dia./Circle/9 MeV	0 (1), 20 (7), 30 (5)
11.	Lumbosacral nerve plexus (L4-S5)	9 cm dia./Circle/11 MeV	0 (3), 20 (4), 25 (4), 30 (3), 35 (3), 40 (4), 50 (2), 54 (2), 70 (2)
12.	Lumbosacral nerve plexus (L4-S5)	9 cm dia/Circle/9 MeV	10 (4), 15 (4), 20 (4)
13.	Graft of infrarenal aorta	3.5 × 15 cm/Rectangle/9 MeV	0 (6), 20 (8), 25 (8), 30 (8)
14.	Spinal cord	3.5 × 15 cm/Rectangle/11 MeV	0 (3), 20 (7), 25 (7), 30 (8)

dia = diameter; cm = centimeter; pulm = pulmonary.

asymptomatic esophageal diverticulum and paraesophageal fibrosis on histologic review. The data (acute plus chronic) suggest that esophageal tolerance to single IOERT doses appears to be limited to 20 Gy for full-thickness portals.

2.2. Esophagus, Partial-Thickness

In a separate NCI study (6), dogs receiving mediastinal IOERT that did not include full-thickness esophageal treatment did not suffer severe clinical or radiographic sequelae at IOERT doses as high as 40 Gy. In many cases of mediastinal disease, esophageal shielding or partial-thickness esophageal inclusion may be possible, thus contributing to few complications at higher doses.

Table 3
IOERT Tolerance for Intact Normal Tissues in Dogs

Tissue	Dose (Gy)	Maximum Follow-up (Months)	Endpoint
Esophagus, full-thickness	20	60	Ulcerations and strictures above this dose
Esophagus, partial-thickness	40	60	No sequelae at this dose
Duodenum, lateral wall	20	60	Ulceration, fibrosis and stenosis
Bile duct	20	60	Fibrosis and stenosis above this dose
Lung	20	60	Fibrosis at this dose
Trachea	30	60	Threshold for submucosal fibrosis
Aorta	30	60	Threshold for fibrosis, patency up to 50 Gy
Vena cava	30	60	Threshold for fibrosis, patency up to 50 Gy
Heart, atrium	20	60	Moderate fibrosis at all dose levels
Bladder	20	60	Ureteral stenosis and possible obstruction above this dose
Ureter	30	60	Threshold for stenosis and obstruction
Kidney	30	60	Threshold for complete intensified fibrosis
Peripheral nerve	15	60	Threshold for sensory-motor neuropathy
Spinal cord	20	18	Threshold for spinal hemorrhage and myelopathy

Table 4
IOERT Tolerance for Surgically-Manipulated Tissues in Dogs

Tissue or Manipulation	Dose (Gy)	Maximum Follow-up (Months)	Endpoint or Result
Intestinal suture line (defunctionalized)	45	60	Threshold for fistula formation
Biliary-jejunal anastomosis	20	18	Threshold for anastomotic disruption
Bronchial stump	40	60	Normal healing at this dose
Aortic anastomosis	45	60	Threshold for late fistula formation
Aortic prosthetic graft	20	60	Threshold for stenotic graft occlusion
Bladder, cystotomy	45	60	Normal healing with no changes in contractility at this dose

2.3. Small Intestine Anastomosis

The NCI instituted large-animal trials involving the IOERT tolerance of defunctionalized anastomosed small intestine (1,7,8). A jejunal blind loop was surgically constructed, with intestinal continuity maintained by an end-to-side jejunojejunostomy. Of 18 dogs treated with doses ranging from 0 to 45 Gy, three developed intussusception of the blind loop requiring surgical intervention. Alteration of surgical technique to include mesenteric fixation of the blind loop corrected the problem in subsequent dogs. Animals sacrificed 1 wk postoperatively showed no histologic differences between irradiated segments and jejunum outside the IOERT field. However, animals receiving 45 Gy were noted to have reduced anastomotic bursting strength with some values less than 10% of those for animals receiving lesser doses. No major histologic differences were noted between 3 and 12 mo of follow-up, except for moderate mural fibrosis in some 45-Gy animals.

After a 5-yr follow-up, surviving animals that received 45-Gy IOERT developed internal interloop fistulas of the irradiated suture line *(9)*. Mucosal atrophy and hyaline necrosis of the intestinal wall was also present. Five-year follow-up of animals receiving 30 Gy showed varying degrees of hyaline degeneration of the muscularis, associated with submucosal fibrosis.

It therefore appears that, whereas acute IOERT tolerance of defunctionalized intestinal anastomoses can be as high as 45 Gy, chronic complications do render this dose excessive. A dose of 30-Gy IOERT did appear to be well tolerated in the long term.

2.4. Intact Bile Duct

Intact canine bile duct radiotolerance was investigated at the NCI *(10)*. Experimental dogs received IOERT to the subhepatic space and hepatoduodenal ligament at doses of 0, 20, 30, or 45 Gy with follow-up to 5 yr *(9,10)*. No perioperative complications were noted in any animal. However, late duodenal obstruction developed in all doses because of inclusion of the lateral duodenal wall in the field. Latency varied from 6 wk at 45 Gy to 8 mo at 20 Gy. Bile ducts remained patent in all but a single 45-Gy animal, although pathologically ductal fibrosis was in evidence, which increased as a function of dose. In irradiated dogs at all doses, changes of periportal inflammation and early fibrosis which appeared within 3 mo were considered to be a function of partial biliary obstruction caused by bile duct fibrosis. Three of six irradiated animals developed frank biliary cirrhosis by 12 mo, presumably from chronic partial biliary obstruction. However, one animal that received 30 Gy to the bile duct, was followed for 5 yr without clinical sequelae. Postmortem examination at the time of elective sacrifice revealed no evidence of obstruction or biliary cirrhosis *(9)*. Atrophy with mild fibrosis was noted in the bile duct wall.

The potential acute toxicities and chronic partial biliary obstruction that can lead to cirrhosis limit IOERT doses above 20 Gy to the bile duct. However, some animals may remain asymptomatic for long periods at higher doses. Duodenal bypass should be considered if any portion of the duodenal wall must be included in IOERT field because of the potential for fibrosis and subsequent stenosis or obstruction.

2.5. Biliary-Enteric Anastomosis

Additionally, IOERT was applied to dogs that had undergone biliary-enteric anastomoses *(8)*. After jejunojejunostomy with formation of a jejunal blind loop, the bile duct was transected and anastomosed to the blind loop in an end-to-side fashion. Doses from 0–45 Gy of IOERT were delivered. One control animal remained clinically well through 18 mo of follow-up. However, all irradiated animals died of complications of therapy. Five animals suffered anastomotic disruption within 3 wk postoperatively. One dog experienced fibrotic anastomotic obstruction after 20-Gy IOERT, which led to cholangitis. Another 45-Gy animal suffered bile-duct necrosis with subsequent bile peritonitis. It was thus apparent that any IOERT to biliary-enteric anastomoses contributed to poor healing and should be avoided clinically.

3. RESPIRATORY SYSTEM

3.1. Lung and Bronchial Stump

IOERT delivery to the lungs and mediastinal structures were investigated at the NCI *(3–6)*. Following pneumonectomy, experimental dogs received IOERT in doses ranging from 0 to 40 Gy to the pleura, mediastinum, intact lung, and to the closed bronchial stump following pulmonary resection. All irradiated animals developed pleural plaques at doses of 20–40 Gy within 12 mo *(3)*. Fibrosis was pathologically evident in the pleura, and fibrotic pulmonary changes became evident in alveolar septa in the surrounding pulmonary vasculature, and in bronchioles. Chronic concurrent pneumonitis appeared within 3 mo in all IOERT fields that included the pulmonary parenchyma. The pneumonitis progressed pathologically to interstitial fibrosis and arteriolar sclerosis by 12 mo.

After a 5-yr follow-up, sharply marginated pulmonary fibrosis was the predominant pathologic change within the IOERT treatment portals *(5,6)*. At pneumonectomy sites, all animals had wound healing of bronchial stumps, observed up to 5 yr, with IOERT doses ranging to 40 Gy *(5)*.

3.2. Trachea

Among dogs receiving radiation to intact tracheal segments during IOERT to the mediastinum, gross specimens of the irradiated trachea revealed no changes *(3–6)*. Nine of 15 dogs receiving doses up to 40 Gy showed no significant histologic changes within the trachea. Three animals had mild focal glandular atrophy with telangiectasia. One animal in each of the 30- and 40-Gy IOERT dose groups showed major tracheal changes at 12-mo follow-up. Squamous metaplasia had replaced the normal columnar respiratory epithelium, widespread mucosal denuding was present, and submucosal fibrosis was prevalent. A 30-Gy animal experienced chondronecrosis of the tracheal rings. Another 40-Gy animal developed carinal necrosis with bronchial obstruction which necessitated compassionate sacrifice 5 mo following therapy *(6)*. On 5-yr follow-up of four surviving animals receiving 20 or 40 Gy, only minimal submucosal fibrosis was noted *(5,6)*.

4. CARDIOVASCULAR SYSTEM

4.1. Heart

The right atria of 18 dogs were irradiated using 5-cm mediastinal portals in an NCI trial *(6)*. IOERT doses of 0, 20, 30, or 40 Gy were delivered. On necropsy 3 and 12 mo after treatment, dense fibrotic replacement of the myocardium was grossly noted after 30 and 40 Gy. Microscopically, changes ranged from mild medial hyaline degeneration to myocardial infarction and coagulation necrosis secondary to radiation vasculopathy. Myointimal proliferation and perivascular sclerosis contributed to epicardial thickening.

At 5-yr follow-up, moderate fibrosis at all dose levels was documented *(5)*. A straightforward dose-response relationship was not observed, although generally worsening histopathologic change occurred at higher IOERT doses *(5,6)*. It appears reasonable to suggest minimizing cardiac inclusion in any IOERT field, but especially when doses greater than 20 Gy are administered.

4.2. Aorta and Vena Cava

The great vessels of dogs received IOERT in doses of 0, 20, 30, 40, or 50 Gy administered in a portal covering the retroperitoneum and encompassing the infrarenal aorta and vena cava to the bifurcation *(7)*. Control sham-irradiated animals had no clinical or pathological abnormalities throughout a 5-yr follow-up period, during which time contrast radiographic evaluations of the great vessels were regularly performed *(9)*. Similarly, no clinical or pathological changes were detected in the aorta or vena cava of any of four dogs receiving 20 Gy. Animals receiving 30 Gy showed minor pathologic changes of subintimal fibrosis, beginning 12 mo following IOERT. Animals receiving 40 Gy had the development of mild-to-moderate intimal and subintimal fibrosis pathologically, but showed no clinical or radiologic vascular abnormalities. Three of four dogs receiving 50 Gy died of treatment-related complications to nonvascular structures within 6 mo of IOERT. A single surviving 50-Gy dog showed aortic and caval patency at 5 yr, with moderate fibrosis in the subintimal and medial regions of both the aorta and vena cava.

The canine experience suggested that large vessels can tolerate large single radiation doses without clinical consequences. Since the canine vessels ranged from 5–10 mm in diameter, some caution must be exercised in extrapolating data to smaller vessels, where a relatively modest degree of mural fibrosis could result in a higher proportionate luminal narrowing than would be observed in larger caliber vasculature.

4.3. Aortic Anastomosis

Aortic anastomoses were constructed in NCI animals by the transection of the midabdominal aorta and end-to-end resuturing *(1,8)*. IOERT doses of 0–45 Gy were delivered to 11 animals. Mild medial thickening with elastic fiber destruction was noted in animals that received 30–45 Gy when sacrificed 7 d postoperatively. Of the remaining animals followed through 14 mo postoperatively, one animal developed anastomotic obstruction with collateralization after 20-Gy IOERT, and another animal developed an anastomotic arteriovenous fistula 2 mo after 45 Gy. No suture line dehiscence was noted at any dose, although the development of the vascular fistula was considered to be dose-limiting.

4.4. Aortic Prosthetic Graft

In another NCI study, 30 animals underwent transection of the infrarenal aorta, with segmental resection and reanastomosis with a polytetrafluoroethylene prosthetic graft *(11)*. IOERT doses of 0, 20, 25, or 30 Gy were administered, after which half of the animals were randomized to 36-Gy external-beam irradiation (EBRT) in 10 fractions of 3.6 Gy over 4 wk. Postoperative anticoagulation was provided with aspirin. The most frequent acute complication was thrombosis at the graft site, which affected 7 of 10 animals followed up to 6 mo. Four dogs developed perioperative thrombi requiring emergent surgical thrombectomy; three had subsequent thrombus recurrence. Thrombosis was unrelated to IOERT dose and was considered to be a complication of surgical technique or manipulation.

On 5-yr follow-up, anastomotic stenosis was the most frequent toxicity, although this was not symptomatic in any animal, because of the formation of collaterals bridging the grafted segment. Graft occlusion occurred in 3 of 14 animals receiving IOERT doses of 20 Gy, whereas graft occlusion occurred in five of six dogs receiving 25 Gy or more. Incidence of graft occlusion was similar in both the IOERT alone and the IOERT and EBRT groups. Histologic changes were generally better correlated with total radiation dose (i.e., IOERT and EBRT), than with IOERT doses alone. Pseudointimal hyperplasia and thrombosis were the most commonly assessed changes on histopathologic review.

It can be concluded that IOERT may be administered to a fresh vascular prosthesis without fear of anastomotic dehiscence. Long-term patency of irradiated grafts, however, is questionable even with doses of <25 Gy.

5. GENITOURINARY SYSTEM

5.1. Ureter and Kidney

The effects of IOERT on the intact ureter were investigated at the NCI in a canine study involving irradiation of retroperitoneal tissues (7). IOERT doses of 0, 20, 30, 40, or 50 Gy were delivered to an area extending from the renal vessels to the aortic bifurcation in 20 dogs. The portal included the inferior pole of one kidney and a segment of ipsilateral ureter. Doses up to 40 Gy produced few clinically apparent toxicities in the acute period, except for a single 30-Gy animal that developed septic hydronephrosis 6 wk post-operatively.

No significant clinical or histopathologically changes were detectable in the nonirradiated control or 20-Gy animals with up to 5 yr of follow-up. At 6 mo following treatment, one 30-Gy and one 40-Gy animal developed changes in the irradiated kidney on intravenous pyelography that were consistent with radiation nephritis. Another 40-Gy dog developed ureteral stenosis with hydronephrosis at 6 mo (Fig. 2). Three of four animals that received 50 Gy suffered acute or chronic clinical complications: Two experienced rectal perforation with purulent peritonitis because of bowel that was inadvertently irradiated; another animal developed septic hydronephrosis and radiation nephritis. Two 30-Gy animals were sacrificed within 12 mo of treatment: One animal developed septic hydronephrosis and had a stenotic ureter; moderate radiation nephritis was noted in another animal that was clinically well. In two 40-Gy animals euthanized within 12 mo postoperatively, moderate-to-severe radiation effects were noted in both the ureter and kidney, with edema and fibrotic inflammation. In all three 50-Gy dogs, ureters in the irradiated fields showed significant stenosis, and both ureteral and renal fibrosis were prominent within 12 mo.

Follow-up at 5-yr of surviving animals revealed dense retroperitoneal fibrosis and encasement of the ureters in all animals receiving doses of 30 Gy or greater (9). A surviving 30-Gy animal developed an osteosarcoma within the radiation field. A 40-Gy dog had chronic right hydronephrosis that had persisted since 6 mo following treatment. A 50-Gy animal required nephrectomy for ureteral obstruction and sepsis several months following IOERT.

These studies suggested that ureteral tolerance to IOERT is 20–30 Gy. Significant fibrosis and resulting stenosis with the possibility of obstruction is likely at higher doses.

5.2. Bladder

Bladder tolerance to IOERT was investigated in a study at the NCI involving 18 dogs (12,13). After laparotomy and cystotomy, a 5-cm circular field was placed on the bladder mucosa and doses of 0, 20, 25, 30, 35, or 40 Gy IOERT were administered. The radiation portal included the trigone and both ureteral orifices. Dogs were followed closely up to 5 yr with clinical evaluation, intravenous pyelography, and cystometry. There were no acute complications in any animal. Animals receiving 25 Gy or more had a 33% likelihood of renal failure secondary to bilateral hydronephrosis within 2 yr (12). Obstruction occurred at the ureterovesical junction.

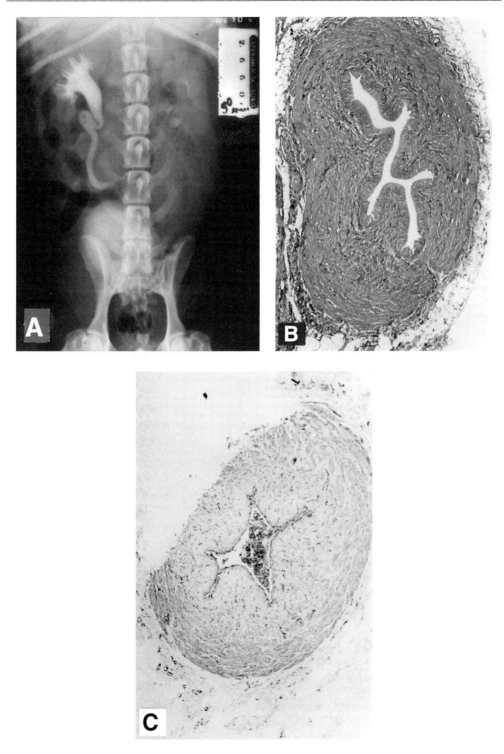

Fig. 2. Experimental animal 6 mo after receiving 40 Gy intraoperative electron beam irradiation (IOERT) to right retroperitoneum, including ureter. (**A**) Right hydronephrosis on excretory urogram. (**B**) Nonirradiated normal left ureter on necropsy (hematoxylin-eosin, magnification 25X). (**C**) Irradiated right ureter showing renal fibrosis and luminal narrowing on necropsy (hematoxylin-eosin, magnification 25X).

Among animals followed for 5 yr, one dog developed a rhabdomyosarcoma in the treatment field *(13)*. Otherwise, there were distinct histopathologic differences between irradiated and unirradiated tissue with mucosal inflammation, edema, and mural fibrosis seen within the IOERT portals. However, no dose-response relationship of severity of damage was noted for the irradiated tissues, with a similar histologic appearance at virtually all doses. On follow-up cystometry, no irradiated animal was noted to have marked changes in contractility from baseline or with respect to control animals.

Extrapolating from this study to clinical bladder preservation trials, 20 Gy IOERT would be expected to contribute little to chronic toxicity. Higher doses carry the risk of ureteral obstruction and consequent renal damage unless ureteral stents are placed, as clinically indicated.

6. NERVOUS SYSTEM

6.1. Peripheral Nerve

Because of clinical reports of toxicities to peripheral nerve in patient trials of IOERT, a canine trial was undertaken at the NCI to determine nerve tolerance *(14)*. The lumbosacral plexus was surgically exposed unilaterally and IOERT doses of 0–75 Gy were delivered. No surgical manipulation of the plexus was performed, and the contralateral nonirradiated lumbosacral plexus served as a control for each dog. Nineteen of 21 irradiated animals developed hind-limb motor changes that varied from mild weakness to complete paralysis. No threshold dose was evident. However, an inverse relationship was apparent between IOERT doses and latency to the onset of symptoms, with higher doses producing neurotoxicity more rapidly.

A subsequent trial was repeated at the NCI in an attempt to better establish a threshold dose *(15,16)*. A similar lumbosacral plexus field was irradiated in canines with doses of 10, 15, or 20 Gy. With a minimum follow-up of 3 yr, no animal receiving 10 or 15 Gy developed clinical neurotoxicity to any degree. All 20-Gy animals developed right hind leg paresis 8–12 mo following treatment. Histologically, nerves showed loss of myelin, fibrosis, and microvascular radiation changes (Fig. 3). The experimental data thus indicated that IOERT of 20 Gy provides a threshold dose for peripheral neuropathy. This closely mirrors data from human trials. Consequently, special care must be taken to shield roots and peripheral nerves incidentally in IOERT portals whenever possible if doses of ≥20 Gy are anticipated. Latency of clinical damage may range up to 24 mo at these doses.

6.2. Spinal Cord

Among a group of beagles (smaller in size than the American foxhound used in other NCI canine trials), the spinal cord received significant radiation exposure because of an oversight in dosimetry *(17)*. No bolus was used for the treatment to retroperitoneal fields. Because of the omission of bolus and the consequent lack of surface-dose absorption with resulting deep penetration, some dogs were treated with nominal IOERT doses of 20 and 30 Gy in such a fashion that the spinal cord was located at the depth of maximum dose. Twenty-two animals were among those exposed to spinal-cord irradiation. Eighteen developed paralysis and incontinence. These animals were sacrificed for compassionate reasons between 6 and 13 mo postoperatively. At necropsy, all animals had severe spinal hemorrhage in the irradiated segments, with consistent demyelination and leukomalacia. There was little surprise that single doses of 20–30 Gy caused significant spinal-cord toxicity. The addition of bolus with IOERT to subsequently treated animals decreased

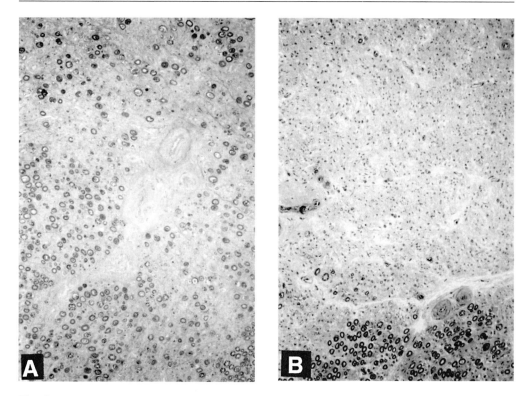

Fig. 3. IOERT to lumbosacral plexus. Histological changes at 3 yr showing loss of some myelinated fibers, fibrosis, necrosis, and myointimal vascular changes. (**A**) 20-Gy dose (silver stain, magnification 50X). (**B**) 40-Gy dose (silver stain, magnification 50X).

spinal-cord dose to approx 10% of nominal levels and totally prevented cord toxicity. This experience emphasized that careful attention to detail and rigorous dosimetry are crucial to maximize potential toxicity to the spinal cord.

7. RADIATION-INDUCED MALIGNANCIES

Several authors have proposed requirements by which tumors may be identified as radiation-induced. The criteria adopted by Powers et al. *(18)* are valid for experimental model systems. These authors consider tumors arising in previously irradiated fields to be radiation induced using the following criteria: the tumors occurred in the radiation portal; they occurred after an appropriate latency period; they were histologically confirmed; and they arose infrequently otherwise in the model species.

Tumor induction in dogs receiving IOERT in various NCI experimental trials has been described *(19,20)*. Forty-six animals that received IOERT were followed clinically for at least 24 mo. Ten tumors developed in nine animals with a median latency of 40 mo. One tumor was a breast cancer developing in a dog that had bladder IOERT and, consequently, this was likely to be a spontaneously-arising neoplasm unrelated to radiation. A benign neuroma arose in one animal on a peripheral nerve IOERT portal, and intraoperative trauma was believed to have contributed to formation of the lesion. A neurofibroma that was histologically benign but was grossly invasive occurred in one peripheral nerve animal. The remaining seven lesions were all malignant. Six of these lesions occurred in fields that contained bone. The tumors were typically associated with bone necrosis in the

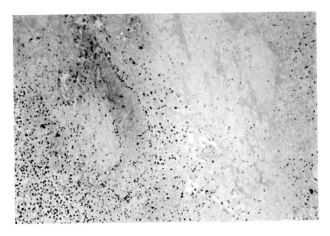

Fig. 4. Rhabdomyosarcoma developing in irradiated bladder (hematoxylin-eosin, magnification 25X).

IOERT portal. The seventh malignancy was a rhabdomyosarcoma occurring in a bladder IOERT field (Fig. 4). All tumors were seen with intraoperative radiation doses of 20–35 Gy.

Collectively, these data suggest that long-term survivors who receive IOERT may be at risk for a late appearing radiation-induced malignancy particularly including bone tumors. To date, human tumor induction has not been noted in the available published clinical trials of IOERT. However, since orthovoltage radiation has higher bone absorption than electron-beam irradiation, techniques for orthovoltage irradiation should be specially designed to minimize the bone dose wherever possible in order to minimize the risk of late bone necrosis with the possibility of tumor induction.

REFERENCES

1. Sindelar WF, Kinsella TJ, Tepper JE, et al. Experimental and clinical studies with intraoperative radiotherapy, *Surg. Gyn. Obstet.,* **157** (1983) 205–219.
2. Sindelar WF, Hoekstra H, Restrepo C, and Kinsella TJ. Pathological tissue changes following intraoperative radiotherapy, *Am. J. Clin. Oncol. (CCT),* **9** (1986) 504–509.
3. Pass HI, Sindelar WF, Kinsella TJ, et al. Delivery of intraoperative radiation therapy after pneumonectomy: experimental observations and early clinical results, *Ann. Thor. Surg.,* **44** (1987) 14–20.
4. Sindelar WF, Hoekstra HJ, Kinsella TJ, et al. Responses of canine esophagus to intraoperative electron beam radiotherapy, *Int. J. Radiat. Oncol. Biol. Phys.,* **15** (1988) 663–669.
5. Tochner ZA, Pass HI, Sindelar WF, et al. Long term tolerance of thoracic organs to intraoperative electron beam radiotherapy, *Int. J. Radiation Oncol. Biol. Phys.,* **22** (1991) 65–69.
6. Barnes M, Pass H, DeLuca A, et al. Responses of the mediastinal and thoracic viscera of the dog to intraoperative radiation therapy (IORT), *Int. J. Radiat. Oncol. Biol. Phys.,* **13** (1987) 371–378.
7. Sindelar WF, Tepper JE, Travis EL, and Terrill R. Tolerance of retroperitoneal structures to intraoperative radiation, *Ann. Surg.,* **196** (1982) 601–608.
8. Tepper JE, Sindelar WF, Travis EL, et al. Tolerance of canine anastomoses to intraoperative radiation therapy, *Int. J. Radiat. Oncol. Biol. Phys.,* **9** (1983) 987–992.
9. Sindelar WF, Tepper JE, Kinsella TJ, et al. Late effects of intraoperative radiation therapy on retroperitoneal tissues, intestine, and bile duct in a large animal model, *Int. J. Radiat. Oncol. Biol. Phys.,* **29** (1994) 781–788.
10. Sindelar WF, Tepper JE, and Travis EL. Tolerance of the bile duct to intraoperative irradiation, *Surgery,* **92** (1988) 533–540.
11. Johnstone PAS, Sprague M, DeLuca AM, et al. Effects of intraoperative radiotherapy on vascular grafts in a canine model, *Int. J. Radiat. Oncol. Biol. Phys.,* **29** (1994) 1015–1025.

12. Kinsella TJ, Sindelar WF, DeLuca AM, et al. Tolerance of the canine bladder to intraoperative radiation therapy: an experimental study, *Int. J. Radiat. Oncol. Biol. Phys.,* **14** (1988) 939–946.

13. DeLuca AM, Johnstone PAS, Ollayos CW, et al. Tolerance of the bladder to intraoperative radiation in a canine model. A five-year follow-up, *Int. J. Radiat. Oncol. Biol. Phys.,* **30** (1994) 339–345.

14. Kinsella TJ, Sindelar WF, DeLuca AM, et al. Tolerance of peripheral nerve to intraoperative radiotherapy (IORT): clinical and experimental studies, *Int. J. Radiat. Oncol. Biol. Phys.,* **11** (1985) 1579–1585.

15. Kinsella TJ, DeLuca AM, Barnes M, et al. Threshold dose for peripheral neuropathy following intraoperative radiotherapy (IORT) in a large animal model, *Int. J. Radiat. Oncol. Biol. Phys.,* **20** (1991) 697–701.

16. Johnstone PAS, DeLuca AM, Bacher JD, et al. Clinical toxicity of peripheral nerve to intraoperative radiotherapy in a canine model, *Int. J. Radiat. Oncol. Biol. Phys.,* **32** (1995) 1031–1034.

17. DeLuca AM, Anderson WJ, Kinsella TJ, and Sindelar WF. Intraoperative radiation therapy produces massive hemorrhage in canine spinal cords, *Soc. Neurosci. Abst.,* **15** (1989) 531–537.

18. Powers BE, Gillette EL, McChesney SL, et al. Bone necrosis and tumors induction following experimental intraoperative irradiation, *Int. J. Radiat. Oncol. Biol. Phys.,* **17** (1989) 559–567.

19. Barnes M, Duray P, DeLuca A, et al. Tumor induction following intraoperative radiotherapy: late results of the National Cancer Institute canine trials, *Int. J. Radiat. Oncol. Biol. Phys.,* **19** (1990) 651–660.

20. Johnstone PAS, Laskin WB, DeLuca AM, et al. Tumors in dogs exposed to experimental intraoperative radiotherapy, *Int. J. Radiat. Oncol. Biol. Phys.,* **34** (1996) 853–857.

9

Studies at Colorado State University of Normal Tissue Tolerance of Beagles to IOERT, EBRT, or a Combination

Edward L. Gillette, Sharon M. Gillette, and Barbara E. Powers

CONTENTS

1. INTRODUCTION

There was renewed interest in IORT (intraoperative irradiation) by radiation oncologists in the United States during the late 1970s. Japanese radiation oncologists had reported some early success particularly treating gastric carcinoma with IORT single doses as large as 50 Gy *(1,2)*.

Following a workshop in Bethesda in 1979, investigators at Colorado State University (CSU) designed experiments to evaluate the response of retroperitoneal tissues in beagles to variable doses of radiation given either in large single-electron doses delivered intraoperatively (IOERT), fractionated doses of external-beam irradiation (EBRT), and the combination of EBRT and IOERT. The trial design was discussed at that workshop and was influenced particularly by Herman Suit who was exploring the potential for IOERT at Massachusetts General Hospital (MGH).

Because the tissues at risk in the para-aortic region were generally considered late responding, it was important to design experiments with long observation times. It was fortunate in those early studies that the experiments could be designed to evaluate tissues for as long as 5 yr following irradiation. Observations were also made at 6 mo and 2 yr. That permitted important observations of late-responding normal tissues irradiated under controlled conditions to variable doses. There were few studies before or since designed to evaluate tissues in that way.

The retroperitoneal field used for the studies at CSU included aorta, vena cava, ureter, vertebral bone, peripheral nerve, and muscle. Initially, a portion of the kidney was

From: *Current Clinical Oncology: Intraoperative Irradiation: Techniques and Results*
Edited by: L. L. Gunderson et al. © Humana Press, Inc., Totowa, NJ

Table 1
Experimental Design

IOERT Only	IOERT Plus 50-Gy EBRT	EBRT only in 30 Fractions
Dose Range 17.5–55 Gy	IOERT Dose Range 10–47.5 Gy	Dose Range 60–80 Gy

Evaluations were made at 6 mo, 2 yr, and 5 yr. Four to six dogs were included for each dose group for each time interval.

included in the field and a separate study of the response of pancreas to IORT was also done. This report is a summary of all those studies except for peripheral nerve which is discussed in Chapter 10.

It became clear that 50-Gy IOERT was not well tolerated by large tissue volumes. Relatively small volumes had been irradiated by the Japanese in their clinical studies, which may have explained the lack of reported complications in their series. It also became apparent that volume would be important in determining the total IOERT dose that might be delivered. Later studies at CSU were designed to evaluate the influence of volume. Those studies are currently being analyzed.

2. METHODS AND MATERIALS

Adult beagle dogs were used in all of the CSU experiments. In the initial studies, there were three treatment groups (Table 1). One group received single IOERT doses of 6-MeV electrons ranging from 17.5–55 Gy. The electrons were delivered through a 5 × 8-cm plexiglas applicator inserted through a midventral celiotomy (Fig. 1A). The moveable abdominal organs were retracted from the field. The electrons were produced by a clinical accelerator with a dose rate of approx 6.5 Gy/min. The right ureter was retracted from the field and only the left ureter was irradiated.

Another group of dogs received variable doses of EBRT delivered in 30 fractions of 2, 2.33, or 2.67 Gy providing a total dose of 60, 70, or 80 Gy delivered over 6 wk. The dose rate was 2.5 Gy/min. Six-MeV photons were delivered to a 5 × 10-cm field through bilaterally opposed portals to the retroperitoneal tissue (Fig. 1B). This volume included the abdominal aorta, vena cava, one ureter, ventral portion of the vertebra, peripheral nerve, and muscle (Fig. 1B).

A third treatment group included dogs receiving 50-Gy EBRT delivered in 25 fractions over 5 wk. This was followed by IOERT doses of 10–47.5 Gy. IOERT was given the week following completion of EBRT.

A variety of radiographic and physiologic studies were done to evaluate the response of the structures irradiated. At the end of prescribed times of observation, or earlier depending on the severity of complications, tissues were taken and evaluated histologically. A variety of semiquantitative and quantitative morphometric analyses were done on the tissues.

3. RESULTS

3.1. Aorta and Vena Cava

The initial studies at CSU were designed to evaluate tissues at 6 mo, 2 yr, and 5 yr following irradiation. At the time the initial studies were done, there was little informa-

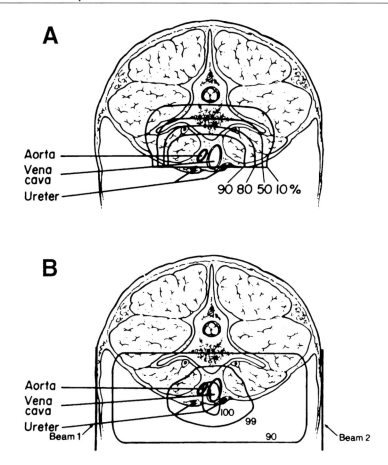

Fig. 1. A clinical accelerator was used to deliver either 6-MeV electrons intraoperatively (**A**) or 6-MeV photons through bilaterally opposed portals (**B**). Bolus was used to ensure that the ureter fell within the 90% isodose line as shown. The electron applicator was offset to the left so that only the left ureter was irradiated (**A**). Reprinted with permission from ref. *9*.

tion available on the response of great vessels to large single doses of irradiation. Currently there is more research because of the interest in prevention of restenosis following surgery of large vessels *(3)*.

3.1.1. AORTA—6-MO EVALUATION

At 6 mo following IORT, there appeared to be little variation in response of the aortas caused by dose *(4)*. At all IOERT doses between 22 and 47 Gy there were occasional small, raised, pale foci in the tunica intima (Fig. 2). The most common lesion was a fibroelastic proliferation that was confined to the subendothelial tunica intima. The intimal proliferations were usually covered by a single lining of endothelial cells. A second observation was focal thinning and architectural disruption of the tunica media that occurred directly beneath the intimal proliferation. There was occasional disorganization and proliferation of smooth muscle and elastic tissue resulting in thickening of the tunica media. Only rarely a proliferation in the tunica media extended through the external elastic membrane into the adventitia. Morphometrically, the thickness of the tunica intima increased approx four-fold after IOERT.

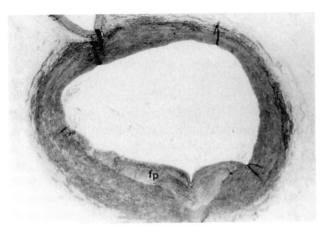

Fig. 2. Mild fibroelastic proliferation (fp) in the tunica intima and thinning of the wall (right) in a canine abdominal aorta 6 mo after 22-Gy IOERT. Verhoff van Geison stain. Magnification 4X. Reprinted with permission from ref. *4*.

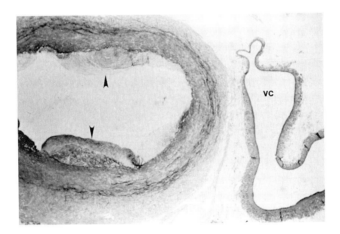

Fig. 3. Extensive fibroelastic proliferation (arrow) in the tunic intima of an abdominal aorta 6 mo after 80 Gy (30 fractions in 6 wk). The vena cava (vc) to this dose showed only mild disruption in the wall. Verhoffs van Geison stain. Magnification 4X. (Used with permission.)

The aortic intimal proliferations at 6 mo were greater in dogs that received EBRT to 60, 70, or 80 Gy over 6 wk (Fig. 3). The proliferations were morphologically similar to those seen after IOERT. The changes in the tunica media were less severe after the fractionated doses. There was a definite dose response following EBRT. The greatest proliferation and narrowing of the lumen of the aorta resulted from 80 Gy given in 30 fractions. Sixty Gy produced little response. When IOERT was combined with fractionated EBRT doses, mild intimal proliferation was observed at all doses. The large single IOERT doses were felt to produce structural alterations in the walls of large blood vessels that were clinically undetectable at early postirradiation times. It was predicted that if these progressed in severity they could lead to late effects such as rupture, fissure, or aneurysm that would be clinically significant.

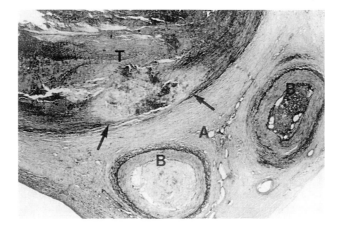

Fig. 4. Aorta 5 yr after 55.0-Gy IOERT. Aneurysm dissecting through the wall of the media (arrows) of the aorta which has a large thrombus (T). Branch arteries (**B**) are also thrombosed and the adventitia (**A**) is markedly thickened. (VVG × 35.) Reprinted with permission from ref. 7.

Findings at the 6-mo evaluation interval suggested that the response in the aorta may have been primarily caused by effects of radiation on the vasa vasorum of the aortic wall and the cells populating the tunica intima layer. It appeared that the fractionated EBRT doses stimulated proliferation of the tunica intima cells and the formation of a generalized thickening or focal plaque in the tunica intima layer. Lindsey had earlier reported similar findings *(5)*. The loss of some of the vasa vasorum could create hypoxic conditions which then could stimulate intimal proliferation. Later hypoxia caused by disruption of the vasa vasorum might increase the probability of serious consequences such as vascular spasm and occlusions. The lack of large proliferations and the focal-wall thinning seen in aortas receiving IOERT could result in focal weakening of the wall and serious later consequences.

The vena cava was studied with the same types of evaluations. No significant alterations in any of the irradiated vena cavae were observed.

3.1.2. Aorta—2- and 5-Yr Evaluations

In a continuation of the first study, aortas were evaluated 2 and 5 yr following irradiation. At that time, dose responses were observed and it was possible to determine a dose with a 50% probability to cause a certain level of injury. The most severe lesions were variably organized thrombi that occupied at least one-third of the luminal area or intimal surface of the aorta (Fig. 4). Six of the dogs with thrombi had dissecting aneurysms. Dissecting aneurysms occurred at doses as low as 25 Gy IOERT plus 50 Gy EBRT. The doses with a 50% probability for causing aueurysms and/or severe thrombi of the aorta were 35-Gy IOERT alone and 27-Gy IOERT plus 50-Gy EBRT (Table 2). No large thrombi or aneurysms were observed 5 yr after EBRT alone to doses as high as 80 Gy. Comparisons of the ED_{50}s for IOERT alone to that of IOERT combined with EBRT indicated that 50 Gy given in 25-Gy fractions had the impact of only approx 8 Gy IOERT. It was suggested at that time that IOERT doses greater than 30 Gy alone or 20-Gy IOERT combined with 50-Gy EBRT would be accompanied by a significant risk of life-threatening lesions of the aorta *(6)*.

Table 2
Tolerance of Canine Retroperitoneal Tissue to IOERT/EBRT.

Tissue	End Point	IOERT ED_{50}	IOERT + EBRT ED_{50}	Estimated MTD IOERT ± EBRT
Aortic wall (6,7)	Aneurysms or thromboses	35.0 Gy (5 yr)	27.0 Gy (5 yr)	30 Gy IOERT
	Narrowing	38.8 Gy (5 yr)	31.0 Gy (5 yr)	20 Gy IOERT + 50 Gy EBRT
Branch arteries		24.0 Gy (5 yr)	19.4 Gy (5 yr)	
Ureter (9)	Radiographic abnormalities	32.5 Gy (5 yr)	29.0 Gy (5 yr)	25 Gy IOERT 17.5 Gy IOERT + 50 Gy EBRT
Muscle (13)	Muscle fibers decrease	21.2 Gy (2 yr) 33.8 Gy (5 yr)	22.9 Gy (2 yr) 25.2 Gy (5 yr)	20–25 Gy IOERT +
	Vessel lesions	19.2 Gy (2 yr) 25.8 Gy (5 yr)	16.0 Gy (2 yr) 18.0 Gy (5 yr)	50 Gy EBRT
Vertebral (17) artery	Fibrosis Hyalinization Necrosis	21.7 Gy (2 yr) 27.0 Gy (5 yr)	20.1 Gy (2 yr) 20.0 Gy (5 yr)	
Bone (17) (Lumbar vertebra)	Bone necrosis	38.2 Gy (2 yr) 28.5 Gy (5 yr)	32.5 Gy (2 yr) 14.4 Gy (5 yr)	15–20 Gy IOERT + 50 Gy EBRT

MTD = maximum tolerated dose; IOERT = intraoperative electron irradiation; EBRT = external beam irradiation.
The estimates for maximum tolerated dose were based on those doses at which minor or no significant injury was observed.

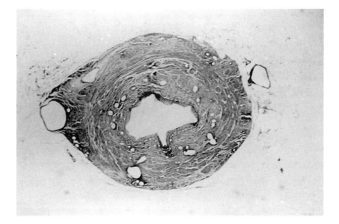

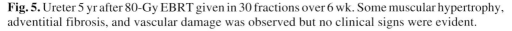

Fig. 5. Ureter 5 yr after 80-Gy EBRT given in 30 fractions over 6 wk. Some muscular hypertrophy, adventitial fibrosis, and vascular damage was observed but no clinical signs were evident.

Other lesions included adventitial fibrosis, which showed a dose response and likely contributed to the severe lesions and thrombosis by causing fibrosis and destruction of the vasa vasorum. Intimal proliferation occurred at low IOERT doses but decreased at higher doses, perhaps because of an inhibition of the proliferative response caused by increased cell kill.

3.1.3. BRANCH ARTERIES

The response of branch arteries was also evaluated *(7)*. The ED_{50} for 50% occlusion of branch arteries was 25-Gy IOERT alone and 19 Gy for IOERT combined with 50-Gy EBRT (Table 1). The conclusion was that 20-Gy IOERT combined with 50-Gy EBRT was near the maximum tolerated dose for aorta and branch arteries. This data on the branch arteries is of special interest currently as these are of similar caliber to coronary arteries and the carotid arteries that are being studied following irradiation for preventing restenosis *(8)*.

3.2. Ureter

3.2.1. EBRT ALONE

The ureters of dogs tolerated doses up to 80-Gy EBRT given in 30 fractions over 6 wk. One dog given 80 Gy had mild ureteral dilatation at 5 yr *(9)*. However, no clinical signs of ureteral injury were seen. Although there were no radiographic changes after EBRT, there was histologic evidence of ureteral damage that included muscular hypertrophy and vascular damage (Fig. 5). There was a decrease in the amount of vasculature in the ureteral wall that could reduce the ability of the ureter to respond to subsequent injury. This had been reported earlier by Albers et al *(10)*. following a study in which ureters were reimplanted after irradiation and showed either marked or moderate obstruction. Ureters reimplanted and then irradiated showed no abnormalities.

3.2.2. IOERT WITH OR WITHOUT EBRT

Mild urographic abnormalities were present following IOERT in only 1 of 5 dogs given 25-Gy IOERT. Severe changes were seen following 32.5 Gy (Fig. 6). It appeared from this study that the ureter might tolerate a single IOERT dose of 25 Gy with little risk

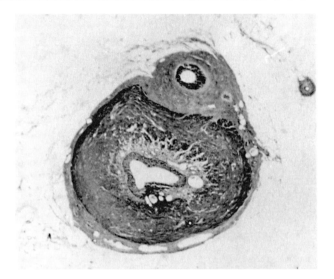

Fig. 6. Left ureter 5 yr after 32.5-Gy IOERT showing decreased lamina propria. Vascular damage characterized by intimal proliferation and perivascular fibrosis were present. Adventitial fibrosis was also present. This dog had grade 6 radiographic changes. Reprinted with permission from ref. *9.*

of complications. When EBRT was combined with IOERT, it appeared that the fraction-ated dose contributed little to the degree of injury.

3.2.3. Influence of Time on Canine Ureteral Changes (Radiographic, Histologic)

Regression of early ureteral changes was observed in this study as well as others *(11,12).* The incidence of radiographic abnormalities following IOERT was less at 5 yr than at 1 yr (Table 3). This occurred at IOERT doses as high as 40 Gy. At IOERT doses above 40 Gy, with or without EBRT, no resolution of strictures was observed. It was felt the damage to the ureter at doses above 40 Gy was likely too severe to allow any recovery. The evidence in this study was that the mucosa was always intact even 5 yr following irradiation. Therefore, the mucosa had the ability to regenerate even in the face of very high doses. Abnormal areas of thinning, hyperplasia, and vacuolization of the transitional epithelium were present. The present lamina propria was decreased with increasing IOERT dose. It was felt that this may have been caused by the loss of vascular endothelial cells and capillaries. Additional injury in the lamina propria was observed following disruption of the mucosa and leakage of urine into the deeper tissues.

The muscular layer was increased in thickness after irradiation. Histologic sections taken at or near the site of stricture showed muscle hypertrophy that may have contributed to partial obstruction of the ureter because of increased peristalsis attempting to maintain urine flow. It appeared from this study that injury was evident 6 mo following irradiation but that some regeneration occurred following that time.

The canine ureter appeared to tolerate 25-Gy IOERT with a low probability for mild dilation. Severe injury occurred at doses greater than 25-Gy IOERT. There was little functional evidence of injury following EBRT. However, the muscular hypertrophy and decrease in percent vasculature as well as the decrease in tolerated IOERT dose can be seen as evidence of residual injury from EBRT. The histologic evidence from this study indicated that chronic injury of the ureter expressed at 5 yr was of vascular etiology.

Table 3
Frequency of Abnormalities on Urograms

	6 mo	1 yr	5 yr
Group I (EBRT)[a]			
60 Gy	0/5	0/5	0/5
70 Gy	0/5	0/5	0/5
80 Gy	0/5	0/5	1/5
Group II (IOERT)			
17.5 Gy	0/5	0/5	0/5
25 Gy	1/5	1/5	1/5
32.5 Gy	3/6	6/6	4/6
40 Gy	2/6	6/6	3/5
47.5 Gy	5/5	4/4	1/1
55 Gy	4/4	4/4	1/1
Group III (EBRT + IOERT)[b]			
60 Gy	0/5	1/5	0/5
67.5 Gy	0/5	3/5	1/5
75 Gy	4/6	6/6	3/3
82.5 Gy	1/6	3/6	1/4
90 Gy	3/5	3/5	3/4
97.5 Gy	3/5	1/4	2/2

[a]EBRT alone—30 fractions over 6 wk.
[b]EBRT—50 Gy in 25 fractions over 5 wk; IOERT—10–47.5 Gy
Total combined doses are shown for EBRT and IOERT.

3.2.4. HUMAN URETERAL TOLERANCE TO IOERT

Studies of ureters of human cancer patients showed a 50% incidence of obstruction following 10 Gy and 70% after doses of 15–25 Gy of IOERT *(11)*. The greater incidence of obstruction than observed in the young beagle dogs may have been caused by the greater age, surgical manipulation, and/or tumor bed effects.

3.2.5. IOERT VOLUME EFFECT ON URETER

Volume has a significant influence on ureteral response to IOERT. Ureters were given variable IOERT dose to lengths of 2, 4, or 8 cm. Ureteral strictures were evaluated with excretory urography. At 3 yr the ED_{50} for the 8-cm length was 22 Gy. The ED_{50} increased to 43 Gy for 4 cm and 85 Gy for 2 cm *(13)*.

3.3. Muscle

The psoas muscles were in the periaortic region irradiated in these studies *(14)*. The left psoas muscle was evaluated. The injury caused in the psoas muscle was characterized by a loss of muscle fibers, atrophy, and fibrosis (Fig. 7). The dose that caused a 50% decrease in muscle fibers 2 yr after irradiation was 21-Gy IOERT (Table 2). The dose to cause a 50% decrease in muscle fibers was 23-Gy IOERT when combined with 50-Gy EBRT. At 5 yr, doses required to cause a 50% decrease in muscle fibers were 34-Gy IOERT only and 25-Gy IOERT when combined with 50-Gy EBRT. The higher doses needed to cause the equivalent effect at 5 yr indicated some regeneration of muscle. Satellite cells or myoblasts have a limited potential for regeneration. It was felt that a more likely explanation in the relative increased volume of muscle at 5 yr compared to

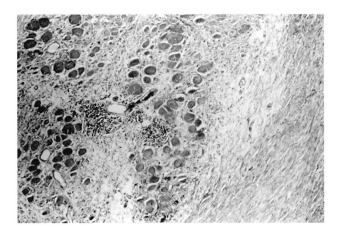

Fig. 7. Muscle atrophy and fibrosis in psoas muscles 2 yr after 25-Gy IOERT.

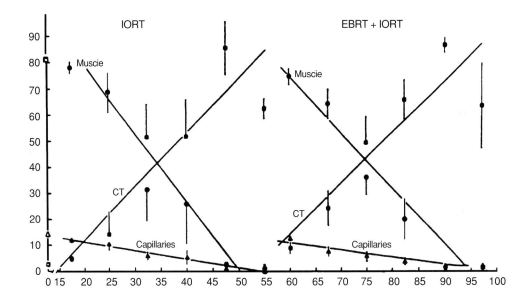

Fig. 8. Graph of percentage of tissue components vs dose 5 yr after irradiation (CT—connective tissue). Mean and standard errors are shown. Control values are open symbols. (Used with permission.)

2 yr was the condensation of the hemorrhage, fibrin, and immature loose connective tissue into a more mature dense connective tissue. Because of the type of morphometry used, the less abundant fibrin and hemorrhage and the more dense connective tissue 5 yr after irradiation would lead to an apparent increase in muscle volume. Some of the remaining muscle fibers may have also undergone hypertrophy.

The results of this study supported a role for vascular damage in causing late muscle atrophy and fibrosis. There was a consistent decrease in the percentage of capillaries with increasing IOERT doses at 2 and 5 yr following irradiation (Fig. 8). The presence of fibrin and hemorrhage within the muscle was an indication of severe vessel injury resulting in vessel rupture. Inflammation was present in most dogs following IOERT, which supports the hypothesis that mediators of inflammation contributed to the fibrosis such as monocytes and macrophages that produced mediators such as TGFβ that induced fibroblast recruitment and proliferation. Radiation-induced muscle atrophy with its associated fibrosis and vascular lesions distinguishes this injury from that which would be caused solely by neurogenic atrophy.

When IOERT was combined with EBRT, there was little additional effect. The lack of effect of 50-Gy EBRT was felt to be because of the response of the IOERT dose obscuring the relatively small contribution of the 50-Gy EBRT given in 2-Gy fractions. At 2 or 5 yr after irradiation, dogs that had received 50–80 Gy of EBRT in 2- to 2.67-Gy fractions, had either none or minimal lesions. It was felt that 20–25 Gy in combination with 50-Gy EBRT would be reasonably well tolerated by the canine sublumbar musculature. Doses above 25-Gy IOERT might lead to significant muscle fibrosis and complications associated with soft-tissue injury.

None of the dogs showed any clinical evidence of damage to the irradiated muscle. The psoas muscle's action is to rotate the thigh medially and to flex the lumbar vertebra. These are subtle movements in the dog and their lack of function would not likely be detected.

Of concern in humans is the possibility of soft-tissue injury complications following abdominal IOERT. These include abscesses, hemorrhages, fibrosis, and pelvic pain *(15)*. This occurred in 24% of 41 MGH patients receiving surgery and IOERT to single doses of 10–20 Gy usually combined with 45–50 Gy of EBRT. A similar 26% incidence of soft-tissue injury was noted in 23 MGH patients who had preoperative EBRT plus resection for clinical fixed tumors in whom no IOERT was given. Two dogs in this study had abscess formation at very high doses 5 yr after 47.5-Gy plus 50-Gy EBRT. It was felt that the doses causing abscesses in humans at much lower doses was likely because of the surgical procedures performed or additional tissue injury caused by the tumor.

3.4. Bone

3.4.1. Empty Lacunae, Bone Necrosis

In the studies done at CSU, the ventral portion of the lumbar vertebra was within the 90% isodose levels. In the study of beagles, the percentage of empty lacunae was used to quantify the effect of IOERT on bone *(16)*. The number of empty lacunae increased from a normal value of 20% to approx 60% after 50-Gy IOERT or 42.5-Gy IOERT in combination with 50-Gy EBRT. This effect was seen 2 yr following irradiation (Fig. 9). The effect was more marked 5 yr after irradiation when the percentage of lacunae increased from 25% in these older dogs to 81% after 55-Gy IOERT and 75% after 47.5-Gy in combination with 50-Gy EBRT (Fig. 10).

Radiation-induced bone necrosis is a late developing and progressive change that may not become significant until more than 2 yr after irradiation (Fig. 11). None of the dogs in these studies developed clinical signs that could be attributed to cortical bone necrosis. However, two dogs had lesions of septic osteoradionecrosis following 47.5-Gy IOERT plus 50-Gy EBRT. Another reason for lack of significant clinical effect is that only part of the vertebra was within the 90% isodose level so the volume of bone effected was quite small. It was felt that this slowly progressive bone necrosis might be more important in older humans who are at risk for age-related and postmenopausal osteoporosis. In addition, the upright posture of humans would add more compressive stress on vertebrae making compression fractures of the vertebrae included in IOERT fields a possibility. Osteonecrosis of the coccyx was described in one patient 7 mo after 25-Gy IOERT *(17)*.

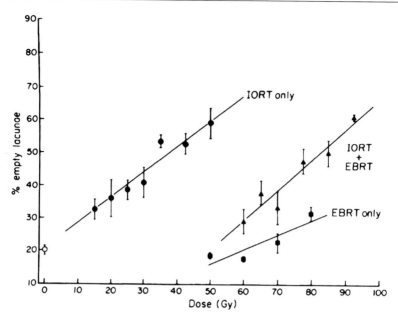

Fig. 9. Dose response graph for percent lacunae 2 yr after irradiation. Means and standard errors are shown. Reprinted with permission from ref. *16.*

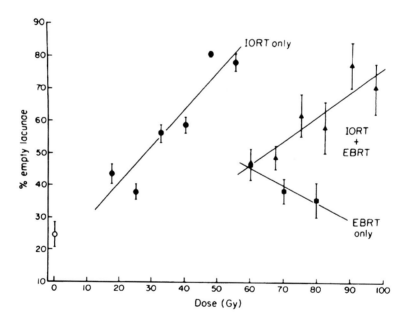

Fig. 10. Dose-response graph for percent empty lacunae 5 yr after irradiation. Means and standard errors are shown. Reprinted with permission from ref. *16.*

The pathogenesis of empty lacunae in bone has been attributed to direct radiation damage to osteocytes or their precursors, the osteoblast, or damage to bone vasculature. In this study, the finding of empty lacunae clustered around Haversian canals devoid of viable capillaries suggested that damage to this vasculature was a likely cause of osteocyte death. The slowly progressive nature of bone necrosis that became most severe 5 yr

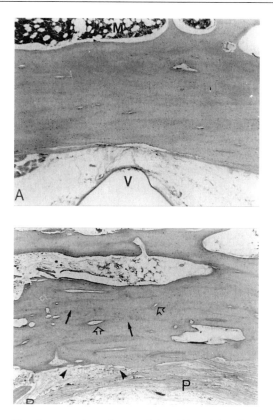

Fig. 11. Ventral cortex of lumbar vertebra of control dog (**A**) and dog 5 years after 32.5-Gy IOERT with 50-Gy EBRT (**B**). Empty lacunae (arrows), Haversian canals devoid of vessels (open arrows), scalloped surfaces (arrowheads), and periosteal inflammation (P) are present in **B**. Normal bone marrow (M), ventral artery (V), and lacunae with osteocytes are in **A**. H&E × 65. Reprinted with permission from ref. *16*.

after irradiation would be consistent with the response of the vasculature. Because of the delivery of the electron beam to the ventral portion of the periaortic region, damage to the ventral vertebral artery which was in the highest dose volume probably contributed to development of bone lesions. Medial necrosis and perivascular fibrosis was observed in that artery 2 yr after irradiation, but did not appear sufficiently significant to effect the function of the artery. These changes progressed to more severe medial necrosis and partial-to-complete thrombosis and disruption of the arterial wall by 5 yr after irradiation. This more severe damage at 5 yr likely accounted for the more severe bone necrosis that was seen. The periosteal lesions of chronic inflammation, edema, and fibrosis were likely secondary to vascular lesions. Vascular leak caused by damaged vessels causes edema that later organizes into fibrous tissue.

Doses required to cause 50% empty lacunae at 2 and 5 yr after irradiation were determined (Table 2). At 2 yr, the dose was 38-Gy IOERT alone and 32.5-Gy IOERT when combined with 50-Gy EBRT. At 5-yr after irradiation, the dose to cause 50% empty lacunae was 28.5-Gy IOERT alone and 14 Gy when combined with 50-Gy EBRT. As might be expected with slowly developing lesions, a much smaller dose was required to cause an isoeffect at 5 yr than at 2 yr. In this study, 80-Gy EBRT given in 30 fractions produced only mild lesions.

3.4.2. OSTEOSARCOMA

Of greater concern than the induction of bone necrosis was the incidence of radiation-induced osteosarcoma *(18,19)*. The incidence of naturally occurring osteosarcomas in dogs is much higher than that in humans *(20)*. However, this is due primarily to the exceptionally high incidence in large breeds that may be 60 times more likely to have osteosarcomas than small breeds. The beagles used in this study are considered a small breed and the natural incidence of osteosarcoma in beagle dogs is very low. In addition, the tumors in this study did not occur at the sites most common for naturally occurring osteosarcoma. Osteosarcomas most frequently occur at the metaphysis of long bones in both humans and dogs. The osteosarcomas in this study developed in the vertebra that was in the IOERT field.

The overall incidence of osteosarcoma in the CSU studies was 8 of 53 dogs evaluated or 15% of all dogs given IOERT and surviving at least 4 yr. The latency time for observing osteosarcomas was 4–5 yr following irradiation. As all dogs were euthanatized at that time, it is not known whether more tumors would have developed with increasing time. No metastasis had developed in those dogs at the time of euthanasia. No osteosarcomas were seen within 5 yr in the 14 beagles given external-beam irradiation at 60, 70, or 80 Gy in 30 fractions. When IOERT was given alone, one osteosarcoma was seen 4 yr after 47.5 Gy. The combination of 50-Gy EBRT followed by IOERT produced the greatest incidence of tumors. Tumor induction appeared to increase within increasing dose between 47.5 and 90 Gy total IOERT and EBRT dose. It was felt that the decreased incidence at 97.5 Gy may have been because of chance, but it also may have been because of increased cell killing that may have reduced the probability of a carcinogenic event occurring. Two of the dogs given 97.5 Gy that did not develop tumors had septic osteo-radionecrosis with very few viable bone cells present. Tumor induction may be caused by malignant change in regenerating cells and to change in the environment leading to expression of that malignant change. The environment was altered because of damage to connective tissues and vessels. The stromal damage was much more severe with large single IOERT doses and that may have contributed to the higher incidence of tumor induction.

The lowest IOERT dose associated with tumor induction in beagles at CSU was 25 Gy. A relatively high incidence of tumor induction was observed in dogs irradiated experimentally at the National Cancer Institute (NCI) *(19)*. It was reported that the frequency of radiation-induced malignancies in dogs receiving IOERT was 15% and was 25% in dogs receiving greater than 25-Gy IOERT. The overall incidence in the CSU study was 15%.

3.5. Kidneys

A separate experiment was done to evaluate the pathogenesis of radiation nephropathy in the dog *(21)*. A single 15-Gy IOERT dose was delivered to the kidneys and biopsies were taken at 2-wk intervals from 3–13 wk. Histologic changes in epithelial cells of the kidney were seen as early as 3 wk after irradiation. The parenchyma decreased to 50% of the preirradiation volume by 9 wk and was repopulated to near normal by 11 wk. A second wave of depopulation, assumed to be caused by beginning perivascular fibrosis, was evident at 13 wk. It was felt that the vascular damage seen 3 wk after irradiation was temporary and may have been related to the parenchymal depopulation. The vessel dimensions returned to near normal as the parenchyma repopulated. However, there was progressively increasing perivascular fibrosis, which caused a reduction in oxygen and nutrient support of the parenchyma and led to a later decrease in parenchymal volume and a permanent loss of renal function.

3.6. Pancreas

In another study, the pancreas and duodenum of 24 beagle dogs were given IOERT with 6-MeV electrons (22). The dose range was 17.5–40 Gy. Billroth II gastrojejunostomy was performed on all dogs prior to irradiation. Two weeks following surgery and IOERT, 50-Gy EBRT was delivered to the pancreas and duodenum. That dose was given in 2-Gy fractions over 5 wk.

There was a significant loss in acinar cells. However, islet cell lesions were not apparent. Pancreatic fibrosis developed and there was damage to blood vessels and the ductular structure of the pancreas with an observation time of 135 d. Twenty-five-Gy IOERT plus 50-Gy EBRT appeared to be tolerated. However, those doses might cause significant later pancreatic injury. It was felt that exocrine pancreatic insufficiency and diabetes mellitus could represent late complications of IOERT for pancreatic adenocarcinoma. The exocrine pancreatic insufficiency could be controlled with replacement therapy but diabetes mellitus would be a more serious complication. The latter complication might be acceptable considering the high fatality rate of pancreatic carcinoma. In addition, most of the pancreas would have to be destroyed to cause diabetes mellitus.

4. DISCUSSION

The interest in IOERT was stimulated because of limitations in delivering adequate EBRT doses to tumors located near critical radiosensitive organs or tissues. Therefore, the objective is to remove sensitive structures such as intestine or kidney from the field and, with direct observation of the tumor bed, deliver a dose of electrons of appropriate energy to limit that dose to the volume of the tumor bed. As the dose is delivered at the time of surgery, the objective was to achieve as high a dose delivered intraoperatively as possible. The limitation of delivery of the EBRT remains the same.

For the studies done on beagles, it was assumed that an EBRT dose of approx 50 Gy could be delivered. Therefore, if an additional IOERT dose could be added, the probability of tumor control would increase. At the time these studies began, there was still uncertainty about the tolerance of normal tissues to large single doses. Although there were indications from Japanese workers that relatively high IOERT doses could be used, most of the radiation oncologists in the United States approached IOERT more conservatively and generally used IOERT doses in the range of 10–20 Gy as a boost to reduced EBRT doses of 45–50 Gy (23).

The tissues at risk for IOERT are late-responding tissues. Those are tissues that have been shown to have an increased risk of injury with larger fraction sizes (24). In all the tissues examined, the principal injury seemed to be the damage to vasculature and connective tissues. Injury to those tissues led to late fibrosis and, if larger vessels were severely injured, necrosis of dependent tissues. In all of the tissues examined, it appeared that 20-Gy IOERT combined with 50-Gy EBRT was reasonably well tolerated. If that total dose is adequate to control the tumor, then the purpose of delivering the IOERT dose would be accomplished.

The influence of volume is critical in IOERT. One of the purposes of doing IOERT is to restrict the volume as much as possible. Later studies at CSU were directed at evaluating the influence of volume and preliminary data indicate that there clearly is a strong volume effect on tissues studied. The tissues in the IOERT field included tubular structures such as the large vessels and ureter, in which the length of the structure irradiated influenced the effect. Other tissues such as nerve, muscle, and bone responded according to the total volume irradiated.

The dogs used for the studies at CSU were healthy, young adults. They were able perhaps to tolerate somewhat higher irradiation doses than human cancer patients. Based on data obtained from those studies and others using similar animal models, it seems likely that meaningful IOERT doses can be delivered in combination with decreased EBRT doses to achieve useful uncomplicated tumor control probabilities *(25)*. As for any treatment plan, due consideration must be given to dose distribution and volume of critical tissues included in the treatment volume.

REFERENCES

1. Abe M, Fakuda M, Yamano K, Matsuda S, and Handa H. Intraoperative irradiation in abdominal and cerebral tumors, *Acta. Radiol.,* **10** (1971) 408–416.
2. Abe M and Takahashi M. Intraoperative radiotherapy: the Japanese experience, *Int. J. Radiat. Oncol. Biol. Phys.,* **7** (1981) 863–868.
3. Rubin P and Waksman R, guest ed. Interdisciplinary radiation medicine for nonmalignant diseases, coronary/vascular restenosis, *Int. J. Radiat. Oncol. Biol. Phys.,* **36(4)** (1996) 763–996.
4. Hoopes PJ, Gillette EL, and Withrow SJ. Intraoperative irradiation of the canine abdominal aorta and vena cava, *Int. J. Radiat. Oncol. Biol. Phys.,* **13** (1987) 715–722.
5. Linsey S, Entenman C, Shumury BU, Ellis EE, Gereci CL, and Skaker R. Aortic arteriosclerosis in the dog after localized aortic irradiation with electrons, *Circ. Res.,* **10** (1962) 61–69.
6. Gillette EL, Powers BE, McChesney SL, and Withrow SJ. Aortic wall injury following intraoperative irradiation, *Int. J. Radiat. Oncol. Biol. Phys.,* **15** (1988) 1401–1406.
7. Gillette EL, Powers BE, McChesney SL, Park RD, and Withrow SJ. Response of aorta and branch arteries to experimental intraoperative irradiation, *Int. J. Radiat. Oncol. Biol. Phys.,* **17** (1989) 1247–1255.
8. Nath R and Roberts KB. Vascular irradiation for the prevention of restenosis after angioplasty: a new application for radiotherapy, *Int. J. Radiat. Oncol. Biol. Phys.,* **36** (1996) 977–979.
9. McChesney Gillette SL, Gillete EL, Powers BE, Park RD, and Withrow SJ. Ureteral injury following experimental intraoperative radiation, *Int. J. Radiat. Oncol. Biol. Phys.,* **17** (1989) 791–798.
10. Albers DD, Dee AL, Kalmon EH, Leverett CL, Brown CH, and Lambird PA. Irradiation injury to the ureter and surgical tolerance: an experimental study, *Invest. Oncol.,* **14** (1976) 229–232.
11. Shaw EG, Gunderson LL, Martin JN, Beart RW, Nagorney DM, and Podratz KC. Peripheral nerve and ureteral tolerance to intraoperative radiation therapy: clinical and dose-response analysis, *Radiother. Oncol.,* **18** (1990) 249–255.
12. Underwood PB, Lutz MH, and Smoak DL. Ureteral injury following irradiation therapy for carcinoma of the cervix, *Obstet. Gynecol.,* **49** (1977) 663–669.
13. Gillette SM, Gillette EL, LaRue SM, Borak TB, and Thames HD. Effects of volume irradiated on canine ureteral function. Accepted, 1998.
14. Powers BE, Gillette EL, McChesney Gillette SL, LeCouteur RA, and Withrow SJ. Muscle injury following experimental intraoperative irradiation, *Int. J. Radiat. Oncol. Biol. Phys.,* **20** (1991) 463–471.
15. Tepper JE, Gunderson LL, Orlow E, et al. Complications of intraoperative radiation therapy, *Int. J. Radiat. Oncol. Biol. Phys.,* **10** (1984) 1831–1839.
16. Powers BE, Gillette EL, McChesney SL, LeCouteur RA, and Withrow SJ. Bone necrosis and tumor induction following experimental intraoperative irradiation, *Int. J. Radiat. Oncol. Biol. Phys.,* **17** (1989) 559–567.
17. Calvo FA, Aristu JJ, Azinovic I, et al. Intraoperative and external radiotherapy in resected gastric cancer: updated report of a phase II trial, *Int. J. Radiat. Oncol. Biol. Phys.,* **24** (1992) 729–736.
18. Gillette SM, Gillette EL, Powers BE, and Withrow SJ. Radiation-induced osteosarcoma in dogs after external beam or intraoperative radiation therapy, *Cancer Res.,* **50** (1990) 54–57.
19. Barnes M, Duran P, DeLuca A, Anderson W, Sindelar W, and Kinsella T. Tumor induction following intraoperative radiotherapy: late results of the National Cancer Institute canine trials, *Int. J. Radiat. Oncol. Biol. Phys.,* **19** (1990) 651–660.

20. Owen LNC. *Bone Tumors in Man and Animal,* Butterworth, London, 1969.
21. Hoopes PJ, Gillette EL, and Benjamin SA. The pathogenesis of radiation nephropathy in the dog, *Radiat. Res.,* **104** (1985) 406–419.
22. Ahmadu-Suka F, Gillette EL, Withrow SJ, Husted PW, Nelson AW, and Whiteman CE. Pathologic response of the pancreas and duodenum to experimental intraoperative irradiation, *Int. J. Radiat. Oncol. Biol. Phys.,* **14** (1988) 1197–1204.
23. Gunderson LL. Past, present and future of intraoperative irradiation for colorectal cancer, *Int. J. Radiat. Oncol. Biol. Phys.,* **34** (1996) 741–744.
24. Withers HR, Thames HD, and Peters LJ. Differences in the fractional response of acutely and late responding tissues, In Karcher K, Kogelnir HD, and Reinartz G, (eds.), *Progress in Radio-Oncology,* vol. II, Raven Press, New York, 1982, pp. 287–298.
25. Gillette EL, McChesney Gillette S, Powers BE, and Thames HD Jr. Potential for a therapeutic gain for IORT combined with EBRT, In Abe M and Takahashi M, (eds.), *Intraoperative Radiation Therapy,* Pergamon, Elmsford, NY, 1991, pp. 12–14.

10 Peripheral Nerve Tolerance
Experimental and Clinical

Edward Gillette, Barbara E. Powers,
Sharon M. Gillette, Leonard L. Gunderson,
and Christopher G. Willett

CONTENTS

INTRODUCTION
ANIMAL STUDIES
CLINICAL DATA
SUMMARY AND FUTURE POSSIBILITIES
REFERENCES

1. INTRODUCTION

Neuropathies are uncommon, but serious, complications following radiation therapy. Radiation therapy of gynecologic tumors in 2410 patients resulted in lumbosacral plexopathies in only four patients *(1)*. It was estimated that the lumbosacral plexus of those patients had received over 70 Gy given by a combination of implants and fractionated external-beam irradiation (EBRT).

Large single irradiation doses as given with intraoperative electron-beam irradiation (IOERT) might be expected to increase the probability of neuropathies. The frequency of peripheral neuropathies following IOERT has been sufficiently great that the tolerance of peripheral nerves appears likely to be dose limiting for many treatment sites. There is relatively little information available in the literature about dose-response relationships or the pathogenesis of peripheral neuropathies following IOERT and even less for IOERT combined with chemotherapy or hyperthermia.

2. ANIMAL STUDIES

Most of the studies of response of peripheral nerves in dogs to IOERT, as for other tissues, were carried out at the National Cancer Institute (NCI) and at Colorado State University (CSU). In 1985, Kinsella et al. *(2)* stated that following 20–26 Gy of IOERT there were clinically detected neuropathies with loss of sensory and motor function in five patients. Kinsella et al. *(3)* reported later that paresis developed in foxhounds following

From: Current Clinical Oncology: Intraoperative Irradiation: Techniques and Results
Edited by: L. L. Gunderson et al. © Humana Press, Inc., Totowa, NJ

Table 1
IOERT-Related Dog Neuropathy: Electrophysiology Abnormalities

NCI (foxhound)		CSU, beagle						
IOERT only		IOERT only		IOERT + 50 Gy EBRT[a]	EBRT only			
Study 1	Study 2	Dose (Gy)	No.	No.	Dose (Gy)	No.	No. Fx/time	
—	0/4	10	—	0/5	0	0/5	—	
—	0/4	15	2/5	1/5	50	0/4	25 Fx 5 wk	
3/4	4/4	20	4/5	2/5	60	0/6	30 Fx 6 wk	
2/2	—	25	4/4	—	70	0/5	30 Fx 6 wk	
—	—	27.5	—	2/5	80	0/4	30 Fx 6 wk	
3/3	—	30	4/4	—				
3/3	—	35	2/2	5/5				
4/4	—	40	—	—				
—	—	42.5	3/3	5/5				
1/1	—	50	2/2	—				
1/1	—	65	—	—				
3/3	—	75	—	—				

[a]50 Gy in 25 fractions over 5 wk.

EBRT = external beam irradiation; IOERT = intraoperative electron irradiation; No. = number; Fx = fraction.

single doses as low as 20 Gy delivered to the lumbosacral plexus and sciatic nerve while surgically exposed. No clinical injury was observed in the foxhounds following doses of 15 Gy or less. The main histologic observation was a loss of predominantly large myelinated fibers. They reported no evidence of vascular occlusion or thrombosis. Fibrosis was present in the endoneurium but not in the perineurium.

The response to large single IOERT doses reported from the NCI was comparable to findings in a study at CSU comparing peripheral-nerve tolerance with fractionated EBRT, IOERT, or EBRT to 50 Gy (25 fractions in 5 weeks) plus variable IOERT doses (4) (Table 1). No clinical signs of neuropathy were observed in the CSU study following EBRT to the lumbosacral plexus with doses of 60, 70, or 80 Gy delivered in 30 fractions over 6 wk (Table 2). Following single IOERT doses of 15 Gy, however, there were significant electrophysiologic changes. Clinical signs of neuropathy were observed at 20 Gy and higher. Histology revealed loss of axons and myelin and an increase in endoneural, perineural, and epineural connective tissue. In the CSU studies, definite vascular lesions were observed and included necrosis and hyalinization of medial small arteries and thrombosis and hemorrhage at high doses. In those dogs, the peripheral nerves in the retroperitoneal area had been irradiated.

In a later CSU study, Vujaskovic et al. (5) reported response of surgically exposed and isolated right sciatic nerve in the midfemoral region and observed similar histologic changes to those reported earlier. That is, whereas no vascular thrombosis or occlusions were observed, there was histomorphometric evidence of a loss of small vessels. It appeared that a dose of greater than 20 Gy would cause some clinically significant peripheral nerve injury as suggested earlier by Kinsella, et al. (3). Clinically significant neurologic or physiologic changes were not present in dogs given 20-Gy IOERT or less.

Table 2
Experimental IOERT Clinical Neuropathies at 4 –5 y, CSU

IOERT		IOERT Plus 50 Gy EBRT		EBRT (30 Fx)	
Dose (Gy)	Incidence	IOERT dose (Gy)	Incidence	Dose (Gy)	Incidence
17.5	0/5	10	0/5	60	0/5
25	1/5	17.5	0/5	70	0/5
32.5	1/5	25	1/6	80	0/6
40	1/5	32.5	1/6		
47.5	3/5	40	3/5		
55	3/5	47.5	3/5		

Fx = fractions; EBRT = external beam irradiation; IOERT = intraoperative electron irradiation.

It appeared that the isolated sciatic nerve irradiated in the midfemoral region, distal to the lumbosacral plexus, was perhaps somewhat less sensitive to IOERT than the nerve or nerve roots irradiated in the lumbosacral plexus or retroperitoneal area. Vujaskovic et al. (5) suggested that the difference might be because neuropathies caused by IOERT of the lumbosacral region resulted from the direct effects of irradiation on nerve and effects of damage to regional muscle and vasculature on the nerve. It was also suggested that severe fibrosis that developed after IOERT to muscle could entrap the nerve and its vasculature causing more severe nerve fibrosis and nerve-fiber loss secondary to the vascular damage. Single doses to the isolated sciatic nerve in the femoral region caused less damage to surrounding tissues and might have prevented some of the secondary effects of irradiation. There is also the possibility that the sciatic nerve in the midfemoral area may be more hypoxic naturally or may be made hypoxic during the isolation procedure and, therefore, less sensitive to irradiation. The main difference is likely to be the time of observation, which was only 1 yr following irradiation of the sciatic nerve.

Kinsella et al. (3) reported time-dose relationships for paresis following experimental IOERT of the lumbosacral plexus and sciatic nerve of the dog. Although paresis was observed as early as 1 yr, it is likely that smaller doses would require a longer period to cause paresis. Neuropathies have been reported to occur as late as 11 yr after EBRT for breast cancer (6). The time course for development of neuropathies after IOERT ranged from 1 to 32 mo with a median of 15 mo (2,7).

It appears that injury to the vasculature is an important factor leading to damage to the nerves. Schwann cells and microvasculature are two critical structures associated with peripheral nerves that are directly affected by irradiation. Clinical tolerance to peripheral nerve injury in the dog appears to be ≤20-Gy IOERT.

2.1. Volume Studies

IOERT in variable doses was given to retroperitoneal field sizes that were 2, 4, or 8 cm long and 5 cm wide (9). The dogs were observed for 3 yr following irradiation. Electrophysiologic procedures were done prior to irradiation and annually following irradiation. Fifteen of 47 dogs treated to an 8-cm field were euthanatized for severe paresis prior to 3 yr. There was a decreasing conduction velocity that correlated with increasing dose for dogs treated to an 8-cm field at 1, 2, and 3 yr following treatment. There was no decrease in mean conduction velocity for dogs treated to either 2 or 4 cm fields. At 3 yr following IORT, the dose for greater than 50% axon and myelin loss was 20 Gy for the 8-cm field, 25 Gy for the 4-cm field, and 26 Gy for the 2-cm field. The latency of injury appeared inversely proportional to dose and to volume treated.

2.2. Hyperthermia

Vujaskovic et al. *(8)* studied the effects of intraoperative hyperthermia combined with intraoperative irradiation. The surgically exposed right sciatic nerves of dogs were given either a range of single IOERT doses of 16–32 Gy or a range of IOERT doses of 12–28 Gy concurrently with 44°C of intraoperatively delivered hyperthermia for 60 min. Heat also was given alone. Two years following treatment, the ED_{50} for limb paresis in dogs exposed to IOERT only was 22 Gy. The ED_{50} for paresis in dogs given IOERT combined with heat was 15 Gy. The thermal enhancement ratio, therefore, was 1.5. The latency for development of peripheral neuropathy was shorter for dogs exposed to the combined treatment.

3. CLINICAL DATA

Peripheral nerve has been defined as the principal dose-limiting normal tissue for IOERT in the pelvis and or retroperitoneum in clinical as well as animal studies. The observations in animal studies from NCI *(3,10)* and CSU *(4,9)* have been presented in detail earlier in this chapter. Clinical analyses from NCI *(2,10–12)* and Mayo Clinic *(7,12,13)* have also delineated peripheral nerve as the primary dose-limiting structure for IOERT. The anatomic location of peripheral nerves often makes it adjacent to or involved by tumor. Even when uninvolved, it is usually impossible to move or shield nerve from the IOERT field.

3.1. NCI Clinical Analyses

3.1.1. GENERAL

In an early report from NCI, Sindelar et al. *(10)* reported mild-to-moderate perineural fibrosis in 7 of 22 patients receiving doses of 20–25 Gy. Kinsella et al. *(2)* reported clinically detectable neuropathy with loss of sensory and motor function in five patients after 20–25 Gy of IOERT. Clinical evidence of neuropathies developed 6–9 mo or later after IOERT.

3.1.2. SARCOMA

NCI conducted a randomized trial from 1980 to 1985 in which 35 patients with retroperitoneal sarcomas were randomized to receive EBRT with or without IOERT *(12)*. All patients had primary lesions; none had prior EBRT or chemotherapy. All had gross total resection, but most had microscopic residual after maximal resection. Patients randomized to EBRT alone received 35–40 Gy to an extended field over 4–5 wk and an additional 15 Gy over 2 wk to a reduced field. The IOERT group received 35–40 Gy in 4–5 wk to an extended field and an IOERT dose of 20 Gy to abutting fields (2–6 abutting fields) plus IV misonidazole. Local control (infield) and small bowel tolerance, both acute and chronic, were statistically better in the IOERT plus EBRT patients ($p < 0.001, < 0.01$, and < 0.05, respectively).

Treatment tolerance, including peripheral neuropathy, was analyzed as a function of treatment method. Neuropathy of any severity was seen in only 1 of 20 patients treated with postoperative EBRT alone vs 9 of 15 treated with IOERT plus postoperative EBRT.

Table 3
Clinical Peripheral Neuropathy Characteristics with Pelvic IOERT, Mayo

Characteristic	Incidence[a]		Severity				Time course (months from IOERT)			
			Mild/mod		Severe		Onset		Resolution	
							Range	Median	Resolved	Range
	No.	%	No.	%	No.	%			No.	%	
Pain	16/50	32	13	26	3	6	1/2–18	15	6/14	42[a]	5–32[c]
Motor	8/50	16	6	12	2	4	3–22	7	1/8	13	20
Sensory	11/50	22	11	22		0	3–22	7	4/11	36	1,7,19,20

[a] 1 patient excluded who died postoperatively.
[b] 2 patients excluded who were lost to follow-up.
[c] Median 15 mo.
Modified from ref. 7.

Seven of 15 patients (47%) with IOERT as a component of treatment had moderate or severe neuropathy vs 0 of 20 with EBRT alone ($p < 0.01$).

3.2. Mayo Clinic Patient Analyses

3.2.1. PELVIC MALIGNANCIES

An initial analysis of nerve and ureteral tolerance with IOERT was published on 51 patients who received IOERT at Mayo as a component of treatment for the management of primary or recurrent pelvic malignancies, initially unresectable for cure (Table 3) (7). Curative surgical alternatives did not exist, or necessitated extensive procedures. Treatment consisted of EBRT (median 50.4 Gy), maximal resection when feasible, and an IOERT boost (range 10–25 Gy) utilizing 9- to 18-MeV electrons. Fifty of the 51 patients were eligible for peripheral neurotoxicity analysis. Complications were scored prospectively on a grade 1–4 basis utilizing criterion developed by the NCI IORT contract group which included NCI, MGH, Howard University, and Mayo Clinic investigators (15,16). Sixteen of the 50 patients (32%) developed grade 1–3 peripheral neuropathy (unilateral pelvic or extremity pain, leg weakness, numbness, or tingling). Pain was severe (grade 3) in only 3 (6%). In the two patients with severe weakness (grade 3), the surgical option for cure was hemipelvectomy and hemicorporectomy. Neuropathy incidence by IOERT location was pelvic sidewall—15 of 32 (47%), presacrum—1 of 12 (8%), central pelvis—0 of 6.

Many patients who are candidates for IOERT present with pain from recurrent tumors caused by neurologic tumor compression or invasion. Whereas all patients are given an informed consent about possible nerve-related side effects, they are aware that with uncontrolled tumor they will often have similar side effects.

3.2.2. COLORECTAL CANCER—GENERAL

In recent Mayo Clinic analyses of IOERT regimens in 178 patients with locally advanced, previously unirradiated, primary (55 evaluable patients) or locally recurrent (123 patients) colorectal cancer (12,13), tolerance data suggests a relationship between IOERT dose and the incidence of grade 2 or 3 neuropathy (Table 4; EBRT factors appeared constant). This trend is consistent with animal data that suggest a correlation

Table 4
Colorectal IOERT, Mayo—IOERT Dose vs Neuropathy

| Disease Presentation | (Ref) | IOERT Dose vs Incidence of Neuropathy (GR 2[a] or 3) | | | | |
| | | ≤12.5 Gy | | ≥15 Gy | | |
		No.	(%)	No.	(%)	P value
Primary[b]	7	1/29	(3)	6/28	(21)	0.03
Recurrent, No Prior EBRT[c]	8	2/29	(7)	19/101	(19)	0.12
Primary + Recurrent		3/58	(5)	25/129	(19)	0.01

[a]Grade 2 neuropathy usually manifest as pain requiring narcotics.
[b]57 IOERT fields in 55 evaluable patients.
[c]130 IOERT fields in 123 patients.

between IOERT dose and the incidence of clinical and electrophysiologic neuropathy in dogs *(3,4,9,10)*. The incidence of grade 3 neuropathy was approx 5% in both primary and locally recurrent patients and the incidence of grade 1–3 neuropathy was approx 32% as in the initial Mayo tolerance analysis by Shaw et al. *(7)* that included noncolorectal plus colorectal sites.

3.2.3. PRIMARY COLORECTAL

In the primary colorectal IOERT analysis from Mayo, symptomatic or objective neuropathy was documented in 18 of 55 evaluable patients or 32% (10 of 18 or 56% had only grade 1 toxicity, usually manifesting as mild or intermittent paresthesia and/or pain not requiring narcotics). Severe neuropathy (grade 3) was documented in only 3 of 55 patients or 5.5%. IOERT factors in the three patients were as follows: dose of 15, 20, and 20 Gy; field size 7.0, 7.5, and 7.5 cm; energy 9, 12, and 18 MeV. One of the three had only microscopic residual disease after resection but received an IOERT dose of 20 Gy since the fractionated EBRT dose was limited to 16.2 Gy in nine fractions because of prior pelvic EBRT in 1966 for a cervix malignancy.

Grade 2 or 3 nerve toxicity was analyzed as a function of disease status and treatment factors (EBRT dose; IOERT dose, field size, and energy; and amount of residual at time of IOERT after maximal resection). Seven of the eight patients with grade 2 or 3 toxicity remained continuously free of disease within irradiation fields, which suggests that their neuropathy was treatment-related. The remaining patient had a $6 \times 5 \times 4$-cm nodal mass that could not be resected after preoperative EBRT of 50.4 Gy in 28 fractions over 5.5 wk. An IOERT dose of 20 Gy was given with 18-MeV electrons, and the patient died 14 mo from initiation of treatment with disease persistence or relapse within EBRT and IOERT fields. In the five patients with grade 2 neuropathy, most had pain requiring narcotics.

Of the seven patients with presumed treatment-related grade 2 or 3 nerve toxicity, incidence vs IOERT dose was as follows—57 fields in 55 patients (Table 5): 1 of 29 (3%) with dose ≤12.5 Gy, 4 of 19 (21%) with dose of 15 or 17.5 Gy, and 2 of 9 (22%) with dose ≥20 Gy (6 of 28 fields or 21%, 6 of 26 patients or 23% incidence with IOERT dose ≥15 Gy; both ≥20 Gy patients had a grade 3 neuropathy). This data suggests a relationship between IOERT dose and the incidence of grade 2 or 3 neuropathy (≤12.5 Gy, 1 of 29 or 3%, ≥15 Gy, 6 of 26 or 23%, $p = 0.03$). Of the five patients with grade 2 intolerance, one received 20 Gy for gross residual ($5 \times 4 \times 1.5$ cm), three received 15 Gy (negative margins—2, microscopic residual—1), and one received 12.5 Gy (negative margins).

Table 5
Primary Colorectal IOERT, Mayo—IOERT Dose vs Grade 2 and/or 3 Neuropathy

IOERT Dose (Gy)	Grade 2[a] or 3 Neuropathy		Grade 3 Neuropathy	
	No.	%	No.	%
≤12.5	1/29	3[b]	0/29	0
15 or 17.5	4/19	21	1/19	5
≥20	2/9	22	2/9	22
Total	7/57[c]		3/57[c]	

[a]Grade 2 neuropathy usually defined as pain requiring narcotics.
[b]P value, log rank = 0.03 with ≤12.5 vs ≥15 Gy for grade 2 or 3 neuropathy.
[c]Grade 3 neuropathy in 3 of 55 evaluable patients (5.5%) treated with 57 IOERT fields.
Modified from ref. 12.

The relative incidence of grade 3 neuropathy by IOERT dose was 0 of 29 for ≤12.5 Gy, 1 of 19 (5%) for 15 or 17.5 Gy, and 2 of 9 (22%) for ≥20 Gy (Table 5).

3.2.4. RECURRENT COLORECTAL

In the recurrent colorectal Mayo Clinic IOERT analysis, symptomatic or objective neuropathy was documented in 42 of 123 patients or 34% (21 of the 42 or 50% had only grade 1 toxicity usually manifesting as mild or intermittent paresthesia and/or pain not requiring narcotics). Severe neuropathy (grade 3) was documented in only 7 of 123 patients or 6%. Two of the seven had local relapse as a potential cause of their neuropathy (IOERT doses of 15 and 20 Gy). IOERT factors in the seven patients included a dose of 15 Gy in three and 20 Gy in four. Three of the seven had microscopic residual disease after maximal resection. Two of the three received 15 Gy but the other received an IOERT dose of 20 Gy for uncertain reasons.

Grade 2 or 3 nerve toxicity was analyzed as a function of disease status and treatment factors (EBRT dose; IOERT dose, field size, and energy; amount of residual at time of IOERT after maximal resection). All of the 14 patients with grade 2 toxicity had remained continuously free of disease within irradiation fields, which suggests that their neuropathy was treatment-related. Incidence of grade 2 or 3 nerve toxicity by IOERT dose was as follows for 130 fields in 123 patients: 2/29 (7%) with dose ≤12.5 Gy and 19/101 or 19% incidence with IOERT dose ≥15 Gy ($p = 0.12$) (Table 4).

4. SUMMARY AND FUTURE POSSIBILITIES

The issue of treatment-related morbidity following aggressive therapy in patients with locally advanced pelvic malignancies is placed into clearer perspective by a consideration of the potential morbidity associated with locally persistent or locally recurrent tumor. When EBRT is used as the main treatment modality for patients with locally advanced primary rectal cancer, the great majority will experience local tumor progression and die within 2 to 3 yr. In the analysis by Schild and colleagues from Mayo (17), for example, the use of EBRT without IOERT following incomplete resection of rectal cancer was associated with a high rate of pelvic relapse (76%) and a 5-yr survival of only 24%. The potential for significant cancer-related morbidity in patients with local tumor persistence or relapse is very significant. Whereas a scientific comparison of morbidity with and without IOERT has not been performed, it is important that patients be informed of the potential for *both* treatment and tumor-related morbidity when obtaining informed consent prior to IOERT. When obtaining informed consent for IOERT in patients with recurrent colorectal cancers, the potential for IOERT-related symptomatic neuropathy must be balanced against the likelihood that local persistence or relapse will result in tumor-related pain. Since many patients with locally recurrent colorectal cancers have moderate or severe pain at the time of presentation, they can usually accept the possibility of temporary pain related to treatment as an alternative to permanent tumor-related pain. Symptomatic pain relief is usually of short duration when EBRT without IOERT is used as the main treatment modality, and >90% of patients have local persistence or progression of disease (most patients are dead by 2 to 3 yr, and 5-yr survival is unusual).

On the basis of both human and animal data, when a full component of irradiation options exists (i.e., can deliver 45–55 Gy of fractionated EBRT), an IOERT dose range of 10–20 Gy should continue to be used for patients with primary colorectal cancer, as determined by the amount of tumor remaining after maximal resection. In patients with gross total resection and microscopic residual disease, the usual IOERT dose of 10–12.5 Gy appears to be quite appropriate. The rate of local failure and grade 2 or 3 neuropathy were both ≤5% in the 56 Mayo IOERT patients with locally advanced primary colorectal cancers.

When a full component of irradiation options exists in patients with locally recurrent colorectal cancers, IOERT doses of 10–20 Gy are again reasonable and are dependent on the amount of tumor remaining after maximal surgical resection. For patients with local recurrence in a previous surgical bed, IOERT doses have often ranged from 15 to 20 Gy, with IOERT doses of 10 and 12.5 Gy used less frequently, even after gross total resection, because of concerns about hypoxia. However, in view of the suggestion of a lower incidence of grade 2 or 3 neuropathy with IOERT doses ≤12.5 Gy, an IOERT dose of 12.5 Gy would be a reasonable compromise instead of a dose of 15 Gy after gross total resection in a patient with locally recurrent disease. If effective local dose modifiers are identified (sensitizers, hyperthermia), it may be possible to use lower IOERT doses combined with dose modifiers in attempts to overcome hypoxic effects of a postsurgical bed. An alternative approach is to evaluate the use of a radiation protector such as Amifostine *(18)* prior to IOERT for patients in whom doses of 15–20 Gy (or higher in patients with prior EBRT) are indicated for unresectable or gross residual disease.

REFERENCES

1. Georgiou A, Grigsby PW, and Perez CA. Radiation-induced lumbosacral plexopathy in gynecologic tumors: clinical findings and dosimetric analysis, *Int. J. Radiat. Oncol. Biol. Phys.*, **26** (1993) 479–482.
2. Kinsella TJ, Sindelar WF, Deluca AM, et al. Tolerance of peripheral nerve to intraoperative radiotherapy (IORT): clinical and experimental studies, *Int. J. Radiat. Oncol. Biol. Phys.*, **11** (1985) 1579–1585.
3. Kinsella TJ, Deluca AM, Barnes M, Anderson W, Terrill R, and Sindelar WF. Threshold dose for peripheral neuropathy following intraoperative radiotherapy (IORT) in a large animal model, *Int. J. Radiat. Oncol. Biol. Phys.*, **20** (1991) 697–701.
4. LeCouteur RA, Gillette EL, Powers EL, Child G, McChesney SL, and Ingram JT. Peripheral neuropathies following experimental intraoperative radiation therapy (IORT), *Int. J. Radiat. Oncol. Biol. Phys.*, **17** (1989) 583–590.
5. Vujaskovic Z, Gillette SM, Powers BE, et al. Intraoperative radiation (IORT) injury to sciatic nerve in a large animal model, *Radiother. Oncol.*, **30** (1994) 133–139.
6. Bentzen SM, Turesson I, and Thames HD. Fractionation sensitivity and latency of telangiectasia after post-mastectomy radiotherapy: a graded-response analysis, *Radiother. Oncol.*, **18** (1990) 95–106.
7. Shaw EG, Gunderson LL, Martin JK, Beart RW, Nagorney DM, and Podratz KC. Peripheral nerve and ureteral tolerance to intraoperative radiation therapy: clinical and dose-response analysis, *Radiother. Oncol.*, **18** (1990) 247–255.

8. Vujaskovic Z, Gillette SM, Powers BE, et al. Effects of intraoperative irradiation and intraoperative hyperthermia on canine sciatic nerve: neurologic and electrophysiologic study, *Int. J. Radiat. Oncol. Biol. Phys.,* **34** (1996) 125–131.

9. Gillete EL, Gillette SM, Vujaskovic Z, et al. Influence of volume on canine ureters and peripheral nerves irradiated intraoperatively. In Schildberg FW, Willich N, and Krämling H (eds.). *Intraoperative Radiation Therapy—Proceedings 4th International IORT Symposium,* Munich, 1992, Essen. Verlag Die Blaue Eule, 1993, pp. 61–63.

10. Sindelar WF, Hoekstra H, Restrepo C, and Kinsella TJ. Pathological tissue changes following intraoperative radiotherapy, *Am. J. Clin. Oncol.,* **9** (1986) 504–509.

11. Johnstone PA, Sindelar WF, and Kinsella TJ. Experimental and clinical studies of intraoperative radiation therapy, *Curr. Probl. Cancer,* **18** (1994) 249–292.

12. Sindelar WF, Kinsella TJ, Chen PW, et al. Intraoperative radiotherapy in retroperitoneal sarcomas: final results of a prospective, randomized trial, *Arch. Surg.,* **128** (1993) 402–410.

13. Gunderson LL, Nelson H, Martenson J, et al. Locally advanced primary colorectal cancer—intraoperative electron and external beam irradiation ± 5-FU, *Int. J. Radiat. Oncol. Biol. Phys.,* **37** (1997) 601–614.

14. Gunderson LL, Nelson H, Martenson J, et al. Intraoperative electron and external beam irradiation ± 5-FU and maximal surgical resection for previously unirradiated locally recurrent colorectal cancer, *Dis. Colon Rectum,* **39** (1996) 1379–1395.

15. Tepper JE, Gunderson LL, Goldson AL, et al. Quality control parameters of intraoperative irradiation, *Int. J. Radiation Oncol. Biol. Phys.,* **12** (1986) 1687–1695.

16. Tepper JE, Gunderson LL, Orlow E, et al. Complications of intraoperative radiation therapy, *Int. J. Radiat. Oncol. Biol. Phys.,* **10** (1984) 1831–1839.

17. Schild SE, Martenson JA, Gunderson LL, and Dozois RR. Long-term survival and patterns of failure after postoperative radiation therapy for subtotally resected rectal adenocarcinoma, *Int. J. Radiat. Oncol. Biol. Phys.,* **16** (1989) 459–463.

18. Peters GJ and VanderVijgh WJF. Protection of normal tissue from the cytotoxic effects of chemotherapy and radiation by amifostine (WR-2721): preclinical aspects, *Eur. J. Cancer,* **31A(Suppl 1)** (1995) 51–57.

IV RESULTS OF IORT WITH OR WITHOUT EBRT BY DISEASE SITE

11 Gastric IORT With or Without EBRT

Rafael Martinez-Monge, Jean P. Gerard,
H. J. Kramling, F. Guillemin, and Felipe A. Calvo

Contents

1. INTRODUCTION

1.1. Epidemiology

Gastric cancer has experienced a marked change in prevalence during the last decades. Although in some countries, as in the Far East, gastric cancer continues to be a national health problem, the incidence in most Western countries is decreasing. Most importantly, whereas the overall incidence of gastric cancer has decreased in Europe and the United States, there has been an increase in the relative percentage of proximal gastric adenocarcinomas and adenocarcinomas arising in the gastroesophageal junction. With the exception of Japan, where mass screening programs have increased the number of patients diagnosed of early gastric cancer, diagnosis at an advanced stage is the rule. Approximately 50–75% of the patients who have gastric resection for cancer have serosal invasion and/or lymph node involvement. This helps to explain why cure rates have remained unchanged for decades in spite of improvements in oncologic therapy. Investigators should consider that both accrual and design of future trials in gastric cancer will probably be affected by these epidemiological trends.

1.2. Staging: AJCC vs JSSS

Japanese intraoperative radiation therapy (IORT) trials for gastric cancer *(1,2)* are reported according to the criteria of the Japanese Surgical Staging System (JSSS) *(3)*. The JSSS and the American Joint Committee for Cancer Staging Classification (AJCC) *(4)*, used in the Western countries, differ substantially. For that reason, results for Japanese and Western IORT trials are not truly comparable. A comparison of the JSSS and the

From: *Current Clinical Oncology: Intraoperative Irradiation: Techniques and Results*
Edited by: L. L. Gunderson et al. © Humana Press, Inc., Totowa, NJ

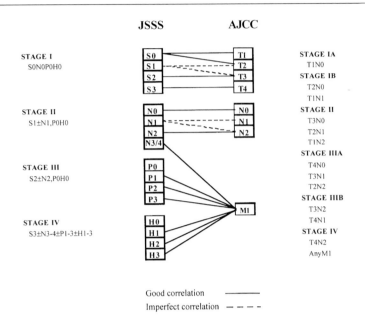

Fig. 1. Correlation between the Japanese Surgical Staging System (JPSS) and the AJCC staging system.

AJCC staging is provided to allow an easier comparison throughout the text (Fig. 1). This comparison contains important flaws, especially in the categorization of Japanese S1 (suspected serosal invasion) which is nonexistent in the AJCC staging and in the equivalence of nodal involvement for both staging systems.

1.3. Surgical Management of Gastric Cancer

Radical surgery remains the only curative option for gastric cancer. Although no randomized trials are available to define the optimal extent of surgery for each disease stage, subtotal gastrectomy with R2 lymphadenectomy is a reasonable alternative for most patients, especially those with distal lesions. Conversely, proximal tumors do functionally better with total gastrectomy and this approach is therefore recommended.

The extent of lymph node dissection is controversial. In general, it varies from limited R2 dissection in Western countries to radical R2 dissection in Japan. This different approach in the treatment of the nodal involvement of gastric cancer has been used to justify the markedly better results reported by Japanese authors. However, it seems that such an extensive nodal dissection is beneficial only to patients with intermediate-stage gastric cancer, with disease involving entire-wall thickness without invading surrounding organs and/or nodal involvement limited to the N1/N2 levels *(15)*. Separate randomized studies from Britain *(6)* and the Netherlands *(7,8)* have not demonstrated survival benefit for routine extended lymphadenectomy to date, but have demonstrated increased morbidity from the more aggressive approach.

1.4. Natural History/Patterns of Failure

1.4.1. After Surgery

Cure rates for resected but high-risk gastric cancer (serosal and/or lymph node involvement) in Western countries have remained uniformly poor for years. This can be

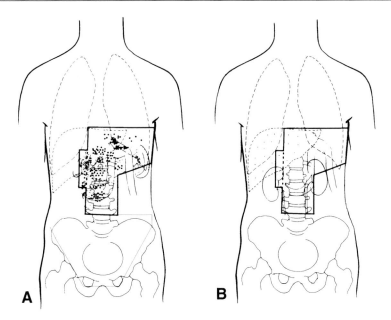

Fig. 2. Patterns of relapse in the University of Minnesota Reoperation Series with superimposed irradiation fields (modified from Gunderson and Sosin, Ref. 11). (**A**) Local regional relapse—tumor bed (●); nodal (o). (**B**) Distant metastases to liver (+) or lung (*); idealized fields superimposed over kidneys.

explained by the inability of surgery to completely eradicate the microscopic component of technically resectable cancers and the inefficacy of chemotherapy and/or radiotherapy as single adjuvants in the adjuvant setting. Nodal involvement and serosal invasion are the two more important prognostic indicators for localized gastric cancer. In Western countries, only patients whose gastric cancer is confined to the gastric wall without invading the serosa can expect cure rates in excess of 50% (9). If, in addition, AJCC N1/N2 involvement occurs (9,10), the survival rates drop to 10–20%.

Survival results of Japanese surgical series appear superior to Western results in some specific disease stages. Noguchi, in a retrospective review of 7220 patients operated for gastric cancer in the Cancer Institute Hospital, Japan between 1949 and 1979, reported a 5-yr survival of 53% for JSSS N1, 26% for JSSS N2, 10% for JSSS N3, and 4% for JSSS N4 (10). The two latter N categories of the JSSS are considered M1 in the AJCC staging system (Fig. 1).

Gunderson and Sosin (11) in their report of the University of Minnesota reoperative series demonstrated that truly complete resection of high-risk resected gastric cancers is difficult to achieve. In this study, 107 patients previously operated with "curative resections" for gastric cancer underwent programmed exploratory laparotomy (at 6–12 mo after the previous surgery, 68 patients) or reoperation because of the development of symptoms suspicious of disease progression (39 patients). In the 105 patients evaluable for relapse patterns, the surgical pathology findings indicated recurrent or persistent tumor in loco-regional areas in 70 patients (88% of the 80 patients who relapsed or 67% of the patients at risk) (Fig. 2). The rate of loco-regional relapse increased by stage, with 43 out of 49 stage C2/C3 patients who developed disease progression relapsing in loco-regional sites. Loco-regional failure was the only manifestation of relapse in 24 patients (29% of those with relapse). Loco-regional sites included the gastric bed in 55% of the cases, regional lymph nodes in 43%, anastomosis/gastric stump in 27%, and other in 5%. The loco-regional relapses were located in more than one site in 60% of patients and were contained in one site in 38%.

These findings were reproduced in an autopsy analysis by Wisbeck et al. *(12)*. In this series, 38 patients with gastric cancer initially confined to the stomach (16 resected, 22 unresectable) were autopsied. Failure in loco-regional sites was observed in 94% of the 16 patients with resected tumors.

However, when patterns of failure are documented by only clinical means, the reported figures are lower than those of reoperative or necropsy series. Landry and Tepper *(9)*, reporting the Massachusetts General Hospital experience on the patterns of failure of completely resected gastric cancer, described an overall loco-regional failure rate in 38% of the 130 patients at risk. In this series, patients were not routinely autopsied, but the failures observed were histologically documented in 69% of the cases.

1.4.2. AFTER SURGERY AND POSTOP EBRT WITH OR WITHOUT CHEMOTHERAPY

Loco-regional relapse rates in series using postoperative external-beam radiation therapy (EBRT) with or without chemotherapy for advanced gastric cancer are in the 8–54% range *(13–20)*. However, when the results of postoperative EBRT have been verified by postmortem examination or laparotomy, a loco-regional recurrence rate as high as 92% has been reported in a National Cancer Institute (NCI) trial *(21)*. Martinez-Monge, University of Navarre *(15)* reported a 20% loco-regional relapse rate in a series of 35 patients with serosal and/or nodal involvement treated with surgery and postoperative EBRT to 45 Gy. The analysis was performed on a clinical basis. The surviving patients were followed up for a median of 7.5 yr, so these results can be rendered as definitive. This discrepancy can be in part explained by the definition of loco-regional sites used in the NCI trial. Loco-regional was censored if relapse occurred in the abdomen, retroperitoneum, thorax, or peritoneal surfaces.

1.4.3. CONCLUSIONS

The reoperation/autopsy series reported by Gunderson and Sosin provided a profound insight in the understanding of patterns of failure for gastric cancer. However, although the population that could benefit from local adjuvant therapy (those patients with isolated loco-regional recurrences, easily encompassable in a tolerable radiation port) ranges from 20 to 30%, single adjuvant studies have failed to improve survival. There are several possible explanations for this finding. First, the areas of failure reported by Gunderson and Sosin may well represent only obvious tumor burden, but not the actual extent of the disease relapse. If the entire tumor burden was located in these areas, an improved loco-regional control could translate into increased survival rates. Second, the actual tumor burden left behind after surgical resection might be larger than estimated and would not be, hence, eradicable by tolerable doses of EBRT. IORT added to standard doses of EBRT could play a role in this setting by improving the therapeutic ratio. Third, IORT plus EBRT but without chemotherapy would likely be inadequate because of the risks of hematological or peritoneal metastases.

1.5. Adjuvant Therapy in Gastric Cancer

Adjuvant therapy for gastric cancer is needed based on the failure patterns and survival results. Unlike other gastrointestinal malignancies, however, no adjuvant therapy has been proven to consistently improve survival in resected high-risk gastric cancer.

Single-agent chemotherapy has been shown to produce clinical responses in the range of 20 to 30% for 5-FU, mitomycin C (MMC), or doxorubicin (ADR). Chemotherapy consisting of 5-FU-based combinations with ADR, MMC, VP16 and/or cisplatin (CDDP) has yielded response rates of 15 to 55% (22). Although some reports have indicated improved survival with the use of adjuvant chemotherapy (23), most studies have failed to demonstrate an overall survival advantage (13,23).

Several randomized trials demonstrate that EBRT with or without chemotherapy improves local control in completely resected (13,16), resected but residual (24–28), or unresectable gastric cancer (24–28) when compared to observation or chemotherapy arms. In resected but residual or unresectable disease, EBRT plus 5-FU prolonged survival when compared to either EBRT alone in a Mayo trial (25–27) or 5-FU and methyl CCNU in a Gastrointestinal Tumor Study Group (GITSG) trial (27,28), but was not clearly superior in terms of survival when compared to chemotherapy alone in additional trials by Eastern Cooperative Oncology Group (ECOG) (14) and GITSG (29). Randomized trials on adjuvant EBRT with or without chemotherapy for resected disease have failed to improve overall survival in several series (13,30), although a small percentage of patients with resected but residual disease were cured with chemoirradiation. To some extent, most of the trials of resected patients have included a variable number of patients with microscopic or gross residual disease. For that reason, it is difficult to ascertain from these studies the real value of adjuvant chemoradiation. In a small randomized Mayo Clinic trial of completely resected patients (16,31), those randomized to receive adjuvant postoperative chemoirradiation had improved 5-yr survival compared to those randomized to a surgery alone control arm at 23 vs 4% ($p < 0.05$). Although 10 patients randomized to receive chemoirradiation refused such, patient outcome by treatment received still revealed a survival trend favoring those who had chemoirradiation (20 vs 12%), but the differences were not statistically significant in view of small patient numbers. Hopefully, the unresolved issue of the true value of adjuvant chemoirradiation will be answered by the phase III United States Intergroup trial 0116/SWOG 9008, that compares surgery alone vs postoperative chemoirradiation (EBRT to 45 Gy in 25 fractions combined with 5-FU/leucovorin-based chemotherapy) in completely resected patients.

2. IORT IN GASTRIC CANCER

2.1. Introduction/Historical Overview

Local relapse or disease remaining in the gastric bed and regional nodes after "curative resections" for patients with serosal invasion and/or lymph node involvement is an almost universal event (11,12). For this reason, techniques that improve loco-regional control are needed in the treatment of gastric cancer patients at high risk for local failure. EBRT is effective in decreasing the local failure rate for resected gastric cancer, but its use is limited by the tolerance of upper abdominal tissues to irradiation.

The pioneering work of Abe of Kyoto University, Japan in the 1970s fostered a renewed interest in the old idea of irradiating tumor-bearing areas under direct vision during laparotomy. Abe described the results of irradiating 14 gastric cancer patients with unresectable lymph nodes after gastrectomy and/or lesions invading the pancreas (32). These lesions were irradiated to 30–35 Gy and no toxicity, such as diarrhea, bloody stool, or abdominal pain was reported. Most interestingly, the lymph node metastases that were smaller than 3 cm in diameter were eradicated. A dose of 40 Gy to the unresected primary tumor was not able to eliminate it, although significant clinical regression was noted.

Based on these results, Abe provided guidelines for treating gastric cancer with IORT alone *(33)*: 30–35 Gy may be curative if the tumor volume is smaller than 3 cm in diameter; for clinically undetectable lesions, a dose of 28 Gy may be optimal; 40-Gy single dose is not effective in eliminating large primary unresected tumors.

Although Abe's work triggered gastric IORT trials around the world, only a few investigators have followed the methodological approach proposed by Abe for gastric cancer *(2,34,35)*. Others have used IORT doses considerably lower than those advised by Abe because of fear of undue severe toxicity. This has followed the tendency in the design of IORT trials for other anatomical locations, in which IORT doses were in the 10–20 Gy range, based on the toxicity patterns of animal studies and preliminary human clinical trials. These latter studies have included the delivery of EBRT with or without chemotherapy postoperatively or preoperatively. Whereas this might compromise the total dose delivered by IORT, it was thought that a wider coverage of the stomach bed and surrounding nodal areas would result in a final advantage because of the knowledge of the patterns of local progression for gastric cancer rendered by the reoperation/necropsy studies.

In summary, IORT for gastric cancer has been used after gross or complete macroscopic resection to boost the surgical bed and/or lymph node areas. Some investigators have favored the use of IORT as the only adjuvant therapy after surgery *(1,2,21,33–35)*, whereas most Western trials have incorporated IORT along with EBRT with or without chemotherapy *(36–40)*.

2.2. Methodology

2.2.1. CANDIDATES FOR IORT PROGRAMS

Although some patients with early gastric cancer have been included in IORT trials *(32,37)*, the excellent cure rates obtained with radical surgery alone do not make this group of patients a good candidate to be enrolled into adjuvant programs. The IORT trial from Kyoto University, reported by Abe, revealed no differences in survival for stage I patients treated with or without IORT *(33)*. Other series also include a small group of early disease-stage patients. This can be attributed more to the limitations of the presurgical clinical staging than to the preferences of the investigators. Patients most likely to benefit from the addition of IORT to resection and EBRT (with or without chemotherapy) include those with positive margins of resection but no evidence of hematogenous or peritoneal spread of disease, or with negative but narrow margins of resection and/or involved lymph nodes.

2.2.2. IORT CHARACTERISTICS

2.2.2.1. Equipment and IORT Target Volume. Most of the research institutions in which gastric IORT trials have been generated have used electron beams generated in linear accelerators. However, there are major differences regarding the technology used. Both docking and nondocking applicators have been used. IORT has been delivered through circular *(36,37)*, pentagonal *(32,35)*, or customized applicators *(2)*. Most institutions have treated a single target volume, whereas others have used multiple abutting fields *(21)*.

A typical IORT target volume for gastric cancer contains the pancreas body and the celiac axis with its branches. Depending on the specific location of the gastric tumor, the head of the pancreas can also be part of the target volume. The distal biliary tract has been usually dissected out to perform the biliary-digestive anastomosis and is not irradiated. Depending on the specific electron-energy selected, the aorta, extrahepatic inferior vena

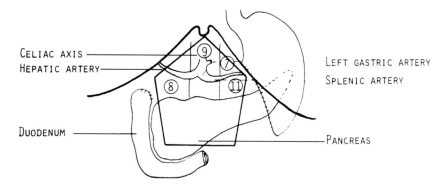

CELIAC AXIS
HEPATIC ARTERY

LEFT GASTRIC ARTERY
SPLENIC ARTERY

DUODENUM

PANCREAS

Fig. 3. Pentagonal IORT field preferred by Abe and colleagues in Kyoto (from Abe et al. Intraoperative radiotherapy of gastric cancer. *Cancer* **34**:2034–2041, 1974, with permission).

Table 1
Technical Characteristics in IORT Trials for Gastric Cancer

Author/Institution	Ref No.	Applicator Shape	Energy	Applicator Size
Abe/Kyoto Univ.	(1,32,33)	Pentagonal	Custom[a]	—
Ogata/Kochi Med. S.	(2)	Lead-shaped	12 MeV	—
Calvo/Univ Navarre	(37)	Circular/elliptical	9–12 MeV	6–9 cm
Sindelar/NCI	(21)	Multiple abutting fields (2–4)	11–15 MeV	—
Coquard/Lyon	(40)	Circular	12 MeV	9 cm (median)
Kramling/Munich[b]	(35)	Pentagonal/circular	—	—
Avizonis/RTOG	(36)	Circular	—	7.5 cm (median)

[a]That which encompasses the target volume thickness within the 90% isodose line.
[b]Abstract information.
 Univ. = University; Med. S. = Medical School; NCI = National Cancer Institute; RTOG = Radiation Therapy Oncology Group.

cava, and the anterior bodies of the underlying T11-L1 vertebrae (anatomical variability exists) are irradiated.

Abe *(1)* recommended the IORT applicator (pentagonal field) be positioned towards the residual tumor or the high-risk lymph node groups along the common hepatic, left gastric and splenic arteries, and around the celiac axis (Fig. 3). In cases in which the posterior wall of the stomach was grossly adherent to the pancreas, this was included in the field. The electron energy was selected to encompass the tumor volume within the 90% isodose line.

Ogata *(2)* used a custom-shaped cone to conform a pentagonal-hexagonal field with 2-mm lead plates aiding to retract and shield radiation-sensitive organs. After 1992, they developed a new surgical technique that provides mobilization of the body and tail of the pancreas for patients with invasion of the pancreas or metastases to the lymph nodes along the splenic artery. Paraortic nodes can also be included after the mobilization of the body of the pancreas.

In general, most groups have used circular cones *(36,37)* centered around the celiac axis and covering a tumor bed 6–10 cm in diameter. Electron energies usually range from 9 to 12 MeV (Table 1).

Table 2
Radiation Characteristics in IORT Trials for Gastric Cancer

Author/Institution	Ref. No.	IORT Dose	EBRT
Abe/Kyoto Univ	(1,32,33)	28–40 Gy	None
Ogata/Kochi Med S	(2)	28–30 Gy	None
Sindelar/NCI	(21)	20 Gy	None
Kramling/Munich[b]	(35)	28 Gy	None
Farthman/Freiburg	(34)	25–28 Gy	None
Avizonis/RTOG	(36)	12.5–16.5 Gy	45 Gy[c]
Dulce/Berlin[b]	(39)	12–16 Gy	24-38 Gy[a]
Coquard/Lyon	(40)	12–15 Gy	46 Gy[a]
Chambert/CHU Bellevue	(38)	15–20 Gy	28-46 Gy
Calvo/Univ Navarre	(37)	15 Gy	40-46 Gy[c]

[a] Four-field technique.
[b] Abstract information.
[c] Field as derived from Univ. Minnesota reoperation data.

2.2.2.2. Implementation and Design. Whereas the initial trials on IORT for gastric cancer called for high IORT doses as the only adjuvant therapy, most subsequent European and United States trials have chosen to reduce the IORT dose and to incorporate EBRT with or without chemotherapy in the adjuvant setting. General characteristics of IORT trials are displayed in Table 2 with regard to the use of IORT with or without EBRT and dose levels.

2.2.3. EBRT Field Design

EBRT is included in IORT trials on the basis that more than 60% of the loco-regional relapses observed in the University of Minnesota reoperative series were multiple (11). Also, the use of EBRT to cover a wide area in the upper abdomen follows the traditional doctrine of designing the radiation fields to treat uninvolved areas with a high probability of containing microscopic disease. However, compared with other anatomical locations, the experience accumulated with radiation therapy for gastric cancer so far is scarce and the optimal radiation management of gastric cancer is still under development.

Gunderson, through the meticulous mapping of areas of relapse following "curative resection" (11) designed a comprehensive radiation portal for EBRT that has been followed by some (Fig. 2) (36,37). This portal design should be considered with the understanding that isolated loco-regional relapses represent only about one third of all loco-regional relapses, according to the Gunderson and Sosin report (11). IORT alone could be inadequate in covering the whole extent of potential microscopic residual disease with a resultant geographical miss. Although many investigators have begun using Gunderson's portal in the postoperative management of high-risk gastric cancer, this idealized design does not represent the only valid approach. EBRT portals should be designed according to the location of the primary tumor, surgical findings, and known patterns of nodal involvement generated from surgical series. A clear example of the need for site-oriented field design is that for proximal gastric tumors that involve the esophagus, the lymphatic drainage places mediastinal nodes at risk. Wisbeek et al., in a autopsy series of 38 patients operated for gastric adenocarcinoma, demonstrated that 69% of the patients with tumors localized in the gastroesophageal junction suffered relapse in extrabdominal sites *(12)*. Their recommendation was to include the mediastinal nodes in the EBRT fields.

Sindelar et al. reported an NCI randomized trial that compared surgery with or without EBRT vs surgery plus IORT, in which the control-arm patients with stages III and IV disease received postoperative EBRT *(21)*. Treatment was performed with computed tomography (CT) assisted planning and 6–10 MV photon beams, usually arranged in a combination of AP/PA and oblique fields, to a total dose of 50 Gy with 1.5- to 1.8-Gy daily fractionation. No details of the criteria for design of the EBRT portals were given.

Calvo and colleagues used 15 MV photon beams, AP/PA fields, and standard 1.8- to 2.0-Gy daily fractionation to deliver a median total EBRT dose of 46 Gy following an IORT dose of 15 Gy (Fig. 4) *(37)*. The idealized fields of Gunderson were modified according to the tumor location, lymph nodes involved in the resected specimen, and most likely patterns of microscopic spread. The mean effective treatment area at midplane after customized blocking was 238.8 cm^2. This did not differ from a control subset of patients treated only with EBRT, with a mean effective area of 243.8 cm^2 *(15)*.

Most authors reporting gastric IORT series have used standard fractionation and varied portals if they decided to treat with EBRT plus IORT. AP/PA ports have been more commonly used *(36,37)*, although a four-field technique has also been reported *(40)*. A three-field technique described by Caudry *(41)* has been used for EBRT alone.

Unfortunately, whereas the characteristics of the IORT part of the treatment are shown meticulously, the EBRT methodology is either omitted or not reported in detail. Another important characteristic of the combined approach IORT plus EBRT is that some patients assigned to receive postoperative EBRT do not receive such because of postoperative complications, death, or refusal. Moreover, the planned EBRT dose is reduced in some additional patients because of gastrointestinal toxicity or to the emergence of late postoperative complications. In general, only 40–90% of the patients included in IORT trials complete the EBRT course as prescribed *(36–38,40)*.

3. IORT CLINICAL RESULTS

3.1. Survival

3.1.1. SURGERY PLUS IORT

Abe *(32)* reported a randomized study of 211 gastric cancer patients with JSSS stages I–IV randomized to either gastrectomy plus IORT (admission on Friday, 101 patients) or gastrectomy alone (admission on Tuesday, 110 patients). The study was conducted between March, 1974 and March, 1984. IORT was delivered to high-risk (28 Gy) or residual tumor areas (30–35 Gy) in the stomach bed and/or upper abdominal nodes. No EBRT was given. The results were updated in 1988 *(33)* with the patients staged according to gross findings during laparotomy and indicated a 5-yr survival advantage for IORT with stages II, III, and IV (Table 3). However, when the results were further updated according to the microscopic findings *(1)*, the differences observed were less and lacked statistical significance (Table 4). When the same analysis was performed by histological features (serosal invasion, nodal station involved), survival trends favored IORT in patients with serosal invasion (S$^+$) and N2/N3 involvement, although these differences were not statistically significant (Table 5).

Ogata *(2)* reported a study from the Kochi Medical School, Japan with 178 gastric cancer patients, JSSS stages II–IV treated with surgery alone (120 patients) or surgery plus IORT (58 patients) during the time period August, 1983 to July, 1992. The patients

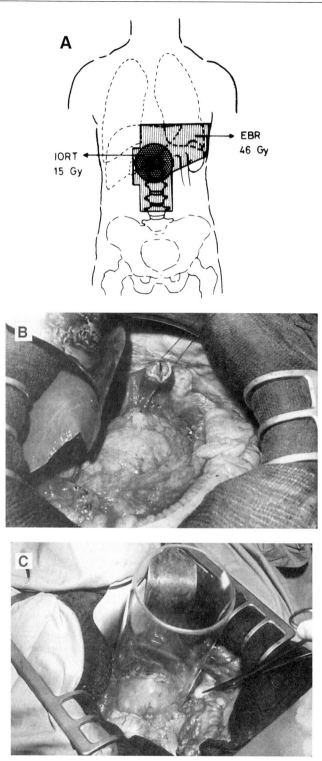

Fig. 4. Integrated program of IOERT (15 Gy) and EBRT (46 Gy) at Pamplona. (**A**) Schematic representation of IOERT plus EBRT (from Calvo, FA, et al. Ref 37, with permission). (**B**) View of tumor bed after resection—note gastric stump with silk suture mobilization superiorly. (**C**) IOERT applicator positioned with visceral structures mobilized from the field.

Table 3
Abe/Kyoto University *(33)*.
Survival Results Based on Gross Histological Findings

| | 5-Yr Survival Rates | |
Surgical Stage	Surgery	Surgery plus IORT
I	93.0%	87.2%
II	61.8%	83.5%
III	36.8%	62.3%
IV[a]	0%	14.7%

[a]In stage IV, patients with peritoneal or visceral metastases were not included (only stage IV H0P0 accepted, mainly patients with direct pancreas invasion, S3 + disease)

Table 4
Abe/Kyoto University *(1)*.
Survival Results Based on Microscopic Histological Findings

| | 5-Yr Cause-Specific Survival Rates | |
Pathological Stage	Surgery Alone	Surgery plus IORT
I	100%	96%
II	66%	78%
III	51%	60%
IV[a]	14%	33%

[a]In stage IV, patients with peritoneal or visceral metastases were not included (only stage IV H0P0 accepted, mainly patients with direct pancreas invasion, S3+ disease).

Table 5
Abe/Kyoto University *(33)*.
Survival Results According to Some Histological Features

| | 5-Yr Cause-Specific Survival Rates | |
Pathology Finding	Surgery Alone	Surgery plus IORT
S-	88.6%	93.8%
S+	50.6%	60.2%
N-	97.4%	100.0%
N1+	67.2%	63.4%
N2/N3+	32.4%	50.8%

S: serosal invasion; N: nodal invasion.

were not randomized. The surgery alone group served as controls. The IORT group presented with more unfavorable features, but the difference was not significant. The results provided by stage demonstrated a slight survival advantage for IORT in stages III and IV that was not statistically significant (Table 6). The best survival advantage for IORT was obtained in stage II patients, but this was not reported to be statistically significant.

Table 6
Ogata/Kochi Medical School Survival Results by Stage

	5-Yr Survival	
Stage	Surgery Alone	Surgery plus IORT
II	63%	100%
III	42%	55%
IV	11%	14%

a Data not contained in journal article and provided through personal communication by the principal author (T.O.).

Chen *(42)* in Beijing reported similar results for stage III gastric cancer treated with IORT. The 5-yr overall survival for the IORT-treated patients was 65% vs only 30% in the surgical group ($p < 0.01$). There was no statistically significant difference in the survival rates for stage IV.

Sindelar *(21)* in an NCI randomized trial, described a 5-yr survival rate of approx 10% for 15 patients with resected gastric cancer stages III–IV treated with radical surgery plus IORT (data not stated in the text and obtained from figures). Median survival time for this subset of patients was 25 mo. There were no differences between the IORT and the EBRT arms regarding survival. The median survival of the 25 patients in the surgery with or without EBRT arm was 21 mo and the 5-yr survival approx 20%. No stage III–IV patient in the control group survived after a median follow-up of 7 yr, whereas 3 out of 15 in the IORT group were alive NED at the time of the analysis ($p = 0.06$).

Finally, two other reports from Germany evaluated the role of gastric surgery plus IORT alone. Farthman *(34)* reported on 36 patients treated with surgery plus IORT 25–28 Gy. The 2-yr overall survival rate was approx 50%. Unfortunately, the characteristics of the patients included in this study are not described in the article. Kramling *(43)* reported a study in which 115 patients with gastric cancer were randomized to IORT or observation. Mean survival time was 26.9 mo for the IORT arm and 30.8 mo for the control group.

3.1.2. Surgery plus IORT plus EBRT

Calvo *(37)* described a 5-yr survival rate of 39% for 48 patients treated with IORT. This study included 16 patients with AJCC stages I–II and 8 patients with anastomotic or nodal recurrences. The percentage of patients with serosal involvement was 70% and 56% had nodal involvement. An update of this series *(15)* included 28 patients with serosal (89%) and/or lymph node involvement (63%), and revealed a 10-yr actuarial overall survival of 38%.

Avizonis *(36)* reported on 27 patients treated with surgery plus IORT of 12.5–16.5 Gy and 45-Gy EBRT. Seventy percent of the patients had AJCC stages III and IV tumors or, similarly, 90% of the patients had JSSS stages III and IV tumors. The 2-yr survival rate was 47% and the 2-yr disease-free survival rate was 27%. Median survival time was 19.3 mo. The 2-yr survival rate for the JSSS stage III patients was 48%.

Coquard *(46)* in a series of 63 patients treated with IORT with or without EBRT in the Centre Hospitalier Lyon, reported a 5-yr overall survival rate of 47%, with a median overall survival of 47 mo. Twenty-eight patients were stages I and II, 29 stages IIIa and

Table 7
Overall Survival in Lyon IOERT Series by Prognostic Factor (40)

Prognostic Factor	12 Months % (#)	24 Months % (#)	60 Months % (#)	p value
Stage				
I	88% (15)	88% (15)	82% (7)	
II	73% (8)	55% (6)	55% (2)	
IIIA	89% (8)	89% (8)	78% (2)	
IIIB	55% (11)	45% (9)	20% (4)	
IV	25% (2)	13% (1)	0%	$p < 0.00001$
pT				
pT1	100% (10)	90% (9)	80% (5)	
pT2	86% (12)	79% (11)	79% (3)	
pT3	58% (20)	52% (17)	32% (7)	
pT4	33% (2)	17% (1)	0%	$p = 0.001$
pN				
pN0	77% (20)	73% (19)	69% (8)	
pN1	100% (5)	100% (5)	100% (2)	
pN2	59% (19)	47% (15)	22% (5)	$p = 0.005$
Residual Disease				
R0	72% (41)	65% (37)	50% (14)	
R1	67% (2)	67% (2)	33% (1)	
R2	33% (1)	0%	0%	$p = 0.04$

IIIb, and 6 patients stage IV. Serosal involvement, with or without adjacent organ invasion (T3 and/or T4) was found in 62% of the cases and N1/N2 nodal involvement in 59%. Most patients were treated surgically with total gastrectomy and proximal (D1) node dissection. A complete resection was performed in 92% of the patients. Thirty patients (48%) received postoperative EBRT through a four-field technique, to a total dose of 44–46 Gy, selected for the patients with poor pathological features in the surgical specimen (serosal and/or nodal involvement). Multivariate analysis demonstrated that the amount of residual disease, TNM stage, pN and pT extent correlated with overall survival (Table 7).

Dulce (39) reported on 26 patients treated with IORT of 12–16 Gy and EBRT of 24–38 Gy. The median survival time for stage III patients was 12 mo. The 2-yr survival rate for stage III patients was 67%.

Chabert (38), CHU Bellevue, reported on 21 patients treated with surgery plus IORT of 15–20 Gy with or without EBRT. Eleven out of 21 patients received EBRT to 28–46 Gy. All but one patient presented with gastric cancer stages II–IV. The 5-yr survival rate was 32% with a median survival time of 19 mo.

3.2. Patterns of Relapse

3.2.1. LOCO-REGIONAL

3.2.1.1. After Surgery plus IORT. Sindelar (21) in an NCI randomized trial, described an overall loco-regional failure rate of 44% for the IORT arm and 92% for the surgery with or without EBRT arm ($p < 0.001$). The time to local failure was longer in the IORT

Table 8
Loco-Regional Failure in IORT Trials for Gastric Cancer

Author/Institution	Ref. No.	IORT Dose	EBRT Dose/% Treated	LRF
Sindelar/NCI[a]	(21)	20 Gy	None	44%
Calvo/Univ Navarre	(37)	15 Gy	46 Gy/89%	10%
Martinez-Monge/Univ Navarre[b]	(15)	15 Gy	46 Gy/100%	11%
Avizonis/RTOG	(36)	12.5–16.5 Gy	45 Gy/85%	37%
Coquard/Lyon	(40)	12–23 Gy	44-46 Gy/48%	24%
Chambert/CHU Bellevue	(38)	15–20 Gy	28-46 Gy/52%	33%

LRF: Loco-regional failure; EBRT: percentage of patients treated with adjuvant external beam radiation therapy.
[a]Nonstandard criteria for definition of loco-regional failure.
[b]Only stages B2 through C3 who completed the radiation course were included.

arm (25 vs 18 mo), but this difference was not significant. However, the time to overall failure was longer in the EBRT arm (16 vs 12 mo) with the differences again lacking statistical significance. The incidence of tumor-bed recurrence was lower in the IORT group, 31 vs 80%. These authors considered loco-regional failures those occurring in the abdomen, retroperitoneum, thorax, and peritoneal surfaces. All relapses were verified by biopsy or laparotomy and all patients who died were autopsied unless a complete verification of the actual extension of the recurrent disease had been carried out within the previous 3 mo. Three noncancer-related deaths in the IORT group at 1, 5, and 32 mo were censored as free of local failure. However, even if these patients had ultimately relapsed, the advantage for the IORT arm would remain considerable (Table 8).

3.2.1.2. After Surgery plus IORT With or Without EBRT. Calvo (37) described a loco-regional failure rate of 10% of 48 patients included in the series at the University of Navarre. This report describes the whole institutional experience, including 16 patients with AJCC tumor stages I–II and 8 patients with recurrent disease (4 anastomotic, 4 nodal). Martinez-Monge (15) updating the previous series for only 28 patients with serosal and/or nodal involvement and treated homogeneously with 15-Gy IORT and EBRT of 40–46 Gy, reproduced the same results with a loco-regional failure rate of 11% projected at 10 yr.

The RTOG trial 85-04 (36) reported a local failure rate of 37% (isolated 15%, combined 22%). The relapses were documented mainly clinically. In this series, 70% of the patients had AJCC stages III and IV. Local failure appeared in 43% of the patients with serosal involvement, in 42% of the node-positive patients and in 63% of the patients presenting with linitis plastica.

Farthman, in a preliminary study at Freiburg University (34), described only one case of local failure among 14 patients dead with disease in a series of 36 patients. Treatment was surgery plus IORT of 25–28 Gy.

Chabert (38), reporting the experience of the CHU Bellevue in the treatment of resected gastric cancer, described a local failure rate of 33%. Patients were treated with surgical resection plus IORT of 15–20 Gy with or without EBRT to 28–46 Gy.

Coquard (40) recently published a series of 63 patients treated with IORT with or without EBRT in the Centre Hospitalier Lyon Sud. The 5-yr local failure rate was 24% and this was not improved with the addition of selective EBRT in patients with the high-risk pathological features of serosal and/or nodal involvement (62% of patients had serosal involvement [T3 or T4] and 59% had N1 or N2 nodal involvement).

3.2.2. Distant Failure

Calvo *(37)* described a rate of distant metastases of 32% (peritoneal carcinomata was included under distant metastases) in a series of 48 patients treated with IORT in the University of Navarre. Martinez-Monge, in an update of the former study reported a distant hematogenous metastases rate of 18.5% and an incidence of peritoneal metastases of 26%. Avizonis reported distant metastases in 48% of the patients (isolated 26%, combined 22%).

Farthman, at Freiburg University *(34)*, described distant metastases and peritoneal dissemination as the main pattern of failure in a series of 36 patients treated with surgery plus IORT of 25–28 Gy. In this series, 13 of 14 patients who died of disease and 2 among 21 alive at the time of analysis had distant and/or peritoneal failure.

Coquard *(40)* reported a 24% incidence of distant metastases in a series of 63 patients treated with IORT with or without EBRT. Thirteen percent of the patients developed peritoneal carcinomata and 11 % developed visceral metastases.

3.3. Preclinical Tolerance Studies

3.3.1. Pancreatic Function

Ahmadu-Suka et al. *(44,45)* described a experiment in which the pancreas and duodenum of beagle dogs were treated with IORT doses of 17.5–40 Gy. Fractionated EBRT was added postoperatively to 50 Gy. Only one dog experienced exocrine pancreatic insufficiency at an IORT dose of 25 Gy. On light microscopy, the number of surviving acinar cells and the degree of pancreatic fibrosis was proportional to the IORT dose.

Heijmans *(46)* described an experimental protocol in which beagle dogs were irradiated with IORT doses of 25, 30, or 35 Gy to the upper abdominal structures. Applicators of 6 to 7 cm in diameter were used with 6- to 8-MeV electron beams. The irradiated structures included the pancreas and the medial wall of the duodenum. Two out of 15 dogs developed toxicity (13%). One had a common bile duct stenosis and the other an enterocolic fistula after 8 and 18 mo follow-up, respectively. No dog developed exocrine insufficiency, diabetes, or pancreatitis. However, subclinical diabetes, manifested by decreased insulin plasma levels and lowered glucose clearance rates, was detected in the dogs irradiated at 30- and 35-Gy IORT ($P = 0.05$) without significant alterations at 25 Gy.

3.3.2. Vascular Tolerance

Johnstone and colleagues *(47)*, reported an NCI study in which 30 dogs were treated with IORT doses of 0–30 Gy immediately after segmental resection of the infrarrenal aorta followed by reconstruction with a prosthetic graft. Half of the dogs received EBRT to 36 Gy. Anastomotic stenosis was observed in most of the animals followed for more than 6 mo. This was correlated with the IORT dose. At an IORT dose of 20 Gy, 3 out of 14 animals developed graft occlusion, whereas at IORT doses of 25 or 30 Gy, five out of six dogs developed late graft occlusion.

Tepper and colleagues *(48)* studied the effect of IORT on aortic anastomoses in dogs. Animals were irradiated with IORT doses of 20, 30, and 45 Gy. There was no evidence of suture-line weakening, regardless of the IORT dose used, but some dogs developed anastomosis obstruction and arterio-venous fistula with IORT doses of between 20- and 45-Gy IORT during the first year of follow-up.

Gillette et al. *(49)* at University of Colorado, studied the response of intact aorta and its branches to IORT, EBRT, or combined IORT and EBRT. IORT doses were from 10 to 47.5 Gy when combined with 50-Gy EBRT (25 fractions/5 wk) and from 17.5–47.5

Gy when delivered alone. Dogs treated with EBRT alone received fractionated EBRT (2–2.67 Gy/fraction) to 60–80 Gy total dose in 6 wk. At 2 yr, there was a high frequency of arteritis and necrosis of the media of branch arteries (only rarely obstructed) at IORT of 20 Gy or IORT of 15 Gy plus 50-Gy EBRT. The ED_{50} for obstruction greater than 50% of the lumen at 5 yr was 24.8 Gy for IORT alone or 19.4 Gy if IORT was combined with 50 Gy EBRT.

3.3.3. GASTRIC MUCOSA TOLERANCE AND GASTRIC-WALL HEALING

Kramling (43) reported the tolerance of gastric mucosa to EBRT using a rabbit model in which animals received IORT to the celiac axis of 0–40 Gy. This was followed by EBRT to 32–52 Gy in 4-Gy fractions. The authors reported an earlier development of gastric ulcers with EBRT in the animals previously treated with IORT. They concluded that IORT to the celiac axis probably produced a reduction in the blood flow of abdominal organs that decreased the tolerance to EBRT.

Grab (50), using the same model, reported the dynamics of wound repair in the stomach of rabbits treated with IORT plus EBRT. At the time of surgery plus IORT, the rabbits underwent full-thickness incision and per prima suture. The success of wound healing was measured using as end points the wound-breaking strength and the collagen types I and III content. All the parameters were found to be lower in the IORT-treated rabbits. The authors concluded that IORT probably produced a reduction in the blood flow of abdominal organs that might be responsible for mucosal, vascular, or anastomotic complications.

3.4. Clinical Tolerance Studies

3.4.1. PANCREATIC FUNCTION

A short-term assessment of pancreatic function after IORT was performed by Abe (32) at the Kyoto University. This author described a temporary increase in the levels of pancreatic amylase and blood glucose after IORT. They returned to normal during the first week after the procedure.

Pancreatic function has been studied also in long-term survivors after IORT. Aristu (51) studied the pancreatic function of 10 patients (minimal follow-up 2 yr) treated at the University of Navarre with gastrectomy, 15-Gy IORT, and EBRT of 45–46 Gy. A healthy control group was used as baseline for comparison. A glucagon test and an iv glucose-tolerance test were performed along with LDH, serum and urine amylase and serum lipase determinations. Basal C-peptide levels were similar between groups, but the incremental and peak values were inferior in the IORT group ($p < 0.01$). Similarly, the basal glycemia and insulinemia did not differ between groups but the 30- and 60-min glycemia were higher in the IORT group and the 30- and 60-min insulinemia were lower. However, exocrine pancreatic function in IORT patients remained similar to controls. These findings indicate that exocrine pancreatic function is not affected by IORT and EBRT, but endocrine pancreatic function appears to be impaired at the subclinical level.

3.4.2. GASTROINTESTINAL BLEEDING; VASCULAR TOXICITY

Calvo (37) reported six cases of gastrointestinal (GI) bleeding among 48 patients treated with gastrectomy and IORT at the University of Navarre. Most received additional EBRT. The incidence rate in this series was 12.5%. In three of the cases, an arterio-enteric fistula could be documented (52). In a subsequent report of this series, in which only patients with serosal and/or nodal involvement were included, the incidence of GI bleeding remained the same *(15)*. Sindelar *(21)*, in an NCI randomized trial, reported two cases of GI bleeding out of 16 patients (12.5%) included in the IORT arm. Kim *(53)* reported 3 cases of GI bleeding in 53 patients (6%) treated with surgery plus IORT and EBRT with chemotherapy. Coquard *(40)* reported two cases (3%) of gastrointestinal bleeding at 3- and 6-mo follow-up in a series of 63 patients treated with IORT with or without EBRT. Both patients were treated with 15-Gy IORT and did not receive any EBRT. Only one of the patients was laparotomized, and no evidence of recurrent tumor was found. Japanese authors *(1,2)* have never reported vascular toxicity in their series.

In a attempt to address the long-term status of upper abdominal vasculature after IORT with or without EBRT, Aristu *(54)* studied 10 long-term survivors (minimal follow-up 2 yr) treated at the University of Navarre with gastrectomy, 15-Gy IORT and EBRT at 45–46 Gy. The study was done performing selective and nonselective angiography of the celiac trunk, mesenteric artery, and renal arteries with late venous phases to visualize the portal vein and its branches. There were no significant changes attributable to IORT. However, six patients developed renal hypoperfusion and four developed left hepatic-lobe hypoplasia. These lesions matched with the shape of the EBRT portal and were attributed to the delivery of EBRT (Fig. 5).

3.4.3. VERTEBRAL TOXICITY

Calvo *(37)* described 6 cases of partial vertebral collapse (vertebrae lying within the IORT/EBRT fields) in a series of 48 gastric patients treated with IORT at the University of Navarre. This clinical finding has also been described in some gynecologic series in which the para-aortic region was treated with IORT because of nodal involvement. Previous clinical reports have also indicated the presence of mild hypocellularity in the vertebrae of patients treated with IORT for upper abdominal malignancies *(55)*.

3.4.4. SOFT-TISSUE TOXICITY

Sindelar *(55)* reported the soft-tissue changes of an overall group of patients treated with IORT to the upper abdomen for miscellaneous malignancies, mainly gastric and pancreatic tumors. They described mild fibrotic changes in the retroperitoneal soft tissues as well as fibrosis in the soft tissues around the porta hepatis and perineural fibrosis.

3.4.5. SMALL-BOWEL TOXICITY

Abe described three cases of small-bowel ulceration, caused by accidental movement into the IORT field during the procedure *(1)*. Small bowel should be always retracted away from the IORT target volume during the IORT procedure because of its limited tolerance. Calvo *(37)* reported 9 cases of enteritis in 48 patients treated with surgery and IORT plus EBRT (19%). Five of them (10%) required surgery. Avizonis *(36)* reported one case of small-bowel obstruction in 27 patients treated with IORT and EBRT (4%). Kim *(53)* reported three cases of small-bowel obstruction in 53 patients treated with IORT and EBRT (5%). No small-bowel complications have been reported in series using IORT alone. The incidence of small-bowel obstruction requiring surgical intervention following surgical procedures alone in the abdomen or pelvis ranges from 5 to 10%, which is similar to the results reported in series combining surgery and IORT/EBRT.

3.4.6. GENERAL TOXICITY

In a randomized gastric trial comparing IORT vs observation, Kramling at the University of Munich *(35)* described enhanced mortality (8 vs 2%) and morbidity (35 vs 28%) in the IORT arm compared to the surgery-alone arm. These differences were not statis-

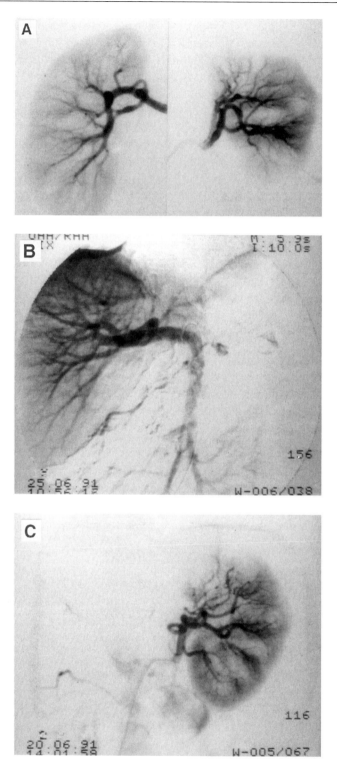

Fig. 5. Upper abdominal vasculature in long-term survivors after IOERT ± EBRT for gastric cancer at the University of Navarre, Pamplona. (**A**) Normal appearance of right kidney but abnormal vessels in the upper pole of the left kidney (within EBRT field). (**B**) Hypoplasia of the left hepatic lobe and left portal vein. (**C**) Hypoperfusion of the upper pole of the left kidney.

tically significant. In another randomized trial by Abe *(1)*, the toxicity results were only scarcely reported. An NCI randomized gastric trial compared surgery and 20-Gy IORT with surgery with or without EBRT *(21)*. The overall incidence of complications was 56%. These complications included 2 fistulae, 1 mesenteric thrombosis, 4 abdominal abscesses, 4 anastomotic strictures, and 1 biliary stricture. Four patients ultimately died of complications. However, the authors did not find a correlation between the observed toxicities and IORT. Moreover, the control group (in which most of the patients received EBRT) suffered a higher rate of complications (72%). This difference was not statistically significant. Avinonis *(36)*, reporting the RTOG gastric trial 85-04, described the toxicity encountered in 27 gastric-cancer patients treated with surgery, IORT of 12.5–16.5 Gy (median 13.75 Gy), and EBRT (85% of the patients). Major postoperative complications were found in 15% of the patients, including 1 pancreatic fistula and 1 postoperative death resulting from necrotizing pancreatitis. Long-term complications were observed in 14% of the patients with one death probably related to necrotizing pancreatitis. Ogata *(2)* reported three cases of wound infection and two of suture leakage in a group of 58 gastric patients treated with surgery and IORT of 28–30 Gy. Kim *(53)* reported two cases of sepsis in a series of patients treated with IORT and EBRT (45-Gy) and chemotherapy. Farthmann *(34)* described a 5% perioperative mortality rate in a series of 36 gastric patients treated with surgery and IORT of 25–28 Gy in the Freiburg University. The morbidity rate was 20%. Postoperative complications in the upper abdominal structures included five cases of anastomotic leakage/gastrointestinal bleeding, four cases of pancreatic fistula/necrosis, and one case of mesenteric vein thrombosis. Chabert *(38)* reported two deaths at 2 and 3 mo after surgery caused by anastomotic leak and sepsis in a series of 21 gastric patients treated with surgery and IORT of 15–20 Gy with or without EBRT. Other complications reported were pancreatic fistula, colic perforation, and sepsis in one patient each. One patient died at 6 mo after surgery due to sepsis and massive hemorrhage.

4. DISCUSSION

4.1. Toxicity

EBRT is a treatment component in the adjuvant setting for some upper gastrointestinal tumors. However, the total dose that can be delivered by EBRT is limited by the presence of surrounding organs or structures including small bowel, stomach, liver, kidney, and spinal cord. As a rule, an EBRT dose of 45–50 Gy delivered with standard fractionation in the postoperative setting controls 80–90% of the patients with a 5–10% small bowel or gastric complication rate *(56)*. If residual disease is left after surgery, the increase in EBRT dose needed to achieve similar control rates will be accompanied by an increase in the small-bowel or gastric complication rates. For most gastrointestinal malignancies, there exists a delicate balance among the EBRT dose required for control of disease and the tolerance dose of the small bowel and stomach.

EBRT portals for gastric cancer, as derived from the University of Minnesota reoperation series, encompass a significant volume of normal tissues. The upper poles of both kidneys and part of the left hepatic lobe are irradiated to doses above their tolerance limits. However, because of the anatomical architecture of these parenchymal tissues, with several units working in an independent fashion, overall renal and liver function are not impaired. The base of the left lung and part of the heart apex are included in the EBRT volume, especially if the portals are designed to treat proximal gastric cancers. However, the volume of these tissues included in the target is usually small, and EBRT doses in the range used for the postoperative management of gastric cancer are well tolerated. The dose to the lower thoracic spinal cord is always restricted to 45–50 Gy, but if it is necessary to increase the dose to the gastric bed, the spinal cord can be spared by a multiple beam arrangement. Small bowel and stomach are the main radiation-limiting structures present in the target volume for gastric cancer. Moreover, the areas in which microscopic or gross residual disease is more likely to remain after cancer surgery are located around the celiac axis, where the bowel mesentery originates. In that specific area, small bowel cannot be spared by field shaping or multiple-beam arrangement and some segments of the small bowel will receive at least the same dose that is prescribed to the target volume. Because of the continuous architecture of the gastrointestinal tract, a blockage at any point will cause an overall failure of the whole system.

The main advantage of using IORT during gastric-cancer surgery is the ability to displace uninvolved stomach and small bowel out of the area to be irradiated. Other additional advantages, such as the ability to treat high-risk areas under direct vision, thus avoiding a geographical miss, are less dramatic, because areas at risk could be marked with clips and treated with EBRT postoperatively. If EBRT doses in the range of 55–70+ Gy are needed to treat the gastric bed, because of residual microscopic or gross disease, combined IORT plus EBRT is probably the only means of achieving local disease control while achieving acceptable gastric and small-bowel tolerance.

However, IORT presents some radiobiological disadvantages. Because IORT is delivered as a large single dose, it does not exploit some of the advantages of fractionated regimens (repair, reoxygenation, and so on) and severe toxicities have been reported in normal tissues that cannot be retracted or shielded during IORT, such as peripheral nerve (57). Although peripheral nerves and vessels tolerate well high doses of fractionated EBRT, peripheral nerve and vessels are dose-limiting structures for IORT. Although peripheral-nerve toxicity is not a matter of concern in gastric IORT, the vascular tolerance (intact vessels and stumps) to IORT has to been considered.

Only an indirect estimation can be obtained from experimental studies with regards to vascular tolerance in the celiac axis region. IORT-related damage to the aorta (intact or surgically manipulated) has been widely studied (47–49), but the conclusions obtained are probably not pertinent to gastric IORT since this vessel may or may not be included in the IORT field. Moreover, the probability of damage is very low at the doses used in clinical practice, with the exception of some Japanese (1,2) and European authors (43) who use IORT doses above 25 Gy. Also, the length of follow-up needed to observe significant damage usually exceeds the life span of the majority of gastric-cancer patients included in IORT trials. However, an interesting extrapolation can be obtained from the University of Colorado experimental studies on aorta branch arteries (49) because these vessels are similar in diameter to the vessels included in the target volume for gastric IORT (celiac axis and its branches). At 2-yr follow-up, most of the animals presented arteritis and necrosis of the media at 20-Gy IORT or 15-Gy IORT plus 50-Gy EBRT. At 5 yr, the ED_{50} for obstruction of more than 50% of the lumen of the aorta branches was estimated to be 24.8 Gy for IORT alone or 19.4 Gy for IORT followed by 50-Gy EBRT. The IORT estimates for more than 50% lumen obstruction are above the doses used in the clinical trials that have reported gastrointestinal bleeding (37,40,55,57). However, IORT doses in the customary range (15-Gy IORT plus 50-Gy EBRT) are able to induce arterial-wall necrosis.

Arterial stumps are included in the IORT volume. The number and localization depends on the type of surgical procedure. However, the radiation tolerance of arterial stumps has not been studied in the experimental setting. Animal studies on large vessels suggest that IORT does not decrease the suture-line strength of anastomosed aortas. However, aortic-wall thrombi formation leading to complete obstruction is a common event during the first months of follow-up at doses as low as 20 Gy with or without additional EBRT. Calvo *(37)* reported six cases of gastrointestinal bleeding among 48 patients treated with gastrectomy plus IORT. Most received additional EBRT. In three of the cases, an arterio-enteric fistula between a vascular stump and the surrounding small bowel could be documented *(52)*. An update of this series included only the IORT patients with serosal and/or nodal involvement that completed EBRT and a group of 35 patients treated with EBRT only that served as a control *(15)*. There were three cases of gastrointestinal bleeding in the IORT plus EBRT group, but none in the EBRT-only group. However, there are other factors to be considered in the genesis of gastrointestinal bleeding. The extent of surgical resection may be a factor. In this latter series *(15)*, the percentage of subtotal gastrectomies in the EBRT-alone group was 40% vs only 18.5% in the IORT plus EBRT group. Gastrointestinal bleeding has been observed in gastric-cancer patients treated with IORT in a percentage ranging from 3 to 12.5%. Most of the observed cases occurred after the perioperative period and within the first year of follow-up *(37)*. It is not possible to make a statement about the role played by IORT in the genesis of this complication because the incidence of gastrointestinal bleeding in surgical series is not well known. However, the results of experimental studies along with clinical data suggest that the combination of radical gastrectomy with R2 lymph-node dissection plus IORT of 10–15 Gy plus EBRT of 40–45 Gy is in the upper limit of vascular tolerance.

The overall complication rate in gastric IORT trials has been reported to be similar to that of EBRT controls *(21)* or registered patients in IORT trials for different anatomical locations serving as controls *(58)*. A recent University of Münich trial reported enhanced mortality and morbidity in the IORT arm vs the surgery-alone arm, but the differences did not reach statistical significance *(43)*. Unfortunately, two other trials *(2,32)* that compare a surgery plus IORT arm vs a surgery-only arm, either do not report the toxicity found in the surgical arm *(2)* or report a negligible overall toxicity *(32)*. Finally, two recent experimental studies reported by Kramling and Grab *(43,50)* demonstrated a decrease in the tolerance of the gastric mucosa to EBRT and an impaired wound healing of the stomach wall after incision and per prima suture in rabbits treated with IORT over the celiac axis region. Although this is an animal study and the doses used are high (20–40 Gy of IORT) compared to most IORT trials, it raises the concern that IORT could disrupt the normal repair mechanisms present in the abdominal tissues through a decrease in the celiac blood flow.

4.2. Local Control

The main goal of IORT in gastric cancer is to increase the local control rates without increasing the complication rates.

A local failure rate of 70% or higher can be expected after surgery alone for gastric cancer patients with serosal and/or lymph-node involvement. The University of Minnesota reoperation series revealed that 67% of the patients at risk developed loco-regional failure, either isolated or combined *(11)*. However, when patterns of failure are documented by clinical means, the figures are lower than those of reoperative or necropsy series. Landry and Tepper *(9)* reported a 38% local failure rate in the Massachusetts General Hospital experience.

The local-failure rates reported in five IORT trials range from 10 to 44% *(15,21,36–38)*. Four of these studies used IORT combined with EBRT and one IORT alone. The actual percentage of patients that received EBRT ranged from 52 to 100%. The results of these IORT series suggest that adjuvant IORT with or without EBRT is superior to surgery alone in terms of local control. Although local control in IORT series can be overscored because of the inherent difficulty in diagnosing local failures in the upper abdomen after surgery and radiation, the number of patients free of local disease present in the IORT with or without EBRT series clearly outweighs the same figures for the historical surgical series.

It is not clear if IORT as the only adjuvant radiation treatment is superior to EBRT alone. Unlike the NCI study, the local control rates obtained in other IORT alone trials have not been reported *(2,32,35)*. In the former study, the overall loco-regional failure rate was 44% for the IORT arm vs 92% for the surgery with or without EBRT arm ($p < 0.001$). The incidence of tumor-bed recurrence was also lower in the IORT than in the EBRT group at 31 vs 80%. This study reports the highest loco-regional failure rate among both IORT trials (44%) and EBRT trials (92%). This can be explained by two reasons: Firstly, these authors considered loco-regional failures as those occurring in the abdomen, retroperitoneum, thorax, and peritoneal surfaces. Secondly, the relapses were verified by biopsy or laparotomy and all patients who died were autopsied unless a complete verification of the actual extension of the recurrent disease had been carried out within the previous 3 mo, thus increasing the number of loco-regional failures diagnosed.

It is not clear if IORT plus EBRT is superior to EBRT alone in terms of local control. The local-failure rates of trials using adjuvant EBRT are in the 8–54% range *(13–19,54)*. Some of these trials incorporate chemotherapy along with EBRT, that can or cannot improve the EBRT results in terms of local control and survival. The EBRT-alone figures almost parallel the local-failure rates in IORT plus EBRT trials, in which a 10–37% range has been reported *(15,36–38)*. However, some patients included in IORT plus EBRT trials did not receive EBRT because of early postoperative death, postoperative complications, poor tolerance to EBRT, or patient refusal, or the patients received EBRT because of high-risk factors. Also, some of the EBRT trials included patients with unresectable disease. In a report that only included patients who completed the prescribed treatment course, Martínez-Monge et al. *(15)* described the experience with EBRT with or without IORT at the University of Navarre during the period 1982–1993. Patients were divided among those treated with IORT plus EBRT or EBRT alone. The EBRT patients were treated before the IORT plus EBRT protocol was active or when it was finished. After a median follow-up of more than 6 yr for the IORT plus EBRT group, and more than 7 yr for the EBRT group, the local-failure rate favored the IORT patients by 11 vs 20% *(15)*. This difference was not statistically significant.

4.3. Survival

Three randomized trials have studied the survival impact of IORT alone when added to surgical resection. A recent update of the University of Kyoto trial *(1)* continued to demonstrate a survival advantage for the IORT arm in the JPSS stages II, III, and IV, although this was not statistically significant. This results were confirmed in a nonrandomized trial from the Kochi Medical School *(2)* in which the IORT patients were compared with a surgery-alone control group and in stage-III patients from the Beijing trial *(42)*. In Western countries, the University of Münich trial *(43)* has not demonstrated any survival advantage between the IORT arm and the surgery-alone arm. In this study, the methodology used was similar to the Japanese trials. Finally, the NCI trial *(21)* compared a surgery plus IORT arm with a surgery with or without EBRT arm and did not find any survival differences. However, in this study, none of the stage III–IV patients in the control group survived after a median follow-up of 7 yr, whereas 3 out of 15 in the IORT group were alive NED at the time of the analysis ($p = 0.06$).

IORT plus EBRT series report 5-yr results in the 10–50% range *(36–40)*. All of these studies are nonrandomized institutional studies, and therefore only an indirect estimation can be made by comparing the survival results of these series with historical surgical results. This is complicated by the fact that some of these studies include patients with either early cancers or recurrent disease. These results are similar to historical surgical series that report 5-yr survival results in the range of 10–40% for patients with serosal invasion and/or lymph node involvement (stages B2 through C3) *(9)*.

CONCLUSIONS

1. IORT is a feasible technique to be incorporated in gastric-cancer surgery. There exists a worldwide experience generated over the last 20 yr in the Far East, Western Europe, and the United States.
2. IORT may produce severe vascular toxicity in the clinical setting at 15 Gy if followed by 45-Gy fractionated EBRT or at a higher dose of IORT alone. A 3–12.5% GI bleeding rate has been reported in several IORT trials.
3. IORT improves local control if added to radical surgery. IORT with or without EBRT trials report local-failure rates in the 10–44% range and is superior to historical surgical controls. It is not clear if IORT plus EBRT is superior to EBRT or IORT alone.
4. Distant and/or peritoneal dissemination is a common pattern of failure in IORT trials for gastric cancer, that is present in 25–31% of the patients. An effective form of systemic adjuvant therapy is needed.
5. IORT for gastric cancer remains an investigational therapy. There is not definitive evidence that IORT alone or combined with EBRT prolongs survival in Western countries.

REFERENCES

1. Abe M, Nishimura Y, and Shibamoto Y. Intraoperative radiation therapy for gastric cancer, *World J. Surg.,* **19** (1995) 544–547.
2. Ogata T, Araki K, Matsuura K, et al. A 10-year experience of intraoperative radiotherapy for gastric carcinoma and a new surgical method of creating a wider irradiation field for cases of total gastrectomy patients, *Int. J. Radiat. Oncol. Phys.,* **32** (1995) 341–347.
3. Nishi M, Nakayima T, and Kajitani T. The Japanese Research Society for gastric cancer—the general rules for the gastric cancer study and an analysis of treatment results based on the rules. In Preece PE, Cuschieri A, Wellwood JM, (eds.) *Cancer of the Stomach,* Grune & Straton, New York, 1986, pp. 107–121.
4. American Joint Committee on Cancer. *Manual for Staging of Cancer,* 4th ed. JB Lippincott, Philadelphia, 1992.
5. Kodama Y, Sugimachi K, Soejima K, et al. Evaluation of extensive lymph node resection for carcinoma of the stomach, *World J. Surg.,* **11** (1981) 127–145.
6. Dent DM, Madden MV, and Price SK. Randomized comparison of R_1 and R_2 gastrectomy for gastric carcinoma, *Br. J. Surg.,* **75** (1988) 110–112.
7. Sasako M, Maruyama K, Kinoshita T, et al. Quality control of surgical technique in a multicenter, prospective, randomized, controlled study on the surgical treatment of gastric cancer, *Jap. J. Clin. Oncol.,* **22** (1992) 41–48.

8. Van de Veide CJH. Surgery of gastric carcinoma R_1 versus R_2 resection. Second International Conference on Biology, Prevention and Treatment of Gastrointestinal Malignancies, Köln, Germany. Symposium Abstracts, p. 21, 1995.

9. Landry J, Tepper JE, Wood WC, Orlow E, Koerner F, and Sullinger J. Patterns of failure following curative resection of gastric carcinoma, *Int. J. Radiat. Oncol. Biol. Phys.,* **19** (1990) 1357–1362.

10. Noguchi Y, Imada T, Matsumoto A, Coit DG, and Brennan MF. Radical surgery for gastric cancer. A review of the Japanese experience, *Cancer,* **64** (1989) 2053–2062.

11. Gunderson LL and Sosin H. Adenocarcinoma of the stomach: areas of failure in a re-operation series (second or symptomatic look) Clinico-pathologiccorrelation and implications for adjuvant therapy, *Int. J. Radiat. Oncol. Biol. Phys.,* **8** (1982) 1–11.

12. Wisbeek WM, Becher EM, and Russell AH. Adenocarcinoma of the stomach: autopsy observations with therapeutic implications for the radiation oncologist, *Radiother. Oncol.,* **7** (1986) 13–18.

13. Allum WH, Hallissey MT, Ward LC, et al. A controlled, prospective, randomised trial of adjuvant chemotherapy or radiotherapy in resectable gastric cancer. Interim report. British Stomach Cancer Group, *Br. J. Cancer,* **60** (1989) 739–744.

14. Klaasen DJ, ManIntyre JM, Catton GE, Engstrom PF, and Moertel CG. Treatment of locally unresectable cancer of the stomach and pancreas: a randomised comparison of 5-fluorouracil alone with radiation plus concurrent and maintenance 5-fluorouracil—An Eastern Cooperative Oncology Group Study, *J. Clin. Oncol.,* **3** (1985) 373–378.

15. Martínez-Monge R, Calvo FA, Azinovic I, et al. Patterns of failure and long-term results in high-risk resected gastric cancer treated with postoperative radiotherapy ± intraoperative electron boost, *J. Surg. Oncol.,* **66** (1997) 24–29.

16. Moertel CG, Childs DS, O'Fallon JR, Holbrook MA, Schutt AJ, and Reitemeier RJ. Combined 5-fluorouracil and radiation therapy as a surgical adjuvant for poor prognosis gastric carcinoma, *J. Clin. Oncol.,* **2** (1984) 1249–1254.

17. Regine WF and Mohiuddin M. Impact of adjuvant therapy on locally advanced adenocarcinoma of the stomach, *Int. J. Radiat. Oncol. Biol. Phys.,* **24** (1992) 921–927.

18. Haas CD, Mansfield CM, Leichman LP, Considine B, and Bukowski RM. Combined nonsimultaneous radiation therapy and chemotherapy with 5-FU, doxorubicin and mitomycin C for residual localized gastric adenocarcinoma; a Southwest Oncology Group Pilot Study, *Cancer Treat. Rep.,* **76** (1983) 421–424.

19. O'Connell MJ, Gunderson LL, Moertel CG, and Kvols LK. A pilot study to determine clinical tolerability of intensive combined modality therapy for locally unresectable gastric cancer, *Int. J. Radiat. Oncol. Biol. Phys.,* **11** (1985) 1827–1831.

20. Slot A, Meerwaldt JH, Van Putten WLJ, and Treurniet-Donker AD. Adjuvant postoperative radiotherapy for gastric carcinoma with poor prognostic signs, *Radiother. Oncol.,* **16** (1989) 269–274.

21. Sindelar WF, Kinsella TJ, Tepper JE, et al. Randomized trial of intraoperative radiotherapy in carcinoma of the stomach, *Am. J. Surg.,* **165** (1993) 178–86.

22. MacDonald JS, Steele G, and Gunderson LL. Carcinoma of the stomach. In DeVita VT Jr, Hellman S, and Rosenberg SA (eds.), *Cancer—Principles and Practice of Oncology,* 2nd ed. Lippincott, Philadelphia, 1989, pp. 765–799.

23. Hermans J, Bonenkamp JJ, Boon MC, et al. Adjuvant therapy after curative resection for gastric cancer: meta-analysis of randomized trials. *J. Clin. Oncol.,* **118** (1993) 1441–1447.

24. Childs DS, Moertel CG, Holbrook MA, Reitemeier RJ, and Colby Jr M. Treatment of unresectable adenocarcinomas of the stomach with a combination of 5-fluorouracil and radiation, *AJR,* **102** (1968) 541–544.

25. Moertel CG, Childs DS, Reitemeier RJ, Colby Jr M, and Holbrook MA. Combined 5-flourouracil and supervoltage radiation therapy of locally unresectable gastrointestinal cancer, *Lancet,* **1** (1969) 865–870.

26. Holbrook MA. Current concepts in cancer—radiation therapy for gastric cancer: treatment principles, *JAMA,* **228** (1974) 1289–1290.

27. Schein PS and Novak J. Gastrointestinal Tumor Study Group: a comparison of combination chemotherapy and combined modality therapy for locally advanced gastric carcinoma, *Cancer,* **49** (1982) 1771–1777.

28. Chevalier TL, Smith FP, Harter WK, and Schein PS. Chemotherapy and combined modality therapy for locally advanced and metastatic gastric carcinoma, *Semin. Oncol.,* **12** (1985) 46–53.

29. Gastrointestinal Tumor Study Group. The concept of locally advanced gastric cancer. Effect of treatment on outcome, *Cancer,* **66** (1990) 2324–2330.

30. Dent DM, Werner ID, Novis B, Cheverton P, and Brice P. Prospective randomized trial of combined oncological therapy for gastric carcinoma, *Cancer,* **44** (1979) 385–392.

31. Gunderson LL, Burch PA, and Donohue JH. The role of irradiation as a component of combined modality treatment for gastric cancer, *J. Infusion Chemo.,* **5** (1995) 117–124.

32. Abe M, Takahashi M, Yabumoto E, Adachi H, Yoshii M, and Mori K. Clinical experiences with intraoperative radiotherapy for locally advanced cancers, *Cancer,* **45** (1980) 40–48.

33. Abe M, Takahashi M, Ono K, Tobe T, and Inamoto T. Japan gastric trials in intraoperative radiation therapy, *Int. J. Radiat. Oncol. Biol. Phys.,* **15** (1988) 1431–1433.

34. Farthmann EH, Kirchner R, Salm R, Strasser C, Frommhold, and Nilles A. Usefulness and limitations of preoperative radiotherapy in association with curative resection in the treatment of gastric cancer, *Chirurgie,* **119** (1993–1994) 565–568.

35. Kramling HJ, Willich N, Cramer C, Wilkowski R, Duhmke E, and Schildberg FW. Early results of IORT in the treatment of gastric cancer. In Vaeth JM (ed.), *Intraoperative Radiation Therapy in the Treatment of Cancer, Front. Radiat. Ther. Oncol.,* **31** (1997) 157–160.

36. Avizonis VN, Buzydlowski J, Lanciano R, Owens JC, Noyes D, and Hanks GE. Treatment of adenocarcinoma of the stomach with resection, intraoperative radiotherapy and adjuvant external beam radiation: a phase II study from Radiation Therapy Oncology Group 85-04, *Ann. Surg. Oncol.,* **2** (1995) 295–302.

37. Calvo FA, Aristu JJ, Azinovic I, et al. Intraoperative and external radiotherapy in resected gastric cancer: updated report of a Phase II trial, *Int. J. Radiat. Oncol. Biol. Phys.,* **24** (1992) 729–36.

38. Chabert M, Schmitt T, Soglu M, et al. Intraoperative radiation therapy (IORT) for locally advanced gastric cancer. Proceedings of the 6th International IORT Symposium and 31st San Francisco Cancer Symposium, San Francisco, September 23–25, 1996.

39. Dulce MC, Kaiser J, Boese-Landgraf J, Scheffler A, Haring R, and Ernst H. Experiences with intraoperative radiotherapy in gastric carcinoma (Berlin method), *Strahlenther, Onkol.,* **167** (1991) 581–591.

40. Coquard R, Ayzac L, Gilly FN, et al. Intraoperative radiation therapy combined with limited lymph node resection in gastric cancer: an alternative to extended dissection? *Int. J. Radiat. Oncol. Biol. Phys.,* **39** (5) (1997) 1093–1098.

41. Caudry M, Escarmant P, Maire JP, Demeaux H, Guichard F, and Azaloux H. Radiotherapy of gastric cancer with a three field combination: feasibility, tolerance and survival, *Int. J. Radiat. Oncol. Biol. Phys.,* **13** (1987) 1821–1827.

42. Chen G and Song S. *Intraoperative Radiation Therapy.* Evaluation of intraoperative radiotherapy for gastric carcinoma—analysis of 247 patients. In Abe M and Takayashi M (eds.), Pergamon, New York, 1991, p. 190.

43. Kramling HJ, Grab J, Zaspel J, et al. Experimental study of vascular sequelae of combined upper abdominal intraoperative and external radiation therapy. In Vaeth JM (ed.), *Intraoperative Radiation Therapy in the Treatment of Cancer, Front. Radiat. Ther. Oncol.,* **31** (1997) 36–40.

44. Ahmadu-Suka F, Gillette EL, Withrow SJ, Husted PW, Nelson AW, and Whiteman CE. Exocrine pancreatic function following intraoperative irradiation of the canine pancreas, *Cancer,* **62** (1988) 1091–1095.

45. Ahmadu-Suka F, Gillette EL, Withrow SJ, Husted PW, Nelson AW, and Whiteman CE. Pathological response of the pancreas and duodenum to experimental intraoperative irradiation, *Int. J. Radiat. Oncol. Biol. Phys.,* **14** (1988) 1197–1204.

46. Heijmans HJ, Mehta DM, Kleibeuker JH, Sluiter WJ, Oldhoff J, and Hoekstra HJ. Intraoperative irradiation of the canine pancreas: short-term effects, *Radiother. Oncol.,* **29** (1993) 347–51.

47. Johnstone PA, Sprague M, DeLuca AM, et al. Effects of intraoperative radiotherapy on vascular grafts in a canine model, *Int. J. Radiat. Oncol. Biol. Phys.,* **29** (1994) 1015–1025.

48. Tepper JE, Sindelar WF, Travis EL, Terrill R, and Padikal T. Tolerance of canine anastomoses to intraoperative radiation therapy, *Int. J. Radiat. Oncol. Biol. Phys.,* **9** (1983) 987–992.

49. Gillette EL, Powers BE, McChesney SL, Park RD, and Withrow SJ. Response of aorta and branch arteries to experimental intraoperative irradiation, *Int. J. Radiat. Oncol. Biol. Phys.,* **17** (1989) 1247–1255.

50. Grab J, Zaspel J, Kallfass E, et al. Reactions of the gastric wall following IORT ± ERT to the upper abdomen in rabbits. In Vaeth JM (ed.), *Intraoperative Radiation in the Treatment of Cancer, Front. Radiat. Ther. Oncol.,* **31** (1997) 36–40.

51. Aristu JJ, Azinovic I, Martinez-Monge R, Tangco E, Yoldi A, and Calvo FA. Pancreatic function following upper abdominal intraoperative and external irradiation. A long-termk clinical analysis. In

Schildberg FW, Willich N, and Krämling H-J (eds.), *Intraoperative Radiation Therapy, Proceedings 4th International Symposium IORT, Munich 1992*. Verlag Die Blaue Eule, Essen, 1993.

52. De Villa VH, Calvo FA, and Bilbao JI. Arteriodigestive fistula: a complication associated with intra-operative and external beam radiotherapy following surgery for gastric cancer, *J. Surg. Oncol.,* **49** (1992) 52–7.

53. Kim MS, Kim SK, Song SK, Kim HJ, Kwon KB, and Kim HD. Complication of intraoperative radiation therapy (IORT) in gastric cancer. *International Congress of Radiation Oncology 1993*. Kyoto, Japan, 1993, p. 357.

54. Aristu JJ, Bilbao JI, Azinovic I, Martinez-Monge R, Tangco E, and Calvo FA. Abdominal vascular changes following gastrectomy, intraoperative and external irradiation: a long-term analysis. In Schildberg FW, Willich N, and Krämling H-J (eds.), *Intraoperative Radiation Therapy, Proceedings 4th International Symposium IORT, Munich 1992*. Verlag Die Blaue Eule, Essen, 1993.

55. Sindelar WF, Hoekstra H, Restrepo C, and Kinsella TJ. Pathological tissue changes following intra-operative radiotherapy, *Am. J. Clin. Oncol.,* **9** (1986) 504–509.

56. Perez CA and Brady LW. Overview. In Perez CA and Brady LW (eds.), *Principles and Practice of Radiation Oncology,* 2nd ed. JB Lippincott, Philadelphia, 1992, pp. 1–63.

57. Sindelar WF, Kinsella TJ, Chen PW, et al. Intraooperative radiotherapy in retroperitoneal sarcomas. Final results of a prospective, randomized, clinical trial, *Arch. Surg.,* **128** (1993) 402–410.

58. Noyes RD, Weiss SM, and Krall JM. Surgical complications of intraoperative radiation therapy: the Radiation Therapy Oncology Group experience, *J. Surg. Oncol.,* **50** (1992) 209–215.

12 IORT in Pancreatic Carcinoma

Paula M. Termuhlen, Douglas B. Evans, and Christopher G. Willett

1. LOCAL CONTROL AND SURVIVAL—NON-IORT RESULTS

1.1. Resectable Pancreas Cancer

Current surgical treatment for adenocarcinoma of the pancreas is based on the surgical procedure of pancreaticoduodenectomy as first described by Whipple et al. *(1)*. However, because of tumor relapse in the liver, peritoneum, and the bed of the resected pancreas, surgery alone cures no more than 25% of patients who undergo resection *(2–5)*. In fact, local recurrence has been documented in 50 to 90% of patients after pancreaticoduodenectomy *(6–10)*. Attempts to improve local control and survival by performing extended lymphatic resection have met with conflicting results *(8,11–14)* and in some centers have been associated with unacceptable morbidity and mortality *(15–17)*. In a series from Japan, extended resection did not prevent local recurrence unless combined with intraoperative irradiation (IORT) *(13,14)*.

1.2. Unresectable Pancreas Cancer

For unresectable pancreas cancer, the use of external-beam irradiation (EBRT) plus 5-fluorouracil (5-FU)-based chemotherapy results in a doubling of median survival when compared with surgical bypass or stents alone (3–6 mo median survival vs 9–13 mo) and an increase in 2-yr survival from 0–5% to 10–20% *(18–20)*. However, 5-yr survival is rare, and local control is low. Even with EBRT doses of 60–70 Gy given in 1.8- to 20.0-Gy fractions over 7–8 wk, local failure was documented in at least two-thirds of the patients in a series from Thomas Jefferson University (TJUH) *(20)*. For those treated with

From: *Current Clinical Oncology: Intraoperative Irradiation: Techniques and Results*
Edited by: L. L. Gunderson et al. © Humana Press, Inc., Totowa, NJ

EBRT alone, local control was achieved in <20% of patients and with EBRT plus chemotherapy local control was achieved in approx 30% of patients.

2. IORT RATIONALE AND GENERAL RESULTS

IORT is a means of delivering a higher dose of irradiation to the pancreas in patients with locally unresectable disease and to the pancreatic bed and high-risk nodal groups in patients following pancreaticoduodenectomy. IORT was initially used in patients with locally advanced, unresectable adenocarcinoma of the pancreas to decrease pain and prevent local-regional tumor progression. Initial studies at the Mayo Clinic involved an intraoperative electron irradiation (IOERT) dose of 20 Gy; after surgical recovery, patients received EBRT with or without concomitant 5-FU *(21,22)*. Median survival was 13 mo and local failure as any component of failure was significantly less common with the addition of IOERT. The experience with IOERT and EBRT at Massachusetts General Hospital (MGH) also yielded a median survival of 12–16 mo with improved pain control and decreased local failure *(23,24)*. IORT has recently been applied to patients with resectable adenocarcinoma of the pancreatic head because of the high incidence of local recurrence with surgery alone. The experience at M.D. Anderson Cancer Center (MDACC) with preoperative 5-FU-based chemoradiation, pancreaticoduodenectomy, and IOERT has decreased local-regional recurrence to 11% *(25)*.

Patient survival depends on the extent of disease and performance status at diagnosis. Therefore, future clinical trials using IORT as one component of a multimodality treatment program will require accurate pretreatment staging. Extent of disease is best categorized as resectable, locally advanced (unresectable), or metastatic. Patients who undergo surgical resection for localized nonmetastatic adenocarcinoma of the pancreatic head have a long-term survival rate of approx 20% and a median survival of 15–22 mo when surgery is combined with adjuvant chemoradiation *(26)*. Disease relapse following a potentially curative pancreaticoduodenectomy remains common, and local recurrence occurs in up to 85% of patients who undergo surgery alone. Local-regional tumor control is maximized with combined-modality therapy in the form of chemoradiation and surgery with or without IORT. Patients with locally advanced, (unresectable) nonmetastatic disease have a median survival of 6–12 mo with chemoirradiation and up to 16 mo with the addition of IORT. Patients with metastatic disease have a short survival (3–6 mo), the length of which depends on the extent of disease and performance status *(26)*.

In the absence of objective, reproducible radiographic criteria for clinical staging, survival statistics are impossible to interpret. The inability of physicians to standardize this important variable is largely responsible for the small amount of data that currently exists on the use of multimodality therapy for pancreatic cancer.

3. IORT PRETREATMENT
EVALUATION AND TREATMENT FACTORS

3.1. Pretreatment Clinical Staging (Radiographic)

Tumors of the pancreas are unlike other solid tumors of the gastrointestinal tract in that accurate diagnosis, clinical staging, and treatment require extensive interaction and cooperation between physicians of different specialties (diagnostic radiologist, interventional upper endoscopist, surgeon, medical oncologist, and radiation oncologist). Accurate clinical staging requires high-quality (helical) computed tomography (CT) to accurately define the relationship of the tumor to the celiac axis and superior mesenteric vessels. In the absence of extrapancreatic disease, the relationship of the low-density tumor mass to the superior mesenteric artery (SMA) and celiac axis is the main focus of preoperative-imaging studies. The current availability of accurate preoperative-imaging studies forms the foundation for two basic principles of clinical research when investigating new therapeutic strategies in patients with pancreatic cancer.

First, local-tumor resectability is most accurately assessed preoperatively; intraoperative exploration is an inaccurate means of assessing critical tumor-vessel relationships *(27,28)*. Objective, reproducible radiographic criteria define potentially resectable disease as: the absence of extrapancreatic disease, the absence of direct tumor extension to the SMA and celiac axis as defined by the presence of a fat plane between the low-density tumor and these arterial structures, and a patent superior mesenteric (SMV)-portal vein confluence. The accuracy of this form of radiographic staging is supported by a recent report by Spitz and colleagues demonstrating a resectability rate of 80% (94/118) and a low rate of microscopic retroperitoneal margin positivity (17%) *(29)*. The accuracy of CT in predicting unresectability and the inaccuracy of intraoperative assessment of resectability are both well established *(26,27)*. Pretreatment staging to exclude patients with locally advanced disease is critical to allow accurate interpretation of results from studies examining the value of multimodality therapy in patients with pancreatic cancer.

Second, published data demonstrate that only patients who undergo a negative-margin pancreaticoduodenectomy receive a survival benefit from surgical resection of the primary tumor *(26,30)*. The median survival of 8–11 mo in patients who undergo pancreaticoduodenectomy and are found to have a positive margin of resection is no different than the median survival reported for patients with locally advanced disease treated with palliative chemoradiation without surgical resection of the pancreas. However, few studies differentiate between grossly positive and microscopically positive margins. The effect of IORT with or without EBRT on microscopically positive margins is not known. The margin most frequently reported as positive in patients who undergo pancreaticoduodenectomy is along the SMV or proximal SMA. Studies that examine the use of IORT following pancreatic resection, in which survival and local control are analysis endpoints should accurately document the pathologic status of the retroperitoneal margin of resection.

3.2. External-Beam Irradiation Factors

The intent of treatment is to use multiple-field, fractionated EBRT techniques with high-energy photons to deliver 45–50 Gy in 1.8-Gy fractions to unresected or residual tumor, or tumor bed (as defined by CT [Fig. 1A] and clips), plus nodal areas at risk (Figs. 1B–E). The spinal cord dose should be less than 35–40 Gy to allow for the option of an IOERT supplement *(19)* (Fig. 1). With pancreatic head tumors, major node groups include the pancreaticoduodenal, porta hepatis, celiac, and suprapancreatic. In patients with unresectable tumor, the latter node group is included in the EBRT field along with the body of pancreas for a 3- to 5-cm margin beyond gross disease. More than two-thirds of the left kidney should be excluded from the AP/PA field since at least 50% of the right kidney is often in the field because of duodenal inclusion (Figs. 1B, D). In patients with lesions of the pancreatic head, the entire duodenal loop (with margin) should be included, because these tumors may invade the medial wall of the duodenum and place the entire circumference at risk. With unresectable tumors of the body-tail, at least 50% of the left kidney may need to be included in order to achieve an adequate pancreatic margin, and

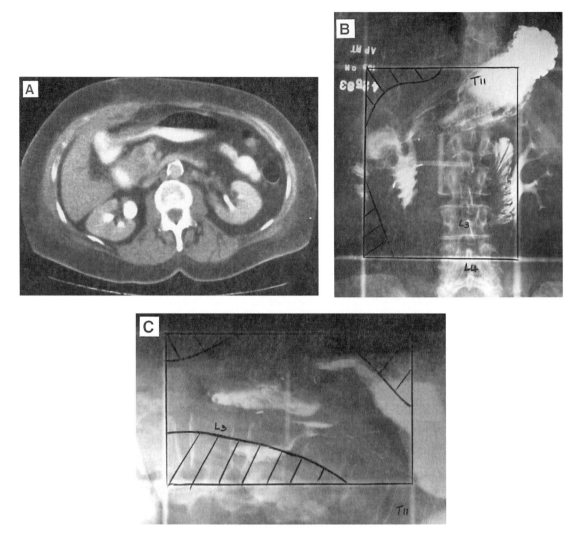

Fig. 1. EBRT four-field technique for pancreatic cancer (Mayo Clinic). (**A**) Mass in head of pancreas on abdominal CT demonstrating relationship to stomach and duodenum. (**B**) AP/PA field with oral contrast to define stomach and duodenum and intravenous contrast to define kidneys. (**C**) Lateral field–posterior aspect includes paraaortic nodes. (**D**) Idealized artists depiction of AP/PA (**D**) and lateral fields (**E**).

to include nodal groups at risk (lateral suprapancreatic and splenic hilum). Since inclusion of the entire duodenal loop is not indicated with tumors of the body or tail, at least two-thirds of the right kidney can be preserved; with tailored blocks, one can usually include pancreaticoduodenal and porta hepatis nodes. For pancreatic head tumors, the superior field extent is at the mid- or upper-T11 vertebral body to achieve an adequate margin on the celiac axis (T12, L1). The upper-field extent is occasionally more superior with tumors of the pancreatic body in order to obtain an adequate margin. With the lateral fields, the anterior field margin is 1.5–2.0 cm beyond gross disease (Figs. 1C,E). The posterior margin is at least 1.5–2.0 cm behind the anterior portion of the vertebral body to allow adequate margins on para-aortic nodes, which are a major lymph-node group at risk with posterior tumor extension from either head or body lesions. The lateral contri-

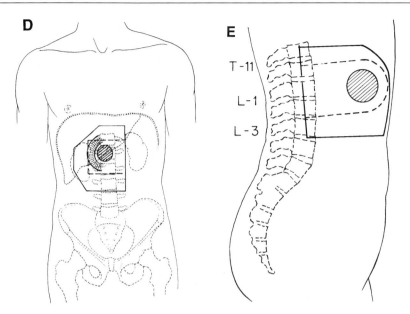

Fig. 1. (*continued*)

bution is usually limited to 18–20 Gy or less, because a moderate volume of kidney or liver may be in the field.

After resection, AP/PA and lateral fields are designed, as for unresected tumors, on the basis of preresection CT tumor volumes, operative clip placement, and postoperative CT nodal volumes. The only border that can perhaps be more restrictive is the anterior border on lateral fields, since the primary tumor has been resected. This border is determined by vascular and nodal boundaries as demonstrated on CT (porta hepatis, superior mesenteric, and celiac) and the anterior margin of the medial portion of the body of the pancreas (after Whipple resection).

3.3. IOERT Equipment and Doses

The Siemens Mevatron ME (magnetron, electrons only) at MDACC was the first linear accelerator designed for dedicated IORT with electrons (IOERT) within the operating room (Fig. 2). It consists of a wall-mounted isocentric gantry with power and control cabinets located in an adjacent room. Radiofrequency energy is generated by a high-power magnetron that can accelerate an electron beam to energies between 6 and 16 MeV. The Mevatron ME can treat at a dose rate of 9 Gy/min to minimize treatment time. The linear accelerator was attached to a 50-cm-thick concrete wall; the other walls were lined with 1.3 cm of lead, as previously described (*31*).

The Mevatron ME utilizes chrome-plated brass treatment applicators with diameters of 5 to 12 cm and straight or beveled ends. The applicator used is optically aligned with a laser projection system and is firmly attached, not to the treatment collimator, but rather to the surgical table using a modified Bookwalter retractor (*32,33*). The surgical table, used for both the operative procedure and patient positioning under the linear accelerator, is a modified Marquet Hiedlberg S couch. Modifications necessary to allow laser-cone alignment include: swivel wheels at both ends of the couch base for ease of mobility; lead screws with hand cranks to provide longitudinal and lateral motion of the table surface; and a covered hand control to prevent folding motions of the table.

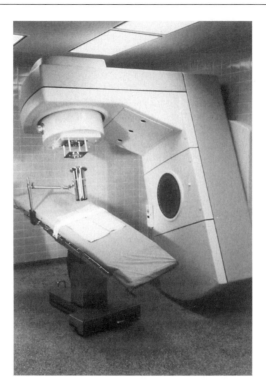

Fig. 2. Photograph of the Siemens Mevatron ME linear accelerator and the surgical table in the dedicated IOERT surgical suite within the operating room complex at the University of Texas M.D. Anderson Cancer Center.

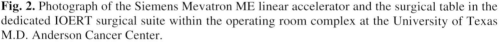

Dosimetry measurements were made for each combination of energy, applicator diameter, and applicator type (flat or beveled end). From these data, depth-dose curves, applicator output factors, and air-gap correction factors were produced that allowed the calculation of monitor settings for delivering a prescribed dose at any selected treatment depth (*33*). Doses of IOERT were prescribed to the 90% isodose depth.

The dose and electron energy of IOERT utilized at MDACC, and other IORT centers, for pancreas cancer is dependent on whether the primary lesion is (locally or advanced) unresectable or is resected with microscopically positive or negative margins. All patients receive EBRT plus concomitant chemotherapy before or after surgery and IOERT. The applicator selected should encompass unresected or residual tumor or tumor bed with ≥1 cm margins (Fig. 3A–D). For unresectable lesions, the IOERT dose is usually 20 Gy with an electron energy of 15–20 MeV. In view of the rapid falloff of electron dosimetry, the spinal cord usually receives only 10–20% of the given dose (Fig. 3E). The use of multiple-field irradiation for the EBRT component of treatment includes lateral fields that exclude spinal cord (*see* Subheading on EBRT Factors). When a gross total resection can be accomplished (Fig. 4), the tumor bed is encompassed within the IOERT applicator (Fig. 5), and a dose of 10–15 Gy is delivered with 9–12 MeV electrons.

3.4. Surgical Factors (Techniques): Pancreaticoduodenectomy

Extended pancreaticoduodenectomy is the term used to describe the operation performed at MDACC for localized adenocarcinoma of the pancreatic head. It incorporates selected aspects of both the traditional Whipple procedure and regional pancreatectomy

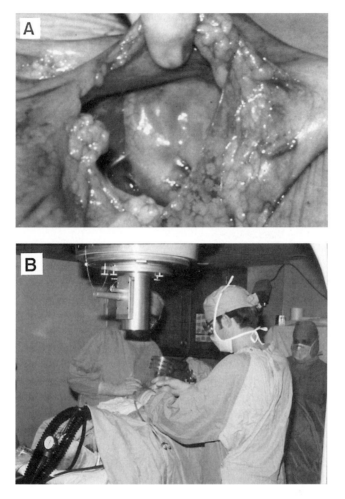

Fig. 3. IOERT technique for unresectable pancreatic cancer (Mayo Clinic). (**A**) Mobilization of stomach. (**B,C**) Inclusion of pancreas mass within IOERT applicator. (**D**) Applicator docked to linear accelerator with suction in place. (**E**) Artists depiction of IOERT dosimetry with 23 MeV beam at MGH. (from Wood WC, et al. *Cancer,* (1982) **49**:1273, with permission).

and has recently been described in detail *(26,28).* The surgical resection differs from standard pancreaticoduodenectomy in three major areas. First, a wide Kocher maneuver is performed, thereby removing all lymphatic tissue over the medial aspect of the right kidney, inferior vena cava, and left renal vein. The rationale for an extended Kocher maneuver is the high incidence of lymph-node positivity in the posterior pancreaticoduodenal region. This maneuver represents a logical strategy to decrease the risk of local tumor recurrence. Second, the retroperitoneal dissection emphasizes clear identification of the superior mesenteric artery and removal of all soft tissue to the right of this vessel (Fig. 4). This requires complete mobilization of the superior mesenteric-portal vein confluence. The retroperitoneal margin is the soft-tissue margin along the right lateral border of the proximal superior mesenteric artery and contains the lateral portion of the mesenteric neural plexus that surrounds the artery. As is true for other solid tumors, adequate local-regional tumor control requires a negative margin of excision and the margin of greatest importance at the time of pancreaticoduodenectomy is the soft-tissue

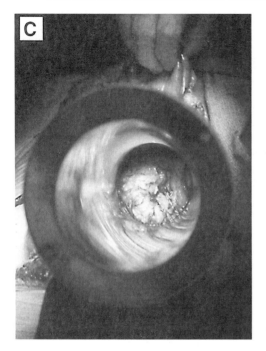

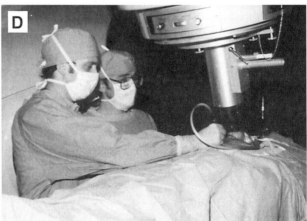

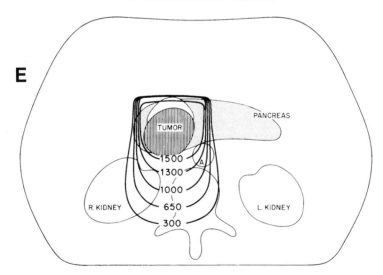

INTRAOPERATIVE ELECTRON BEAM IRRADIATION
Carcinoma, Head of Pancreas
7 cm LUCITE CONE 23 MeV

Fig. 3. (*continued*)

margin along the proximal superior mesenteric artery. Third, segmental resection of the superior mesenteric-portal vein confluence is performed when the tumor is inseparable from the lateral wall of the superior mesenteric vein or portal vein. Presently available data suggest that invasion of the superior mesenteric vein or portal vein is a function of tumor location and size, rather than an indicator of more aggressive tumor biology.

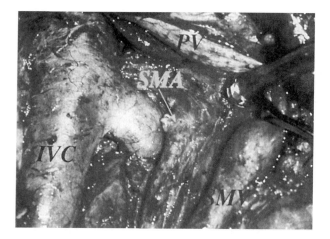

Fig. 4. Operative photograph following pancreaticoduodenectomy. The superior mesenteric vein-portal vein confluence is retracted medially revealing the extent of dissection along the SMA. A wide Kocher maneuver was performed to remove all lymphatic tissue over the medial aspect of the right kidney, inferior vena cava, and left renal vein. A wide retroperitoneal dissection is performed with complete exposure of the SMA and ligation of the inferior pancreaticoduodenal artery. Following pancreatic transection, the SMV-PV confluence is completely mobilized off the uncinate process of the pancreas and retracted medially to the patient's left, allowing exposure of the SMA approx 6 to 8 cm from its origin. The specimen is separated from the SMA using sharp dissection in a distal-to-proximal direction. The tissue adjacent to the proximal 3–4 cm of SMA is labeled as the retroperitoneal margin. IVC, inferior vena cava; PV, portal vein; SMV, superior mesenteric vein.

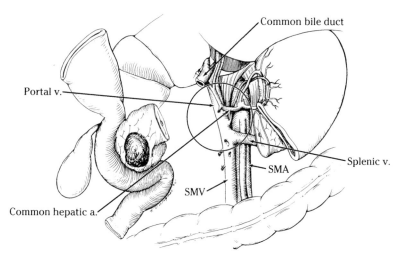

Fig. 5. Electron-beam intraoperative irradiation (IOERT) treatment field included in the circular chrome-plated brass treatment applicator. SMA = superior mesenteric artery; SMV = superior mesenteric vein.

Regional pancreatectomy for adenocarcinoma of the pancreatic head unlike extended pancreaticoduodenectomy, involves removal of lymphatic tissue to the left of the celiac axis and superior mesenteric artery with circumferential skeletonization of these vessels. Regional pancreatectomy as performed in the United States and Japan assumes that a wider lymphadenectomy will increase rates of long-term patient survival. However, evidence for this is lacking *(26)*. There are three principle concerns over the use of regional pancreatectomy for adenocarcinoma of the pancreatic head *(15–17):* the high morbidity and mortality of the procedure; the long-term complications related to poor gastrointestinal function leading to weight loss and chronic debilitation; and the application of such an extensive local-regional therapy, with its associated sequelae, to a disease with such a dominant site of distant organ metastasis (liver). The high morbidity and mortality historically associated with regional pancreatectomy may have been caused by poor patient selection (i.e., the inappropriate application of a bigger operation to patients with advanced disease), as recent reports of regional pancreatectomy demonstrate its safety in the hands of experienced surgeons *(26)*. However, in patients who survive the operation, skeletonization of both sides of the celiac axis and superior mesenteric artery deinnervates the proximal gastrointestinal tract, resulting in rapid gastrointestinal transit and chronic nutritional depletion. Therefore, dissection to the left of the superior mesenteric artery and celiac axis with the intent of removing possible micrometastatic disease within lymph nodes in patients with adenocarcinoma of the pancreatic head has little justification.

In contrast, extended pancreaticoduodenectomy applies basic principles of oncologic surgery to the removal of the pancreatic head, with no additional perioperative morbidity or blood loss *(29)*. The extended lymphadenectomy and retroperitoneal dissection described in extended pancreaticoduodenectomy are done to improve local-regional control by achieving negative retroperitoneal excision margins and adequate regional lymphadenectomy. Prospective data from MDACC have demonstrated improved local-regional control when extended pancreaticoduodenectomy is performed as part of a multimodality treatment program *(25)*. This has resulted in a shift in patterns of disease recurrence from a predominance of local recurrence to a predominance of liver metastases.

4. IORT FOR LOCALLY ADVANCED DISEASE

IORT in patients with locally advanced unresectable disease is well tolerated; the only recognized early complication is prolonged gastric emptying. Since prolonged gastric emptying is a common complication of gastrojejunostomy in this patient population, it is difficult to determine the contribution of IORT to the problem. Duodenal stenosis resulting in gastric outlet obstruction after IOERT was seen in the early experience at Massachusetts General Hospital, so gastrojejunostomy is now standard practice when the IOERT treatment field for unresectable pancreatic head tumors includes the adjacent duodenum (most commonly the medial wall of part two of the duodenum) *(23)*. Late complications of IORT include exocrine pancreatic insufficiency, retroperitoneal fibrosis leading to gastric-outlet obstruction or extrahepatic biliary obstruction, and upper gastrointestinal tract hemorrhage. These complications are uncommon and rarely of major clinical significance.

The published experience with IORT for locally advanced adenocarcinoma of the pancreas appears in Table 1 *(22–24,34–51)*. Median survival ranges from 8–16.5 mo by series (four series included patients with metastases). Recent reports from the MGH and Mayo Clinic with expanded follow-up are reviewed below.

4.1. Mayo Clinic Experience

A recent review from the Mayo Clinic compared survival results with IOERT (20 Gy) plus preoperative or postoperative EBRT with or without 5-FU *(46)*. Fifty-one patients

Table 1
Intraoperative Irradiation for Locally Advanced Pancreatic Cancer

Author	Ref No.	Year	No.	Dose of IORT (Gy)	No. Receiving		No. Treatment Related Deaths	% Pain Relief	Median Survival (mo)
					EBRT	Chemotherapy			
Abe	34	1981	108	15–40	18	47	NA	80	NA
Wood	23	1982	12	15–18	11	6	0	NA	15
Shipley	24	1984	29	15–20	27	20	0	75	16.5
Tepper	35	1987	41	15–20 + Miso	41	41	NA	NA	12
Tuckson	36	1988	35[a]	15–30	14	2	8[b]	57	8.5[a]
Roldan	22	1988	37	20	37	24	0	NA	13.4
Manabe	37	1988	5	30–36.5	8	0	0	100	11.3[c]
Nishimura	38	1988	72	10–40	37	0	NA	76	8.8
Willich	39	1989	30[a]	15–20	11	8	NA	80	8[a]
Cromack	40	1989	29	25	25	25	1	NA	NA
Gilly	41	1990	14	12–25	9	0	0	89	8.9[e]
Abe	42	1991	69	25–40	20	0	1	80	12
Calvo	43	1991	25	15–20	25	0	NA	80	10
Dobelbower	44	1991	27[a]	20–30	19	NA	1	NA	NA[a]
Kojima	45	1991	9	25–30	7	9[d]	0	80	8
Garton	46	1993	27	20	27	25	0	NA	15
Okamoto	47	1994	45	20–30	29	0	1	57	11.1[e]
Kasperk	48	1995	14	10–20	0	0	1	NA	3
Fossati	49	1995	21[a]	20–30	NA	21	1	85	8[a]
Mohiuddin	50	1995	49	10–20	49	49	0	NA	16
Shibamoto	51	1996	29	30–33	29	0	NA	NA	8.5[e]

[a] Includes patients with metastases.
[b] 5 delayed deaths.
[c] Mean.
[d] Mitomycin C used instead.
[e] Survival of patients who received IORT and EBRT.

Table 2
Mayo Clinic Experience with Preoperative or Postoperative
External-Beam Irradiation and IOERT, Locally Unresectable Pancreatic Cancer (46)

Treatment sequence	No. of patients at risk	Median survival (mo)	Overall survival, %	
			2 yr	5 yr
High-dose preop EBRT (±5-FU) and IORT	23[a]	14.9[b]	28	7[b]
IOERT and high-dose postop EBRT (±5-FU)	56	10.5	6	0

[a] Four patients with tumors > 7 cm in diameter were excluded from this comparison because all 56 patients in the high-dose postoperative group had tumors ≤7 cm in diameter.
[b] $p = 0.001$.

with locally advanced pancreatic adenocarcinoma received preoperative standard-fractionation (1.8 Gy/fraction) EBRT, usually with concomitant bolus 5-FU (500 mg/m^2 for three successive days, weeks 1 and 5 of EBRT). Patients were restaged following induction therapy at which time tumor progression (14 patients), or a decrease in performance status (6 patients) prevented reoperation and IOERT in 20 patients (39%). At reoperation, 3 patients were found to have extrapancreatic disease and 1 patient was found to have neuroendocrine carcinoma, leaving 27 patients available for analysis.

Results in the 27 patients treated with preoperative EBRT (plus concomitant 5-FU in 25 patients) and IOERT were compared to 56 patients treated with IOERT and postoperative EBRT with or without 5-FU (45–54 Gy; 1.8 Gy/fraction). Median and actuarial overall survival at 2 and 5 years favored patients treated with preoperative vs postoperative irradiation (Table 2). Actuarial local control at 2 years was 65% in the postoperative group and 68% in the preoperative group. The incidence of liver or peritoneal relapse was the same in both groups of patients at 52% and 54%, respectively.

The authors suggested that the survival advantage seen in patients treated with preoperative chemoradiation and IOERT probably reflects patient selection. Thirty-nine percent of the patients who completed preoperative chemoradiation did not receive IOERT (and were not included in the survival analysis) largely because of disease progression detected at the time of restaging prior to planned operation and IOERT. The ability to avoid the potential morbidity (and duration of recovery) of a major abdominal laparotomy in patients with advanced pancreatic cancer represents a distinct advantage of preoperative over postoperative chemoradiation. When delivering multimodality therapy for any disease, it is beneficial, when possible, to deliver the most toxic therapy last, thereby avoiding morbidity in patients who experience rapid disease progression not amenable to currently available therapies.

4.2. Massachusetts General Hospital Experience

The radiation oncology group at MGH has one of the largest and most mature experiences with IORT for locally advanced tumors of various types (23,24,35). In 1987, Tepper and colleagues reported their experience with 63 patients with locally advanced and nonmetastatic pancreatic cancer (35). The rationale for the updated report was to evaluate the effect of the radiosensitizer misonidazole given in an attempt to decrease the hypoxic fraction of tumor cells. Careful preoperative evaluation was performed including abdominal CT scan, laparoscopy, and in some cases, celiac angiography to ensure the absence of metastatic disease and to document locally advanced, unresectable primary tumors. Preoperative EBRT (10 Gy) was administered during the week prior to IOERT in an effort to prevent peritoneal tumor-cell contamination secondary to surgical manipulation. The IOERT treatment field encompassed the entire tumor with an average applicator diameter of 6–9 cm. The dose of IOERT was 20 Gy. Forty-one patients received the radiosensitizer misonidazole at a dose of 3.5 g/m^2 in a nonrandomized fashion. Treatment was consolidated with postoperative chemoirradiation consisting of 39.6 Gy of EBRT in 22 fractions of 18 Gy, and bolus 5-FU (500 mg/m^2 for 3 d of week 1 of EBRT). Local control was assessed at 3-mo intervals with CT scans.

There was no difference in local tumor control or survival duration in patients treated with or without misonidazole. Local control at 1 yr was 67% in those patients treated with misonidazole and 55% in those who received IORT alone. Median survival was similar for both groups at 12 and 16.5 mo, respectively. Intra-abdominal relapse in the liver or peritoneal cavity was common as in the Mayo analyses. Palliation of pain in the entire group was deemed acceptable with 50% of patients having permanent pain control.

5. IORT FOLLOWING PANCREATIC RESECTION

5.1. Rationale

The effectiveness of IORT plus EBRT (with or without 5-FU) in controlling the primary tumor in patients with unresectable disease (22,24,35), combined with early results from Japan utilizing IORT after pancreaticoduodenectomy (14,52), prompted investigators to combine pancreaticoduodenectomy with adjuvant IORT as a means of decreasing rates of local-regional recurrence in patients with resectable disease. The dose of IORT delivered varied from 10 to 30 Gy (Table 3) (14,25,37,38,40,41,44,47,49,53–58). The majority of studies used doses of 20 Gy or less based on preclinical and clinical studies demonstrating the safety of this dose of IORT (59–63). The major retroperitoneal blood vessels (aorta, celiac axis, SMA, SMV, portal vein, and inferior vena cava) included in the IORT field are not as susceptible to radiation injury, as hollow viscera and solid organs are, although long-term follow-up will be necessary to determine the true extent of vascular injury (62,63).

5.2. IORT Field

The IORT treatment field includes the retroperitoneum and tumor bed extending from the transected bile duct superiorly, to the right kidney laterally, and to the pancreatic remnant medially (Fig. 5) (64). Based upon a previous study in which one patient experienced fatal pancreatic necrosis after IORT (52), the pancreatic remnant is usually excluded from the IORT field. However, in a recent study at the University of Milan, 43 patients underwent adjuvant IORT following pancreaticoduodenectomy with inclusion of the pancreatic remnant in the radiation field (56). One patient died of massive intra-abdominal hemorrhage secondary to a pancreaticojejunal leak, leading the authors to inject the pancreatic duct with neoprene and not anastomose it to the gastrointestinal tract. With this technique, three patients experienced pancreatic fistulas, only one of which subsequently required reoperation because of septic erosion of the left gastric artery.

Table 3
Intraoperative Irradiation for Resectable Pancreatic Cancer

Author	Ref No.	Year	No. Patients	Dose of IORT (Gy)	No. Receiving EBRT	Adjuvant Chemotherapy	Treatment Related Deaths	No. with Local Recurrence	Median Survival (mo)
Manabe	37	1988	4	25–30	4	none	1	2/4	9.5[a]
Nishimura	38	1988	11	10–40	11	none	NA	NA	5
Cromack	40	1989	10	20	0	none	4	NA	NA
Gilly	41	1990	8	12–25	0	none	0	NA	12.6[a]
Hiraoka	14	1990	29	30	0	none	2	1/7	8–14
Ozaki	53	1991	19	30	0	Mitomycin C	0	NA	28%[b]
Dobelbower	44	1991	11	12.5–15	7	5-FU	0	NA	10.5
Gotoh	54	1992	17	30	0	none	1[c]	NA	NA
Johnstone	55	1993	7	20	0	none	NA	NA	NA
Okamoto	47	1994	11	18–30	10	none	0	2/6	39
Zerbi	56	1994	43	12.5–20	0	5-FU + epiadriamicin	1	10/37	NA
Fossati	49	1995	33	12.5–20	9	5-FU	1	7/33	19
Staley	25	1996	39	10–20	39	5-FU	1	4/38	19
Farrell	57	1997	14	12–15	14	5-FU	0	NA	16
Coquard	58	1997	25	12–25	20	5-FU	2	9/25	15

[a] Mean.
[b] 5-yr survival.
[c] Delayed death.

5.3. M.D. Anderson Series

5.3.1. Treatment Factors (EBRT/IOERT)

In contrast to the Milan experience, more than half of the patients in the MDACC experience who have undergone pancreaticoduodenectomy and IORT received preoperative chemotherapy and radiation therapy *(25,29,65)*. The preoperative irradiation field included the primary tumor and pancreaticoduodenal, porta hepatis, and celiac axis lymph-node groups with a field size of 10–15 cm^2. In these patients, the pancreas received 50.4 Gy of EBRT (28 fractions of 1.8 Gy over 5.5 wk) plus infusional 5-FU before surgery. Contrary to what one might expect, it has been suggested that preoperative irradiation decreases the potential for pancreaticojejunal leak because pancreatic exocrine function is decreased after EBRT *(66,67)*. Most of the pancreaticojejunal anastomoses in the MDACC experience were performed over a small silastic stent in two layers using the duct-to-mucosa technique *(68)*. The sides of the IOERT treatment applicator prevented the gastric remnant, small bowel, and colon from entering the treatment field. Extrinsic compression of the superior mesenteric-portal vein confluence and inferior vena cava was avoided by careful applicator placement. IOERT fields ranged from 5 to 10 cm in diameter.

Investigators at MDACC recently reported the outcome of 41 consecutive patients who underwent IOERT following pancreaticoduodenectomy (39 patients) or total pancreatectomy (2 patients) *(64)*. Laparotomy with biopsy and/or biliary or gastric bypass had been performed at other institutions in 19 patients prior to referral. IOERT was delivered in a dedicated operating suite, making patient relocation unnecessary. Twenty-four patients were treated as part of a protocol of preoperative EBRT (45–50.4 Gy given in 1.8-Gy fractions on Monday through Friday) and concomitant protracted-infusion 5-FU; 300 mg/m^2/d; 5–7 d/wk) *(65)*. Eight of the remaining 17 patients received postoperative EBRT and concomitant 5-FU. Thirty-six patients had adenocarcinoma (pancreatic head, 34; distal bile duct, 1; ampulla, 1), four patients had nonfunctioning islet-cell tumors of the pancreatic head, and one patient had small-cell carcinoma of the pancreatic head. No patient during the 3-yr study period failed to receive IOERT because of operative complications. The median applicator diameter (treatment field) was 7 cm (range, 5–10 cm). Four patients had a grossly positive retroperitoneal margin and received 20 Gy of IOERT; 12 patients had an unsuspected microscopic focus of carcinoma within 2 mm of the retroperitoneal resection margin on frozen section analysis and received 15 Gy; and the remaining 25 patients had a negative retroperitoneal margin and received 10 Gy. The additional time required to deliver IOERT, from completion of tumor resection to initiation of reconstruction, averaged 50 minutes.

Early in the M.D. Anderson experience with segmental resection of the SMV or portal vein, surgeons were hesitant to proceed with IOERT immediately following venous reconstruction. Similar to the experience in Japan *(14,54)*, they have since proceeded directly with IOERT following completion of the venous anastomosis *(30,68)*. Gotoh et al. *(54)* have reported on the use of a heparinized bypass catheter between the SMV and portal vein placed just prior to resection of the pancreas and utilized during IOERT so as not to decrease the size of the treatment field, as would occur when the root of the mesentery is displaced cephalad for completion of a primary end-to-end anastomosis between the SMV and portal vein. In contrast, surgeons at MDACC utilize interposition grafts for reconstruction of the SMV, thereby avoiding cephalad displacement of the mesentery and obviating the need for bypass catheters *(69)*.

5.3.2. RESULTS—LOCAL CONTROL, TOLERANCE, SURVIVAL

Local recurrence within the IOERT treatment field was been suggested by CT scan in 4 of 25 patients who had histologically negative retroperitoneal margins following pancreaticoduodenectomy for adenocarcinoma of the pancreatic head; the median time to recurrence was 10 mo (range, 6–14 mo) *(64)*. A typical low-density lesion in proximity to the SMA origin on CT scans was considered a local recurrence, regardless of clinical symptoms; histologic or cytologic confirmation of recurrent disease was not required for a patient to be classified as having local or distant recurrence. Only one patient had a clinically symptomatic local recurrence, manifested by ascites resulting from portal vein thrombosis and progressive carcinomatosis. At a median follow-up of 8 mo (range, 2–31 mo), no patient has developed clinical signs or symptoms of mesenteric vascular thrombosis or has died of an acute unexplained abdominal catastrophe. Only one patient developed portal vein thrombosis identified on follow-up CT scan. This patient had extensive carcinomatosis with tumor recurrence at the level of portal vein occlusion.

The survival advantage for the combination of chemoradiation and pancreaticoduodenectomy compared with pancreaticoduodenectomy alone for resectable pancreas cancer (Table 4) *(25,70–76)* likely results from improved local-regional tumor control. Because of the poor rates of response to 5-FU-based systemic therapy in patients with measurable metastatic disease, it is unlikely that current chemoradiation regimens significantly impact the development of distant metastatic disease. Recent data from Staley and colleagues at MDACC support this belief *(25)*. Thirty-nine patients received preoperative 5-FU based chemoirradiation, pancreaticoduodenectomy, and IOERT for potentially resectable adenocarcinoma of the pancreatic head. Thirty-eight of the 39 patients were evaluable for patterns of treatment failure; there was one perioperative death. Overall, there were 38 relapses in 29 patients: 8 (21%) were local-regional (pancreatic bed and/or peritoneal cavity), and 30 (79%) were distant (lung, liver, and/or bone). The liver was the most frequent site of tumor relapse, and liver metastases were a component of treatment failure in 53% of patients (69% of all patients who had relapse). Fourteen patients (37% of all patients; 48% of patients who had relapse) had liver metastases as their only site of recurrence. Isolated local or peritoneal relapse was documented in only four patients (11%). In contrast, previous reports of pancreaticoduodenectomy for adenocarcinoma of the pancreas have documented local recurrence in 50 to 80% of patients *(26)*. This improvement in local-regional control was seen despite the fact that 14 of 38 evaluable patients had undergone laparotomy with tumor manipulation and biopsy prior to referral for chemoirradiation and reoperation. If these 14 patients were excluded, only two patients (8%) would have experienced local or peritoneal recurrence as any component of treatment failure.

The first report of standard-fractionation chemoirradiation (50.4 Gy over 5.5 wk with concomitant 5-FU) from MDACC documented gastrointestinal toxic effects (nausea, vomiting, and dehydration) that required hospital admission in one-third of patients *(65)*. The recently reported multicenter Eastern Cooperative Oncology Group (ECOG) trial documented the need for hospital admission in 51% of patients during or within 4 wk of completing chemoirradiation *(75)*. The gastrointestinal toxicity of standard-fractionation (5.5 wk) preoperative chemoirradiation prompted a change in the chemoirradiation program at MDACC in an effort to decrease length of treatment and thereby reduce cost, toxicity, and patient inconvenience while attempting to maintain therapeutic efficacy *(26,29,76)*. Chemoradiation is currently delivered using a rapid-fractionation schedule over 2 weeks to a total dose of 30 Gy, at 3 Gy/fraction (10 fractions), 5 d/wk. This program

Table 4
Recent Chemoradiation Studies in Patients with Resectable Pancreatic Cancer

Author (Institution or Group)	Ref No.	Year	No. Patients	Dose of EBRT (Gy)	Chemotherapy Agents	Median Survival (mo)
Postoperative EBRT ± 5FU (adjuvant)						
Kalser (GITSG)	70	1985	21	40	5-FU	20 $p < 0.05$
Surgery alone		1985	22	0	none	11
GITSG (GITSG)	71	1987	30	40	5-FU	18
Whittington (U. Penn)	72	1991	28	45–63	5-FU, mitomycin C	16
Foo (Mayo)	73	1993	29	35–60	5-FU	23
Surgery alone			89	0	none	12
Yeo (J. Hopkins)	74	1997	120	>45	5-FU	20 $p = 0.003$
Surgery alone		1997	53	0	none	14
Preoperative EBRT + 5FU (neoadjuvant)						
Hoffman (ECOG)	75	1998	24	50.4	5-FU, Mitomycin C	16
Staley (MDACC)	25	1996	39[a]	30–50.4	5-FU	19
Pisters (MDACC)	76	1998	20	30	5-FU	25

All patients underwent a pancreatectomy with curative intent.

GITSG: Gastrointestinal Tumor Study Group; MDACC: M. D. Anderson Cancer Center.
[a] IORT (10–15 Gy) given following resection of the pancreatic tumor.
Adapted from Spitz FT, et al.

is based on the principle that the total radiation dose required to obtain a given biological effect decreases as the dose per fraction increases *(26)*. The lower total dose of irradiation (30 Gy) is one part of a treatment program that also includes the concurrent infusion of chemotherapy, and an additional 10 Gy of radiation administered as IOERT. The 10 Gy administered during IOERT, in addition to the 30 Gy (3 Gy/fraction) preoperatively results in a 53% higher biologically equivalent dose (BED) to the tumor bed than that administered with conventional fractionation. Furthermore, the potential risk for late effects with the schedule of 30 Gy is actually 20% less than that with the conventional radiation schedules of either 50 Gy using 2 Gy/fraction or 50.4 Gy using 1.8 Gy/fraction *(77)*. The BED for late radiation effects is 50 at 2 Gy/fraction, 46.9 using 1.8 Gy/fraction, and only 39.9 with the rapid-fractionation schedule. The reason that the BED for late radiation effects with the rapid-fractionation schedule is lower than that with conventional treatment schedules is because of the lower total radiation dose administered with EBRT. Furthermore, the BED for late radiation effects does not reflect the IOERT and EBRT components combined as the risk for late radiation effects is reflected only by the EBRT component of the therapy.

5.4. Thomas Jefferson University Hospital Series

Other investigators have also recently reported their experience with IORT following pancreatic resection. Farrell and colleagues from TJUH reported 14 patients treated between 1987 and 1994. Six patients had AJCC stage I disease, two had stage II disease, and six had stage III disease *(57)*. All patients had ductal adenocarcinoma and were treated with either total pancreatectomy (2), distal pancreatectomy (2), or pancreaticoduodenectomy (10). These patients were compared to a control group of 11 patients treated for various pancreatic neoplasms who underwent pancreatic resection without IOERT IORT (12–15 Gy) was delivered with electrons from a linear accelerator in the irradiation facility immediately adjacent to the operating room. Patients did require movement from one room to another through a sterile corridor. Postoperatively, the IOERT group received an additional 60 Gy of fractionated EBRT with or without 5-FU as a radiosensitizer.

The authors concluded that IOERT contributed to improved survival without additional morbidity as demonstrated by a median survival of 16 mo (5-yr survival of 15.5%) in patients treated with combined modality therapy to include IOERT compared to a median survival of 12 mo in patients treated with pancreatectomy alone. Interestingly, there were fewer operative complications in the IORT group despite longer operative times. The median operative time for the patients receiving IORT was 8 h, 15 min compared to a median of 5 h, 50 min in the surgery-alone group. Postoperative stay and duration of ileus were also shorter in the IORT group in contrast to other studies.

5.5. Lyon Series

Coquard and colleagues from Lyon, France reported their experience with 25 patients who underwent pancreatic resection and IORT between January, 1987 and March, 1995. Nine patients were stage I, five were stage II, and 11 were stage III *(58)*. No patients had evidence of distant metastases at the time of resection. The following surgical resections were performed with curative intent: pancreaticoduodenectomy in 22 patients, distal pancreatectomy in 2 patients, and total pancreatectomy in 1 patient. An IORT dose of 12–20 Gy was delivered to the tumor bed, upper mesenteric vessels, and the left portion of the portal vein. Seventeen patients received postoperative fractionated EBRT (46 Gy); seven with concurrent 5-FU. The median survival for this group was approx 14 mo with a 5-yr survival of 10%, including patients who died in the postoperative period. Local control was evaluated in 23 patients either radiographically or by reoperation. Nine patients had local-regional recurrences—two associated with distant or peritoneal metastases. Coquard and colleagues concluded that IORT is feasible and safe but its contribution to survival duration remains to be determined.

6. CONCLUSIONS AND FUTURE POSSIBILITIES

Studies have documented the safety and improved pain control from the use of IORT in patients with locally advanced pancreatic cancer. The goal of IORT as part of a multimodality treatment program involving pancreaticoduodenectomy is also improved local-regional tumor control; only through this mechanism do these local treatment modalities have potential to increase quality and length of patient survival. Accurate pretreatment staging is essential for future studies attempting to document the effect of IORT combined with novel systemic therapies directed at distant-organ metastases. Future multimodality treatment strategies will combine local-regional therapies such as IORT with systemic therapies directed at newly discovered molecular targets. Gene therapy to include restoration of wild-type p53, or members of the bcl-2 family of antiapoptotic proteins may be combined with irradiation to accentuate local tumor effects (78). It is clear that a multifaceted approach will be required if we hope to impact the quality of life and ultimate survival of patients with pancreatic cancer.

REFERENCES

1. Whipple AO, Parsons WV, and Mullin CR. Treatment of carcinoma of the ampulla of vater, *Ann. Surg.,* **102** (1935) 763–779.
2. Crist DW, Sitzman JV, and Cameron JL. Improved hospital mobidity, mortality, and survival after the Whipple procedure, *Ann. Surg.,* **206(3)** (1987) 358–365.
3. Martin FM, Rossi RL, Dorrucci V, Silverman ML, and Braasch JW. Clinical and pathologic correlations in patients with periampullary tumors, *Arch. Surg.,* **125(6)** (1990) 723–726.
4. Pellegrini CA, Heck CF, Raper S, and Way LW. An analysis of the reduced morbidity and mortality rates after pancreaticoduodenectomy, *Arch. Surg.,* **124(7)** (1989) 778–781.
5. Trede M, Schwall G, and Saeger HD. Survival after pancreaticoduodenectomy, 118 consecutive resections without an operative mortality, *Ann. Surg.,* **211(4)** (1990) 447–458.
6. Andrèn-Sandberg A, Ahren B, Tranberg KG, and Bengmark S. Surgical treatment of pancreatic cancer. The Swedish experience, *Int. J. Pancreatology,* **9** (1991) 145–151.
7. Griffin JF, Smalley SR, Jewell W, et al. Patterns of failure after curative resection of pancreatic carcinoma, *Cancer,* **66** (1990) 56–61.
8. Ishikawa O, Ohhigashi H, Sasaki Y, et al. Practical usefulness of lymphatic and connective tissue clearance for the carcinoma of the pancreas head, *Ann. Surg.,* **208(2)** (1988) 215–220.
9. Ozaki H, Kinoshita T, Kosuge T, Egawa S, and Kishi K. Effectiveness of multimodality treatment for resectable pancreatic cancer, *Int. J. Pancreatology,* **7(1–3)** (1990) 195–200.
10. Tepper J, Nardi G, and Suit H. Carcinoma of the pancreas: review of MGH experience from 1963 to 1973. Analysis of surgical failure and implications for radiation therapy, *Cancer,* **37(3)** (1976) 1519–1524.
11. Fortner JG. Regional pancreatectomy for cancer of the pancreas, ampulla, and other related sites. Tumor staging and results, *Ann. Surg.,* **199(4)** (1984) 418–425.
12. Gall FP and Kockerling F. The problem of radical surgery in pancreatic cancer and its implications for a combined-treatment approach, *Recent Results Cancer Res.,* **110** (1988) 79–86.
13. Hiraoka T. Extended radical resection of cancer of the pancreas with intraoperative radiotherapy, *Baillieres Clin. Gastroenterol.,* **4(4)** (1990) 985–993.
14. Hiraoka T, Uchino R, Kanemitsu K, et al. Combination of intraoperative radiation with resection of cancer of the pancreas, *Int. J. Pancreatology,* **7** (1990) 201–207.

15. Fortner JG, Kim DK, Cubilla A, Turnbull A, Pahnke LD, and Shils ME. Regional pancreatectomy: en bloc pancreatic, portal vein and lymph node resection, *Ann. Surg.,* **186(1)** (1977) 42–50.

16. Nagakawa T, Konishi I, Ueno K, et al. Surgical treatment of pancreatic cancer. The Japanese experience, *Int. J. Pancreatology,* **9** (1991) 135–143.

17. Sindelar WF. Clinical experience with regional pancreatectomy for adenocarcinoma of the pancreas, *Arch. Surg.,* **124(1)** (1989) 127–132.

18. Gunderson LL, Nagorney DM, Martenson JA, et al. External beam plus intraoperative irradiation for gastrointestinal cancers, *World J. Surg.,* **19** (1995) 191–197.

19. Gunderson LL, Willett C. Pancreas and hepatobiliary tract cancer. In Perez CA and Brady LW, (eds.), *Principles and Practice of Radiation Oncology,* 3rd ed. J.B. Lippincott, Philadelphia, 1997, pp. 1467–1488.

20. Whittington R, Solin L, and Mohiuddin M. Multimodality therapy of localized unresectable pancreatic adenocarcinoma, *Cancer,* **54** (1984) 1991–1998.

21. Gunderson LL, Martin JK, Kvols LK, et al. Intraoperative and external beam irradiation ±5-FU for locally advanced pancreatic cancer, *Int. J. Radiat. Oncol. Biol. Phys.,* **13(3)** (1987) 319–329.

22. Roldan GE, Gunderson LL, Nagorney DM, et al. External beam versus intraoperative and external beam irradiation for locally advanced pancreatic cancer, *Cancer,* **61** (1988) 1110–1116.

23. Wood WC, Shipley WU, Gunderson LL, Cohen AM, and Nardi GL. Intraoperative irradiation for unresectable pancreatic carcinoma, *Cancer,* **49** (1982) 1272–1275.

24. Shipley WU, Wood WC, Tepper JE, et al. Intraoperative electron beam irradiation for patients with unresectable pancreatic carcinoma, *Ann. Surg.,* **200** (1984) 289–296.

25. Staley CA, Lee JE, Cleary KA, et al. Preoperative chemoradiation, pancreaticoduodenectomy, and intraoperative radiation therapy for adenocarcinoma of the pancreatic head, *Ann. Surg.,* **171(1)** (1996) 118–125.

26. Evans DB, Abbruzzese JL, and Rich TA. Cancer of the pancreas, in DeVita VT, Hellman S, and Rosenberg SA, (eds). *Cancer, Principles and Practice of Oncology,* J.B. Lippincott, Philadelphia, 1997, pp. 1054–1087.

27. Fuhrman GM, Charnsangavej C, Abbruzzese JL, et al. Thin-section contrast-enhanced computed tomography accurately predicts the resectability of malignant pancreatic neoplasms, *Am. J. Surg.,* **167(1)** (1994) 104–113.

28. Robinson EK, Lee JE, Lowy AM, Fenoglio CJ, Pisters PW, and Evans DB. Reoperative pancreaticoduodenectomy for periampullary carcinoma, *Am. J. Surg.,* **172(5)** (1996) 432–438.

29. Spitz FR, Abbruzzese JL, Lee JE, et al. Preoperative and postoperative chemoradiation strategies in patients treated with pancreaticoduodenectomy for adenocarcinoma of the pancreas [Review], *J. Clin. Oncol.,* **15(3)** (1997) 928–937.

30. Fuhrman GM, Leach SD, Staley CA, et al. Rationale for en-bloc vein resection in the treatment of pancreatic adenocarcinoma adherent to the superior mesenteric-portal vein confluence. Pancreatic Tumor Study Group, *Ann. Surg.,* **223(2)** (1996) 154–162.

31. Mills MD, Almond RR, Boyer AL, et al. Shielding considerations for an operating room based intraoperative electron radiotherapy unit, *Int. J. Radiat. Oncol. Biol. Phys.,* **18(5)** (1990) 1215–1221.

32. Hogstrom KR, Boyer AL, Shiu AS, et al. Design of metallic electron beam cones for an intraoperative therapy linear accelerator, *Int. J. Radiat. Oncol. Biol. Phys.,* **18(5)** (1990) 1223–1232.

33. Nyerick CE, Ochran TG, Boyer AL, and Hogstrom KR. Dosimetry characteristics of metallic cones for intraoperative radiotherapy, *Int. J. Radiat. Oncol. Biol. Phys.,* **21(2)** (1991) 501–510.

34. Abe M and Takahashi M. Intraoperative radiotherapy: the Japanese experience, *Int. J. Radiat. Oncol. Biol. Phys.,* **7** (1981) 863–868.

35. Tepper JE, Shipley WU, Warshaw AL, Nardi GL, Wood WC, and Orlow EL. The role of misonidazole combined with intraoperative radiation therapy in the treatment of pancreatic carcinoma, *J. Clin. Oncol.,* **5(4)** (1987) 579–584.

36. Tuckson WB, Goldson AL, Ashayeri E, Halyard-Richardson M, DeWitty RL, and Leffall LD. Intraoperative radiotherapy for patients with carcinoma of the pancreas. The Howard University Hospital experience, 1978–1986, *Ann. Surg.,* **207(6)** (1988) 648–654.

37. Manabe T, Baba N, Nonaka A, et al. Combined treatment using radiotherapy for carcinoma of the pancreas involving the adjacent vessels, *Int. Surg.,* **73** (1988) 153–156.

38. Nishimura A, Sakata S, Iida K, et al. Evaluation of intraoperative radiotherapy for carcinoma of the pancreas: prognostic factors and survival analyses, *Radiat. Med.,* **6(2)** (1988) 85–91.

39. Willich N, Denecke H, Krimmel K, and Grab J. The Munich experience in intraoperative irradiation therapy of pancreatic cancer, *Ann. Radiol.,* **32(6)** (1989) 484–486.

40. Cromack DT, Maher MM, Hoekstra H, Kinsella TJ, and Sindelar WF. Are complications in intraoperative radiation therapy more frequent than in conventional treatment?, *Arch. Surg.*, **124** (1989) 229–234.

41. Gilly FN, Romestaing PJ, Gerard JP, et al. Experience of three years with intraoperative radiation therapy using the Lyon intra-operative device, *Int. Surg.*, **75** (1990) 84–88.

42. Abe M, Shibamoto Y, Ono K, and Takahashi M. Intraoperative radiation therapy for carcinoma of the stomach and pancreas. In Vaeth JM and Meyer JL, (eds.), *The Role of High Energy Electrons in the Treatment of Cancer, Front. Radiat. Ther. Oncol.*, **25** (1991) 258–269.

43. Calvo FA, Santos M, Abuchaibe O, et al. Intraoperative Radiotherapy in gastric and pancreatic carcinoma: a European experience. In Vaeth JM and Meyer JL, (eds.), *The Role of High Energy Electrons in the Treatment of Cancer Front. Radiat. Ther. Oncol.*, **25** (1991) 270–283.

44. Dobelbower RR Jr, Konski AA, Merrick HW III, Bronn DG, Schifeling D, and Kamen C. Intraoperative electron beam radiation therapy (IOEBRT) for carcinoma of the exocrine pancreas, *Int. J. Radiat. Oncol. Biol. Phys.*, **20** (1991) 113–119.

45. Kojima Y, Kimura T, Yasukawa H, et al. Radiotherapy-centered multimodal treatment of unresectable pancreatic carcinoma, *Int. Surg.*, **76** (1991) 87–90.

46. Garton GR, Gunderson LL, Nagorney DM, et al. High-dose preoperative external beam and intraoperative irradiation for locally advanced pancreatic cancer, *Int. J. Radiat. Oncol. Biol. Phys.*, **27** (1993) 1153–1157.

47. Okamoto A, Tsuruta K, Isawa T, Kamisawa T, Tanaka Y, and Onodera T. Intraoperative radiation therapy for pancreatic carcinoma: the choice of treatment modality, *Int. J. Pancreatology*, **16(2–3)** (1994) 157–164.

48. Kasperk R, Klever P, Andreopoulos D, and Schumpelick V. Intraoperative radiotherapy for pancreatic carcinoma, *Br. J. Surg.*, **82** (1995) 1259–1261.

49. Fossati V, Cattaneo GM, Zerbi A, et al. The role of intraoperative therapy by electron beam and combination of adjuvant chemotherapy and external radiotherapy in carcinoma of the pancreas, *Tumori*, **81** (1995) 23–31.

50. Mohiuddin M, Regine WF, Stevens J, et al. Combined intraoperative radiation and perioperative chemotherapy for unresectable cancers of the pancreas, *J. Clin. Oncol.*, **13(11)** (1995) 2764–2768.

51. Shibamoto Y, Nishimura Y, and Abe M. Intraoperative radiotherapy and hyperthermia for unresectable pancreatic cancer, *Hepato-Gastroenterology*, **43** (1996) 326–332.

52. Shibamoto Y, Manabe T, Baba N, et al. High dose, external beam and intraoperative radiotherapy in the treatment of resectable and unresectable pancreatic cancer, *Int. J. Radiat. Oncol. Biol. Phys.*, **19** (1990) 605–611.

53. Ozaki H, Kinoshita T, Kosuge T, Shimada K, Yamamoto J, and Egawa, S. Evidence of effective multidisciplinary treatment for resectable pancreatic cancer from the viewpoint of the CA19-9 level, *Int. J. Pancreatology*, **9** (1991) 159–163.

54. Gotoh M, Monden M, Sakon M, et al. Intraoperative irradiation in resected carcinoma of the pancreas and portal vein, *Arch. Surg.*, **127** (1992) 1213–1215.

55. Johnstone PA and Sindelar WF. Patterns of disease recurrence following definitive therapy of adenocarcinoma of the pancreas using surgery and adjuvant radiotherapy: correlations of a clinical trial, *Int. J. Radiat. Oncol. Biol. Phys.*, **27** (1993) 831–834.

56. Zerbi A, Fossati V, Parolini D, et al. Intraoperative radiation therapy adjuvant to resection in the treatment of pancreatic cancer, *Cancer*, **73** (1994) 2930–2935.

57. Farrell TJ, Barbot DJ, and Rosato FE. Pancreatic resection combined with intraoperative radiation therapy for pancreatic cancer, *Ann. Surg.*, **226(1)** (1997) 66–69.

58. Coquard R, Ayzac L, Gilly F-N, et al. Intraoperative radiotherapy in resected pancreatic cancer: feasibility and results, *Radiother. Oncol.*, **44** (1997) 271–275.

59. Goldson AL, Ashaveri E, Espinoza MC, et al. Single high dose intraoperative electrons for advanced stage pancreatic cancer: phase I pilot study, *Int. J. Radiat. Oncol. Biol. Phys.*, **7** (1981) 869–874.

60. Ohara K and Takeshima T. Tolerance of canine portal vein anastomosis to intraoperative X-irradiation, *Acta. Oncol.*, **26(6)** (1987) 459–462.

61. Sindelar WF, Hoekstra H, Restrepo C, and Kinsella TJ. Pathological tissue changes following intraoperative radiotherapy, *Am. J. Clin. Oncol.*, **9(6)** (1986) 504–509.

62. Ahmadu-Suka F, Gillette EL, Withrow SJ, Husted PW, Nelson AW, and Whiteman CE. Exocrine pancreatic function following intraoperative irradiation of the canine pancreas, *Cancer*, **62(6)** (1988) 1091–1095.

63. Poulakos L, Elwell JH, Osborne JW, et al. The prevalence and severity of late effects in normal rat duodenum following intraoperative irradiation, *Int. J. Radiat. Oncol. Biol. Phys.*, **18(4)** (1990) 841–848.

64. Evans DB, Termuhlen PM, Byrd DR, Ames FC, Ochran TG, and Rich TA. Intraoperative radiation therapy following pancreaticodudenectomy, *Ann. Surg.,* **218(1)** (1993) 54–60.

65. Evans DB, Rich TA, Byrd DR, et al. Preoperative chemoradiation and pancreaticoduodenectomy for adenocarcinoma of the pancreas, *Arch. Surg.,* **127(11)** (1992) 1335–1339.

66. Ishikawa O, Ohigashi H, Imaoka S, et al. Concomitant benefit of preoperative irradiation in preventing pancreas fistula formation after pancreatoduodenectomy, *Arch. Surg.,* **126(7)** (1991) 885–889.

67. Lowy AM, Lee JE, Pisters PWT, et al. Prospective, randomized trial of octreotide to prevent pancreatic fistula following pancreaticoduodenectomy for malignant disease, *Ann. Surg.,* **226** (1997) 632–641.

68. Evans DB, Lee JE, and Pisters PWT. Pancreaticoduodenectomy (Whipple Operation) and total pancreatectomy for cancer. In Nyhus LM, Baker RJ, and Fischer JF, (eds.), *Mastery of Surgery,* Little, Brown, Boston, 1997, pp. 1233–1249.

69. Leach SD, Lee JE, Charnsangavej C, et al. Patient survival following pancreaticoduodenectomy with resection of the superior mesenteric-portal vein confluence for adenocarcinoma of the pancreatic head, *Br. J. Surg.,* **85** (1998) 611–617.

70. Kalser MH and Ellenberg SS. Pancreatic cancer. Adjuvant combined radiation and chemotherapy following curative resection, *Arch. Surg.,* **120** (1985) 899–903.

71. Gastrointestinal Tumor Study Group. Further evidence of effective adjuvant combined radiation and chemotherapy following curative resection of pancreatic cancer, *Cancer,* **59** (1987) 2006–2010.

72. Whittington R, Bryer MP, Haller DG, Solin LJ, and Rosato EF. Adjuvant therapy of resected adenocarcinoma of the pancreas, *Int. J. Radiat. Oncol. Biol. Phys.,* **21** (1991) 1137–1143.

73. Foo ML, Gunderson LL, Nagorney DM, et al. Patterns of failure in grossly resected pancreatic ductal adenocarcinoma treated with adjuvant irradiation +/– 5 fluorouracil, *Int. J. Radiat. Oncol. Biol. Phys.,* **26(3)** (1993) 483–489.

74. Yeo CJ, Abrams RA, Grochow LB, et al. Pancreaticoduodenectomy for pancreatic adenocarcinoma: postoperative adjuvant chemoradiation improves survival. A prospective, single-institution experience, *Ann. Surg.,* **225(5)** (1997) 621–633.

75. Hoffman JP, Lipsitz S, Pisansky T, Weese J, Solin L, and Benson AB. Phase II trial of preoperative radiation therapy and chemotherapy for patients with localized, resectable adenocarcinoma of the pancreas: an Eastern Cooperative Oncology Group study, *J. Clin. Oncol.,* **16** (1998) 317–323.

76. Pisters PWT, Abbruzzese JL, Janjan NA, Cleary KR, Charnsangavej C, Goswitz MS, Rich TA, Raijman I, Wolff RA, Lenzi R, Lee JE, Evans D. Rapid-fractionation preoperative chemoradiation, pancreaticoduodenectomy, and intraoperative radiation therapy for resectable pancreatic adenocarcinoma. *J. Clin Oncol.,* in press.

77. Barton M. Tables of equivalent dose in 2 Gy fractions: a simple application of the linear quadratic formula, *Int. J. Radiat. Biol. Phys.,* **31(2)** (1995) 371–378.

78. Meyn RE. Apoptosis and response to radiation: implications for radiation therapy, *Oncology,* **11** (1997) 349–356.

13 Biliary Tract IORT
Bile Duct and Gallbladder

Takeshi Todoroki, Leonard L. Gunderson, and David Nagorney

CONTENTS

1. RESULTS OF STANDARD TREATMENT

1.1. Surgical Considerations

Many patients with gallbladder and extrahepatic biliary-duct lesions have either technically unresectable lesions or have gross or microscopic residual disease after attempts at resection because of anatomic location and technical limitations (1–3). Surgical removal of a malignant gallbladder lesion often necessitates blunt dissection from the liver with narrow or nonexistent margins unless a wedge of liver is removed.

A larger percentage of patients with proximal lesions are undergoing curative resections in modern series (2,4–6). In an early Mayo analysis, only 5% of 78 patients with Klatskin tumors had curative resection, and there were no long-term survivors (1). In a recent analysis of 171 patients with surgical exploration at Mayo Clinic from 1976 to 1985 for extrahepatic cholangiocarcinoma, the rate of curative resection with negative margins by site of primary was 15% for proximal lesions, 33% for mid-ductal, and 56% for distal lesions (6). Five-year survival rates as high as 40% have been reported in patients with proximal lesions who have negative resection margins (5,6). Many patients with proximal lesions, however, are not candidates for resection because of both extent and location. For such patients, orthotopic liver transplantation is being evaluated in selected centers with 5-yr survival rates of 15 to 20% (5,7,8).

From: Current Clinical Oncology: Intraoperative Irradiation: Techniques and Results
Edited by: L. L. Gunderson et al. © Humana Press, Inc., Totowa, NJ

Lesions in the periampullary region or distal common duct have a uniformly better prognosis. Resection with a Whipple procedure is usually feasible and results in long-term survival in 30 to 40% of patients *(5,6)*.

1.2. Patterns of Relapse After Standard Surgical Resection

Local relapse in the tumor bed or regional nodes (LF-RF) is common in spite of "curative resection" for both gallbladder and extrahepatic biliary-duct lesions *(3,5)*. With mid and proximal bile duct cancer, proximal and distal margins of resection are often narrow; radial margins are usually narrow if the primary lesion extends beyond the entire duct wall. With ductal lesions, loco-regional relapse is a common cause of death. In combined series with "curative" simple cholecystectomy for gallbladder cancer, 95 of 110 or 86% of patients with early relapse died with or because of local recurrences, and 11 of 25 or 48% of patients alive at 5 yr had local recurrence *(9)*. Twelve of 16 or 75% of patients with radical "curative" cholecystectomy, died with or because of local recurrence *(9)*. Hepatic metastases can occur with gallbladder and ductal tumors, but with gallbladder primary lesions, it may be difficult to differentiate liver metastasis from direct extension. Peritoneal involvement is more common with gallbladder cancer than with ductal primary tumors.

Kopelson et al. *(3)* analyzed patterns of relapse after curative resection in a Massachusetts General Hospital (MGH) series of 28 patients with complete resection of gallbladder or ductal lesions. In the 25 postoperative survivors, distant metastases occurred in nine (36%) as a component of relapse. Loco-regional relapse occurred in 13 patients (52%) as the major mode of relapse. Initial spread through the wall of the organ seemed to be the best predictor of loco-regional relapse—4 of 11 patients (36%) with lesions confined to the wall vs 9 of 14 or 64% with lesions extending beyond the wall.

Willett et ai. analyzed patterns of relapse in 41 MGH patients with ampullary carcinomas *(10)*. In 12 patients with low-risk pathologic features (limited to the ampulla or duodenum, well- or moderately differentiated histology, uninvolved resection margins and nodes), 5-yr actuarial local control and survival rates were 100 and 80%, respectively, with surgery alone. In 17 high-risk patients treated with surgery alone, those rates were 50 and 38%, respectively, $p < 0.05$ (high risk was defined as tumor invasion of the pancreas, poorly differentiated histology, involved nodes or resection margins).

1.3. External Irradiation With or Without Chemotherapy

Although areas of malignant obstruction can be decompressed with placement of percutaneous transhepatic catheters, retrograde endoscopic stents, or by performing a surgical bypass such as a segment 3 Roux-y hepaticojejunostomy, none of these procedures actively treat the tumor. Therefore, the addition of external-beam radiation therapy (EBRT) with or without chemotherapy to palliative drainage is reasonable. Significant palliation and occasional long-term survival can be obtained with EBRT to doses of 40–60 Gy in 4.5–7 wk for unresectable or recurrent bile-duct cancers, but permanent local control is uncommon *(9,11–14)*. In view of the presence of multiple dose-limiting organs including liver, stomach, duodenum, kidneys, and spinal cord, EBRT doses higher than 40–45 Gy can be obtained with acceptable morbidity only if tumor extent is carefully defined with imaging studies and surgical clips, and the patient is treated with sophisticated multiple-field EBRT techniques that may include noncoplanar beams using three dimensional (3D) treatment planning *(11)*.

Combinations of EBRT and chemotherapy need to be evaluated more extensively in view of survival trends seen in an early analysis by Kopelson et al. *(9),* and more recent series from Thomas Jefferson *(15),* Sloan Kettering *(16),* and the University of Pennsylvania and Fox Chase *(17).* In the latter series, 1- and 3-yr survival appeared to be better in patients with gross residual disease who received both modalities vs EBRT alone (1-yr survival of 65 vs 17%; 3-yr 26 vs 8%, $p = 0.02$).

In bile-duct patients with subtotal resection and residual disease, an EORTC analysis suggests that the addition of EBRT may improve survival. The EORTC group *(18)* analyzed a series of 55 patients in whom 17 were treated with surgery alone and 38 received postoperative irradiation (52 of 55 had pathologically positive margins). The irradiated patients had a median survival of 19 vs 8.3 mo with surgery alone (1 yr 85 vs 36%, 2 yr 42 vs 18%, 3 yr 31 vs 10%; $p = 0.0005$).

Investigators from Johns Hopkins reported a series of 50 patients with localized proximal bile-duct cancers who had exploration with or without resection and were potential candidates for postoperative irradiation *(2,19).* A gross total resection with positive or negative margins was performed in 21 patients (42%), and partial resection in 10 (20%). An additional 12 patients (24%) were unresectable and had stents placed. Twenty-three patients received postoperative EBRT to a mean dose of 46 Gy in 5 wk for the 14 resected patients and 50 Gy for the 9 patients with unresected lesions (target volumes were not defined in the manuscript). Eight of 14 resected patients received a transcatheter iridium boost to an average dose of 13 Gy at an unspecified depth. The addition of irradiation in this very mixed group of patients, neither improved nor detracted from duration or quality of survival, with duodenal and hepatic toxicity the same in irradiated and nonirradiated patients. Strategies suggested by the authors to improve outcome included adding 5-FU with or without cisplatin to irradiation, increasing dose of irradiation ± field size and considering altered sequencing with preoperative irradiation with or without chemotherapy instead of postoperative treatment.

In the MGH ampullary-cancer series reported by Willett et al. *(10),* 29 of 41 patients had high-risk pathologic features (17 were treated with surgery alone and 12 received postoperative EBRT with or without 5-FU). Although the adjuvant treatment appeared to improve both 5-yr local control and survival rates with values of 83 vs 50% and 51 vs 38%, respectively, these differences were not statistically significant in view of the small patient numbers and distant risks (liver, peritoneum, pleura).

2. SPECIALIZED IRRADIATION MODALITIES

The usual tumor-related cause of death after EBRT, with or without chemotherapy, for locally unresectable biliary-tract cancers is local persistence of disease. In view of the proximity of dose-limiting organs and structures to the malignancy, improvements in local control may be feasible with the addition of specialized boost techniques including brachytherapy via transhepatic catheters or retrograde endoscopic stents or intraoperative radiation therapy (IORT) with electrons, orthovoltage, or HDR brachytherapy (with or without irradiation dose modifiers).

2.1. Transcatheter Brachytherapy With or Without External Irradiation

The temporary insertion of sealed radioactive sources via transhepatic catheters or stents placed endoscopically can deliver localized high-dose irradiation. This method of

Table 1
Irradiation for Locally Advanced (Usually Unresected) Primary Bile-Duct Cancer

| Investigation (ref. no.) | No. Pts. | Median (mo) | Survival | | | | | Local Relapse no. (%) | Septic Death no. (%) |
			12 mo no. (%)	18 mo no. (%)	24 mo no. (%)	36 mo no. (%)	60 mo no. (%)		
External Irradiation with or without Chemotherapy									
Buskirk et al. (12)	11	12.0	–(55)	0	–	–	–	6/11/(55)	0
Fields and Emami (13)	9	7.0	1 (11)	1 (11)	0 (0)	–	–	6/9 (67)	–
Hanna and Rider (14)	14	12.3	–	–	–	–	–	–	–
Alden and Mohuidden (15)	8	13.5	–	–	–(25)	–	–	–	–
Fogel and Weisberg (42)	34	11.0	–(48)	–(30)	–(18)	–(12)	–(6)	9/10 w/autopsies	–
Transcatheter alone									
Fletcher et al. (43)	8	11+	4 (50)	3 (38)	–	–	–	3/8 (38)	–
Karani et al. (44)	30	not given	21 (70)	–	5 (17)	–	–	–	–
Transcatheter plus External with or without Chemotherapy									
Fields and Emami (13)	8	15	5 (63)	–	2 (25)	1 (13)	–	4/8 (50)	2/8 (25)
Alden and Mohuidden (15)	13	24	–	–	–(40)	–	–	–	–
Minsky et al. (16) (brachy boost 6 of 10)	10	16	–(80)	–(50)	–(50)	–(50)	NA	5/10 (50)	–
Hayes et al. (20)	8	13.4	4 (50)	2 (25)	1 (13)	–	–	–	1/8 (13)
Johnson et al. (21)	7	12.5	4 (57)	2 (29)	2 (29)	–	–	–	1/7 (14)
Foo et al. (22)	24	12.8	16 (67)	9 (38)	–(19)	–(14)	–(14)	8 (33)	–
Fritz et al. (23)	30	10	–(34)	–(20)	–(18)	–(18)	–(8)	14/27 (52)	–
Veeze-Kuypers (24)	42	10	–(46)	–(27)	–(18)	–(13)	–	–	–
Herskovic et al. (45) (additional 4 no EBRT)	12	–	5 (42)	–	–	–	–	3/16 (19)	3/16 (19)
IORT									
Todoroki et al. (34)	5	8.0	2 (40)	1 (20)	0 (0)	–	–	4/4 evaluable	–
Iwasaki et al.[a] (34)	12	15.0	7 (58)	–	–	–	–	–	–
IORT plus External									
Mayo Clinic (27,28)	14[b]	18.5	10 (71)	6 (43)	4 (29)	2 (14)	1 (7)	6 (43)	–
Deziel et al. (32)	9[c]	13	2 (40)	2 (40)	1 (20)	1 (20)	–	–	–
Bussee et al. (33)	12	14.0	–	–	1 (8)	–	–	5/10 evaluable	–
Iwasaki et al.[a] (35)	7	7.0	1 (14)	–	–	–	–	–	–

[a] 13 of 19 had noncurative resection before IORT; 6 were unresected; mo = months, no = number, pts = patients, w = with.
[b] If an additional patient treated with palliative intent is included, median SR = 16.5 mo.
[c] Data includes 4 patients with gallbladder cancer and 5 with bile duct.
Modified from ref. 11.

boost treatment is attractive because of its potentially wide applicability (as opposed to that of IOERT). Deaths from sepsis are reported more commonly than in EBRT only series, however, which is a reflection of the need for transhepatic catheters in all patients with inherent risks.

There is a suggestion of improved survival in patients with unresectable bile-duct cancers treated with EBRT plus brachytherapy when compared with either method alone *(11,20,21)*, but no randomized trials have been performed to test these possible differences. In view of short follow-up and a low incidence of survival beyond 1 yr, the exact incidence of loco-regional failure is difficult to discern in many of the published series.

In a recent Mayo Clinic series *(12,22)*, 24 patients received EBRT to 45–50.4 Gy with or without 5-FU (9 patients) followed in 2–4 wk by a transcatheter iridium boost of 20–25 Gy (calculated at a 1.0-cm radius in 20 of the 24). Local failure was documented in eight patients or 33%. Five-year overall and disease-free survival were 14% in the total group (3 survivors ≥ five years; five-year survival (SR), 2 of 9 or 22% in patients who received 5-FU with EBRT vs 8% in the 15 with no 5-FU during EBRT).

Data from a 48-patient single-institution analysis from Thomas Jefferson University Hospital (TJUH) *(15)* suggest a positive impact of increased irradiation dose on median and 2-yr survival in 24 patients treated with EBRT with or without chemotherapy and transcatheter iridium. Higher doses were usually achieved by combining EBRT doses of 44–46 Gy with a brachytherapy boost dose of 25 Gy calculated at a 1-cm radius. Two-year SR for all 48 patients was 18% with median survival of 9 mo. Patients treated with irradiation vs those without radiation had 2-yr SR of 30 vs 17% and median SR of 12 vs 5.5 mo ($p = 0.01$). Irradiated patients treated to a dose of >55 Gy vs <55 Gy had 2-yr SR of 48 vs 0% and median SR of 24 mo vs 6 mo ($p = 0.0003$). Radiation dose response was also suggested by an increase in median survival with an increase in irradiation doses from <45, 45–54, 55–65, and 66–70 Gy, respectively (4.5, 9, 18, and 25 mo).

Results in two European series suggest a potential advantage of combining EBRT plus brachytherapy with a noncurative resection. In the Fritz et al. analysis of 39 patients treated at the University of Heidelberg with EBRT plus high-dose-rate brachytherapy with or without noncurative resection *(23)*, those with noncurative resection vs no resection had a suggestive increase in survival (median: 12 vs 8 mo; 3 yr: 32 vs 5%, 5 year: 32 vs 0%, $p = 0.004$). In a Rotterdam series by Veeze-Kuypers et al., of 42 patients treated with EBRT plus ^{192}Ir with or without resection *(24)*, the 11 patients with noncurative resection had improved median survival of 15 vs 8 mo, and 3-yr SR of 36 vs 6% ($p = 0.06$) when compared to results in the 31 patients without resection.

3. TREATMENT FACTORS (EBRT, SURGERY, IORT)

3.1. Preoperative Staging

Surgical unresectability of bile duct cancer is based on a predetermined sequence of imaging studies obtained preoperatively in patients with obstructive jaundice. A chest X-ray is obtained to exclude pulmonary metastases. Once extra-abdominal metastases are excluded, abdominal imaging is performed to assess the local and regional extent of the tumor. Abdominal ultrasonography is generally used initially to determine the site of the bile duct obstruction, the tumor morphology (papillary, nodular, or sclerotic) and whether regional lymph node metastases or intrahepatic metastases are present. Additionally, ultrasonography with Doppler capacity can determine whether hepatic arterial or portal venous blood flow has been affected. If no obvious metastases are identified, percutaneous transhepatic cholangiography is performed. Complete visualization of both the right and left intrahepatic ductal systems is essential for assessment of bile duct resectability. Cholangiography should demonstrate both the proximal and distal extent of the tumor. In general, multicentric tumors or tumors with bilateral intrahepatic segmental ductal extension preclude resection. If cholangiography shows only unilateral segmental extension or less proximal extension, resection is possible. Computed tomography (CT) of the abdomen is performed to further exclude regional and intrahepatic metastases and assess for hepatic lobar atrophy. If metastases are excluded and the atrophy exists only on the side of the intrahepatic segmental extension, angiography is performed to assess vascular involvement. Angiography should demonstrate both the hepatic arterial and portal venous anatomy clearly. Bile duct cancers are resectable if the blood supply to the liver can be maintained. If hepatic resection is undertaken, angiography should demonstrate the ability to preserve or at least to reconstruct the vasculature to the postresection liver remnant. Other imaging studies that may be used to assess resectability include magnetic resonance imaging (MRI) and 3D functional imaging by GSA scintigraphy.

Staging of proximal bile duct cancers has been based on the Bismuth system. Bismuth classification of proximal bile duct tumors is as follows:

Type 1: Confined to bile duct 2 cm or more below confluence.
Type 2: Ductal confluence involved but no intrahepatic segmental extension.
Type 3A: Ductal confluence involved with right unilateral segmental extension.
Type 3B: Ductal confluence with left intrahepatic segmental extension.
Type 4: Bilateral intrahepatic segmental extension.

In general, Bismuth Types 2 and 3 require hepatic resection. Implicit in all resections of bile duct cancer is a thorough regional lymphadenectomy with skeletalization of the hepatic artery and portal venous systems. Bilioenteric continuity is restored via a Roux-en-Y hepaticojejunostomy.

3.2. Irradiation Techniques—EBRT

3.2.1. Dose-Limiting Structures

A major deterrent to improved results with EBRT with or without bradytherapy for technically unresectable lesions is the limited irradiation tolerance of the liver, duodenum, stomach, and spinal cord and the lack of clear definition of the lesion's location and extent relative to the liver *(25)*. Although the superior and inferior extent of bile-duct malignancies can often be outlined by a percutaneous cholangiogram or endoscopic retrograde cholangiopancreatography (ERCP), the degree of extraductal invasion is poorly defined by current diagnostic-imaging procedures. Clip placement at the time of surgical exploration or resection is useful in outlining the extrahepatic component of ductal cancers and in defining the bed of the gallbladder. Shaped, multiple fields, and shrinking-field techniques should be used to spare as much normal tissue as possible *(12,20,25,26)*.

3.2.2. EBRT Treatment Volume and Dose

Areas at risk for local relapse or progression include the tumor bed or unresected tumor and nodes along the porta hepatis, pancreaticoduodenal system, and celiac axis. An excretory urogram should be done at time of simulation to confirm left renal function as one-half to two-thirds of the right kidney is often included in the anteroposterior (AP/PA)

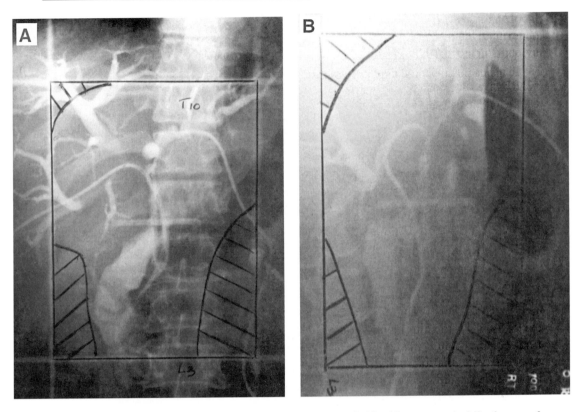

Fig. 1. EBRT treatment fields (Mayo Clinic). (**A**) APPA field with contrast in bile ducts and duodenum; (**B**) lateral field.

component of treatment. An initial set of AP and cross-table lateral simulation films can identify surgical clips and renal position relative to the field center. Contrast is injected into the transhepatic catheter to define the extent of ductal tumor, and the location of pancreaticoduodenal nodes is determined with contrast agent in the stomach and duodenum (nodes lie adjacent to medial wall).

The initial large-field treatment volume for EBRT fields can be treated to 40–45 Gy in 1.8-Gy fractions given 5 d/wk via a multiple-field plan (AP and laterals or AP/PA and laterals) using shaped blocks to exclude unnecessary normal stomach, small intestine, kidney, and liver (Fig. 1) *(12,20,25,26)*. Use of lateral fields for a portion of the treatment allows a reduction in dose to the spinal cord, right kidney, and portions of the liver. Wedge-pair or arc techniques may be utilized for either large or boost fields to alter dose distribution. Liver intolerance to irradiation may necessitate an initial field reduction after 30–36 Gy and a second reduction after 45–50 Gy if unresected or residual gross disease exists. For bile-duct primary lesions, the preferred initial intrahepatic field margin beyond gross ductal disease is 3–5 cm because of the tendency for submucosal spread within lympatics; these margins often need to be reduced to 2–3 cm after a dose of 30–36 Gy. The upper dose level within the second boost field is 55–70 Gy delivered over 6.5–8 wk with EBRT alone. The higher doses are used only if the boost volume is carefully defined, but could possibly be used more frequently with the advent of 3D techniques and noncoplanar beams *(11)*. If boost-dose irradiation is feasible with brachytherapy techniques, the tumor-nodal dose is carried to 45–50 Gy with EBRT techniques and 20–30

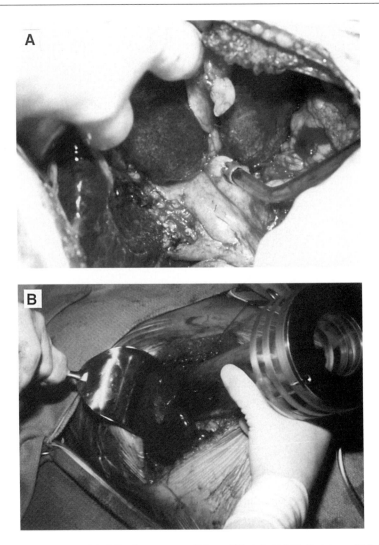

Fig. 2. IOERT for unresectable bile duct cancer (Mayo Clinic). (**A**) Definition of klatskin tumor. (**B**) placement of IOERT applicator. (**C**) IOERT treatment field at liver hilum. (**D**) IOERT applicator "docked" to accelerator.

Gy is delivered to a 1-cm radius with transcatheter ^{192}Ir *(12,20,22)*. If extraductal extent can ultimately be defined more precisely with transcatheter ultrasound or coil magnetic resonance imaging (MRI) imaging studies, both 3D and brachytherapy boost techniques can be enhanced.

3.3. Surgical and IORT Factors

3.3.1. UNRESECTABLE BILE DUCT

In most reported bile duct series, IORT has been used as a supplement to EBRT for unresectable lesions. Exploratory laparotomy is performed to rule out occult peritoneal seeding, and intraoperative liver ultrasound is done to rule out undiscerned small liver metastases. The hilar component of the unresectable cancer is then surgically exposed, and titanium or small vascular clips are placed to mark the medial, lateral, and inferior

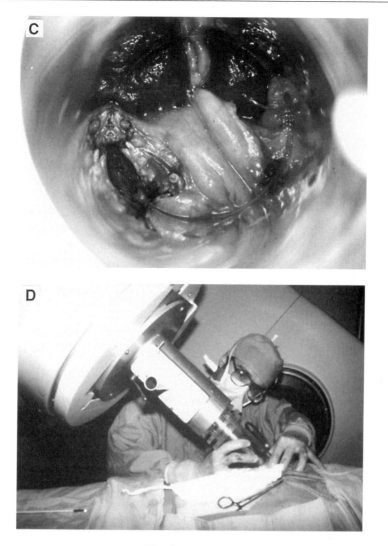

Fig. 2. (*continued*)

extent of disease for purpose of postoperative EBRT field design. Duodenum and stomach can usually be mobilized out of the intended IOERT field.

The surgeon and radiation oncologist then determine the appropriate size IORT applicator to encompass both the palpable and radiographic tumor with at least a 1 cm margin (i.e., 4 cm diameter lesion requires ≥6 cm diameter applicator) (Fig. 2). For unresectable lesions, the depth of the malignancy relative to the surgically exposed hilar lesion has to be estimated from preoperative imaging studies for purpose of determining IOERT energy (PTHC, ERCP, CT abdomen). In the reported Mayo series (*27,28*), IOERT energies ranged from 9 to 18 MeV. Since lesions are usually unresectable, IOERT doses commonly range from 15–20 Gy depending on the planned EBRT dose.

3.3.2. Major Resection Procedures and Indications, University of Tsukuba

In locally advanced biliary tract cancers, the extension mode of the tumor has a very wide range, and the surgical procedure should coordinate to the variety of tumor spread.

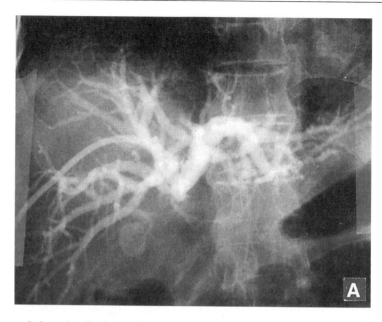

Fig. 3. Diagnostic imaging findings of patient with locally advanced stage IV gallbladder cancer, Tsukuba University. (**A**) Cholangiogram. Hepatic ducts were completely obstructed at the confluence of main hepatic ducts. Tumor extension reached to the bifurcation of anterior and posterior segmental duct branches (↑). Gallstone (★). (**B**) Computed tomography (CT). Gallbladder cancer with extension to the liver (↑) and massive lymph node metastases (↑) were demonstrated. (**C**) Angiogram showed ill-marginated staining of the gallbladder, encasement of the cystic artery and neovascularity of the epicholedochal plexus. (**D**) Portograph revealed remarkable involvement of the truncus of the portal vein (from Todoroki et al. *World J. Surg.* **15** (1991) 357–366, 1991, with permission).

Practically, liver resections of various extent, hepaticocholedocus resection with chole-cystectomy, pancreatoduodenectomy, reconstruction of portal vein and/or hepatic arteries following resection, and systematic node dissection are a basic component of resection surgery. For selecting resection procedures, tumor invasion to the (a) hepatic parenchyma, (b) intra- and extrahepatic bile ducts, (c) hepatic arteries, (d) portal veins, and (e) lymph node metastasis will be taken into account based on preoperative imaging studies (Fig. 3). Furthermore, a majority of patients with locally advanced disease require percutaneous transhepatic cholangio-drainage (PTC-D) for their associated obstructive jaundice to avoid unfavorable postresection complications. At Tsukuba University, PTC-D is performed to relieve jaundice for every patient with a serum total bilirubin level higher than 10 mg/dL or for patients with less than that level to clarify the exact location and pattern of the bile duct obstruction. In order to predict the functional volume and configuration of the liver remaining after resection, the new technology of 3D-functional liver imaging by GSA scintigraphy is applied routinely for patients with jaundice in whom extended hemilobectomy or hepatopancreatoduodenectomy would be inevitable.

The criteria for (1) hepaticocholedochus resection (HCR), (2) liver resection, and (3) systematic node dissection are as follows:

(1) HCR is defined as a bile duct resection of the main hepatic ducts up to above the primary bifurcation and down to the intrapancreatic portion. HCR is essential for patients

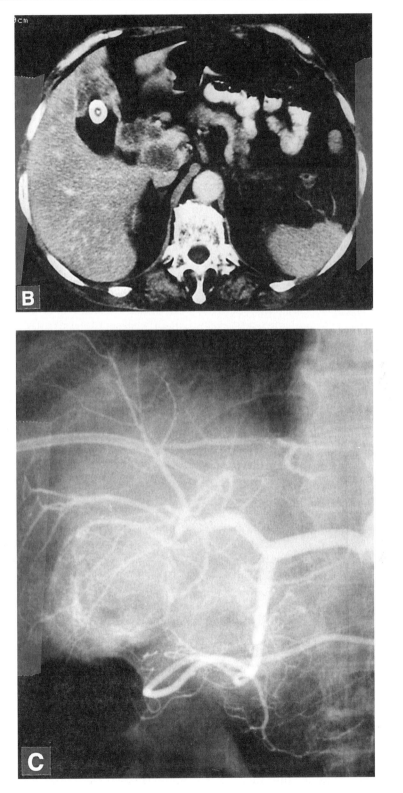

Fig. 3. (*continued*)

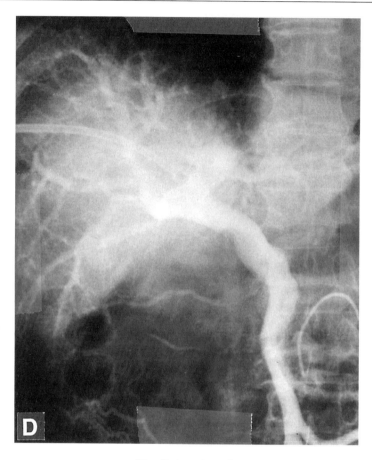

Fig. 3. (*continued*)

with bile duct cancer that has originated from or extends to the major hepatic bile ducts, or for gallbladder cancer that extends to the bile duct. From a view point of preoperative imaging studies, HCR should be considered when cholangiography revealed obstructive or narrowing changes of the main hepatic ducts and/or extrahepatic bile duct.

(2) Liver resections of various extents—major hepatectomies, bisegmentectomies (S4 and S5), and wedge resections of the gallbladder fossa—are performed alone, or with HCR according to the location of involved bile ducts. Furthermore, pancreaticoduodenectomy (PD) should be applied to patients with heavily metastasized peripancreatic lymph nodes and/or direct tumor extension to the head of the pancreas via the hepatoduodenal ligament. Hepatic bisegmentectomy will be carried out when the tumor extends less than 2 cm into the liver parenchyma in patients with gallbladder cancer, or when the tumor extends bilaterally to the main hepatic bile ducts with or without hepatic parenchymal involvement in patients with bile duct cancer. Hepatic lobectomy should be done when the apparent tumor invasion extends beyond the scope of bisegmentectomy, or, regardless of the extent of parenchyma invasion, when the tumor involvement in the portal vein precluded its reconstruction after resection. Resection of the spigelian lobe is essential when the tumor extension on the left hepatic duct reaches the bifurcation of the branch to the spigel lobe. Wedge resection of the gallbladder fossa is

selected when the tumor is located on the fossa without evident invasion into the hepatic parenchyma.

(3) The procedure of systematic node dissection is divided into three categories. The first category or grade involves dissection of nodes in the hepatoduodenal ligament including cystic duct, pericholedochal and hilar lymph nodes. The second category includes nodes in the first grade dissection, but in addition, lymph nodes of the right side of the celiac, around the common hepatic artery, periportal portion beneath the neck of the pancreas, and the right side of the superior mesenteric artery. The nodes of the right side of the aorta up to beneath the spigelian lobe and down below the bifurcation of the left renal vein are extirpated as a sample to check for metastasis. The third grade or category involves dissection of the para-aortic nodes together with the first and second category dissection.

3.3.3. GALLBLADDER

The largest experience using surgical resection and IOERT for locally advanced gall-bladder cancers has been described by Todoroki et al. *(29)*. From October 1970 to May 1997, 93 patients with stage IV cancers had surgical resection alone or in combination with EBRT, IORT, or IORT with EBRT at Tsukuba University. Resection procedures for stage IV disease varied due to the extent and mode of tumor invasion as previously discussed. Seventy-two of the 93 patients underwent some type of liver resection: major hepatectomy in 17 patients, hepatic bisegmentectomy (segment IV and V) in 43, and 12 had wedge resection of the gallbladder fossa. Of the 72 with liver resection, 68 had additional hepaticocholedochus resection (HCR) as previously described. Pancreatic-oduodenectomy (PD) was also performed in 31 of the 72. Major vessels were reconstructed following resection of the portal vein and/or hepatic artery in 22 patients.

After en bloc resection of the cancerous lesion (Fig. 4A,B), alone or combined with portal vein resection, IOERT was delivered to the liver hilum, including left and right intrahepatic ducts and Gleason's capsule in 40 of the 93 patients (mean dose 20.9 Gy, range 15 to 30 Gy). After IOERT delivery, lymphadenectomy was performed, as indicated, around the aorta and inferior vena cava. The irradiated intrahepatic ducts were then anastomosed to nonirradiated jejunum (Fig. 4C). Postoperative EBRT was given to 21 of the 40 IORT patients and an additional 10 received postoperative EBRT alone without IORT. The mean EBRT dose was 40 Gy in 1.8 to 2.0 Gy fractions with a range of 12 to 54 Gy. The EBRT field included the periportal, celiac, and superior mesenteric nodal regions as well as the IOERT field.

The rationale for combining maximum resection with IOERT with or without EBRT in the Tsukuba series is based on an evaluation of X-ray sensitivity of human biliary-tract cancer lines by investigators from the University of Tsukuba and Harvard School of Public Health *(30)*. Although a number of clinical studies have indicated the efficacy of resection combined with IORT for advanced biliary-tract cancer, the in vitro radiosensitivity of cells from this type of cancer has not been well described. The study from Tsukuba and Harvard Public Health was designed to examine both the sensitivity of human biliary-tract cancer cells to ionizing radiation and the combined effects of radiation and 5-FU in these cells. Five of the six cell lines examined that were derived from biliary-tract cancers were significantly more resistant to radiation than two unrelated tumor cell lines, MCF-7 and Tera-2. The mean D_0, D_{10}, and SF_2 values for the five biliary-cancer cell lines were 2.45 ± 0.23, 6.46 ± 0.41, and 0.60 ± 0.04 Gy, respectively. The sixth

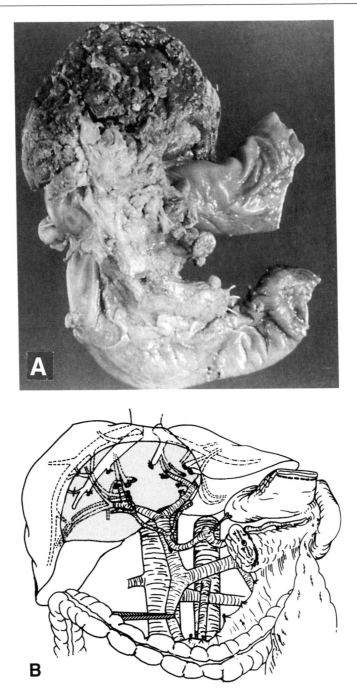

Fig. 4. Surgical specimen and operative procedures for the patient in Fig. 3. (**A**) Surgical specimen of hepatic segmentectomy (SIVb, SV) with hepaticocholedochus resection and pancreaticoduodenectomy. Gallbladder cancer had directly extended to the omentum, hepatic parenchyma, duodenum, head of the pancreas, and transverse colon. (**B**) Schematic view after the hepatic segmentectomy (SIVb, SV) with hepaticocholedochus resection, pancreaticoduodenectomy and colon resection (p: portal vein, s: stomach, pn: pancreas). (**C**) Photograph of the completed hepaticojejunostomies following IORT after hepatic segmentectomy (SIVb, SV) (from Todoroki T et al., *World J. Surg.* 1991, with permission). (**D**) Cholangiogram on postoperative day 14.

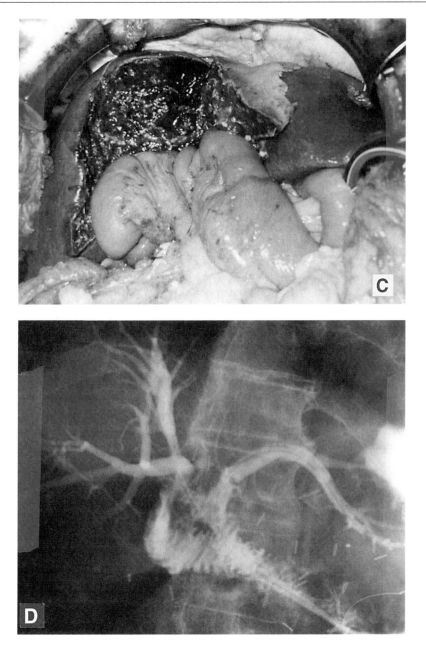

Fig. 4. (*continued*)

cell line was considerably more radiosensitive than the others ($D_0 = 0.77 \pm 0.02$; $D_{10} = 2.95 \pm 0.06$; $SF_2 = 0.35 \pm 0.03$). The results suggested that bile-tract cancers as a group may be relatively radioresistant. Thus, tumor control may not be readily achieved by radiation alone. Combining IORT with maximal tumor resection can potentially improve tumor control and minimize the radiation dose to normal tissue, including grossly normal liver. Ongoing studies are being conducted of the combined effects of irradiation and 5-FU in biliary tract cancer cells.

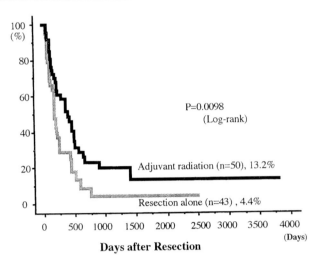

Fig. 5. Survival rate in Tsukuba series following resection of Stage IV gallbladder cancers treated with resection alone (*n* = 43) versus resection plus adjuvant irradiation (*n* = 50); IOERT with or without postoperative EBRT (*n* = 40) or postoperative EBRT without IOERT (*n* = 10).

4. IORT WITH OR WITHOUT EBRT RESULTS

4.1. United States Series

In the United States series, both electrons and orthovoltage have been used as the method of IORT for primary biliary lesions. Many patients received both EBRT and IORT.

In the Rush Presbyterian IOERT series of nine patients, four had gallbladder cancer and five had extrahepatic bile-duct cancers. Five received EBRT, and four had chemotherapy. IOERT doses ranged from 15–22 Gy in the seven patients with unresectable lesions or partial resection with gross residual disease. Two of five bile-duct patients and one of four gallbladder patients survived ≥18 mo *(31)*. Median survival for that group was 13 mo with 1-yr survival of 56%. The single disease-free survivor at >40 mo had bile-duct cancer and was the only patient in the series to receive concomitant chemotherapy during the EBRT component of treatment.

In a Joint Center analysis *(32)*, 15 patients received IORT doses of 5–20 Gy with orthovoltage for either primary (12 patients) or locally recurrent disease (3 patients). Thirteen also received postoperative EBRT. Median survival of the 12 patients with primary disease was 14.0 mo, and local progression or persistence was documented in 50% of evaluable patients (5 of 10). The three patients with locally recurrent cancers survived 2, 9, and 11 mo.

Mayo Clinic investigators reported an IOERT series of 15 unresectable patients at risk ≥1 yr *(27,28)*. Of 15 patients, 14 received EBRT doses of 45–50 Gy in 1.8-Gy Fx (before IOERT in 2 patients and after IOERT in 13) and 12 of 15 received IOERT doses of 20 Gy (15, 17.5, and 19 Gy in the other 3 patients). Median survival was encouraging at 16.5 mo for the entire group and 18.5 mo in the 14 patients treated with curative intent (one patient was a 5-yr survivor). Five of the 14 curative patients (36%), were alive at 2 yr. Local tumor persistence or relapse was diagnosed in 6 of 14 treated with curative intent (43%), but in 3 who died of noncancer causes, it was documented only at autopsy (15, 21.5, and 37 mo). Only three patients received concomitant 5-FU during EBRT.

4.2. Japan IORT Series

In an early report of 11 patients treated in Japan at the Universities of Tsukuba and Chiba with 25–30 Gy IORT alone for biliary-tract cancer (6 gallbladder, 5 bile duct), Todoroki and coworkers *(33)* noted local persistence or progression in 9 patients (82%). This was documented at autopsy in 8 patients. Of the 5 patients with bile-duct cancers, the four postoperative survivors died with a local component of disease.

4.2.1. BILE DUCT

In a recent update from the University of Tsukuba by Todoroki and colleagues *(34)*, 81 patients were treated for bile-duct cancer between 1976 and 1986. Fifty had curative or noncurative resection (no further treatment, 33; IOERT boost, 14; EBRT, 3), and 31 had no tumor resection (biliary drainage alone, 21; IOERT, 6; EBRT, 4). Before 1983, IOERT doses ranged from 20 to 35 Gy, and no EBRT was given (12 patients; 9 with resection). Since 1983, the IOERT dose was limited to 20 Gy, and fractionated EBRT doses of 30–40 Gy in 4–5 wk were usually added (7 patients received both; 4 had resection). The decision to decrease the IOERT dose was based on an excessive incidence of complications. Impact of treatment method on duration of survival in that series is seen in Table 2. There is a suggestion of an impact on interval survival at 18 and 24 mo with the addition of IOERT. With biliary drainage alone, survival at 6 mo was approx 20% with a 1-yr survival rate of ≤5% and no 18-mo survivors. Only one patient (8%) with noncurative resection alone was alive at 18 and 24 mo vs 38% and 17% with IORT plus noncurative resection and 42 and 21% with biliary drainage plus IORT. Only 1 of 6 patients (17%) without any resection survived beyond 15 mo vs 5 of 13 (38%) with subtotal resection.

4.2.2. GALLBLADDER CANCER

Stage IV gallbladder cancer has a distressingly dismal prognosis with a predominant local-regional failure problem after radical resection. The intent of Todoroki et al. in combining resection and IOERT at the University of Tsukuba *(29,30)* was to prolong survival by decreasing local relapse together with minimizing the sacrifice of normal tissues and structures surrounding the tumor. From October 1976 to May 1997, 93 patients with a Stage IV gallbladder cancer underwent resection at Tsukuba University *(30)*. Resection procedures varied by the extent and mode of tumor extension and were discussed earlier in the chapter.

Survival results were compared in the various treatment groups *(30)*. For the 43 patients treated by resection alone, only one patient survived more than 26 months. Median survival was 6 months, and five-year survival was only 4.4%. Of the 50 patients who received IOERT with or without EBRT or postoperative EBRT alone, 5-yr survival was 13.2% and median survival was 13 mo, $p = 0.0098$. Of the 52 patients with microscopic residual after resection, 22 had resection alone and 30 received IOERT with or without postoperative EBRT. Median and 5-yr survival rates favored those who received irradiation at 16 vs 8 mo and 20% vs 0% ($p = 0.005$). The surgical mortality rate as a whole was quite reasonable at 5.4%.

In an earlier analysis of 87 patients with Stage IV gallbladder cancer, local-regional control rates in patients who were M0 at time of resection were 28.7% with resection alone *(29)*. When resection was combined with IOERT with or without postoperative EBRT, local regional control was achieved in 73.6% of patients.

Table 2
Potential Impact of Treatment Intensification on Duration of Survival in Locally Advanced Bile Duct or Gallbladder Cancer

Series/Treatment Method (ref. no.)	No.	Median (Mo.)	Survival (%)						p
			12 mo	18 mo	24 mo	36 mo	48 mo	60 mo	
Bile-Duct EBRT with or without Resection									
EORTC (18)									
Noncurative resection alone	17	8.3	36	—	18	10	—	—	p = 0.0005
Noncurative resection plus EBRT	38	19	85	—	42	31	—	—	
Lyon Sud and Centre Léon Berard (38)									
Palliative treatment—RT alone	51	12	55	—	29	15	—	—	
	25	10	40	—	5	0	—	—	0.03
Curative treatment—RT plus resection	26	22	—	—	48	32	—	—	0.05
Microscopic residual (10 of 14)	14	27.5	86	—	62	55	—	—	
Gross residual	12	13	57	—	30	10	—	—	
University of Pittsburgh (39)									
EBRT ± 5-FU ± resection	55	9	32	20	10	6	4	—	
Transplant + EBRT ± 5-FU	9 (of 55)	12	50	32	22	22	22	—	
Bile-Duct EBRT with or without Brachytherapy									
Mayo Clinic									
Unresected									
EBRT ± 5-FU *(12)*	11	12	55	0	—	—	—	—	
EBRT ± 5-FU + IOERT *(27,28)*	14	18.5	71	43	29	14	7	7	
EBRT ± 5-FU + 192Ir *(22)*	24	12.8	67	38	19	14	14	14	
EBRT + 5-FU + 192Ir	9	13	67	44	22	22	22	22	
EBRT + 192Ir	15	12	67	32	16	8	8	8	
Noncurative resection + EBRT ± 5-FU *(12)*	6	12	50	33	33	33	0	—	
Thomas Jefferson University Hospital (15)									
No Irradiation	48	9	—	—	18	—	—	—	p = 0.01
Irradiation ± 5-FU ± 192Ir	24	5.5	—	—	17	—	—	—	
	24	12	—	—	30	—	—	—	
<55 Gy	—	6	—	—	0	—	—	—	
>55 Gy	—	24	—	—	48	—	—	—	p = 0.0003

continued

240

Table 2
(*continued*)

Series/Treatment Method (ref. no.)	No.	Median (Mo.)	Survival (%)						
			12 mo	18 mo	24 mo	36 mo	48 mo	60 mo	p
University of Heidelberg (23)									
EBRT + HDR brachy ± resection	30	10	34	20	18	18	8	8	
No resection	21	7.9	38	8	5	5	5	0	
Resection, noncurative	9	12.1	64	42	32	32	32	32	0.004
Rotterdam (24)									
EBRT + [192]Ir ± resection	42	10	46	27	18	13	—	—	
No resection	31	8	40	26	18	6	—	—	
Resection, noncurative	11	15	65	36	36	36	—	—	p = 0.06
Bile-Duct IOERT with or without EBRT									
Mayo Clinic - unresected									
EBRT ±5-FU (12)	11	12	55	0	—	—	—	—	
EBRT ±5-FU + IOERT (27,28)[a]	14	18.5	71	43	29	14	7	7	
Rush Presbyterian (31)									
No irradiation	6	(4.6)[b]	0	—	—	—	—	—	
EBRT ±5-FU + [192]Ir	13	(11)[b]	46	—	—	—	—	—	p = 0.03[c]
IOERT ± EBRT	9	13 (16.8)[b]	56	—	—	—	—	—	
Iwasaki et al. (Japan) (34)									
Noncurative resection—alone	13	—	44	8	8	8	—	—	
Noncurative resection—plus IORT	13	—	46	23	15	8	—	—	
Unresected—biliary drainage only	21	—	≤5	0	—	—	—	—	
—plus IORT	6	—	33	17	17	0	—	—	
Gallbladder Surgery with or without EBRT, IORT, Both									
Todoroki et al., Japan (29,30)									
Surgery alone	43	6	—	—	4	—	—	4	
Surgery + IORT, EBRT, or both	50	13	—	—	22	—	—	13	p = 0.0098[c]

RT = irradiation; EBRT = external beam irradiation; IOERT = intraoperative electron irradiation; HDR brachy = high dose rate brachytherapy.

[a] Single 5-yr survivor died at 60 mo with progression within EBRT field.

[b] Survival data in parenthesis represents mean survival in months, p value listed is for irradiation vs no irradiation.

[c] p value is for irradiation vs. no irradiation.

4.2.3. SUMMARY

Although the method of treatment was not randomized in the Tsukuba series, their results indicate that aggressive resection combined with IORT with or without EBRT may be an efficient modality for improving the prognosis of locally advanced gallbladder cancer. Whether results could be improved further by delivering EBRT plus infusion 5-FU prior to resection in patients with negative laparoscopy remains to be determined.

4.4. European IOERT Bile Duct Series

4.4.1. METHODS

Since 1991, 24 patients with carcinoma of the extrahepatic bile ducts including 17 with proximal third lesions were treated by surgery and IOERT in the University Hospital in Essen, Germany *(36)*. IOERT was applied with energies of 6–15 MeV and total doses of 12–20 Gy. Resection was complete in 6 patients, 11 had microscopic residual disease, and 7 had gross residual disease. Ten patients received postoperative EBRT; 8 received postoperative EBRT to a total dose of 45 Gy in 25 fractions over 5 wk in combination with continuous infusion 5-FU (300 mg/m^2/d), and two received EBRT without 5-FU. Two patients who were functionally inoperable were assigned to subsequent liver transplantation. In these two cases, IORT was applied to avoid tumor growth and tumor spread while the patients awaited transplant.

4.4.2. RESULTS

Median survival of the 22 nontransplant patients was 8.6 mo *(35)*. Six patients were still alive at 1–18 mo, 4 of them with no evidence of disease. Two patients had received their planned liver transplant and were alive without tumor at 38 and 43 mo, respectively.

4.4.3. SUMMARY

IORT followed by postoperative EBRT and continuous infusion 5-FU is a promising combination of therapeutic modalities in the treatment of carcinoma of the extrahepatic bile ducts. In inoperable cases, subsequent liver transplantation may improve the overall survival and offer an additional option for cure.

5. POTENTIAL IMPACT
OF TREATMENT INTENSIFICATION ON SURVIVAL

The potential impact of treatment intensification on duration of survival is seen in separate series from Japan, Mayo Clinic, TJUH, Rush Presbyterian, EORTC, University of Heidelberg, Rotterdam, Lyon, and the University of Pittsburgh (Table 2). Many of the survival trends seen, however, may be caused by patient selection rather than treatment method, and randomized trials will be needed to test some of the issues.

In the bile-duct series from Japan by Iwasaki and colleagues *(35)*, with biliary drainage alone (21 patients), SR at 6 mo was only 20%, with a 1-yr survival rate of ≤5% and no 18-mo survivors. With noncurative resection with or without IORT (13 patients each group) or biliary drainage plus IORT (6 patients), SR appeared to be better (1-yr SR 44, 46, and 33%; 2-yr SR 8, 15, and 17%).

In the Japan gallbladder analysis from the University of Tsukuba by Todoroki et al. *(29,30)*, with surgery alone for stage IV disease (*n* = 43), median survival was 6 mo and survival at 2 and 5 yr was only 4.4%. When surgery was supplemented by either EBRT only (10 patients) or IOERT with or without EBRT (*n* = 40), median and 5-yr survival were 13 mo and 13.2%, respectively ($p = 0.0098$, log rank). Of the 52 patients with microscopic residual after resection, 5-yr SR was better in the 30 patients who received IORT with or without EBRT than those with surgery alone at 2% vs 0% ($p = 0.005$).

In data from Mayo Clinic (12,22,26,28), survival ≥18 mo was 0% with external irradiation with or without 5-FU for 11 patients with unresectable bile-duct lesions, 33% with gross total or subtotal resection before EBRT in 6 patients, and 38 and 43% respectively in patients with unresectable lesions treated with EBRT plus a specialized boost with [192]Ir (24 patients) or IOERT (14 patients). There were four 5-yr survivors in the latter group of 38 patients (10.5%). Nine of the 24 patients with an ^{192}Ir boost received 5-FU during EBRT and two (22%) were 5-yr disease-free survivors vs 8% 5-yr SR in the 15 patients with no 5-FU during EBRT (81).

The TJUH series of 48 patients was previously discussed with regard to the suggested impact on survival of irradiation vs none and increase in irradiation dose (15). The 2-yr SR was 48 vs 30% with an increase in median survival of 24 vs 6 mo with >55 vs <55 Gy, $p = 0.0003$.

In the Rush Presbyterian analysis (32), treatment combinations of EBRT with IOERT or brachytherapy appear to have improved SR when compared to patients who received no irradiation. For the six patients with no irradiation, mean and 1-yr SR were, respectively, 4.6 mo and 0% vs 11 mo and 46% in 13 patients who received EBRT with or without [192]Ir. For the nine patients who received IOERT with or without EBRT, median SR was 13 mo, mean SR 17 mo, and 1-yr SR 56%. Survival trends for patients without vs with irradiation achieved statistical significance ($p = 0.03$).

At least four series suggest that palliative resection plus irradiation give additive benefit over either alone, and one series suggests a liver transplant may be additive to EBRT. In the EORTC series previously discussed (18,37), irradiation appeared to improve survival in patients with resection but positive margins (median SR 19 vs 8.3 mo, 2 yr SR 42 vs 18%, 3-yr 31 vs 10% $p = 0.0005$). In the Fritz et al. analysis (23) of 39 patients treated at the University of Heidelberg with EBRT plus high-dose-rate bradytherapy with or without noncurative resection, those with noncurative resection had a suggestive increase in survival (median: 12 vs 8 mo; 3-yr: 32 vs 5%, 5-yr: 32 vs 0%, $p = 0.004$). In a Rotterdam series by Veeze-Kuypers et al. (24) of 42 patients treated with EBRT plus ^{192}Ir with or without resection, the 11 with noncurative resection had improved median SR at 15 vs 8 mo, and 3-yr SR of 36 vs 6% ($p = 0.06$) when compared to the 31 patients with no resection. In a Lyon series by Mahe et al. (38), patients with a curative vs palliative treatment approach appeared to do better (3-yr SR of 32 vs 0%, $p = 0.03$) as well as those with gross total resection (10 of 14 had positive resection margins) vs gross residual (3-yr SR of 55 vs 10%, $p = 0.05$). In a University of Pittsburgh analysis by Flickenger et al. (39), the best long-term survival in 55 patients with EBRT with or without 5-FU and resection was seen in 9 patients with transplant plus EBRT with or without 5-FU (4-yr SR 22 vs 4%).

6. SEQUELAE OF TREATMENT (SURGERY, EBRT, IORT)

6.1. Gastric and Duodenal Tolerance

A good analysis of gastric and duodenal tolerance with EBRT exists in the biliary-duct analysis from Mayo by Buskirk et al. (12). For locally unresectable or resected but residual biliary cancer, three aggressive treatment regimens were used: EBRT alone or combined with 5-FU (45 Gy in 25 fractions in 5 wk to a tumor and nodal field, with a reduced field boost for 10–20 Gy in 2-Gy fractions) or similar EBRT to a tumor and nodal field combined with IOERT or transcatheter brachytherapy. The distal stomach and duodenal C-loop were usually within the EBRT field to a dose of 45 Gy. With brachytherapy, patients received doses of 15–30 Gy, usually calculated at a 1-cm radius from the transcatheter iridium. With IOERT patients, the duodenum and stomach were usually surgically excluded.

An analysis comparing dose with complications was performed for patients who received EBRT alone or EBRT combined with IOERT electrons. With EBRT doses of 55 Gy or less to the duodenum or stomach, the risk of severe GI complications varied from 5 to 10%, depending on which parameter was evaluated. At doses greater than 55 Gy, one-third of the patients developed severe GI problems. In patients who received EBRT plus iridium, the dose to the EBRT field was limited to 50.4 Gy, but most received additional radiation dose to duodenum and/or stomach from the iridium boost (higher doses with distal lesions). There was a 30 to 40% incidence of severe complications in the duodenum or stomach in this group of patients.

6.2. Biliary-Duct Tolerance

Biliary-duct tolerance to EBRT with or without transcatheter or IORT boosts has been evaluated in animal models as well as in clinical pilot studies. Todoroki (40) studied the effects of large single doses of irradiation to the liver hilum in rabbits and found hepatic parenchymal atrophy, significant biliary fibrosis, and necrosis at doses greater than 30 Gy. Sindelar and coworkers (41) investigated the effects of IORT on the extrahepatic bile duct in dogs and noted dose-related fibrosis and duct stenosis at doses of 30 Gy or greater. Duct stenosis resulted in secondary hepatic changes of biliary cirrhosis that developed with time.

At the radiation-dose levels used in the aggressive treatment combinations at Mayo Clinic (i.e., EBRT plus transcatheter or IOERT boost), temporary fibrosis and duct stenosis have not been unexpected or uncommon (12,25,26). Transhepatic catheters or U-tubes were previously left in place in these patients until the degree of stenosis had stabilized or lessened on serial cholangiograms, which usually occurs within 12–18 mo of treatment. In view of stent-related morbidity, we now attempt to remove transhepatic catheters or endoscopic stents within 3–6 mo of the brachytherapy boost if imaging techniques of the biliary tree suggest this is medically feasible.

6.3. Hepatic Artery Tolerance

In the series reported by Iwasaki and colleagues (35), the IOERT dose for bile duct malignancies had been reduced to a maximum of 20 Gy following curative or noncurative resection because of an excess incidence of severe complications. When IOERT doses of 20–35 Gy were used, four of seven patients with IOERT after surgical manipulation of the hepatic artery developed stenosis, obstruction, or aneurysm. In five patients treated subsequently with IOERT doses of 20 Gy or less after resection, no severe vascular complications occurred.

7. FUTURE POSSIBILITIES

In an attempt to improve survival and disease control for patients with biliary-tract malignancies, it would be of interest to combine the various modalities that appear to impact those endpoints. For lesions that are unresectable with standard or extended surgical procedures, these options include EBRT, simultaneous or maintenance chemo-therapy, a specialized irradiation boost with transcatheter iridium or IOERT with or without liver transplant. Improved imaging techniques would be helpful in defining both surgical resectability and tumor/target volumes for EBRT (standard and 3D conformal) and specialized boosts with IOERT or brachytherapy.

The increased utilization of simultaneous EBRT plus chemotherapy is indicated in view of results in single-institution studies in patients with bile-duct cancers and randomized single institution and group trials in other GI sites (unresectable pancreas; unresected or residual gastric and large bowel; resected but high-risk rectal and pancreas with or without gastric; unresected esophagus). The use of low-dose infusion 5-FU instead of bolus 5-FU during EBRT may be safer and more efficacious as it would be less apt to result in severe leukopenia in a patient at risk for tube-related sepsis.

With regard to the use of IOERT vs brachytherapy for a specialized boost, this is dependent on whether the patient is a potential candidate for resection. If the primary lesion appears to be surgically unresectable on the basis of imaging studies and the specialized irradiation boost can safely be given via the transcatheter approach, this is a more cost efficacious method of delivery. If stomach or duodenum cannot be excluded from a brachytherapy field, however, it may be reasonable to reoperate for the purpose of giving the boost with IOERT while displacing those structures.

For patients who present with surgically unresectable lesions, it would be reasonable to initiate treatment with EBRT plus 5-FU infusion and plan to re-evaluate 3–4 wk after completion of such for the option of attempted gross total resection with or without specialized IORT boost. This approach is supported by results in bile-duct series from Heidelberg *(23)*, Rotterdam *(24)*, and Lyon *(38)* that show a survival advantage for patients with resection vs no resection and the excellent 5-yr results with resection plus IOERT and EBRT in locally advanced gallbladder cancers demonstrated by Todoroki et al. in Tsukuba *(29,30)*. Both Mayo Clinic and the University of Pittsburgh are conducting pilot studies in which patients with proximal lesions are candidates for liver transplant following preoperative EBRT plus concomitant 5-FU with or without brachytherapy (Mayo) for lesions that are unresectable by standard surgical criterion.

For patients in whom microscopic or gross residual disease remains after an attempt at resection, the addition of EBRT with or without chemotherapy seems reasonable on the basis of bile-duct analyses by Gonzalez et al. for the EORTC group *(18,37)* and Weiss et al. for Fox Chase/University of Pennsylvania *(17)* and the use of IOERT (plus EBRT and resection) is supported by the excellent long-term results achieved in locally advanced gallbladder cancers by Tsukuba *(29,30)*. The availability of IOERT or HDR-IORT may allow delivery of a localized boost dose of irradiation after resection but before reconstruction as in the Tsukuba gallbladder series by Todoroki et al. *(29,30)* (i.e., IOERT for positive radial or circumferential margins because of adherence to porta hepatis structures that could not be boosted with postoperative transcatheter iridium; HDR-IORT for microscopically positive ductal margins). It would be of interest to investigate sequencing issues in patients with potentially or borderline resectable lesions (give EBRT plus 5-FU before instead of after resection to alter implantability of cells that may be shed at the time of resection).

REFERENCES

1. Adson MA and Farnell MD. Hepatobiliary cancer—surgery considerations, *Mayo Clinic Proc.,* **56** (1981) 686–699.
2. Cameron JL, Pitt HA, Zinner MJ, et al. Management of proximal cholangiocarcinoma by surgical resection and radiotherapy, *Am. J. Surg.,* **159** (1990) 91–97.

3. Kopelson G, Galdabini J, Warshaw A, and Gunderson LL. Patterns of failure after curative surgery for extrahepatic biliary tract carcinoma, *Int. J. Radiat. Oncol. Biol. Phys.,* **7** (1981) 413–417.

4. Hadjis NS, Blenkhart JI, Alexander N, Benjamin IS, and Blumgart LH. Outcome of radical surgery in hilar cholangiocarcinoma, *Surgery,* **107** (1990) 597–604.

5. Lai ECS and Lo CM. Cholangiocarcinoma, *GI Cancer,* **1** (1996) 163–170.

6. Nagorney DM, Donohue JH, Farnell MB, Schleck CD, and Ilstrup AM. Outcomes after curative resection of cholangiocarcinoma, *Arch. Surg.,* **128** (1993) 871–879.

7. Goldstein RM, Stone M, Tillery W, et al. Is liver transplantation indicated for cholangiocarcinoma, *Am. J. Surg.,* **166** (1993) 768–772.

8. Starzl TE, Todo S, Tzakis A, et al. Abdominal-organ cluster transplantation for the treatment of upper abdominal malignancies, *Ann. Surg.,* **210** (1989) 374–386.

9. Kopelson G, Harisiadis L, Tretter P, and Chang CH. The role of radiation therapy in cancer of the extrahepatic biliary system: an analysis of thirteen patients and a review of the literature of the effectiveness of surgery, chemotherapy, and radiotherapy, *Int. J. Radiat. Oncol. Biol. Phys.,* **2** (1977) 883–894.

10. Willett C, Warshaw AL, Convery K, and Compton CC. Pattern of failure after pancreatoduodenectomy for ampullary carcinoma, *Surg. Gynecol.,* **176** (1993) 33–38.

11. Gunderson LL and Willett CG. Pancreas and hepatobiliary tract. In Perez C and Brady L (eds.), *Principles and Practice of Radiation Oncology,* 3rd ed., J. B. Lippincott, Philadelphia, PA, 1997, pp. 1467–1488.

11. Robertson JM, Marsh L, Tenhaken RK, and Lawrence TS. The clinical application of a non-axial treatment plan for pancreatic and biliary malignancies, *Radiother. Oncol.,* **24** (1992) 198–200.

12. Buskirk SJ, Gunderson LL, Schild SE, Bender CE, et al. Analysis of failure following curative irradiation of extrahepatic bile duct carcinoma, *Ann. Surg.,* **215** (1992) 125–131.

13. Fields JN and Emami B. Carcinoma of the extrahepatic biliary system: results of primary and adjuvant radiotherapy, *Int. J. Radiat. Oncol. Biol. Phys.,* **13** (1987) 331–338.

14. Hanna SS and Rider WD. Carcinoma of the gallbladder or extrahepatic bile ducts: the role of radiotherapy, *Can. Med. Assoc. J.,* **118** (1978) 59–61.

15. Alden ME and Mohiudden M. The impact of radiation dose in combined external beam and intraluminal Ir-192 for bile duct cancer, *Int. J. Radiat. Oncol. Biol. Phys.,* **28** (1994) 945–951.

16. Minsky BD, Wessan MF, Armstrong JG, et al. Combined modality therapy of extrahepatic biliary system cancer, *Int. J. Radiat. Oncol. Biol. Phys.,* **18** (1990) 1157–1163.

17. Weiss MC, Whittington R, Schultz D, Jardines L, et al. Extrahepatic biliary carcinoma: primary treatment and patterns of failure, *Int. J. Radiat. Oncol. Biol. Phys.,* **24** (1992) 213.

18. Gonzalez DG, Gerald JP, Maners AW, De La Lande-Guyauz B, et al. Results of radiation therapy in carcinoma of the proximal bile duct (Klatskin tumor), *Sem. Liver Dis.,* **10** (1990) 131–141.

19. Pitt HA, Nakeeb A, Abrams RA, et al. Perihilar cholangiocarcinoma: postoperative radiotherapy does not improve survival, *Ann. Surg.,* **221** (1995) 788–798.

20. Hayes JK, Sapozink MD, and Miller JF. Definitive radiation therapy in bile duct carcinoma, *Int. J. Radiat. Oncol. Biol. Phys.,* **15** (1988) 735–744.

21. Johnson DW, Safai C, and Goffinet DR. Malignant obstructive jaundice: treatment with external beam and intracavitary radiotherapy, *Int. J. Radiat. Oncol. Biol. Phys.,* **11** (1985) 411–416.

22. Foo M, Gunderson LL, Bender C, and Busbirk S. External radiation therapy and transcatheter iridium in the treatment of extrahepatic bile duct cancer, *Int. J. Radiat. Oncol. Biol. Phys.,* **39** (1997) 929–935.

23. Fritz P, Brambs HJ, Schraube P, et al. Combined external beam radiotherapy and intraluminal high dose brachytherapy on bile duct carcinomas, *Int. J. Radiat. Oncol. Biol. Phys.,* **29** (1994) 855–861.

24. Veeze-Kuypers B, Meerwaldt JH, Lameris JS, et al. The role of radiotherapy in the treatment of bile duct carcinoma, *Int. J. Radiol. Biol. Phys.,* **18** (1990) 63–67.

25. Gunderson LL, Martenson JA, Smalley SR, and Garton GR. Upper gastrointestinal cancers: rationale, results and techniques of treatment. In Meyer J and Vaeth J (eds.), *Lymphatics and Cancer: Controversies in Oncology Management, Front Radiat. Ther. Oncol.,* **28** (1994) 121–139.

26. Buskirk SJ, Gunderson LL, Adson MA, et al. Analysis of failure following curative irradiation of gallbladder and extrahepatic bile duct carcinoma, *Int. J. Radiat. Oncol. Biol. Phys.,* **10** (1984) 2013–2023.

27. Gunderson LL, Nagorney DM, Garton GR, Donohue JA, and McIlrath DR. Pancreas and bile duct cancer results of IORT. In Abe M and Takahashi M (eds.), *Intraoperative Radiation Therapy,* Pergamon, New York, 1991, pp. 212–214.

28. Monson JRT, Donohue JH, Gunderson LL, Nagorney DM, Bender CE, and Wieand HS. Intraoperative radiotherapy for unresectable cholangiocarcinoma: the Mayo Clinic experience, *Surg. Oncol.,* **1** (1992) 283–290.
29. Todoroki T, Kawamoto T, Otsuka M, Takada Y, et al. IORT combined with resection for stage IV gallbladder carcinoma. In Vaeth JM (ed.), *Intraoperative Radiation Therapy in the Treatment of Cancer.* Karger, Basel, *Radiat. Ther. Oncol.,* **31** (1997) 165–172.
30. Todoroki T, Takahashi H, Koike N, et al. Outcomes of aggressive treatment of stage IV gallbladder cancer and predictors of survival. Hepatogastroenterology, in press.
31. Moon Y, Nagasawa H, Dahlberg WK, Todoroki T, and Little JB. Enhanced x-ray sensitivity of human biliary tract cancer lines by 5-fluorouracil, *Int. J. Oncol.* **10** (1997) 545–551. *Int'l IORT Conference Abstracts,* San Francisco, CA, 1996.
32. Deziel DJ, Kiel KD, Kramer TS, Doolas A, and Roseman DL. Intraoperative radiation therapy in biliary tract cancer, *Am. Surg.,* **54** (1988) 402–407.
33. Busse PM, Stone MD, Sheldon TA, Chaffey JT, et al. Intraoperative radiation therapy for biliary tract carcinoma: results of a five-year experience, *Surgery,* **105** (1989) 724–733.
34. Todoroki T, Iwasaki Y, Okamura T, et al. Intraoperative radiotherapy for advanced carcinoma of the biliary system, *Cancer,* **46** (1980) 2179–2184.
35. Iwasaki Y, Todoroki T, Fukao K, O'hara K, Okamura T, and Mishimura A. The role of intraoperative radiation therapy in the treatment of bile duct cancer, *World J. Surg.,* **12** (1988) 91–98.
36. Willborn K, Sauerwein W, Erhard J, et al. IORT of carcinoma of the extrahepatic bile ducts. In Vaeth JM (ed.), *Intraoperative Radiation Therapy in the Treatment of Cancer,* Karger, Basel, *Front. Radiat. Ther. Oncol.,* **31** (1997) 173–176.
37. Verbeck PCM, Van Leeuwen DJ, Van DerHeyde MN, and Gonzalez DG. Does adjuvant irradiation after hilar resection improve survival of cholangiocarcinoma, *Ann. Chir.,* **45** (1991) 350–354.
38. Mahe M, Romestaing P, Talon, et al. Radiation therapy in extrahepatic bile duct carcinoma, *Radiother. Oncol.,* **21** (1991) 121–127.
39. Flickenger JC, Epstein AH, Iwatsuki S, et al. Radiation therapy for primary carcinoma of the extrahepatic biliary system, *Cancer,* **68** (1991) 289–294.
40. Todoroki T. The late effects of single massive irradiation with electrons of the liver hilum of rabbits, *Jap. J. Gastroenterol. Surg.,* **11** (1978) 169.
41. Sindelar WF, Tepper J, and Travis EL. Tolerance of bile duct to intraoperative irradiation, *Surgery,* **92** (1982) 533–540.
42. Fogel TD and Weissberg JB. The role of radiation therapy in carcinoma of the extrahepatic bile ducts, *Int. J. Radiat. Oncol. Biol. Phys.,* **10** (1984) 2251–2258.
43. Fletcher MS, Dawson JL, Wheeler PG, et al. Treatment of high bile duct carcinoma by internal radiotherapy with Iridium-192 wire, *Lancet,* **2** (1981) 172–174.
44. Karani J, Fletcher M, Brinkley D, et al. Internal biliary drainage and local radiotherapy with Ir-192 wire in the treatment of hilar cholangiocarcinoma, *Clin. Radiol.,* **36** (1985) 603–606.
45. Herskovic AM, Engler MJ, and Noell KT. Radical radiotherapy for bile duct carcinoma, *Endocurie Ther. Hyper. Oncol.,* **1** (1985) 119–124.
46. Farley DR, Weaver AL, and Nagorney DM. "Natural history" of unresected cholangiocarcinoma: patient outcome after noncurative intervention, *Mayo Clin. Proc.,* **70** (1995) 425–429.

14 Primary Colorectal EBRT and IOERT

Christopher G. Willett, Paul C. Shellito, and Leonard L. Gunderson

CONTENTS

1. INTRODUCTION

Carcinoma of the rectum is a heterogeneous disease. At one end of the clinical spectrum, a small number of patients present with superficially invasive cancers who are well served by limited procedures, such as local excision or endocavitary irradiation. The great majority of patients with rectal cancer, however, have mobile but more deeply invasive tumors that require low anterior or abdominoperineal resection. At the other and less favorable end of the clinical spectrum, a subset of patients present with locally advanced tumors that are adherent or fixed to adjoining structures such as the sacrum, pelvic sidewalls, prostate, or bladder.

Within this last group of patients categorized as "locally advanced," there is also variability in disease extent with no uniform definition of resectability. Depending on the report, a locally advanced lesion can range from a tethered or marginally resectable tumor to a fixed cancer with direct invasion of adjacent organs or structures. The definition will also depend upon whether the assessment of resectability is made clinically or at the time of surgery. In some cases, tumors thought to be unresectable at the time of initial clinical or radiographic examination may be found to be more mobile when the patient is examined under anesthesia. With these caveats, a good working definition of a locally advanced tumor is a tumor that cannot be resected without leaving microscopic or gross residual disease at the resection site because of tumor adherence or fixation to that site. Figure 1 shows the computed tomography (CT) scan of a patient with a "locally advanced" rectal cancer invading the posterior and left pelvic side wall tissues. At surgery, it was adherent

From: *Current Clinical Oncology: Intraoperative Irradiation: Techniques and Results*
Edited by: L. L. Gunderson et al. © Humana Press, Inc., Totowa, NJ

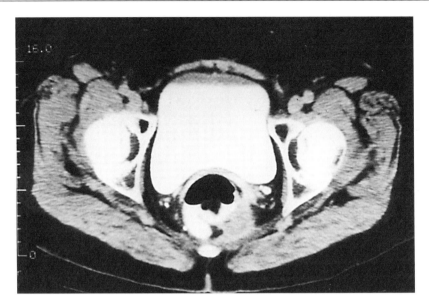

Fig. 1. Preoperative staging. Preoperative pelvic CT demonstrating mass in the left posterior lateral rectum with lack of free space posteriorly relative to pelvic structures.

to the sidewall and pathological review of the resection specimen showed that the radial soft-tissue margins were positive for carcinoma. Since these patients do poorly with surgery alone, irradiation and chemotherapy have been added to improve the outcome. This chapter will summarize the evolution of treatment and the role of intraoperative irradiation in this group of patients.

2. EXTERNAL-BEAM IRRADIATION

In the past, the management of locally advanced rectal cancer has been variable. Some patients have had incomplete surgical resections alone, whereas others have had radiation alone or surgery combined with post- or preoperative irradiation. The results of high-dose external-beam irradiation (EBRT) as a primary curative treatment have been unsatisfactory with local failure rates of at least 90% or greater and 5-yr survivals of less than 10%. Wang and Schulz reported that of 58 patients with recurrent, inoperable, or residual rectosigmoid carcinoma treated at Massachusetts General Hospital (MGH) with 35–50 Gy in 4–5 wk, six patients survived 5 yr disease free *(1)*. O'Connell et al. noted that 37 of 44 patients with locally unresectable or recurrent rectal carcinoma treated at Mayo Clinic with 50 Gy in a split-source fashion over 7 wk with and without adjuvant immunotherapy had progression of disease *(2)*. Median survival was approx 18 mo in both groups of patients. Of 31 patients assessable for sites of initial tumor progression, 17 had local progression only, 11 had concurrent local progression and distant metastases only, and 3 developed only distant metastases (28 of 31 or 90% had progression within EBRT field). Brierley and Cummings reported that of 77 patients with clinically fixed tumors who were treated at Princess Margaret Hospital with 50 Gy in 20 fractions over 4 wk, local control was 3% and survival was 4% *(3)*. Unless the patient is not a candidate for surgery, EBRT alone has no role as definitive treatment.

Table 1
Preoperative Radiation Therapy and Resection of Locally Advanced Rectal Cancer

	# of Patients	Resectable for Cure (%)	Local Control of those Resected (%)	5-Yr Survival of those Resected, (%)
Tufts University (7)	28	50	—	41
Massachusetts General Hospital (8)	25	72	62	43[a]
University of Florida (9)	23	48	45	18
University of Oregon (10)	72	39	32	10
Brigham and Women's Hospital (11)	20	65	77	53

[a]6-yr survival rate of 26%.

3. EXTERNAL BEAM IRRADIATION AND SURGERY

3.1. Postoperative EBRT

Combinations of EBRT and surgical resection have been used to improve local control and survival. When radiation therapy is given after subtotal resection, local control and survival is better in patients treated for residual microscopic disease compared to patients treated with gross residual disease.

Allee et al. reported the results of 31 patients with residual microscopic cancer treated at MGH with 45 Gy in 25 fractions over 5 wk followed by additional boost-field irradiation to as much as 60–70 Gy if small bowel could be moved from the radiation field (4). Local-control rate and 5-yr disease-free survival rates were 70 and 45%, respectively. In contrast, these figures were 43 and 11% for 25 patients treated for gross residual disease. A possible dose-response correlation was seen in patients with microscopic residual disease; the risk of local failure was 11% (1 of 9) with doses of 60 Gy or greater vs 40% (8 of 20) if the boost dose was less than 60 Gy. There was no clear dose-response relationship in patients with gross disease.

Of 17 Mayo Clinic patients receiving EBRT after subtotal resection, Schild et al. observed that local control was achieved in 3 of 10 patients (30%) with microscopic residual cancer and one of seven patients (14%) with gross remaining cancer (5). Four of the 17 patients (24%) have remained disease-free for more than 5 yr, and median survival was 18 mo.

Ghossein et al. treated patients at Albert Einstein to 46 Gy in 1.8-Gy fractions followed by a field reduction to the area of persistent disease which received 60 Gy (6). The incidence of local failure and survival for patients treated with microscopic disease was 16 and 84%, whereas for patients with gross disease, these figures were 50 and 39%, respectively.

3.2. Preoperative EBRT

For patients presenting with locally advanced disease (unresectable for cure because of tumor fixation), the use of high-dose preoperative EBRT (45–50 Gy in 1.8- to 2.0-Gy fractions) has been used to reduce tumor size and facilitate resection (Table 1). Emami et al. reported that the rate of resectablity of 28 Tufts University patients after full-dose preoperative EBRT was 50% (7).

Dosoretz et al. reported MGH results in 25 patients with unresectable tumors in the rectum or rectosigmoid treated with 40–52 Gy preoperative EBRT *(8)*. Sixteen of the 25 patients underwent potentially curative resection and the 6-yr survival was 26% (with 3 postoperative deaths). Total pelvic failure after curative resection was 39% (5 of 13 patients).

Mendenhall et al. reviewed 23 patients with locally advanced carcinoma who received 35–60 Gy of preoperative irradiation at the University of Florida *(9)*. Eleven patients were able to undergo complete resection with a 5-yr absolute survival of 18% and a local failure of 55%.

As reported by Stevens and Fletcher, 28 of 72 patients (39%) with locally advanced carcinoma of the rectum or rectosigmoid who received 50–60 Gy preoperatively were resectable in a series from the University of Oregon *(10)*. However, tumor recurred locally in nine of 28 (32%) of these patients and the 5-yr survival was only 10%.

Of 20 Brigham and Women's Hospital patients with unresectable rectal cancer undergoing 43–55.8 Gy preoperative irradiation reported by Whiting et al., 13 patients (65%) underwent resection with curative intent *(11)*. Three of thirteen (23%) subsequently developed a local failure. The 5-yr survival was 40%.

There has been one randomized prospective study examining the merits of preoperative irradiation in patients with locally advanced rectal cancer. Under the auspices of the Northwest Rectal Cancer Group (Manchester, United Kingdom), 284 patients with tethered or fixed rectal cancer were entered into a prospective randomized trial between 1982 and 1986 assessing the effects of preoperative irradiation given 1 wk before surgery *(12)*. One hundred and forty one patients were allocated to undergo surgical treatment alone and 143 were allocated to receive 20 Gy in four fractions before surgery. This study showed a marked reduction in local recurrences in the irradiated group (12.8%) vs surgery-alone group (36.5%). Although there was no significant difference in either overall survival or cancer-related mortality between the two treatment groups, subset analysis of the patients who underwent curative surgery reveals an overall mortality of 53.3% for patients allocated to surgery alone and 44.9% for patients allocated to preoperative radiotherapy. This was a significant reduction in mortality.

In summary, following full-dose preoperative irradiation, most series report that one-half to two-thirds of patients with locally advanced rectal cancers will be converted to a resectable status. However, despite a complete resection and negative margins, the local failure rate depending on the degree of initial tumor fixation varies from 23 to 55%.

4. PREOPERATIVE EBRT WITH
CHEMOTHERAPY AND SURGERY WITH OR WITHOUT IOERT

Because of the efficacy of postoperative irradiation and 5-FU in the adjuvant treatment of rectal cancer, there has been interest in examining this approach preoperatively. These investigations have studied combinations of moderate- to full-dose preoperative irradiation (45–50.4 Gy) with 5-FU-based chemotherapy for patients with clinical T3 and T4 rectal cancer. Comments in this chapter will be limited to analyses of patients with clinical T4 or tethered T3 tumors *(13)*. The endpoints of these studies have included not only resectability, local control, and survival but pathological downstaging and sphincter preservation rates.

In a report from the MD Anderson Hospital (MDAH), 38 patients with locally advanced rectal cancer (T4 or tethered T3) received 45 Gy in 25 fractions of preoperative EBRT with continuous infusion chemotherapy of 5-FU and/or cisplatin and surgery. Eleven of

Table 2
Preoperative Chemotherapy, Radiation Therapy, and Resection of Locally Advanced Rectal Cancer

Study	# Pts.	Drugs	EBRT Dose	Complete Resection Rate	Local Failure	Survival
MD Anderson (13)	38[a]	5-FU Infusion $\pm$ CDDP	45 Gy	84%	Crude - 3%	3 Yr - 82%
MSKCC (14)	36	5-FU/ Leucovorin	50.4 Gy	97%	4 Yr. Act. 30%	4 Yr - 67%
Tom Baker Cancer Ctr (16)	46	5-FU/Mit-C	40 Gy	89%	2 Yr. Act. 16%	3 Yr - 31%
Thomas Jefferson (17)	31	C.I. 5-FU	55.8 Gy	94%	Crude - 16%	3 Yr - 68%
Emory (18)	20	5-FU Bolus	50 Gy	N.S.	Crude - 10%	3 Yr - 82%

[a]Tethered T3 and T4 tumors: 11 of 38 received IOERT supplement to site of adherence at time of resection.
MSKCC = Memorial Sloan Kettering Cancer Center; pts = patients; EBRT = external beam irradiation, IOERT = intraoperative electron irradiation, 5-FU = 5 fluorouracil, CDDP = cisplatin, Mit-C = mitomycin C, CI = continuous infusion, N.S. = not stated, yr = year.

the 38 received an IOERT supplement to the site of adherence at time of resection. Three-year survival and local recurrence rates were 82 and 3%, respectively. These results contrasted to a 3-yr survival and local recurrence rate of 62 and 33% for 36 similarly staged patients undergoing preoperative irradiation without chemotherapy or IOERT at MDAH. Although there was a higher rate of sphincter-preserving procedures in patients receiving chemoirradiation (35%) vs patients undergoing irradiation only (7%), there were no differences in rates of resectability or pathological downstaging between these groups of patients receiving chemotherapy vs no chemotherapy.

Other investigations, however, have reported higher resectability and pathological downstaging rates with the use of preoperative chemoirradiation schedules. In an analysis of 36 patients (30 primary and 6 recurrent) with locally advanced/unresectable disease who were treated with 50.4 Gy of pelvic irradiation and concurrent 5-FU and leucovorin at Memorial Sloan Kettering Cancer Center (MSKCC), the resectability rate with negative margins was 97% and the total complete pathologic response rate was 25% (14). Similarly, a Swedish study reported an enhanced resectability rate in patients with unresectable rectal cancer who received preoperative irradiation, 5-FU, methotrexate, and leucovorin rescue compared with 38 patients who received radiation alone (71 vs 34%) (15). Investigators from Tom Baker Cancer Centre reported an 89% complete resection rate in 46 patients with tethered and fixed rectal cancer treated with 40 Gy and 5-FU infusion and mitomycin-C (16). Of 31 patients receiving continuous 5-FU infusion throughout irradiation at Thomas Jefferson University Hospital (TJUH), 29 patients (94%) underwent complete resection with negative margins (17). Enhanced resectability is an important endpoint since patients with initially unresectable rectal cancer who have microscopic or gross residual disease have higher local failure and lower survival rates compared with those patients who undergo a complete resection.

Analyses of local control and survival following treatment programs of preoperative chemoirradiation and surgery for locally advanced rectal cancer are limited by small patient numbers and short follow-up. Nevertheless, preliminary results suggest improved outcomes in patients receiving chemoirradiation compared to prior studies evaluating patients undergoing irradiation only (Table 2) (13–18). Based on this data, combinations of moderate- to high-dose preoperative irradiation with concurrent 5-FU-based chemotherapy appear to result in improved rates of resectability and possibly local control and survival.

Although the dose and techniques of irradiation are similar in these studies (45–50.4 Gy in 25 to 28 fractions to the pelvis via a three or four-field arrangement), there is marked variability in 5-FU administration. Some studies employ a schedule of 5-FU administered as a bolus for three consecutive days during weeks 1 and 5 of irradiation, whereas other investigators have utilized a continuous infusion approach throughout irradiation. Additionally, several investigators have used other agents such as leucovorin, cisplatinum, and mitomycin-C in combination with 5-FU. Because of the Intergroup trial showing a survival advantage for patients treated with continuous-infusion 5-FU throughout irradiation compared to patients treated with bolus 5-FU in the postoperative setting *(19)*, it would seem appropriate that this approach should be adopted for preoperative irradiation programs in rectal cancer. The value of additional agents such as leucovorin, levamisole, cisplatinum, and mitomycin-C in combination with 5-FU is under investigation. It is becoming clear from the adjuvant rectal cancer trials that more chemotherapy with irradiation is not necessarily better. In the adjuvant postoperative chemoirradiation rectal-cancer trials, it appears that the three-drug combination of 5-FU, levamisole, and leucovorin is more toxic and no more efficacious than 5-FU only or the two-drug regimen of 5-FU and leucovorin *(20)*.

At present, investigators at both MGH and Mayo are using a 5-FU schedule of 225 mg/m^2/24 h for 5 d (MGH) or 7 d (Mayo) per week throughout the 5.5-wk to 6-wk course of preoperative irradiation (45 Gy to the pelvis followed by a tumor boost of 5.4–9.0 Gy in 1.8-Gy fractions). In our experience, this 5-FU schedule with preoperative pelvic irradiation has been well tolerated.

5. INTRAOPERATIVE ELECTRON-BEAM IRRADIATION (IOERT)

Despite full-dose preoperative irradiation and complete resection of locally advanced rectal cancer, local failure occurs in at least one-third of patients. These local failure rates are even higher in patients undergoing subtotal resection. At MGH, Mayo Clinic, and other centers in the United States, Europe, and Asia, intraoperative electron-beam irradiation (IOERT) has been used in combination with preoperative EBRT (with and without 5-FU) and maximal surgical resection for patients with gross residual cancer, microscopically positive resection margins, or simply a site of tumor adherence.

5.1. Treatment Factors

5.1.1. EBRT

Patients with locally advanced primary rectal cancer have been evaluated in aggressive local strategies including EBRT, IOERT, and maximal resection at MGH since 1978 *(21,22)*. Such patients currently receive full-dose preoperative EBRT with infusional 5-FU (225 mg/m^2/d 5 d/wk throughout irradiation). Four-field techniques are used to carry extended pelvic fields to 45 Gy in 25 fractions over 5 wk and boost fields to tumor plus 2–2.5 cm are carried to 50.4–54 Gy (Figs. 2A–E).

5.1.2. SURGERY

Following a course of preoperative chemoirradiation, surgical exploration is undertaken 4–6 wk later. The delay allows ongoing tumor shrinkage after the cessation of preoperative treatment as well as resolution of treatment-induced acute inflammation.

Accurate preoperative staging is important since IOERT benefits primarily those patients who can undergo a grossly complete tumor resection. Ideal patients are in reasonably good health and are willing to undergo major surgery that may include stoma

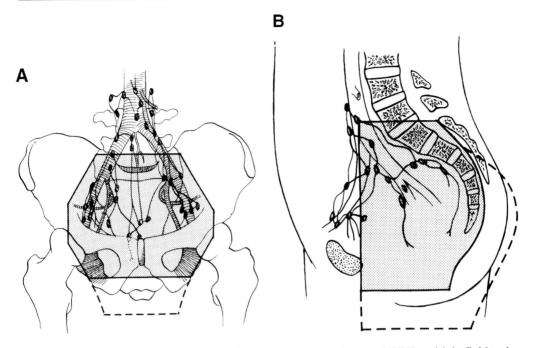

Fig. 2. EBRT techniques. (**A–E**) Idealized artist's depiction of pelvic EBRT multiple field techniques using AP/PA and lateral fields for rectal cancer (**A–C**) or sigmoid cancer (**D, E**). (Modified from L. L. Gunderson, et al., *Front Rad Ther Oncol* **28:**140–154, 1997.)

creation and possible pelvic exenteration. There should be no distant metastases to liver, lungs, or peritoneum, and no adenopathy of the para-aortic area, or groins. There should be no invasion of pelvic nerves or the sciatic notch (i.e., no sciatica or sacral/buttock pain), and, no evidence of tumor invading or wrapped around the iliac vessels or ureters. In order to assess the extent of tumor, preoperative evaluation ordinarily includes: abdominal and rectal exam, sigmoidoscopy and/or colonoscopy, abdominal plus pelvic CT scan (Fig. 1), and chest X-ray (sometimes chest CT scan). Transanal ultrasound usually adds little to the evaluation since tumors appropriate for IOERT are large and advanced on clinical exam alone. If there is any question of involvement of the urologic system, iv urogram, and possibly urology consult and cystoscopy, may be required. If a colostomy is possible, preoperative evaluation by an enterosomal therapist can be very helpful, not only to begin stroma counseling and teaching but also to mark the optimal site on the abdomen for the stroma.

Surgery is usually best carried out via a midline incision that allows extension as necessary and permits multiple stomas. Adhesions are completely taken down, and the abdomen is carefully evaluated for liver and peritoneal metastases. If metastases are found that are not resectable with curative intent (i.e., solitary liver metastasis), intraoperative irradiation is not performed, and treatment ends with palliative resection (or only EBRT).

If no metastases are evident, or are limited and can be resected for cure, the patient undergoes abdominoperineal resection, low anterior resection, or pelvic exenteration, depending upon the extent and location of the tumor (Figs. 3A–D). *En bloc* wide resection is the goal; at least a grossly complete resection of the tumor is desirable, but if that cannot be done, as much of the cancer as possible is removed. Early intraoperative rectal irriga-

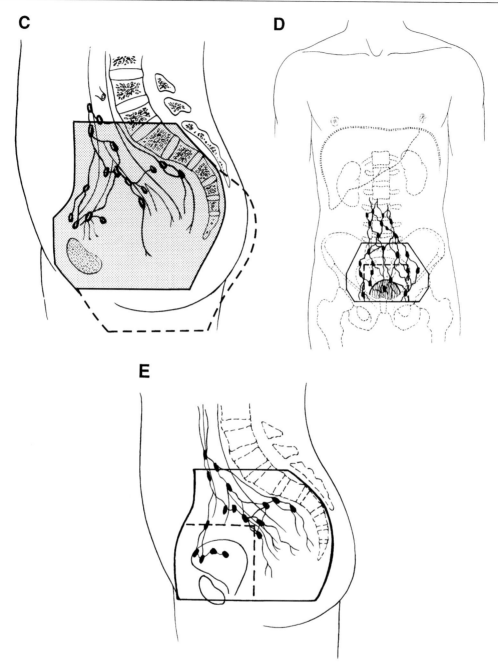

Fig. 2. (*continued*)

tion with sterile water is helpful to eliminate residual stool and possibly exfoliated cancer cells from the rectal stump in preparation for anastomosis (usually with a circular stapler passed via the anus). Lavage is worthwhile even if abdominoperineal resection is planned because the tumor may be fractured or the rectum perforated during a difficult dissection. For any resection of locally advanced primary rectal or sigmoid cancer, mobilization of the tumor off the sacrum (Figs. 3A,B) and pelvic sidewall can be difficult. Sometimes a

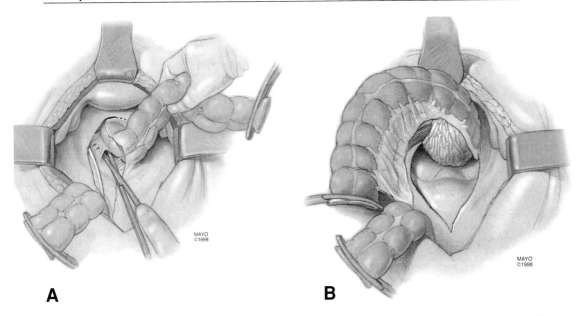

Fig. 3. Surgical techniques. (**A**) Sharp dissection of rectum and tumor out of pelvis. (**B**) Rectal mobilization completed (mesorectal excision). (**C**) Following preoperative chemoirradiation, use unirradiated large bowel for the proximal end of the anastomosis. The left side of the figure depicts resection of the large bowel from the level of proximal descending colon to retro or infraperitoneal rectum. On the right is the reconstructed large bowel with anastomosis. (**D**) Placement of vascularized omental pedicle in the pelvis after rectal resection and re-anastomosis.

large periosteal elevator (e.g., Cobb elevator) functions well for this. Hemostasis after resection is important since pooled blood over the tumor bed could decrease the IOERT dose at depth.

If an anastomosis is to be done, it is completed after the delivery of IOERT. To minimize the likelihood of complications, it is preferable to mobilize the left colon completely and use unirradiated bowel (descending colon) for the proximal end of the anastomosis (Fig. 3C). Placement of pedicled omentum in the pelvis at the end of the procedure (Fig. 3D) is often beneficial; it may decrease the risk of a leak from an anastomosis, it minimizes the risk of malignant small-bowel obstruction if pelvic recurrence later occurs after abdominoperineal resection, it keeps small bowel out of the pelvis in case postoperative EBRT is necessary, and it helps prevent pelvic sepsis by eliminating dead space (which is a substantial risk especially after pelvic exenteration).

5.1.3. IOERT FACTORS

The decision to treat with IOERT is based upon the operative findings, pathologic margin status, and pretreatment physical exam and imaging studies, and is an intraoperative collaborative judgment made by the surgeon and the radiation oncologist. It is critical to define the area at highest risk for subsequent local relapse in order to determine the optimal position for the IOERT field. Margins of resection are determined by frozen section pathologic analysis of the surgical specimen and sometimes the tumor bed. If no tumor adherence exists after preoperative chemoirradiation and adequate soft-tissue radial margins are present (>1 cm), IOERT was often not delivered at MGH until recent analyses suggested a high risk for relapse in patients with pretreatment adherence who had T3 or

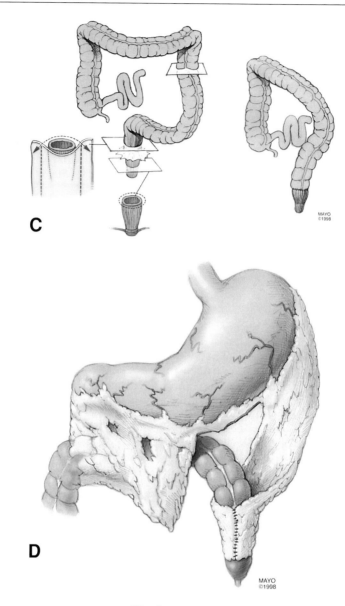

Fig. 3. (*continued*)

N(+) disease after preoperative treatment (*see* subheading 5.2). Patients with gross residual cancer, with microscopically positive margins, or with close (≤5mm) radial soft-tissue margins have always been candidates for IOERT. The tumor bed is marked with sutures to facilitate later positioning of the IOERT applicator and to direct the IOERT.

An IOERT applicator is selected according to the location and size of the area to be irradiated. The internal diameters of circular applicators range from 4–9 cm at MGH and from 4–9.5 cm at Mayo. Applicator size is selected to allow full coverage of the high-risk area that is generally on the presacrum or pelvic sidewall. Usually, the largest applicator that will fit into the area is best. The applicator's shape is chosen so that the geometry fits the specific situation of tumor vs normal tissue. The applicator must abut the site being treated, which can be difficult if the high-risk area is located in an anatomically confined

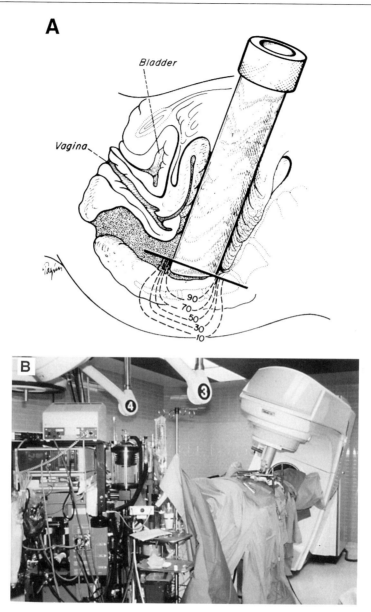

Fig. 4. IOERT techniques (MGH, Mayo Clinic). (**A**) Artist's rendition of IOERT to the *presacrum* via an *abdominal approach*. (**B,C**) Treatment of the pelvic sidewall with either minimal gantry angle (**B**) or > 45° (**C**). (**D**) IOERT treatment of the *distal presacrum* coccygeal region via perineal approach with gantry angle exceeding 45°. (**E,F**) Treatment of the *prostate, base of bladder* via the *perineal approach* with the patient supine (**E**). Note gantry angle exceeding 90° (**F**).

region such as the pelvis. Some have beveled ends of 15° or 30°, enabling good apposition of the applicator to sloping surfaces in the pelvis in order to maximize dose homogeneity (Fig. 4A; also see Chapters 3 and 4). It is important that the applicator be placed so that the tumor or tumor bed is fully covered, that sensitive normal tissues are not included in the beam, and that there is no fluid buildup in the treatment area. The applicator not only directs the electron beam accurately to the high-risk area, but it also serves to retract

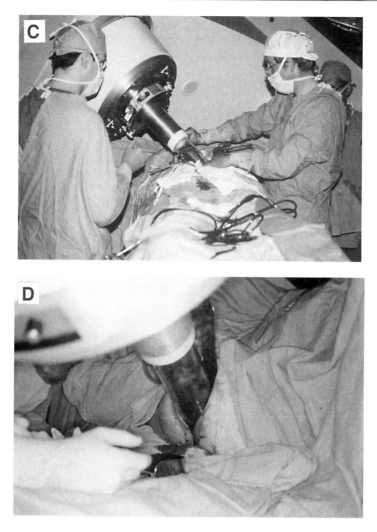

Fig. 4. (*continued*)

sensitive normal tissues out of the way, especially small bowel and ureter. Visceral retraction and packing are usually necessary also. If a distal rectal stump remains for later anastomosis, it should also be excluded from the IOERT field by retraction outside the applicator with the applicator and packing or with the use of lead sheets that can be cut out to block sensitive normal tissues that cannot be removed from the path of the beam. During treatment, suction catheters are positioned to minimize fluid buildup within the applicator.

Most IOERT treatments in rectal cancer are given via a transabdominal approach since the area of concern is usually posterior presacrum or posterolateral pelvic sidewall (Figs. 4A–C; also see Chapters 4 and 7). A perineal port is occasionally used after abdomino-perineal resection to treat a very low-lying tumor involving the coccyx or distal presacrum, distal pelvic sidewall, or portions of the prostate and base of the bladder when an exenteration is not performed (Figs. 4D–F; also see Chapters 4 and 7). The perineal approach is technically more difficult. Rarely it may be impossible to abut the applicator to the tumor bed if the lesion is located very low in the pelvic sidewall in an obese male with a narrow pelvis.

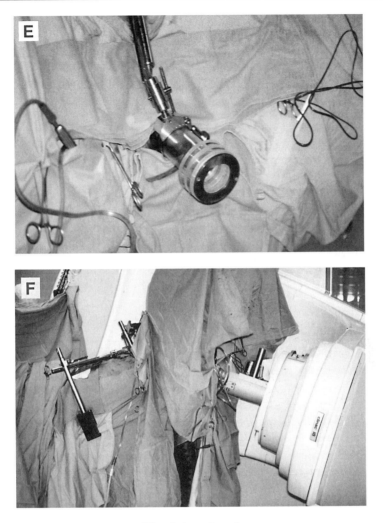

Fig. 4. (*continued*)

After positioning the IOERT applicator, it is docked to the linear accelerator, and IOERT is delivered. Typical doses of radiation delivered intraoperatively are in the range of 10–20 Gy with the lower doses being given for minimal residual disease (narrow or microscopically positive margins) and the higher doses for gross residual disease after maximal resection. For patients undergoing complete resection with negative but narrow margins, the IOERT dose is usually 10–12.5 Gy, whereas for patients undergoing subtotal resection with microscopically positive margins, the dose is 12.5–15 Gy. For patients with macroscopic or gross residual after resection, the dose is 17.5–20 Gy. Typical electron energies used are 9–15 MeV, depending on the thickness of residual tumor. The dose is quoted at the 90% isodose.

5.2. MGH Results (EBRT With or Without 5-FU, Resection, IOERT)

The IOERT program at MGH began in 1978 (*21,22*). Sixty-four patients with locally advanced primary rectal cancer have undergone full-dose preoperative irradiation (with or without 5-FU) and resection with IOERT. The 5-yr actuarial local control and disease-

Table 3
MGH Primary Rectal IOERT Series—5-Yr Actuarial Local Control
and Disease-Specific Survival by Degree of Resection

Degree of Resection	# Pts.	LC (%)	DSS (%)
Complete Resection	40 (12)	91	63
Partial Resection	24 (5)	63	35
Microscopic residual	17 (4)	65	47
Macroscopic residual	7 (1)	57	14

LC - local control; DSS - disease specific survival.
Number in parenthesis indicates number of patients at risk at 5 yr.

Table 4
MGH Primary Rectal IOERT Series—5-Yr Actuarial Local Control and
Disease-Specific Survival of Completely Resected Patients by Pathological Stage

Pathologic Stage	# Pts	LC (%)	DSS (%)
No Tumor or Intramural Tumor Only	6 (3)[a]	100	63
Transmural, and/or Lymph Node Positive	34 (10)[a]	88	64

LC - local control; DSS - disease specific survival.
[a]Number in parenthesis indicate number of patients at risk at 5 yr.

specific survival for 40 patients undergoing complete resection with IOERT was 91 and 63%, respectively (Table 3). For 24 patients undergoing partial resection, local control and disease-specific survival correlated with the extent of residual cancer: 65 and 47%, respectively, for microscopic residual disease, and 57 and 14%, respectively, for gross residual disease.

Local control and disease-specific survival of the completely resected patients are correlated to the post-EBRT pathologic findings (Table 4). Although there was a trend of improved local control in patients with intramural tumors compared to patients with transmural tumors after irradiation, these differences were not statistically significant.

5.2.1. TREATMENT TOLERANCE

The 5-yr actuarial risk of complications of the 64 patients receiving IOERT was 16% (Table 5). Two patients developed osteoradionecrosis of the sacrum requiring surgical intervention. No deaths were seen as a consequence of these complications.

5.2.2. LOCAL RELAPSE VS STAGE OF DISEASE AFTER PREOP EBRT: IOERT SELECTION ISSUES, MGH

An important issue in the use of IOERT in rectal cancer is the selection of patients for this modality. After moderate- to high-dose preoperative irradiation (45–50.4 Gy), tumor regression or pathological downstaging is observed. The question arises whether patients with locally advanced rectal cancers exhibiting marked regression after preoperative treatment are at lower risk for local recurrence than patients with tumors not exhibiting this response. If so, IOERT would be of limited value in the subset of patients with downstaged tumors and probably should not be administered.

Table 5
Complications in MGH IOERT
Series of 64 Primary Rectal Patients

Pelvic Abscess	1
Sepsis (from central line)	1
Wound Dehiscence	1
Small Bowel Obstruction	1
Small Bowel Fistula	5
Delayed Perineal Wound Healing	2
Sacral Osteoradionecrosis	2
Ureteral Obstruction	2
Total	15

The incidence of local relapse as a function of stage of disease after preoperative irradiation with or without concomitant 5-FU has been evaluated in three separate MGH analyses. For 11 patients with locally advanced (T4) rectal cancer treated with preoperative irradiation and simple curative resection in the original MGH series, five of eight patients (62.5%) that had persistent tumor extension grossly beyond the bowel wall failed in the pelvis vs none of three patients with tumor confined to the wall or only microscopic extra rectal extension (8). In an analysis of 28 patients with *tethered* (T3) rectal cancers treated with preoperative irradiation and resection at MGH, the 5-yr actuarial local recurrence and disease-free survival was 24 and 66%, respectively. No correlation between local control and posttreatment extent of tumor penetration through the rectal wall and/or lymph node involvement was observed.

In the most recent MGH analysis, the outcome of 47 patients with locally advanced rectal cancer receiving 45–50.4 Gy preoperative irradiation and complete resection with clear resection margins by pathological stage was evaluated (unpublished results). These patients did not receive IOERT because it was judged not indicated because of the favorable response to preoperative irradiation or IOERT was not technically feasible. For 24 patients with no residual tumor or tumor confined to the rectal wall after preoperative EBRT, the 5-yr actuarial local control rate was 87%. In contrast, the 5-yr actuarial local failure rate was 68% for 27 patients with transmural tumors and/or lymph-node metastases. Despite a favorable response to preoperative irradiation and no clearly defined indication for IOERT at surgery (tumor adherence or compromised soft-tissue margins), the local failure rates were high in this group of patients, especially for patients with tumors exhibiting transmural penetration and/or lymph node metastases. The extent of tumor regression after preoperative irradiation is no longer used as an absolute guide to the need for IOERT at MGH.

5.3. Mayo IOERT Series

At the Mayo Clinic, the treatment approach of primary locally advanced rectal carcinoma has been similar to MGH combining EBRT (with or without 5-FU) with surgery and IOERT to high-risk regions (24,25). From April, 1981 through August, 1995, 61 patients with primary locally advanced primary colorectal cancer received an IOERT dose of 10–20 Gy, usually combined with 45–55 Gy of fractionated EBRT. Concomitant 5-FU was delivered during EBRT in 40 patients (71%), but only 3 (5%) received maintenance chemotherapy. The amount of residual disease remaining at IOERT after

Table 6
Primary Colorectal IOERT: 5-Yr Actuarial Local Control, Distant Failure,
And Overall Survival by Degree of Resection and Amount of Residual Disease, Mayo Analysis

Degree of Resection, Amount Residual	5-Yr Actuarial Results			
	# Pts	LC (%)	DF (%)	O.S. (%)
No Tumor	2	100	0	100
Complete Resection	18	93	54*	69
Partial (Subtotal) Resection				
Microscopic residual	19	86	50*	55
Macroscopic residual	16	73	83*	21
No Resection	1	—	—	0
All Patients	56	84	59	46

LC - Local Control, DF - Distant Failure, OS - Overall Survival
*3-yr actuarial DF of 43%, 38%, and 66% for complete resection, microscopic residual or gross residual.

exploration and maximal resection in the 56 patients with ≥18 mo of follow-up was gross residual in 16, microscopic or less in 39 and unresected in 1.

5.3.1. Disease Control and Survival, Mayo Analysis

The impact of degree of resection and amount of residual disease on disease control and survival is seen in Table 6 and Fig. 5A. The 5-yr survival for the entire group of patients was 46%. Patients with microscopic or less residual fared better than those with gross residual with a 5-yr actuarial overall survival of 59 vs 21% ($p = 0.0005$). Failures within an irradiation field have occurred in 4 of 16 patients (25%) who presented with gross residual after partial resection vs 2 of 39 (5%) with microscopic or less residual after gross total resection ($p = 0.01$). Within the more favorable group, patients with negative margins or no residual tumor did somewhat better than those with positive margins, with regard to local control and survival, but with no statistical significance.

The impact of other treatment and disease prognostic factors on disease control is seen in Table 7. The factors other than amount of residual with a statistical trend for improved local control were grade 1, 2 vs grade 3, 4 (LF rate of 7 vs 17% and actuarial 3- and 5-yr rates of 4 vs 32%, $p = 0.09$) and nodal status of negative vs positive (LF 4 vs 19%; 3- and 5-yr rates of 4 and 23%, $p = 0.11$). Additional factors with statistical impact on distant relapse included EBRT and 5-FU (vs EBRT alone, $p = 0.013$) (Fig. 5B) and colon primary (vs rectal, $p = 0.03$). Nodal status had no impact on distant relapse rates (nodes-negative: 12 of 24 or 50%; nodes positive: 14 of 27 or 52%). Because of the high rates of distant metastases in these patients, (absolute 27 of 56 or 48%; 3- and 5-yr actuarial of 45% and 59%), more routine use of systemic chemotherapy was advised.

The influence of other prognostic factors on survival is seen in Table 8. Treatment factors that influenced survival included EBRT plus 5-FU vs EBRT alone (Fig. 5B) (favorable trends but p-value NS) and treatment sequence in those with EBRT plus 5-FU (Fig. 5C). Preoperative EBRT plus 5-FU had improved survival when compared with postoperative EBRT plus 5-FU with median survival of 81 vs 25 mo and 3- and 5-yr survival of 62 vs 17%, $p = 0.005$. There was a nonsignificant trend in survival favoring patients with grade 1 or 2 lesions vs those with grade 3 or 4 lesions and for patients with nodes negative vs positive. Prognostic factors that appeared to impact disease-free sur-

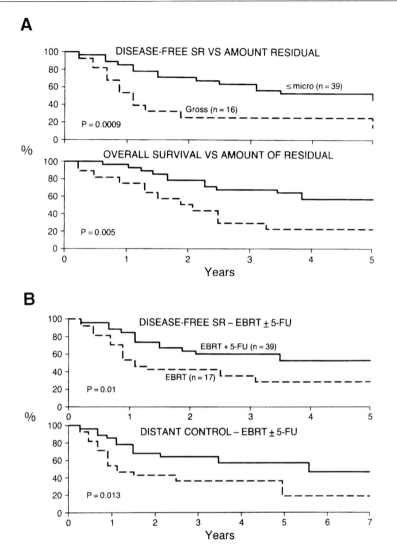

Fig. 5. Impact of prognostic factors on distant control and survival, Mayo Clinic analysis of 56 patients with EBRT with or without 5-FU, resection, and IOERT for locally advanced primary colorectal cancer. (**A**) Amount of residual. (**B**) EBRT ± 5-FU. (**C**) Treatment sequence of pre versus postoperative EBRT in the 38 patients with EBRT plus concomitant 5-FU. (**D**) Site of primary-colon versus rectum. (Modified from L.L. Gunderson et al. [25].

vival (SR) included EBRT plus 5-FU vs EBRT alone (3-yr SR 59 vs 28% and 5-yr SR 54 vs 9%, $p = 0.01$) (Fig. 5B), colon vs rectal primary (3-yr SR 71 vs 37%, 5-yr SR 71 vs 16%, $p = 0.009$) (Fig. 5D), and amount of residual (≤ microscopic vs gross, 3-yr SR 58 vs 25%, 5-yr SR 46 vs 13%, $p = 0.0014$) (Fig. 5A).

5.3.2. Treatment Tolerance, Mayo Analysis

An in-depth analysis of peripheral nerve tolerance following IOERT was also performed (Table 9). Symptomatic or objective neuropathy was documented in 18 of 56 patients (32%). Ten of 18 (56%) had only grade 1 toxicity, usually manifesting as mild or intermittent paresthesis and/or pain not requiring narcotics. Of the 7 patients with

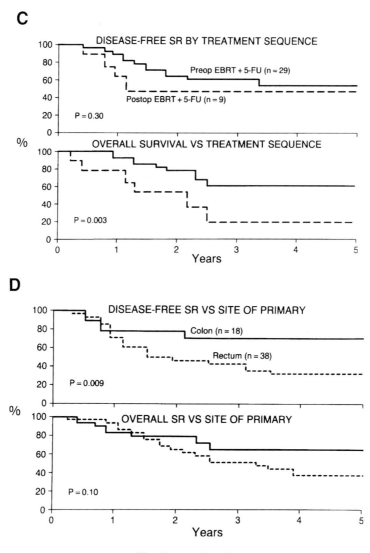

Fig. 5. (*continued*)

presumed treatment-related grade 2 (usually pain requiring narcotics) or grade 3 nerve toxicity, the data suggested a relationship between IOERT dose and the incidence of grade 2 or 3 neuropathy ($\leq$12.5 Gy: 1 of 29 or 3%; $\geq$15 Gy: 6 of 26 or 23%, $p = 0.03$). The relative incidence of grade 3 neuropathy by IOERT dose for 57 fields in 55 evaluable patients was 0 of 29 for $\leq$12.5 Gy, 1 of 19 (5%) for 15 or 17.5 Gy and 2 of 9 (22%) for 20 Gy.

The incidence of other treatment-related side effects including ureter is seen in Table 9. The IOERT boost field encompassed 10 ureters in 9 of the 56 patients (solitary ureter: 8 patients, bilateral ureters: 1 patient). Subsequent ureteral narrowing with hydronephrosis (grade 2) or obstruction requiring a stent (grade 3) occurred in five patients who had a ureter within IOERT fields (five of nine—56%) and in five patients in whom the ureter was not included in the field (includes one patient with bilateral ureteral obstruction: one

Table 7
Primary Colorectal IOERT: Impact of Treatment
and Disease Prognostic Factors on Disease Relapse, Mayo Analysis

Prognostic Factor	# at Risk	Local Relapse (EBRT) (%)			Distant Metastases (%)			
		No. (%)	3 and 5 yr	p^a	No. (%)	3 yr	5 yr	p
EBRT +/- 5-FU (n = 56)								
EBRT + 5-FU	39	4 (10)	11	0.54	14 (36)	35	41	0.013
EBRT	17	3 (18)	24	—	13 (77)	66	83	—
Treatment sequence (n = 38)								
Preop EBRT+5-FU[b]	29	4 (14)	14	—	10 (35)	32	39	0.18
Postop EBRT+5-FU	9	0	0	0.37	4 (44)	53	53	—
Site of Primary (n = 56)								
Colon	18	1 (6)	6	0.20	5 (28)	29	29	0.03
Rectum	38	6 (16)	21	—	22 (58)	53	75	—
Grade (n = 56)[c]								
1,2	27	2 (7)	4	0.09	15 (56)	43	43	0.83
3,4	29	5 (17)	32		12 (41)	45	45	
Nodal status (n = 51, unk - 5)								
Negative	24	1 (4)	4	0.11	12 (50)	50	62	0.95
Positive	27	5 (19)	23		14 (52)	48	63	
Total group	56	7 (13)	16	—	27 (48)	45	59	—

[a] Log rank p value.
[b] Central failure in IOERT field occurred in only 1 patient (preoperative EBRT + 5-FU, rectal, no resection).
[c] Time to relapse by grade: grade 2 LF range 1.0–5.5 yr, DF range 0.5–5.5 yr, grade 3 all *LF* by 3 yr, DF by 1.5 yr; grade 4 all LF by 2 yr, DF by 1.5 yrs.
EBRT = external beam irradiation; IOERT intraoperative electron irradiation; LF = local failure in EBRT field; DF = distant failure, 5-FU = 5-Fluorouracil, unk = unknown. Modified from ref 21.

ureter was within the IOERT field, the other was surgically dissected). Pelvic relapse was the probable cause of ureteral obstruction in only one patient.

5.4. MD Anderson IOERT Series

In the MD Anderson study, 11 of 38 patients (29%) with primary locally advanced rectal cancer received IOERT to high-risk regions in the pelvis because of persistent tumor adherence or residual tumor following preoperative irradiation and infusional chemotherapy *(13)*. No local failures were seen in these patients although 7 of 11 patients developed distant metastases. One patient developed a sensory neuropathy following 20 Gy of IOERT.

5.5. Pamplona IOERT Series

In Europe, the Pamplona group has been investigating IOERT in a variety of disease sites, including rectal cancer *(26)*. From March, 1986 to October, 1993, 59 patients with primary locally rectal cancer received IOERT as a treatment component in multimodal strategies including surgery and postoperative EBRT (13 patients, group I) or preoperative chemoirradiation followed by planned surgery (46 patients, group II). Pelvic recurrence has been identified in only one patient (simultaneously with lung and liver

Table 8
Primary Colorectal IOERT - Survival by Prognostic Factor, Mayo (September, 1995)

Prognostic Factor	# at Risk	Overall Survival %					Disease-Free Survival %			
		Median	2 yr	3 yr	5 yr	p[a]	2 yr	3 yr	5 yr	p[a]
EBRT ± 5-FU (n = 56)										
EBRT + 5-FU	39[b]	81 mo	72	53	53	0.39	59	59	54	0.01
EBRT alone	17	40 mo	64	58	35	—	41	28	9	—
Treatment Sequence (n = 38)										
Preop EBRT + 5-FU	29	81 mo	77	62	62	0.003	61	61	54	0.30
Postop EBRT + 5-FU	9	25 mo	52	17	17	—	47	47	47	—
Site of Primary (n = 56)										
Colon	18	81 mo	77	63	63	0.10	71	71	71	0.009
Rectum	38	37 mo	65	51	38	—	46	37	16	—
Grade (n = 56)										
1,2	27	67 mo	73	60	54	0.28	62	57	57	0.32
3,4	29	37 mo	68	51	36	—	46	37	37	—
Nodal status (n = 51)										
Negative	24	45 mo	79	67	47	0.34	58	50	38	0.67
Positive	27	28 mo	59	46	41	—	51	45	29	—
Total group	56	40 mo	70	55	46		54	48	35	

[a] Log rank p value, univariate.

[b] 1 of 39 had chemotherapy prior to but not concomitant with EBRT.

EBRT = external beam irradiation; IOERT = intraoperative electron irradiation; 5-FU = 5-fluorouracil; mo = months

Modified from ref 21.

Table 9
Primary Colorectal IOERT Peripheral Nerve
and Ureter Toxicities—Treatment or Tumor Related, Mayo Analysis

	Grade of Toxicity				
	1 No. (%)	2 No. (%)	3 No. (%)	4 No. (%)	Total n=56
Peripheral nerve	10 (18)	5 (9)	3 (5)[a]	0	18 (32)
Ureter	0	3 (5)	6 (11)	0	9 (16)

[a] IOERT dose of 15, 20, 25 Gy: (≤12.5 Gy: 0 of 29, 15 or 17.5 Gy: 1 of 19 or 5%, ≥20 Gy: 2 of 9 or 22%).

metastasis) and distant dissemination, as the only site of progression, in 9 (42% in group I and 9% in group II). Cause-specific survival projected over 80 mo was 52 and 77% in group I and II, respectively. Toxicity attributable to IORT consisted of pelvic pain (delayed neuropathy) observed in four patients (9%) and ureteral stenosis in five patients (11%).

5.6. New England Deaconess Orthovoltage IORT Series

The New England Deaconess Hospital has recently analyzed their orthovoltage IORT experience for locally advanced rectal cancer (27). Between 1982 and 1993, 33 patients with locally advanced rectal cancer (primary: 22 patients and recurrent: 11 patients) received preoperative irradiation with 5-FU-based chemotherapy and curative resection. Intraoperative irradiation through a 300-kVp orthovoltage unit was given to 26 patients. The median dose of IORT was 12.5 Gy (range 8–20 Gy). The 5-yr actuarial overall survival and local control rates for patients undergoing gross complete resection and IORT were 64 and 75%, respectively. The crude local-control rate for patients following complete resection with negative margins was 92% for patients treated with IORT. IORT was ineffective for gross residual disease with all four patients progressing locally despite therapy. Seventeen patients (65%) developed pelvic soft-tissue complications and were treated successfully by posterior thigh myocutaneous flap. The incidence of complications was similar in the patients with primary or recurrent disease.

6. CONCLUSIONS AND FUTURE POSSIBILITIES

The treatment of locally advanced or clinical stage T4 primary rectal cancer has evolved over the past 20 years. In the 1980s, treatment programs of moderate- to high-dose preoperative EBRT followed by surgery were carried out at several centers in the United States. These studies showed that a complete resection was possible in one-half to two-thirds of patients with locally advanced rectal cancer after full-dose preoperative EBRT. Despite irradiation and complete resection, local failure occurred in at least one-third of these patients. Recent efforts to improve local control have included the administration of concurrent chemotherapy with preoperative irradiation and the use of IOERT at resection.

Because of the efficacy of postoperative irradiation and 5-FU in the adjuvant treatment of rectal cancer, there has been interest in investigating this approach neoadjuvantly. These investigations have studied combinations of moderate- to full-dose preoperative EBRT (45–50.4 Gy) with 5-FU-based chemotherapy. Although limited by small patient numbers and short followup, the data from these studies show improved rates of resectability and possibly local control and survival. Concurrent 5-FU-based chemotherapy should be utilized with moderate- to high-dose preoperative irradiation programs.

To further improve local control in patients with locally advanced rectal cancer, investigators from the United States and Europe have studied IOERT in combination with treatment programs of EBRT, surgery, and more recently chemotherapy. The data from these studies is compelling that local control is improved in patients receiving IOERT compared to patients not receiving this therapy. The result is most beneficial in patients undergoing complete resection vs patients undergoing partial resection. Disease persistence or relapse within the IOERT and EBRT fields is higher when the surgeon is unable to accomplish gross total resection. Therefore, it seems reasonable to consistently add 5-FU (infusion vs bolus with or without other drugs) during EBRT and to evaluate the use of dose modifiers in conjunction with IOERT (sensitizers, hyperthermia, and so on).

Patient selection for IOERT following preoperative chemoirradiation for patients with pretreatment T4 lesions varies somewhat by institution and investigator. In both the initial MGH IOERT program and the current Mayo IOERT program, an attempt was made to reconstruct the site of pretreatment tumor fixation on the basis of pretreatment imaging and physical exam and treat the area with IOERT. In an attempt to exclude patients from the potential side effects of IOERT, Tepper and Willett appropriately attempted to exclude from IOERT those patients with lack of adherence following preoperative irradiation (with or without concomitant 5-FU) or with a good radial margin (≥1 cm). On the basis of the recent updated MGH analysis, it now appears that in any patient with T3 disease following preoperative treatment, an attempt should be made to define and treat the area of pretreatment fixation (i.e., using pretreatment physical exam and imaging studies in addition to operative findings). In patients with tumor regression to a T0–2 extent after preoperative treatment, it may be reasonable to withhold IOERT on the basis of a 5-yr actuarial local control rate of 87% in 20 patients followed at MGH. It will be of interest to have other institutions analyze their data in similar fashion.

The treatment-related morbidity of IOERT in patients with primary locally advanced rectal cancer has been minimal. It should be remembered, however, that the incidence of grade 2 or 3 peripheral neuropathy appears to be related to an increase in the IOERT dose as seen in the in-depth analysis from Mayo investigators (≤12.5 Gy, 1 of 29 or 3%, ≥15 Gy, 6 of 26 or 23%, $p = 0.03$). These trends are consistent with animal data that suggest a correlation between IOERT dose and the incidence of clinical and electrophysiologic neuropathy in dogs (*see* Chapter 10 text and references). In spite of the potential for ureteral toxicity with IOERT-containing regimens (*see* Chapters 8 and 9 for animal data), ureter is not dose limiting for IOERT because stents can be inserted to mitigate obstruction and preserve renal function as indicated. Therefore, when tumor is adherent to ureter, it should be included in the IOERT boost. Animal studies at Colorado State University suggest that the incidence of IOERT-related ureteral changes is related to the length of ureter within the field *(28)*.

In this disease site, IOERT has been integrated successfully into treatment programs utilizing EBRT, chemotherapy, and surgery. However, in view of the high metastatic potential of approx 50% in patients with locally advanced colorectal cancer, 4–6 mo of systemic chemotherapy should be evaluated as a component of the aggressive treatment approaches discussed in this chapter. Several trials reveal a significant improvement in tumor response rates and median survival for 5-FU plus leucovorin when compared with 5-FU alone in the treatment of advanced metastatic large-bowel cancer *(29,30),* and 5-FU plus leucovorin has demonstrated a survival advantage over surgery alone in an adjuvant colon setting *(31,32)*. On the basis of the intergroup rectal adjuvant study 86-47-51, the use of continuous infusion 5-FU-based chemotherapy should be evaluated as systemic therapy because of its potential to decrease distant metastases and thereby improve survival *(19)*.

REFERENCES

1. Wang CC and Schulz MD. The role of radiation therapy in the management of carcinoma of the sigmoid, rectosigmoid, and rectum, *Radiol. Soc. N. Am.,* **79** (1962) 1–5.
2. O'Connell MJ, Childs DS, Moertel CG, et al. A prospective controlled evaluation of combined pelvic radiotherapy and methanol extraction residue of BCG (MER) for locally unresectable or recurrent rectal carcinoma, *Int. J. Radiat. Oncol. Biol. Phys.,* **8** (1982) 1115–1119.
3. Brierley JD, Cummings BJ, Wong CS, Keane TJ, et al. Adenocarcinoma of the rectum treated by radical external radiation therapy, *Int. Radiat. Oncol. Biol. Phys.,* **31** (1995) 255–259.
4. Allee PE, Tepper JE, Gunderson LL, et al. Postoperative radiation therapy for incompletely resected colorectal carcinoma, *Int. J. Radiat. Oncol. Biol. Phys.,* **17** (1989) 1171–1176.
5. Schild SE, Martenson JA, Gunderson LL, et al. Long-term survival and patterns of failure after postoperative radiation therapy by subtotally resected rectal adenocarcinoma, *Int. J. Radiat. Oncol. Biol. Phys.,* **16** (1988) 459–463.
6. Ghossein NA, Samala EC, Alpert S, et al. Elective postoperative radiotherapy after incomplete resection of colorectal cancer, *Dis. Colon. Rectum,* **24** (1981) 252–256.
7. Emami B, Pilepich M, Willett CG, Munzenrider JE, and Miller HH. Effect of preoperative irradiation on resectability of colorectal carcinomas, *Int. J. Radiat. Oncol. Biol. Phys.,* **8** (1982) 1295–1299.
8. Dosoretz DE, Gunderson LL, Hedberg S, et al. Preoperative irradiation for unresectable rectal and rectosigmoid carcinomas, *Cancer,* **52** (1983) 814–818.
9. Mendenhall WM, Bland KI, Pfaff WW, et al. Initially unrsectable rectal adenocarcinoma treated with preoperative irradiation and surgery, *Ann. Surg.,* **205** (1987) 41–44.
10. Stevens KR and Fletcher WS. High dose preoperative pelvic irradiation for unresectable adenocarcinoma of the rectum or sigmoid, *Int. J. Radiat. Oncol. Biol. Phys.,* **9** (1983) 148.
11. Whiting JF, Howes A, and Osteen RT. Preoperative irradiation for unresectable carcinoma of the rectum, *Surgery (Gynecology & Obstetrics),* **176** (1993) 203–207.
12. Marsh PJ, James RD, and Scholfield PF. Adjuvant preoperative radiotherapy for locally advanced rectal carcinoma, *Dis. Colon. Rectum,* **37** (1994) 1205–1214.
13. Weinstein GD, Rich TA, Shumate CR, Skibber JM, et al. Preoperative infusional chemoradiation and surgery with or without an electron beam intraoperative boost for advanced primary rectal cancer, *Int. J. Radiat. Oncol. Biol. Phys.,* **32** (1995) 197–204.
14. Minsky BD, Cohen AM, Enker WE, Saltz L, et al. Preoperative 5-FU, low-dose leucovorin, and radiation therapy for locally advanced and unresectable rectal cancer, *Int. J. Radiat. Oncol. Biol. Phys.,* **37** (1997) 289–295.
15. Frykolm G, Glimelius B, and Pahlman L. Preoperative irradiation with and without chemotherapy (MFL) in the treatment of primary non-resectable adenocarcinoma of the rectum. Results from two consecutive studies, *Eur. J. Cancer Clin. Oncol.,* **25** (1989) 1535–1541.
16. Chan A, Wong A, Langevin J, and Khoo R. Preoperative concurrent 5-fluorouracil infusion, mitomycin C and pelvic radiation therapy in tethered and fixed rectal carcinoma, *Int. J. Radiat. Oncol. Biol. Phys.,* **25** (1992) 791–799.
17. Chen ET-TSU, Mohiuddin M, Brodovsky H, Fishbein G, and Marks G. Downstaging of advanced rectal cancer following combined preoperative chemotherapy and high dose radiation, *Int. J. Radiat. Oncol. Biol. Phys.,* **30** (1994) 169–175.
18. Landry G, Koretz MJ, Wood WC, Bahri S, et al. Preoperative irradiation and fluorouracil chemotherapy for locally advanced rectosigmoid carcinoma: phase I–II study, Radiology, **188** (1993) 423–426.
19. O'Connell MJ, Martenson JA, Wieand HS, et al. Improving adjuvant therapy for rectal cancer by combining protrated-infusion 5-FU with radiation therapy after curative surgery, *N. Engl. J. Med.,* **331** (1995) 502–507.
20. Tepper JE, O'Connell M, Petroni G, et al. Toxicity in the adjuvant therapy of rectal cancer, *Proceedings of ASCO,* **15** (1996) 210.
21. Gunderson LL, Cohen AM, Dosoretz DE, Shipley WU, et al. Residual, unresectable, or recurrent colorectal cancer: external beam irradiation and intraoperative electron beam boost ± resection, *Int. J. Radiat. Oncol. Biol. Phys.,* **9** (1983) 1597–1606.

22. Willett CG, Shellito PC, Tepper JE, Eliseo R, Convery K, and Wood WC. Intraoperative electron beam radiation therapy for primarily locally advanced rectal and rectosigmoid carcinoma, *J. Clin. Oncol.,* **9** (1991) 843–849.

23. Willett CG, Shellito PC, Rodkey GV, and Wood WC. Preoperative irradiation for tethered rectal cancer, *Radiother. Oncol.,* **21** (1991) 141–142.

24. Gunderson LL, Martin JK, Beart RW, Nagorney DM, et al. External beam and intraoperative electron irradiation for locally advanced colorectal cancer, *Ann. Surg.* **207** (1988) 52–60.

25. Gunderson LL, Nelson H, Martenson JA, Cha S, et al. Locally advanced primary colorectal cancer: intraoperative electron and external beam irradiation ± 5-FU, *Int. J. Radiat. Oncol. Biol. Phys.,* **37** (1997) 601–614.

26. Azinovic I, Calvo FA, Aristu JJ, Martinez R, et al. Intraoperative radiation therapy as a treatment component in primary rectal cancer: ten-year experience, (Personal Communication).

27. Kim HK, Jessup M, Beard CJ, Bornstein B, et al. Locally advanced rectal carcinoma: pelvic control and morbidity following preoperative radiation therapy, resection and intraoperative radiation therapy, *IJROBP,* **38** (1997) 777–783.

28. Gillette SM, Gillette EL, Vujaskovic Z, Larua SM, and Park RD. Influence of volume on intraoperatively irradiated canine ureters. Fifth international IORT abstracts, *Hepatol. Gastroenterol.,* **41** (1994) 28.

29. Erlichman C, Fine S, Wong A, and Elhakeim T. A randomized trial of 5-fluorouracil (5-FU) and folinic acid (FA) in metastatic colorectal carcinoma, *J. Clin. Oncol.,* **6** (1988) 469–475.

30. Poon MA, O'Connell MJ, Moertel CG, Wieand HS, et al. Biochemical modulation of fluorouracil: evidence of significant improvement of survival and quality of life in patients with advanced colorectal carcinoma, *J. Clin. Oncol.,* **7** (1989) 1407–1418.

31. O'Connell M, Mailliard J, Kahn MJ, MacDonald J, et al. An intergroup trial of intensive 5-FU and low dose leucovorin as surgical adjuvant therapy for high risk colon cancer, *J. Clin. Oncol.,* **15** (1997) 246–250.

32. Wolmark N, Rockette H, Fisher B, Wichersham DL, et al. The benefit of leucovorin-modulated 5-FU (LV-5-FU) as postoperative adjuvant therapy for primary colon cancer: results from NSABP C-03, *J. Clin. Oncol.,* **11** (1993) 1879–1887.

15 Recurrent Colorectal

EBRT With or Without IOERT or HDR-IORT

*Leonard L. Gunderson, Christopher G. Willett,
Michael G. Haddock, Heidi Nelson,
Ignacio Azinovic, Subir Nag, Felipe A. Calvo,
Kjell M. Tveit, Ralph Dobelbower,
and Hollis W. Merrick*

CONTENTS

1. INTRODUCTION

Aggressive treatment approaches in patients with local or regional relapse after resection of primary rectal or colon cancers is often not considered. For those institutions that favor an aggressive approach in such patients by combining external irradiation with or without chemotherapy, resection and intraoperative irradiation (IORT), justification is found in series that use only the non-IORT components. Data will be presented in this chapter from United States and European non-IORT vs IORT series to allow comparisons of disease control and survival. IORT tolerance and future potential as a component of treatment will be discussed.

From: *Current Clinical Oncology: Intraoperative Irradiation: Techniques and Results*
Edited by: L. L. Gunderson et al. © Humana Press, Inc., Totowa, NJ

2. RESULTS WITH NON-IORT TREATMENT APPROACHES

2.1. Surgery Alone

A majority of patients who develop local or regional recurrence after curative resection of primary rectal or colon cancers are treated with palliative intent in most institutions in the United States and worldwide. Exceptions include patients with a true anastomotic recurrence or female patients with a limited vaginal recurrence. In either instance, complete resection with negative margins may be feasible, and postoperative external-beam radiation therapy (EBRT) plus chemotherapy can be given as indicated. Patients with prior resection of rectal or sigmoid cancers often present with pelvic pain, which is a manifestation of local recurrence involving nerve in the presacrum or pelvic sidewalls. Presentation with pain usually indicates that a surgical approach will be unlikely to yield negative resection margins. Distal sacrectomy with negative resection margins can occasionally be performed in patients with a central, distal pelvic relapse. If relapse develops after abdominoperineal resection, male patients may also require a pelvic exenteration in view of bladder or prostate involvement. Most patients, however, either have no surgical resection or a subtotal resection with gross or microscopic residual in view of tumor fixation to presacrum, pelvic sidewalls, or both.

In a recent Mayo Clinic analysis of 106 patients with subtotal resection of a localized pelvic recurrence from rectal cancer, 12 patients were treated with surgery alone, and the remainder had some type of irradiation *(1)*. Of the 12 with no irradiation, 3- and 5-yr overall survival rates were 8 and 0%, respectively. If eight patients who received EBRT with no planned spatial relationship to surgery are included, 3-yr survival increases to 15%, but 5 yr was still 0%.

2.2. External Irradiation With or Without Chemotherapy

External irradiation and chemotherapy has definite palliative symptomatic benefit for locally recurrent lesions but long-term survival is infrequent *(2–10)*. Relief of pain and/ or bleeding is achieved in approx 75% of patients with doses as low as 20 Gy in 10 fractions over 2 wk, but doses in most series vary from 40–60 Gy in 1.8- to 2.5-Gy fractions. Median duration of symptom relief is only 6–9 mo, and long-term survival is infrequent (0–5% in most series).

Some data suggest a correlation between irradiation dose and duration of palliation *(7,11–13)*. In an analysis by Wang and Schulz *(7)* for residual, inoperable, or recurrent lesions, the percentage of patients who received palliation for 6 mo or more increased with doses beyond 41 Gy (21–30 Gy: 3 of 24 or 12%, 31–40 Gy: 5 of 28 or 31%, 41–50 Gy: 7 of 12 or 58%). Correlation of response and irradiation dose level was also seen in series reported by Hindo et al. *(11)*, Rao et al. *(12)*, and Overgaard et al. *(13)* on groups of patients treated for palliation. In 110 patients, Hindo et al. reported successful response in 20% of patients treated with a nominal single dose (NSD) of 400–700 ret, 67% with 701–1000 ret, and 82–89% in the other three dose divisions (1001–1300, 1301–1500, and 1501–1750 ret). Rao et al. treated 92 patients with successful palliation in only 12% with an NSD of 1000 ret or less, 49% with 1000–1200 ret, 59% with 1200–1400 ret, and 87% with 1400–1700 ret.

Lybeert et al. *(14)* published data from a group of 95 locally recurrent rectal cancer patients in the Netherlands treated with EBRT with or without 5-FU for relapse after radical surgery. Seventy-six patients presented with loco-regional relapse only (Table 1), and 19 presented with loco-regional relapse and concomitant distant metastases. The

Table 1
Locally Advanced Recurrent or Primary Colorectal Cancer Survival And Disease Relapse with EBRT with or without IOERT, Various Series

Disease Category and Treatment	Ref. No.	No. Pts at Risk	Overall Survival (%) Median (mo)	2 yr	3 yr	5 yr	Local Relapse (EBRT) No. (%)	Actuarial (%) 3 yr	Distant Relapse No.(%)	Actuarial (%) 3yr
PRIMARY - EBRT ± IOERT										
Mayo Clinic[a]	51									
EBRT		17	18	35	24	24	13 (76)	76	10 (59)	59
EBRT + IOERT		56	40	70	55	46	7 (13)	16	27 (48)	45
RECURRENT + PRIMARY - EBRT										
Mayo Clinic - Moertel	5	65								
EBRT alone		—	10.5	24	9	—	—	—	—	—
EBRT + 5-FU		—	16	38	19	5	—	—	—	—
RECURRENT - EBRT										
Netherlands - Lybeert et al.	14	76	14	25	13	5	43/63 (68)	—	26/63 (41)	—
EBRT < 50 Gy		—	12	20	6	0	—	—	—	—
EBRT ≥ 50 Gy		—	20	40	18	10	—	—	—	—
Australian - EBRT	15	135	15	—	—	—	—	—	—	—
Low dose palliative		16	9	13	6	—	— (94)	—	—	—
High dose palliative										
(45 Gy/3 Gy Fx)[c]		80	15	26	12	4	— (94)	—	— (38)[c]	—
Radical (50-60 Gy/2 Gy Fx)[c]		39	18	31	28	≤9	— (82)	—	— (49)[c]	—
RECURRENT-IOERT										
Mayo Clinic - Suzuki et al.	1									
No IOERT		64	17	26	18	7[b]	54 (84)	93	29 (45)	54
IOERT ± EBRT		42	30	62	43	19[b]	16 (38)	40	24 (57)	60
Mayo Clinic - Gunderson et al.	24, 25									
EBRT + IORT										
No prior EBRT		123	28	62	39	20	24 (20)	25	65 (53)	64
Prior EBRT		51	23	48	28	12	18 (35)	55	26 (51)	71

[a]All deaths within 30 mo. Local failure range of 3–15 mo. Distant failure range of 3–17 mo. IOERT patients with ≥18 mo FU.

[b]Survival advantage for IOERT vs no IOERT, $p = 0.0006$ (log rank univariate analysis).

[c]High-dose palliative patients had 1 wk treatment break after 30 Gy in 10 Fx; incidence of metastasis underestimated as patients were only investigated as warranted by symptoms.

IOERT = intraoperative electron irradiation; EBRT = external beam irradiation; DM = distant metastasis; FU = follow-up; mo = months; No = number; Pts= patients, yr = year.

275

total dose of EBRT was 44 Gy median (range 6–66 Gy) and 40 Gy median (range 6–50 Gy), respectively. Twelve of 76 with localized relapse received concomitant 5-FU with EBRT. In the patients with loco-regional relapse only, recurrence-free and overall survival rates after EBRT were, respectively, 23 and 61% at 1 yr, and 6 and 13% at 3 yr. Recurrent or persistent disease inside the EBRT volume was an important clinical problem in 43 of 63 evaluable patients or 68% (42 of 43 were diagnosed within 2 yr). In the 76 patients with loco-regional relapse only, using recurrence-free survival as the endpoint, dose of EBRT was a significant multivariate prognostic factor ($p = 0.01$); using survival as the endpoint, dose of EBRT ($p = 0.005$) and grade of tumor differentiation ($p = 0.002$) were significant.

Investigators at Peter MacCullum Cancer Institute *(15)* retrospectively analyzed a group of 135 patients with locally recurrent, nonmetastatic rectosigmoid cancer treated from 1981 to 1990 with three different dose ranges of radiotherapy: 50–60 Gy (radical group: 2-Gy fractions, no split), 45 Gy (high-dose palliative group: 3-Gy fractions with 1 wk split after 30 Gy in 10 fractions) and <45 Gy (low-dose palliative group). Symptomatic response rates of 85, 81, and 56% were achieved in the radical, high-dose palliative, and low-dose palliative groups, respectively. Objective response rates were assessed only in the radical and high-dose palliative groups and were 44 and 37%, respectively. Estimated median survival times were 17.9 mo, 14.8 mo, and 9.1 mo for the radical, high-dose, and low-dose palliative groups, respectively (Table 1).

2.3. Mayo Analyses: EBRT
With or Without Chemotherapy or Immunotherapy

External irradiation has been used alone or in combination with chemotherapy, immunotherapy, surgical resection, or IOERT at Mayo Clinic for locally advanced colorectal cancers. Earlier Mayo analyses did not analyze results separately as a function of locally recurrent vs primary locally advanced cancers. Two of the analyses that included patients with locally recurrent lesions were small, single-institution randomized trials *(5,9)*.

In the first randomized trial, a group of 65 patients with locally unresectable or recurrent colorectal carcinoma was treated with 40 Gy in 2-Gy fractions over 4 wk plus placebo or 5-FU (15 mg/kg on the first 3 d of EBRT) *(5)*. Median survival time was 10.5 mo in the placebo group vs 16 mo in those receiving 5-FU concomitant with EBRT ($p < 0.05$) (Table 1). Two-year survival was 24 vs 38% and 3-yr survival was 9 vs 19%.

In a later trial, 44 patients with locally advanced rectal cancer (unresectable 7, resected but residual 7, locally recurrent 30) received 50 Gy split-course pelvic irradiation with or without adjuvant immunotherapy *(9)*. Site of initial tumor progression could be evaluated in 31 patients, and local progression within the radiation field was diagnosed in 28 (90%). In 17 (55% of evaluable patients), it was the only site of disease. Median survival time in both groups of patients was approx 18 mo. In this trial, 36 of 44 patients were experiencing significant pelvic or perineal pain prior to EBRT. Although 94% of patients experienced temporary improvement in pain following treatment, median duration of pain relief was only 5 mo.

3. PATIENT SELECTION AND TREATMENT FACTORS—IOERT
3.1. Patient Selection and Evaluation

Appropriateness for an IOERT boost should be determined by the surgeon and radiation oncologist in the setting of a joint-preoperative consultation, whenever feasible. This allows input from both specialties with regard to studies that would be helpful for IOERT and EBRT planning as well as whether IOERT is appropriate. An informed consent can be obtained with regard to potential benefits and risks, and optimal sequencing of surgery and EBRT can be discussed and determined.

General criterion for evaluation and selection of patients with recurrent colorectal cancers have been detailed previously in publications from both Mayo Clinic and MGH *(8,16–24)*. By definition, there must be no contraindications for exploratory surgery. In a majority of patients treated at both institutions, surgery alone would not achieve local control, and EBRT doses needed for local control following subtotal resection or with EBRT alone would exceed normal tissue tolerance. An IOERT approach should permit direct irradiation of unresected or marginally resected tumor with single or abutting IORT fields while allowing the ability to surgically displace or shield dose-limiting normal organs or tissue. Patients with documented distant metastases are not usually candidates, since life span is not adequate to evaluate treatment-related effectiveness or tolerance. Exceptions are considered for the following situations: surgical resection of solitary liver or lung metastasis is feasible and planned, or metastases have been stable for ≥1 yr.

The pretreatment patient workup should include a detailed evaluation of the extent of the locally recurrent lesion combined with studies to rule out hematogenous (liver/lung) or peritoneal spread of disease. In addition to history and physical exam, the routine evaluation includes complete blood count (CBC), liver and renal chemistries, chest film, and CEA. If the rectum is still present, the local evaluation includes digital exam, proctoscopy, and/or colonoscopy, and a barium enema study including cross-table lateral views. When low- or mid-rectal lesions are immobile or fixed or symptoms suggest pelvic recurrence following abdominoperineal resection, computed tomography (CT) of the pelvis and abdomen can confirm lack of free space between the malignancy and a structure that may be surgically unresectable for cure (i.e., presacrum, pelvic sidewall) in whom preoperative irradiation plus 5-FU-based chemotherapy should be given prior to an attempt at resection. Extrapelvic spread to para-aortic nodes or liver and the pretreatment status of ureters with regard to presence or absence of obstruction can also be determined from a CT of the abdomen and pelvis. If hematuria is present or findings on CT or excretory urogram suggest bladder involvement, cystoscopy is done prior to or on the day of surgical confirmation. In patients with cutaneous or perineal fistulae, fistulography may be helpful in determining both size and depth for purpose of treatment planning.

3.2. Sequencing of Treatment Modalities

For most patients with locally recurrent colorectal cancers, delivery of 45–55 Gy plus concomitant 5-FU-based chemotherapy preoperatively with reoperation in 3–5 wk offers the following theoretical advantages over the sequence of resection and IOERT followed by postoperative EBRT plus chemotherapy.

1. Potential alteration of implantability of cells that may be disseminated intra-abdominally or systemically at the time of marginal or partial surgical resection.
2. Deletion of patients with metastases detected at the restaging work-up or laparotomy thus sparing the potential risks of aggressive surgical resection with or without IOERT.
3. Possible tumor shrinkage with an increased probability of achieving a gross total resection.
4. Reduction of treatment interval between the EBRT and IOERT components of irradiation (if surgical resection and IOERT are done initially and postoperative complications ensue, the delay to the EBRT plus chemotherapy component of treatment may be excessive).

If patients present with locally recurrent colorectal cancer after adjuvant treatment that included 45–50 Gy of EBRT, full doses of preoperative EBRT will not be feasible *(25)*. In such instances, we usually deliver 10–30 Gy in 1.8- to 2.0-Gy fractions with surgical exploration and attempted resection in 1 d to 3 wk (advantages #1 and 4 still exist).

There would appear to be no tumor-related advantages in having surgical resection and IOERT precede the external component of treatment. For patients with locally recurrent pelvic lesions, the altered sequencing may, however, provide an advantage for normal tissue tolerance *(2,8,26–29)*. If fixed loops of small bowel were found at exploratory laparotomy, they could be mobilized out of the pelvis. Pelvic reconstruction could be performed with omentum or mesh to allow displacement of small bowel during subsequent EBRT plus chemotherapy. As we enter an era of decreasing health-care finances, however, the idea of performing two surgical procedures may be difficult to justify (exploration and reconstruction; exploration, resection, and IORT after preoperative irradiation plus chemotherapy). An alternate approach would be to keep the planned preoperative dose at a level of 40–45 Gy, instead of a higher dose of 50.4–54 Gy, if fixed loops of small bowel were adjacent to the recurrent disease and could not be excluded after a dose of 40–45 Gy.

At the present time, chemotherapy is instituted simultaneously with EBRT for locally advanced primary and locally recurrent colorectal cancers. The advantage of starting irradiation and chemotherapy simultaneously is that effective local and systemic treatment are instituted simultaneously *(30–34)*. There is less danger, therefore, that one component of disease will become uncontrollable because of progression during single-modality treatment. The disadvantage of starting chemotherapy simultaneously with EBRT is that full-intensity chemotherapy may never be feasible. For tolerance reasons the intensity of chemotherapy during EBRT is usually less than if chemotherapy precedes EBRT. If further cycles of chemotherapy are given after pelvic EBRT, full-intensity chemotherapy may not be feasible because of alterations in bone-marrow reserve.

A potential advantage of altered sequencing of chemotherapy and EBRT (i.e., deliver two cycles of multiple-drug chemotherapy before starting combined irradiation/chemotherapy) would be the ability to give full-intensity chemotherapy for at least two cycles. This may have increased impact on occult systemic disease and thereby improve the ultimate rates of systemic disease control. The danger of starting chemotherapy before EBRT, however, is that the local component of disease may continue to progress and subsequent resection may never be feasible.

3.3. Irradiation Factors

3.3.1. EBRT WITH OR WITHOUT CONCOMITANT CHEMOTHERAPY

The method of EBRT in previously unirradiated patients has been fairly consistent in most single-institution and group colorectal IOERT studies. In the Mayo and MGH trials, doses of 45–55 Gy (100 cGy = 1 Gy; 1 cGy = 1 rad) are delivered in 1.8-Gy fractions, 5 d/wk over 5–6 wk in previously unirradiated patients. For pelvic lesions, treatments are given with linear accelerators ≥10-MV photons and four-field-shaped external-beam techniques *(16,19,21,23,24)* (*see* Chapter 14). With extrapelvic lesions, unresected or residual disease plus 3- to 5-cm margins of normal tissue are included to 45 Gy, usually with parallel-opposed fields *(22,24,26,35)* (Fig. 1). Reduced fields with 2- to 3-cm margins are treated to 50–55 Gy. When chemotherapy is given during EBRT, 5-FU is either given as a single drug in protracted daily venous infusion (225 mg/m^2/24 h; 7 d/wk or until

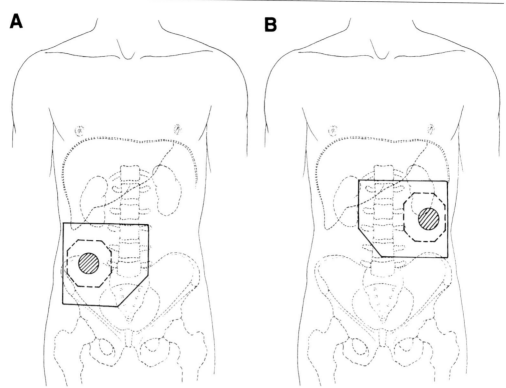

Fig. 1. EBRT technique for extrapelvic lesions presented as idealized fields for right colon or left colon lesions: (**A**) cecum; (**B**) mid-descending colon. [With permission from Gunderson LL and Martenson JA. *Front. Radiat. Ther. Oncol.*, **28** (1994) 140–154.]

intolerance; ref. *33*) or in combination with leucovorin in bolus injections (5-FU 400 mg/m² plus leucovorin 20 mg/m² iv push for four consecutive days during the first week of EBRT and 3–4 d during the last week) *(34)*.

In previously irradiated patients only partial dose EBRT can be given as a component of treatment *(25)*. Since marginal resection is usually the surgical option, it is preferable that low-dose EBRT be given prior to an attempt at resection unless the patient presents with fixed small-bowel loops within a prior high-dose EBRT field. Initially Mayo patients in retreatment situations received EBRT alone or EBRT plus bolus 5-FU with or without leucovorin. Currently, patients receive 20–30 Gy in 1.8- to 2.0-Gy fractions plus protracted venous infusion 5-FU (225 mg/m²/24 h). With concomitant bolus 5-FU plus EBRT, surgery would need to be delayed for ≥2 wk after delivery of the bolus 5-FU to allow the WBC and platelet nadirs to have been reached. With infusion 5-FU at 225 mg/m², patients can proceed directly to surgical resection after completion of the combined EBRT plus concomitant chemotherapy, if indicated or desired.

3.3.2. IOERT

EBRT is supplemented by intraoperative electron irradiation (IOERT) at the joint discretion of the surgeon and radiation oncologist as discussed previously. The radiation oncologist joins the surgeon at the time of surgical exploration or resection to help determine feasibility of a subsequent IOERT boost and size and shape of the IOERT applicator. If surgical exploration precedes EBRT and residual or unresectable disease remains after an attempt at resection, a similar intraoperative assessment for IOERT can be performed.

After abdominoperineal resection, optimal IOERT field exposure is determined with regard to an abdominal (Figs. 2A–D) vs perineal approach (Fig. 2E), and prone vs supine or lithotomy patient position (16,19,21,23,24). If an exenteration is necessary, the prostatic fossa in the retropubic region can be treated through an abdominal (Figs. 2B–D) incision. Tumor adherence to anterior pelvic structures including the prostate or base of bladder can produce a technical challenge, as a perineal approach for IOERT is usually necessary. Patients can be treated in either the prone or supine position. Before the Maquet table became available at Mayo Clinic, patients were usually placed in the prone position for IOERT after colostomy formation and abdominal closure (see Chapter 7, Fig. 3). With the availability of the Maquet table, patients remain in the supine surgical position for IOERT (Fig. 2E). The main technical challenge is the need for greater exposure and increased hip abduction. The small size of the pelvic inlet between ischial tuberosities in males can occasionally prevent use of an adequate-sized applicator.

Since April, 1989, both the operative procedure and delivery of IOERT at Mayo Clinic in Rochester are performed in a dedicated IORT suite within a hospital operating room and a similar facility became available at MGH in June, 1996 (see Chapter 3). The operating rooms were designed to allow complete OR capabilities as well as delivery of IOERT with or without dose modifiers. The linear accelerator at Mayo is a refurbished Clinac 18 that provides variable electron energies from 6 to 18 MeV, and MGH uses the Siemens nonmobile dedicated IOERT linear accelerator with variable electron energies of 6–18 MeV.

The IOERT dose is calculated at the 90% isodose line and is dependent on the amount of residual disease remaining after maximal resection and the amount of EBRT that has or can be delivered as a component of treatment. For patients in whom 45–50 Gy of fractionated EBRT is feasible, the following IOERT guidelines apply: negative margins or microscopic residual, 10–12.5 Gy; gross residual ≤2 cm in largest dimension, 15 Gy; unresected or gross residual ≥2 cm, 17.5–20 Gy. In retreatment situations in which fractionated EBRT doses are restricted to 0–30 Gy, IOERT doses usually range from 15–20 Gy, but doses as high as 25 Gy may have to be considered.

Electron energies are chosen on the basis of maximum thickness of disease after maximal resection and the ability to achieve complete hemostasis after surgical resection. The lower energies of 6, 9, and 12 MeV are used after gross total resection or with minimal residual disease. If the 6-MeV energy is chosen, 0.5–1.0 cm of bolus material may need to be used to improve the surface dose. If surgical hemostasis is incomplete and suction drainage is not functioning properly, choice of either 6 or 9 MeV electrons could result in underdosage at depth. The 15–18 MeV energies and doses of 20 Gy are used more commonly in patients in whom gross residual or unresectable disease exists after attempts at resection.

The size and shape of the IOERT lucite applicators used are dependent on tumor location. For pelvic tumors, circular applicators with 15° or 30° bevels are usually needed to conform to the anatomy of the presacrum, pelvic sidewall, or anterior pelvis. With the 30° bevel, the depth of isodose curves is more shallow at the heel end of the applicator than the toe end (17) and should be considered when placing the treatment applicator relative to the tumor bed or residual tumor. For extrapelvic lesions, rectangular and elliptical applicators with flat or 20° bevel ends are occasionally used (Fig. 2E), in institutions in which they are available, in addition to circular applicators (Fig. 2F).

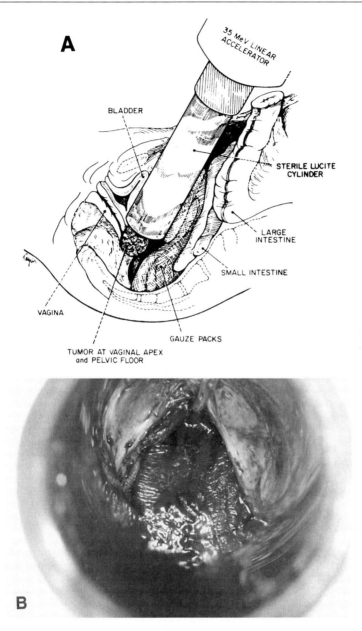

Fig. 2. IOERT techniques. (**A**) Artists idealized depiction of IOERT applicator in position to include relapse at vaginal apex and pelvic floor. (**B–D**) Prostatic fossa in the retropubic region is included in the IOERT field (8.0 cm applicator with 30° bevel) after an exenterative procedure—gantry angle exceeds 45°. (**E**) Treatment of low-lying pelvic tumor or tumor bed via the perineal incision with the patient supine - gantry angle approaches 90°.

3.3.3. IOERT vs HDR-IORT (*see* Chapter 7)

Since February, 1992 IOERT has been performed at Ohio State University (OSU) using a dedicated Siemens linear accelerator with electron energies of 6–18 MeV (36). In addition, sites that are nonaccessible for IOERT have been treated intraoperatively using a HDR afterloader (HDR-IORT) that is transported to the shielded operating room

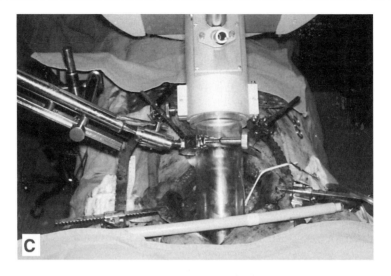

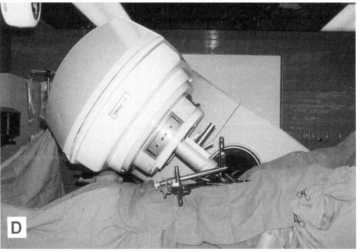

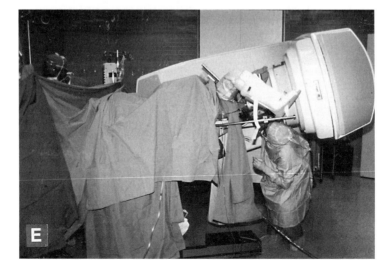

Fig. 2. (*continued*)

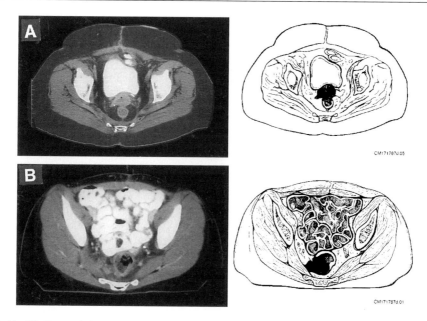

Fig. 3. (A–D). Potential resectability of locally recurrent pelvic lesions as based on pretreatment imaging studies. (**A**) This case illustrates a fixed, but resectable lesion involving *anterior* structures. The primary T3N0M0 rectal cancer was managed with low anterior resection, without postoperative chemotherapy or radiation therapy. The recurrence was fixed to the bladder and was treated with preoperative EBRT plus chemotherapy followed by resection and IOERT. (Reprinted with Permission from Churchill Livingstone.) (**B**) In this case, a fixed, but resectable *lateral* pelvic recurrence was diagnosed following a low anterior resection for a T2N0M0 primary rectal carcinoma. No adjuvant therapy had been administered; therefore, a full course of external beam plus chemotherapy was delivered followed by complete abdominal perineal resection with negative margins. (Reprinted with permission from Churchill Livingstone.) (**C**) *Posterior* recurrence involving the sacrum was diagnosed in this patient who had initially presented with a T3N0M0 lesion of the rectum, treated with resection and adjuvant chemoradiation. After a second course of external beam radiation plus chemotherapy, an en bloc resection of the tumor and sacrum accomplished negative margins. IOERT was administered to the surgical site at risk for recurrence. (Reprinted with Permission from Churchill Livingstone.) (**D**) This case illustratets a locally recurrent lesion that is *fixed* and *not resectable.* The primary, a T3N1M0 tumor, was treated with abdominal perineal resection and a full course of adjuvant radiation and chemotherapy. Recurrent tumor was found to involve the bladder, sacrum, and lateral pelvic sidewall and was not amenable to resection. (Reprinted with Permission from Churchill Livingstone.)

from the radiation oncology department (*see* Subheading 7.0 and Chapter 7 for an expanded presentation of HDR-IORT technique).

3.4. Surgical Considerations

The intent of surgery is to accomplish a gross total resection if technically feasible and safe. Although palliation may be a secondary benefit from reresective surgery for local recurrence, extensive surgical procedures are not advised for purposes of palliation alone, unless disabling complications of sepsis or bleeding are an issue. Patients should, therefore, be evaluated for the possibility of curative-intent surgery, with the possibility of extrapelvic disease excluded and the potential resectibility of local disease determined on the basis of preoperative imaging studies (Fig. 3A–D). Finally, with regard to preop-

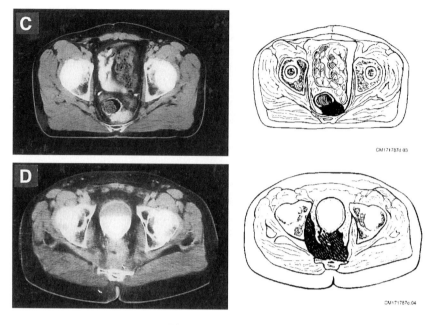

Fig. 3. (*continued*)

erative selection, patients must be of suitable general health and must be counseled on the extensiveness of the multimodality therapy.

Pelvic recurrences are typically amenable to reresection if they are strictly posterior or anterior (Fig. 3A,C). Evidence of lateral pelvic sidewall involvement diminishes the chance of complete resection (Fig. 3B,D); however, operative assessment and at least an opportunity for resection and IOERT is warranted, providing no other contraindications are identified. Although loco-regional recurrences that occur above or below S2 of the sacrum are amenable to resection using anterior-table sacral resection or distal sacrectomy, respectively, the presence of tumor both above and below S2 precludes curative surgery. Similarly, although vascular tumor involvement of either the arterial or venous structures at or distal to the aorta may be resectable, involvement of both structures contraindicates curative surgery in most if not all cases.

At the time of surgery, careful assessment for extrapelvic disease is essential. If possible it is preferable to determine resectability before critical structures are sacrificed or injured. Adjacent involved organs should be removed *en bloc* with the specimen if the associated morbidity is acceptable to the patient and physician. When the recurrent tumor is locally adherent to the prostate or base of the bladder (Fig. 3A,D), since the side effects of pelvic exenteration are excessive, it may be preferable to deliver preoperative EBRT and infusional 5-FU (or bolus 5-FU plus leucovorin) followed by gross total resection, with organ preservation, and supplemental IOERT to the site of adherence (may be able to spare the organ involved by adherence). However, in view of severe adhesions caused by prior surgery and/or adjuvant EBRT, organ preservation is often not technically feasible in the setting of recurrent lesions, and exenterative procedures may be necessary to accomplish a gross total resection. The option to spare the bladder should be reserved for those cases in which present function is good and there is minimal adherence, such that comparable loco-regional control could be accomplished with exenteration vs organ-preserving resection plus IOERT.

In the setting of pelvic recurrence of rectal cancer, it is rarely possible or reasonable to restore intestinal continuity. Most often a previous low anterior resection is being converted to an abdominal perineal resection (APR), or a previous APR to a sacrectomy or exenteration. In the face of local relapse, it is usually ill advised to place another anastomosis in this heavily treated field that is at risk for subsequent local relapse. Rarely, in a highly motivated patient with good sphincter function and a very proximal anastomotic recurrence, it may be reasonable to perform a coloanal anastomosis. Following moderate doses of preoperative EBRT (45–50 Gy) with or without 5-FU-based chemotherapy, anterior resection and primary anastomosis may be safely accomplished if an unirradiated loop of large bowel can be used for the proximal limb of the anastomosis. Temporary diverting colostomies need be done only if surgical indications exist.

If at the end of resection it is decided that postoperative EBRT is indicated, small titanium or vascular clips should be placed around areas of adherence or residual disease for the purpose of boost-field EBRT. The pelvic floor should be reconstructed after resection to minimize the amount of small bowel within the true pelvis, and primary closure of the perineum should be performed after APR to hasten healing (2–6 wk vs 2–3 mo) and decrease the interval to postoperative EBRT and chemotherapy, if indicated. In patients who have been heavily pretreated or those with large defects, vascularized myocutaneous flap closure should be strongly considered. The muscle closes the dead space of the pelvis, which is typically fibrotic and prone to small-bowel adhesion formation, and the fresh nonirradiated skin ensures perineal healing. For posterior sacrectomy wounds, myocutaneous flap closure has become the standard at Mayo Clinic.

If patients develop locally recurrent disease following prior adjuvant EBRT, preoperative and postoperative EBRT options are limited at the time of retreatment unless pelvic reconstruction can be accomplished to displace small bowel (omentum, mesh, other). In previously irradiated patients, IOERT as salvage is usually feasible only in the setting of gross-total resection of disease, and extended organ resection (anterior exenteration, distal sacrectomy, and so on) may be necessary to achieve total resection.

4. UNITED STATES RESULTS—IOERT WITH OR WITHOUT EBRT, PREVIOUSLY UNIRRADIATED PATIENTS

4.1. Local Control and Survival with IOERT Regimens

IOERT has been used at MGH for both locally advanced primary and recurrent colorectal cancers as a component of an aggressive combined approach with EBRT with or without 5-FU and maximal resection (8,16,17,20,21,23,37). Willett et al. (21) reported 5-yr actuarial survival of 19% in 32 patients who received EBRT (with or without 5-FU), IOERT, and maximal resection at MGH for locally recurrent rectal lesions. Prognostic factors that appeared to alter local control and survival are discussed in the next section.

In the Mayo Clinic analysis by Suzuki et al. (1), of 106 patients with subtotal resection of a localized pelvic recurrence from rectal cancer, 42 received IOERT as a component of treatment (41 of the 42 received EBRT; ≥45 Gy in 38). EBRT was the only method of irradiation in 37 patients, and 29 of the 37 received the EBRT in close approximation to subtotal resection in a planned adjuvant role. The 3-yr survival rate was only 18% in the 29 adjuvant EBRT patients vs 42.5% in patients with IOERT as a component of treatment, and 5-yr survival was 7 (EBRT) vs 19% (IOERT) ($p = 0.005$ in a pair-wise com-

Table 2
Colorectal IOERT—Locally Recurrent, No Prior EBRT
Disease Relapse By Prognostic Factor, Mayo

Prognostic Factor	No. at Risk	Local (EBRT) (%)				Distant (%)			
		No.	(%)	3 yr	p[a]	No.	(%)	3 yr	p[a]
EBRT +/– 5-FU									
EBRT	32	5	(16)	16	.46	20	(63)	69	—
EBRT + 5-FU	91	19	(21)	29	—	45	(50)	63	.32
Treatment Sequence									
Preop EBRT + 5-FU	78[b]	17	(22)	31	—	36	(46)	61	.36
Postop EBRT + 5-FU	13[b]	2	(15)	17	.43	9	(69)	71	—
Site of Primary									
Colon	43	6	(14)	20	.51	24	(56)	76	—
Rectum	80	18	(23)	26	—	41	(51)	60	.19
Amount of Residual[c]									
Gross	65	16	(25)	32	—	37	(57)	64	—
≤Microscopic	57	8	(14)	16	.30	27	(47)	64	.84
Margin (+)	40	7	(18)	19		24	(60)	71	
Margin (–)	14	0	(0)	0		3	(21)	43	
No tumor	3	1/3		0		0	(0)	0	
Grade (n = 121, unk-2)									
1,2	69	15	(22)	24	.81	41	(59)	66	.98
3,4	52	9	(17)	28	—	24	(46)	63	—
Total Group	123	24	(20)	25		65	(53)	64	

[a]Log rank p value.
[b]1 patient each group with EBRT dose <40 Gy.
[c]1 patient with no resection—developed distant relapse.
Modified from ref. 24.

parison) (Table 1). Disease control within irradiation fields also appeared to be better in IOERT patients. In previous Mayo Clinic EBRT analyses that included both locally advanced primary and recurrent lesions and in the Suzuki analysis *(4,8)*, local progression was documented in 90% of EBRT patients vs 40% in the 42 IORT patients in the Suzuki analysis. Although differences seen from series to series may reflect selection bias in nonrandomized series instead of treatment effect, it is possible that improvements in control of loco-regional component of disease with the addition of IOERT may translate into improved short-term, if not long-term survival.

In the most recent Mayo analysis *(24)*, 123 colorectal patients with local or regional recurrence and no previous EBRT for their large-bowel cancer were treated with an aggressive multimodality approach including EBRT with or without 5-FU, maximal surgical resection, and IOERT (Tables 2 and 3). Median survival and 2-yr survival rates appeared better than two prior Mayo Clinic EBRT trials that contained a large percentage of patients with recurrence *(5,9)* (IOERT median survival 28 vs 16 and 18 mo with EBRT plus 5-FU or EBRT plus immunotherapy). Five-year actuarial survival was seen in 20% of patients in the current IOERT series (Fig. 4A) vs 5 *(5)* to 7% *(1)* in earlier Mayo Clinic EBRT analyses that noted 5-yr results.

Table 3
Colorectal IOERT—Locally Recurrent, no prior EBRT, Survival By Prognostic Factor, Mayo

Prognostic Factor	No. at Risk	Overall Survival %					Disease-Free Survival %			
		Median	2 yr	3 yr	5 yr	p[a]	2 yr	3 yr	5 yr	p[a]
EBRT +/- 5FU (n = 123)										
EBRT alone	32	25 mo	55	29	16	—	37	27	18	—
EBRT + 5-FU	91	31 mo	65	43	22	.14	49	35	26	.22
Treatment Sequence (n = 91)										
Preop EBRT + 5-FU	78[b]	31	66	44	19	.91	49	37	27	.50
Postop EBRT + 5-FU	13[b]	28	56	38	28[c]	—	49	29	19	—
Site of Primary (n = 123)										
Colon	43	27	59	26	21	—	34	21	21	—
Rectum	80	31	64	43	20	.60	52	39	26	.12
Amount of Residual (n = 123)										
Gross	65	27	60	36	18	—	47	34	24	.91
≤ Microscopic	57	29	64	41	24	.56	45	33	24	—
Margin (+)	40	29	65	41	27		40	26	21	
Margin (−)	14	30	44	44	—		57	57	—	
No tumor	3	20	100	50	—		100	100	—	
Grade (n = 121, unk-2)										
1,2	69	29	65	39	19	.65	44	31	19	.82
3,4	52	27	56	38	22	—	45	36	30	—
Total Group	123	28	62	39	20		46	33	24	

[a] Log rank p value.
[b] 1 patient each group with EBRT dose <40 Gy.
[c] Survival decreased to 19% at 5.5 yr.
[d] No resection - 1 patient, expired ≥2 yrs but <3 yrs.
Modified from ref. 24.

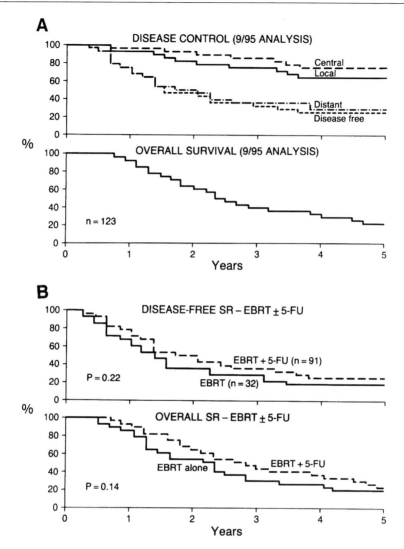

Fig. 4. Impact of prognostic factors on disease control and survival in Mayo Clinic analysis of 123 patients with locally recurrent colorectal cancer and no prior EBRT. (Reprinted from LL Gunderson et al. *(24)* with permission.) (**A**) Disease control and survival for entire patient group (*n*=123). (**B**) EBRT with or without concomitant 5-FU. (**C**) Amount of residual disease after maximal resection.

4.2. Prognostic Factors for Disease Control and Survival with IOERT Regimens

Both 5-yr actuarial local control (LC) and disease-free survival (DFS) were improved in Massachusetts General Hospital (MGH) analyses if the surgeon was able to perform a gross total resection prior to IOERT. In the initial analysis of 32 patients by Willett et al. *(21)*, 5-yr LC and DFS were 42 and 33% with negative resection margins after gross total resection vs 11 and 6% with any degree of residual disease, microscopic or gross. In the most recent MGH analysis of 41 recurrent IOERT patients *(23)*, 5-yr actuarial LC and DFS were 47 and 21%, respectively in the 27 patients with gross total resection with negative but narrow or microscopically positive margins vs 21 and 7% in the 14 patients with gross residual disease (Table 4). Five-year DFS in all 41 patients was 16% and the

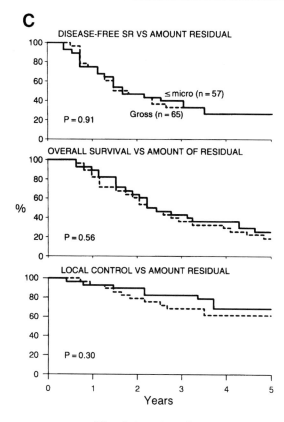

C

DISEASE-FREE SR VS AMOUNT RESIDUAL

≤ micro (n = 57)

Gross (n = 65)

P = 0.91

OVERALL SURVIVAL VS AMOUNT OF RESIDUAL

%

P = 0.56

LOCAL CONTROL VS AMOUNT RESIDUAL

P = 0.30

Years

Fig. 4. (*continued*)

5-yr overall survival rate was 30% (5 of 41 received no or limited EBRT because of prior EBRT—4 of 5 failed locally and died of disease). Data from Rush-Presbyterian Hospital *(38)* Radiation Therapy Oncology Group (RTOG) *(39)* and the University of Navarra *(40)* also support the correlation between local tumor control and amount of residual disease after resection (Table 4). Patients with gross total resection and only microscopic residual had better in-field disease control than those with unresected or gross residual disease.

In the most recent Mayo Rochester IOERT series of 123 patients with locally recurrent colorectal cancer and no prior EBRT for their malignancy *(24)*, the amount of residual after maximal resection had no statistically significant impact on either disease control or survival (Tables 2 and 3) (Fig. 4C), although there were slight improvements in local control favoring the 57 patients with microscopic residual after maximal resection vs the 65 with gross residual. Lack of difference in central control is possibly accounted for by the differential IOERT dose used at Mayo Clinic Rochester on the basis of amount of residual after maximal resection. Local relapse, both absolute and actuarial, was slightly higher in patients with gross residual disease after resection with absolute rates of 25 vs 14% and 3- and 5-yr figures of 32 vs 16% and 40 vs 33% ($p = 0.30$). Overall survival in the 65 IOERT patients with gross residual vs the 57 with microscopic residual was similar, however, with a median of 28 vs 30 mo, 3 yr: 36 vs 41% and 5-yr: 18 vs 24% ($p = 0.56$). Disease-free survival curves were superimposable at 2, 3, and 5 yr. IOERT results in patients with gross residual disease after maximal resection in the most recent

Table 4
Colorectal IOERT—Tumor Failure
in IOERT (CF) or EBRT Field (LF) vs Amount of Residual

| | | | CF or LF (%) | | Residual vs CF or LF (%) | | |
Series	Ref. No.	No. Pts.	Pri	Rec	None	Res (m) or none	Unresect or Res(g)
MGH (5-yr actuarial)							
Primary	37	42	23	—	12	31	50
Recurrent	21,23	41	—	70	—	53	79
Rush Presbyterian	38						
Primary		9	33	—	—	14	100
Recurrent		35	—	54	—	39	64
RTOG–Recurrent	39	37	—	62	—	33	89
Pamplona–Recurrent	40	27	—	74	—	50	84

Pri = primary; Rec = recurrent; No = number; Pts = patients; CF = central failure (IOERT field); LF = local failure (external beam field); Res(m)(g) = microscopic and gross residual; unresect = unresectable.

Mayo series appear better than in other series. However, this may be a function of different patient selection, standardly higher IOERT doses, and the ability to deliver EBRT doses ≥ 45 Gy in 1.8-Gy fractions (or the TDF equivalent) in 119 of 123 patients. In addition 91 of 123 patients received concomitant 5-FU with EBRT with trends for improvements in disease control and survival when compared to the 32 patients with no concomitant 5-FU (Fig. 4B) (median survival 32 vs 26 mo, overall survival: 3 yr, 43 vs 29% and 5-yr 22 vs 16%, $p = 0.14$; disease-free survival rate: 3-yr 35 vs 27%, and 5-yr 26 vs 18%, $p = 0.22$).

4.3. Distant Control—Implications for Chemotherapy

Since the risk of subsequent distant metastases exceeds 50% in patients who present for IOERT at the time of local recurrence, effective systemic therapy will be needed as a component of aggressive treatment approaches including IOERT. In the most recent Mayo series (24), 65 of 123 patients (53%) developed distant metastases with a 3-yr rate of 64%. Although 91 of the 123 patients (74%) received 5-FU-based chemotherapy simultaneously with EBRT, only 2 patients received maintenance chemotherapy after resection and IOERT. For patients who did or did not receive chemotherapy, the absolute rate of distant metastases was 45 of 91 or 50% vs 20 of 32 or 63%, respectively ($p = 0.32$).

4.4. Tolerance of IOERT

Structures at major risk with the use of IOERT for recurrent colorectal cancers include primarily ureter and peripheral nerve (17,19,41–51). Although ureteral narrowing or obstruction as a result of IOERT has been demonstrated in both animal (17,19,43–47) and clinical studies (19,42–44), the ureter is not dose-limiting for IOERT as stents can be placed to overcome obstruction and preserve renal function as indicated. Peripheral nerve is the main dose-limiting structure for IOERT as judged from data generated from both clinical and animal studies (19,42–44,48–51). In an early Mayo Clinic IOERT tolerance analysis by Shaw et al. (42), symptomatic or objective neuropathy occurred in 12 of 37 (32%) pelvic IOERT colorectal patients at risk ≥12 mo (pain in 12 patients, severe in 3 of 37 at risk or 8%; motor in 7 patients, severe in only 1 of 37 or 3%; sensory in 8, none severe). When obtaining informed consent for IOERT, the potential for IOERT-related symptomatic neuropathy must be balanced against the likelihood that local persistence or relapse will result in tumor-related pain. Because many patients with locally recurrent colorectal cancers have moderate or severe pain at time of presentation, they can usually accept the possibility of temporary pain related to treatment as an alternative to permanent tumor-related pain.

In the recent Mayo analysis of 123 patients with IOERT as a component of treatment for locally recurrent colorectal cancers (24), the incidence of peripheral neuropathy of any degree was 34% (42 of 123 patients), as in the prior analysis by Shaw et al. (42). The incidence of severe neuropathy was also similar at 6% (7 of 123 patients had grade 3 toxicity). Twenty-one of 42 patients had only a grade 1 neuropathy (mild paresthesia or pain not requiring narcotics). Data in the updated Mayo analysis suggested a relationship between IOERT dose and grade 2 or 3 neuropathy. The incidence of grade 2 or 3 neuropathy by IOERT dose level was as follows (130 fields in 123 patients): ≤12.5 Gy: 2 of 29 or 7% vs ≥15 Gy: 19 of 101 patients or 19%. If data from the 55 evaluable patients with 57 IOERT fields in the primary colorectal IOERT Mayo analysis (51) were combined with the recurrent colorectal series, incidence of grade 2 or 3 neuropathy by IOERT dose was as follows: ≤12.5 Gy: 3 of 58 or 5%; ≥15 Gy: 25 of 129 or 19%, ($p = 0.01$). This trend is consistent with animal data that suggest a correlation between IOERT dose and incidence of clinical and electrophysiologic neuropathy in dogs (48–50).

The ureter can become narrowed or obstructed as a result of IOERT. In the prior published Mayo Clinic analysis of 51 patients with pelvic IOERT for primary or recurrent malignancies, 44% of previously unobstructed ureters became partially or totally obstructed when included in the IOERT field (42). In the updated Mayo recurrent colorectal IOERT analysis (24), 7 of 123 patients (6%) developed partial ureteral obstruction, and 12 developed an obstruction requiring stents (10%). IOERT was a potential contributing factor to obstruction in 12 of the 33 patients with ureter in an IOERT field (36%). The ureter has also been shown to have IOERT-related toxicity in animal studies evaluating IOERT with or without EBRT (43–47).

Ureter is not dose limiting for IOERT since stents can be inserted to overcome obstruction and preserve renal function as indicated. Therefore, when tumor is adherent to ureter, it should be included in the IOERT boost. In most institutions, ureteral stents are placed only if subsequent obstruction develops since stent-related problems are not infrequent. Animal studies from Colorado State University (CSU) suggest that the incidence of IOERT-related ureteral changes is related to the length of ureter within the IORT field (47). Data concerning length of ureter within IOERT fields have not been correlated with subsequent intolerance in clinical series.

The issue of morbidity following aggressive treatment approaches is placed into perspective by an evaluation of tumor-related morbidity. As noted initially, when EBRT is used as the main treatment modality for locally recurrent rectal cancer, symptomatic pain relief is usually of short duration, >90% of patients have local persistence or progression of disease, most are dead by 2–3 yr, and 5-yr survival is unusual.

On the basis of both human and animal data, when a full component of irradiation options exists (i.e., can deliver 45–55 Gy fractionated EBRT), IOERT doses of 10–20 Gy continue to be practical, dependent on the amount of tumor remaining after maximal surgical resection. For patients with local recurrence in a previous surgical bed, IOERT doses of 15–20 Gy have been used by many investigators even after gross total resection,

Table 5
Colorectal IOERT, Norwegian Experience[a]—
Local Tumor Failure (in EBRT Field) with Primary or Recurrent Disease
and Gross (Macroscopic) Residual Tumor or Not After Maximal Resection

Series	No. Pts.	Local failure (%)	Residual vs Local Failure (%)	
			No gross residual	Gross residual
Primary	32	28	24	32[b]
Recurrent	83	31	28	36[b]

[a]IORT was given to 66 of the 115 patients (54)
[b]Local progressive disease

because of concerns about hypoxia. However, in view of the suggestion of a lower incidence of grade 2 or 3 neuropathy with IOERT doses ≤12.5 vs ≥15 Gy in updated Mayo analyses, an IOERT dose of 12.5 Gy would be a reasonable compromise after a gross total resection. If effective local dose modifiers are identified (sensitizers, ref. 52; hyperthermia, ref. 53), it may be possible to use lower IOERT doses combined with dose modifiers in attempts to overcome hypoxic effects of a postsurgical bed. IOERT doses >20 to ≤25 Gy should be considered only when external doses must be limited because of prior EBRT in view of an increased risk of neuropathy in animal studies *(48–50)*.

5. EUROPEAN AND NORWEGIAN RESULTS—IORT WITH OR WITHOUT EBRT

5.1. Norwegian Results

One hundred and fifteen patients, 75 males and 40 females, were treated between 1990 and 1995 with preoperative EBRT followed by attempts at radical surgery and IOERT *(54)*. The preoperative EBRT dose was, in general, 46 Gy. Thirty-two patients (28%) had locally advanced unresectable primary tumors, usually because of fixation to bony structures. The majority of patients (83 patients, 72%) had locally recurrent cancer. Of these, 47 were located perirectally, 7 were classified as anastomotic, and 10 were perineal (19 were difficult to localize anatomically). There was no macroscopic (gross) residual tumor left after maximal resection in 65% of the patients (75 patients) and 35% had gross residual tumor.

IOERT was given to 66 patients (57%). In 49 cases, IOERT was not given for various reasons. In the group of patients given IOERT, the fraction of patients with no gross residual disease after resection was 74%, compared to 53% in the group of patients not receiving IOERT. In 76% of the patients an IOERT dose of 15 Gy was given, and most of these had microscopic residual tumor remaining. In patients with gross residual tumor, a dose of 20, 18, 17.5, or 15 Gy was used, depending mainly on the amount of residual disease. No chemotherapy was given either concomitant with EBRT or as maintenance therapy.

Table 5 gives information on local recurrence rates for patients treated for either primary or locally recurrent cancers, in relation to whether or not gross residual tumor was present after maximal resection. Of the 83 patients with locally recurrent disease, 26 (31%) have developed a local recurrence at a median observation time of 4 yr. Sixteen of the recurrences were found in patients with no gross residual tumor (28%). In 10 patients with gross residual tumor, tumor progression was found locally (36%). The local recurrence rate in patients with primary tumors was 9 of 32 (28%). The local recurrence rate was about the same in patients treated with IOERT and in patients who did not receive IOERT; however, the groups are not directly comparable.

The 4-yr survival rate was 40% in the entire series, 55% in the primary cases, and 34% in the recurrent cases. The survival rate (SR) was highly dependent on whether gross residual tumor was left or not (in recurrent cases, 4-yr SR of 50% in patients with no gross residual and 0% in patients with gross residual tumor; in primary cases 60 vs 0%). The effect of IOERT on survival cannot be determined in this study as the groups of patients given IOERT or not are not directly comparable.

A randomized trial to investigate the relative merits of IOERT and chemotherapy in locally advanced primary and recurrent rectal cancer is ongoing in Scandinavia. The calculated accrual necessary to address both questions was for 200 patients, and the trial opened for accrual in early 1997.

5.2. European Results—IORT With or Without EBRT

The current philosophy in Europe is closely related to the United States concept that utilizes IORT as a segment of a multidisciplinary approach in cancer management. Either before or after surgery, a component of EBRT with or without 5-FU-based chemotherapy is always attempted, if no previous EBRT has been delivered. Maintenance 5-FU-based chemotherapy or new chemotherapeutic regimens (oxaliplatin, CPT-11) are also recommended since local relapse is often the prelude of distant disease even after thorough staging is performed. Published results from Pamplona (40) are in concordance with the experience from United States institutions.

5.2.1. PAMPLONA EXPERIENCE

In a recent update from the Pamplona series (data not previously published), 37 patients have been treated with IOERT for locally advanced recurrent colorectal carcinoma with lesions fixed to the presacral space or pelvic side walls. In this set of patients, 12 were treated with an IOERT boost alone since they had received previous EBRT for their primary disease. Of 37 patients, 25 were treated with EBRT, 11 with postoperative EBRT and 14 with preoperative chemoradiation. In the preoperative approach, carboplatin (55 mg/m^2) plus 5-FU (1 gm/m^2, maximum tolerated dose of 1.5 gm) were given as a continuous infusion for 3–5 d concurrently with the initiation and ending of the EBRT course. Current doses of EBRT are in the range of 40–50 Gy using standard techniques and fractionation schemes. Four to six weeks after EBRT, patients are restaged with CT scan (abdominopelvic and thorax) and surgery is performed if no systemic disease is found.

IOERT has been performed using a nondocking system in a nondedicated area. The methodological aspects of the Pamplona IOERT procedure have been described previously (40). IOERT doses of 10–15 Gy are used for microscopical residual disease and 15–20 Gy for macroscopic (gross) residue. The treatment area is defined mutually by the surgeon and radiation oncologist, and in most cases the presacral space is included in the IOERT field. Two or more IOERT fields may be used preferentially after pelvic exenterations with careful attention to avoid overlapping fields.

Results from the Pamplona update show local recurrence in 50% of the 34 evaluable patients. Among the three different treatment groups of IORT alone or with postoperative EBRT or preoperative EBRT plus chemotherapy, local relapse rates are almost identical at 55, 44, and 50%, respectively. The actuarial local control rate at 26 mo was increased

Table 6
Summarized European Results with IORT with or without EBRT for Locally
Recurrent Colorectal Cancer with Regard to Local Control Rates and Actuarial 3-Yr Survival

Institution	Ref. No.	No. Patients	LC[a]	Survival[b]
Pamplona	40, 55			
IOERT+EBRT		25	30%	38%
IOERT alone		12	0%	12%
France	56			
IORT + EBRT		16	61%	68%
IORT alone		30	0%	24%[c]

[a]LC: actuarial local control rates
[b]Survival: 3-year actuarial survival rates
[c]No long-term survivors beyond 42 months

in patients treated with EBRT plus IOERT vs IOERT alone at 40 vs 0% ($p = 0.03$). Residual disease after surgery seems to be another factor related to local relapse. Crude rates decreased with a smaller amount of residual disease after surgery, being 56% after incomplete resections vs 22% when microscopic residual remained after gross total resection ($p = $ ns).

Systemic failure is also considerable, showing crude rates for the three treatment groups of 45, 56, and 29%, being slightly better for those patients treated with preoperative radiotherapy. However, this could be explained as the majority of the patients treated with the preoperative sequence regularly received concomitant chemotherapy.

Long-term survival in this group is dismal, with a median survival time from initiation of treatment for patients treated with IORT alone of 15 vs 22 mo for those treated with EBRT plus IORT ($p = 0.03$). In patients treated with adjuvant EBRT, the preoperative sequence seems to have better disease survival rates than postoperative EBRT at 23 vs 10 mo, respectively ($p = 0.01$).

Toxic events related to the treatment consisted of neuropathy in 11 patients (30%); pelvic infection, 4 patients (11%); fistula, 11 patients (30%); severe hemorrhage, 3 patients (8%); and ureteral stenosis in 7 patients (19%). Although toxicity seems to be increased in this group of patients, all patients had received previous treatment.

5.2.2. FRENCH IORT GROUP

Similar findings have been observed by investigators from the French IORT group as seen in Table 6 (55). In 73 patients treated with an IORT boost, only 50 had localized pelvic relapse (36 of 50 patients had received prior EBRT). Long-term survival for the entire series is 30% at 3 yr with an actuarial local control rate of 31% at 3 yr. In the 30 patients treated with IORT alone, no long-term survivors were found after 42 mo vs 70% for the 16 patients treated with IOERT plus EBRT. Actuarial local control was 60% for EBRT plus IORT vs 0% with IORT alone.

5.2.3. SUMMARY

In view of the patterns of failure in recurrent colorectal carcinoma patients treated with IORT, additional efforts to increase the intensity of treatment strategies should be explored in order to improve disease control rates. As both local and distant failure are important events in the clinical evolution of these patients, systemic therapy should routinely be integrated into the current management of locally recurrent colorectal carcinoma. Since patients who had received previous radiation therapy with their primary disease have a worse prognosis, novel therapeutics should be considered, including reirradiation using modern radiotherapeutic techniques (EBRT with or without brachytherapy) combined with concomitant and maintenance systemic therapy to achieve both radiosensitization and to decrease distant metastases.

6. RESULTS WITH IOERT WITH OR WITHOUT EBRT IN PREVIOUSLY IRRADIATED PATIENTS

6.1. Non-IORT Salvage Results

There is very little information in the literature regarding salvage therapy for patients with locally recurrent colorectal cancer who have previously received high- or moderate-dose irradiation. Previously irradiated patients who develop local recurrence appear to have a worse prognosis than those with local recurrence following surgical resection who have not received prior irradiation. In the series of Frykholm et al. *(56)*, the 5-yr survival rate following local recurrence was 6% in patients treated initially with surgical resection alone vs 0% for previously irradiated patients. Nearly one-fourth (23%) of the previously irradiated patients died with local disease and no known distant metastases. In a randomized Swedish study *(57)* comparing preoperative radiation to surgical resection alone, 15% of irradiated patients suffered local recurrence and were treated with a variety of combinations of surgery, radiation, and chemotherapy that resulted in a median survival time of 11 compared to 15 mo for locally recurrent patients treated initially on the surgery alone arm ($p = 0.0002$). The 5-yr survival rate was 5% among previously unirradiated patients, and there were no 5-yr survivors in the previously irradiated group *(58)*.

6.2. Salvage IOERT Without EBRT, Miscellaneous United States and European Series

Because of dose-limiting peripheral nerve toxicity, palliative resection plus IOERT without additional EBRT is unlikely to result in acceptable local control in previously irradiated patients. Wallace et al. *(23)* treated five previously irradiated patients with IOERT and limited or no additional EBRT; four of five had subsequent local relapse. In the updated Pamplona series of 37 patients discussed in Subheading 5.2.1. of this chapter *(40)*, 12 previously irradiated patients received IOERT without additional EBRT. The reported local recurrence rate was 100% with 3- and 5-yr actuarial survival rates of 12 and 0%, respectively. Similar results were reported in the French analysis *(55)* in which 30 patients received IOERT alone because of prior EBRT (100% local relapse, no long-term survivors beyond 42 mo).

6.3. Salvage IOERT Without EBRT, Medical College of Ohio Series

6.3.1. METHODS

Merrick et al. reported the Medical College of Ohio (MCO, Toledo) experience with 38 patients who were treated for locally recurrent rectal cancer after prior adjuvant EBRT for the primary lesion. These patients underwent re-exploration with maximal surgical excision and IOERT in an attempt to achieve palliation and improve survival. All patients had extensive preoperative evaluations including CT scans of the abdomen and pelvis.

At the time of surgery, three patients were excluded from the study because of extensive disease outside the pelvis (*n* = 2) or absence of local recurrence on exploration (*n* = 1). The remaining 35 patients underwent surgery with IOERT. The type of surgical procedure was determined by the extent and location of the tumor and the nature of prior surgery: 16 patients had excision of a perineal mass, 10 had abdominoperineal resection, 4 pelvic exenteration, 4 sacrectomy, 2 partial vaginectomy, 1 low anterior resection, and 5 exposure only (some patients had multiple procedures). All operations were performed with the intent of complete resection, but in 15 of the 35 cases, this could not be achieved because of extensive local disease.

IOERT was delivered via a Varian Clinac 18 linear accelerator in doses ranging from 10 to 25 Gy to a variety of sites within the pelvis: 14 patients received IOERT to the sacral hollow, 9 to the lateral pelvic wall, 4 to the rectum, 3 to the prostate and bladder, 1 to the vagina, and 4 to multiple areas.

6.3.2. MCO RESULTS

Most of the 35 patients in the MCO study group tolerated the treatment well. There was one significant short-term complication: occlusion of an external iliac artery, which required surgical treatment. Long-term complications included permanent leg and back pain (2 of 9 patients with IOERT to the lateral pelvic sidewall), urinary incontinence, and persistent perineal sinus (2 patients). There were no deaths within 30 d of surgery.

The 3-yr actuarial survival rate from the time of IOERT and surgical resection of recurrence was 20%. In the group of 20 patients in whom complete resection of gross disease was achieved, the 2-yr survival rate was 45% and the 3-yr survival rate was 30%; in the 15 patients with incomplete resection, the 2-yr survival rate was only 27%. Ten of the 35 patients (29%) in this group again developed local disease. Most patients reported at least partial pain relief.

6.4. Salvage IOERT With or Without Limited EBRT, Mayo Analysis

IOERT following maximal surgical resection and selective EBRT has been utilized as attempted salvage therapy at Mayo Clinic in patients with locally recurrent colorectal cancer following previous high- or moderate-dose irradiation *(25)*. In a series of 51 previously irradiated patients who received IOERT, additional EBRT with or without chemotherapy was delivered to 37 of 51 (75%). The median EBRT dose was 25.2 Gy (range 5–50.4 Gy), and care was taken not to exceed small-bowel tolerance doses.

Survival and disease control data in the Mayo IOERT series of previously irradiated patients are presented in Table 6. The median survival was 23 mo, with 3- and 5-yr actuarial survival rates, of 28 and 12%, respectively. Subsequent local rerecurrence was noted in 18 patients (absolute rate of 35%; 3-yr actuarial, 55%) and distant metastasis in 26 patients (absolute rate of 51%; 3-yr actuarial, 71%). These results appear to be an improvement over the historically reported nearly uniform disease relapse and death reported in this group of patients.

6.4.1. PROGNOSTIC FACTORS

Because of the limited number of previously irradiated patients who have been treated with IOERT, no clear prognostic factors for survival and disease control have been identified. In the Mayo analysis *(25)* there was a nonstatistically significant trend toward improved local control and central control within the IOERT field with the use of EBRT retreatment doses ≥30 Gy.

The amount of residual disease after surgical resection may also be an important prognostic factor. Median survival in the Mayo series was 34 mo for patients with close but negative margins, 21 mo for those with microscopically positive margins, and 16 mo for those with gross residual disease *(25)*. There were no 5-yr survivors in the Mayo patients with gross residual tumor at the time of IOERT. In the MCO analysis *(58)*, similar trends were seen with an improvement in survival in the 20 patients with gross total resection vs the 15 patients with an incomplete resection (2-yr SR 45 vs 27%).

6.4.2. DISTANT RELAPSE

Although aggressive local therapy with EBRT, surgery, and IOERT may control local disease in a significant number of patients who develop local relapse in spite of adjuvant treatment, long-term survival is limited by the high rate of distant relapse despite careful clinical staging at the time of local relapse in an attempt to detect occult distant disease. In the Mayo series *(25)*, the actuarial rate of distant relapse was 71% at 3 yr. Improvements in survival will require the addition of effective systemic therapy to aggressive local therapy. Potential systemic therapies that should be explored in this group of patients might include 6 mo adjuvant 5-FU plus leucovorin, which has been shown to improve survival in high-risk colon-cancer patients following surgical resection *(59–61)* or with metastatic cancer *(63–68)* or monoclonal antibody therapy with murine 17-1a monoclonal antibodies, which have been shown to improve survival in Dukes' C colon-cancer patients in one randomized trial *(69)*.

Although distant relapse has limited the number of long-term survivors, the palliative benefits of aggressive local therapy should not be overlooked. Nearly all patients with locally recurrent rectal cancer experience severe tumor-related morbidity. Nonaggressive local therapy is largely ineffective. For instance, although EBRT may temporarily alleviate symptoms of local recurrence in 80–90% of patients, the median duration of pain relief is only 5–6 mo and the average symptom-free interval is only one-third of the patient's remaining lifespan *(70–72)*.

6.4.3. TOLERANCE ISSUES WITH RETREATMENT

Aggressive salvage therapy is often not offered to previously irradiated patients with local recurrence because of the potential for severe treatment-related morbidity. Reirradiation with EBRT can be accomplished with acceptable toxicity if small-bowel tolerance doses are not exceeded. Simulation films with small-bowel contrast must be used to determine the dose of EBRT that can be safely administered preoperatively. Mohiuddin et al. *(73)* have reported the results of preoperative reirradiation to a median dose of 36 Gy using lateral fields to exclude small bowel and reduce bladder volumes in a group of 39 previously irradiated patients with recurrent rectal cancer. Subsequent small-bowel obstruction was noted in 15% of patients, gastrointestinal fistula in 8%, and chronic severe diarrhea in 8%. In the Mayo IOERT series of previously irradiated patients *(25)*, severe complication rates were similar to those seen in previously unirradiated patients *(24)* who received EBRT plus surgery and IOERT with the exception of severe wound complications, which were observed in 20% of previously irradiated patients vs 7% of those without prior irradiation. Bowel obstruction was observed in 16% of previously irradiated patients and 20% of patients not previously irradiated.

6.5. Future Possibilities

Future studies in previously irradiated colorectal patients with advanced locally recurrent disease should focus on the addition of systemic therapies to aggressive local therapy, which includes reirradiation plus concurrent 5-FU-based chemotherapy, surgical resection, and IOERT. Further improvements in local and central disease-control rates are also necessary, and the use of tumor radiosensitizing agents and/or normal tissue radioprotectants during EBRT and IOERT should be explored.

7. RESULTS WITH IOERT OR HDR-IORT WITH OR WITHOUT EBRT— OHIO STATE EXPERIENCE

7.1. Patient Group

Nag (36) reported the OSU IORT experience with 45 patients (28 males, 17 females) ranging in age from 16 to 77 yr (mean 56.2 yr) who were treated between March, 1992 and November, 1994. All but one had recurrent colorectal cancers. Forty-four of the 45 had adenocarcinoma; one had a low-grade rectal liposarcoma. Initial presenting stage was Dukes B or C in 29 of 39 cases in which stage was reported. All but one patient, who refused surgery, had a prior curative resection, usually low anterior resection (LAR), abdominoperineal resection (APR), or hemicolectomy. Twenty-six of 45 cases had prior EBRT, mostly 45–50 Gy at 1.8-Gy fractions; one person received prior ^{125}I brachytherapy to a minimal peripheral dose of 160 Gy. Thirty-three of 42 cases received prior 5-FU-based chemotherapy.

7.2. Surgical and Irradiation Factors

The types of tumor resection at time of relapse included exenteration - 10, APR - 8, liver resection -11, retroperitoneal resection - 8, pelvic mass resection - 9, small bowel resection - 1. The sites of IORT were the liver, retroperitoneum, and presacrum. The target area to be irradiated varied from 20–96 cm^2 with IOERT and from 9–120 cm^2 for HDR-IORT.

If the target area was accessible to the IOERT applicator, a dedicated Siemens linear accelerator installed in a shielded operating room was used to deliver IOERT (in 27 patients). An intraoperative applicator of 5–11 cm in diameter (to cover the entire tumor bed plus 1–2 cm margin) was selected to deliver 6–15 MeV electrons (usually 6 or 9 MeV). A wet gauze bolus of 0.5–1.0 cm was used in 7 patients to either improve surface dose or decrease depth dose.

HDR-IORT was used in 18 patients at OSU when the tumor bed was inaccessible to the IOERT applicator. The target area in the tumor bed was measured, and an HDR-IORT applicator that adequately encompassed the target area was selected. Various sized, presterilized applicators, made of silicone, foam, or Delrin were available to fit different-sized tumor beds. The rigid Delrin applicators were used for flat surfaces. Silicone applicators, having limited flexibility, were used on gently sloping surfaces. The very flexible foam applicators were used for irregular or curved surfaces. Four to 10 (median 6) hollow plastic catheters were inserted parallel and 1 cm apart in the selected applicator. The applicator was then placed over the tumor bed and secured by gauze packing or suturing to the underlying tissues. In unusual circumstances, the catheters were individually sutured (at two sites) to the tumor bed. Adjacent normal tissues (e.g., bowel) were retracted with a retractor and/or by packing with gauze. Tissues that could not be retracted (e.g., nerves or kidneys) were shielded by pliable lead sheets whenever possible. With dummy sources in the catheters, a radiograph was obtained to verify catheter position.

Various preplanned treatment programs corresponding to each applicator and prescribed dose were available. Equal dwell times were used instead of an optimizing program, as it was thought that the higher central dose achieved with equal dwell times was an advantage. Furthermore, errors were less likely using equal dwell times. The appropriate treatment program was then retrieved from the planning computer and transferred to the treatment control panel. The catheters were connected to a mobile high-dose rate remote afterloading machine that was brought to the shielded operating room from the radiation oncology department. Then, treatments proceeded without delay since new dosimetry was not required. The actual treatment time ranged from 2.4–39.3 min (median 15.8 min) with the patient under general anesthesia.

Radiation doses delivered (at 90% isodose for IOERT or at 0.5 cm depth for HDR-IORT) varied from 10–20 Gy, depending on the volume of residual disease and whether the patient had been previously irradiated. Previously irradiated patients ($n = 26$) received an IORT dose of 10 Gy *(3)*, 15 Gy *(15)*, 17.5 Gy *(3)*, or 20 Gy *(5)*, previously unirradiated patients ($n = 19$) received intraoperative doses of 10 Gy *(15)* or 15 Gy *(4)*. Because of the rapid fall-off in dose from brachytherapy, stating doses to normal tissues was not very meaningful since these were quite variable. Eight previously unirradiated patients received postoperative EBRT, usually to 45 Gy in 25 fractions; one received 36 Gy to the periaortic region. Another 10 previously unirradiated patients did not receive the planned postoperative radiotherapy, because of either patient refusal in 3 instances or poor medical condition in 7. Three previously irradiated patients received postoperative EBRT of 30–36 Gy. Two patients were subsequently retreated with IORT for rerecurrent disease.

7.3. Results

The overall local control rate was 56%, with a mean follow-up time of 18.4 mo. Local control in the various groups is given in Table 7. The overall median survival was 20 mo, with 71, 35, and 17% actuarial survival rates at 12, 24, and 36 mo, respectively. Major morbidity occurred in 19 of 45 patients (42%) including one patient who died intraoperatively of a myocardial infarction. All patients had undergone prior abdominal surgery and an attempt at radical resection at the time of IORT, whereas 11 had received prior radiotherapy. The combination of repeat radical abdominal surgery and prior EBRT made this a high-risk group for major morbidity.

Subset analysis of local control, major morbidity, and overall survival failed to identify any statistically significant variable or subgroup by age, prior radiotherapy, intraoperative site, or whether the patient received postoperative EBRT. However, patients with microscopic residual disease after maximal resection had better local control (48%) than patients with gross residual disease (25%), approaching statistical significance ($p = 0.19$).

7.4. Future Possibilities

The experience of OSU is unique in that whereas most institutions deliver IORT (to accessible sites) using IOERT, the additional availability of HDR-IORT at OSU allows the delivery of radiation to sites (e.g., pelvic side wall, retropubic areas) that may be less accessible by IOERT. Ideally both HDR-IORT and IOERT should be available for optimal management of patients with locally recurrent colorectal cancers.

Table 7
Locally Advanced Recurrent Colorectal Cancer in Previously Irradiated Patients:
Survival and Disease Control in Mayo IOERT Series by Prognostic Factor (25)

Prognostic Factor	No. at risk	Overall Survival (%)				Local Relapse		Central Relapse		Distant Relapse	
		Median (mo.)	2 yr	3 yr	5 yr	No. (%)	Actuarial 3 yr (%)	No. (%)	Actuarial 3 yr (%)	No. (%)	Actuarial 3 yr (%)
EBRT dose											
<30 Gy	35	23	49	23	—	15 (43)	61	10 (29)	41	17 (49)	76
≥30 Gy	16	18	43	34	17	3 (19)	37	2 (13)	25	9 (56)	64
Residual											
Gross	17	16	42	21	—	4 (24)	57	3 (18)	54	8 (47)	—
≤Microscopic	34	27	52	27	17	14 (41)	57	9 (26)	36	18 (53)	65
(+) margin	21	21	40	27	—	10 (48)	65	7 (33)	43	12 (57)	62
(−) margin	13	34	73	25	25	4 (31)	45	2 (15)	24	6 (46)	69
Primary Site											
Colon	7	21	43	29	14	2 (29)	17	2 (29)	17	3 (43)	72
Rectum	44	23	49	27	11	16 (36)	63	10 (23)	41	23 (52)	71
Grade											
1,2	22	19	45	31	10	10 (45)	55	8 (36)	45	12 (55)	60
3,4	29	31	51	26	13	8 (28)	55	4 (14)	29	14 (48)	80
All Patients	51	23	48	28	12	18 (35)	55	12 (24)	36	26 (51)	71

EBRT = External beam irradiation; IOERT = intraoperative electron irradiation; mo = months; yr = year; No = number.

Table 8
Local Control With IOERT or IOHDR—OSU Experience *(36)*

	Previously Unirradiated	*Previously Irradiated*	*Total*
Overall	12/19 (63%)	13/26 (50%)	25/45 (56%)
Completed Postop EBRT	3/6 (50%)	0/2 (0%)	3/8 (37.5%)
No Postop EBRT	9/13 (69%)	13/24 (54%)	22/37 (59%)

8. FUTURE POSSIBILITIES

Encouraging trends exist in colorectal IOERT analyses with regard to improvement in local control and possibly survival of patients with locally recurrent colorectal lesions when compared to non-IOERT series, and continued evaluation of IOERT approaches seems warranted. Disease persistence or relapse within the IOERT and EBRT fields is higher, however, when the surgeon is unable to accomplish a gross total resection. In the MGH analysis of locally recurrent rectal cancer, failure within irradiation fields was excessive even with gross total resections if margins were microscopically positive. Therefore, a protracted venous infusion of 5-FU (with or without other drugs) should consistently be considered during EBRT *(33)*, and dose modifiers should be evaluated in conjunction with IOERT (sensitizers, hyperthermia, and so on). To maximize the percentage of patients who can technically receive an IORT component of treatment, it would be reasonable for large institutions to have both IOERT and HDR-IORT capability in an operating room setting, because certain technical factors can result in inability to treat with either method (inaccessible location for IOERT, residual disease >1 cm thickness for HDR-IORT).

Since the incidence of distant metastases exceeds 50% in patients with locally recurrent colorectal cancer in this and other series, 4–6 mo of systemic chemotherapy should be evaluated as the systemic component of the aggressive treatment approaches discussed in this chapter. A number of randomized trials reveal a significant advantage in tumor response rates for 5-FU plus leucovorin when compared with 5-FU alone in the treatment of advanced metastatic large-bowel cancer *(62–68)*. Improvements in median survival were observed in two trials *(64,66)* when compared with single-agent 5-FU and in a third trial when compared with 5-FU plus high-dose methotrexate *(65)*, but this has not translated into improved long-term survival beyond 2-yr. A meta-analysis of multiple 5-FU-leucovorin studies in advanced colorectal cancer demonstrated a highly significant benefit over single agent 5-FU in terms of tumor response rates, but this did not result in a discernible improvement in overall survival *(68)*. In addition, in an adjuvant colon cancer setting, 5-FU plus leucovorin has demonstrated survival advantages over a surgery alone control arm in an North Central Cancer Treatment Group (NCCTG) coordinated intergroup study *(59)* and vs MOF chemotherapy in a National Surgical Adjuvant Breast and Bowel Project (NSABP) trial *(60)*. Finally, it would be reasonable to evaluate continuous infusion 5-FU alone or combined with other agents as systemic therapy for locally recurrent colorectal cancers in view of its statistically significant impact on survival and distant metastasis in the Mayo Clinic NCCTG 86-47-51 randomized adjuvant rectal trial *(33)*.

In view of the extremely high rates of distant metastasis seen in these patients and the fact that many patients will have received adjuvant 5-FU-based chemotherapy, further 5-FU-based chemotherapy may be insufficient as the systemic modality of treatment. CPT-11 (irinotecan) is being evaluated in depth both as a single agent and in combination with other drugs *(74)*. On the basis of both laboratory and preliminary clinical data, interest exists in further evaluations of the use of antibodies as a component of treatment alone or in conjunction with chemotherapy. As previously noted, monoclonal antibody therapy with 17-1a has demonstrated survival benefits in resected node-positive colon-cancer patients similar to 5-FU leucovorin or 5-FU levamisole in one randomized European trial *(69)*. Most patients who present with recurrent colon cancer will have already received adjuvant 5-FU leucovorin or 5-FU levamisole. Those who present with local recurrence of rectal cancer after adjuvant EBRT will usually have received 5-FU-based chemotherapy both concomitant with EBRT and as maintenance therapy. In such patients, the evaluation of alternative systemic agents including antibody treatment and CPT 11 will be of importance.

REFERENCES

1. Suzuki K, Gunderson LL, Devine RM, et al. Intraoperative irradiation after palliative surgery for locally recurrent rectal cancer, *Cancer*, **75** (1995) 939–52.
2. Gunderson LL and Martenson JA. Irradiation of adenocarcinomas of the gastrointestinal tract, *Front. Radiat. Ther. Oncol.*, **22** (1988) 127–48.
3. Williams IG. Radiotherapy of carcinoma of the rectum. In Dukes C (ed.), *Cancer of the Rectum.* E&S Livingston, Edinburgh, 1960, pp. 210–219.
4. Whitely HW, Stearns MW Jr, Leaming RH, and Deddish MR. Radiation therapy in the palliative management of patients with recurrent cancer of the rectum and colon, *Surg. Clin. North. Am.*, **49** (1969) 381–7.
5. Moertel CG, Childs DS Jr, Reitemeier RJ, Colby MY, and Holbrook MA. Combined 5-fluorouracil and supervoltage radiation therapy of locally unresectable gastrointestinal cancer, *Lancet*, **2** (1969) 865–7.
6. Urdaneta-Lafee N, Kligerman MM, and Knowlton AH. Evaluation of palliative irradiation in rectal carcinoma, *Radiology*, **104** (1972) 673–7.
7. Wang CC and Schulz MD. The role of radiation therapy in the management of carcinoma of the sigmoid, rectosigmoid, and rectum, *Radiol.*, **79** (1976) 1–5.
8. Gunderson LL, Cohen AM, and Welch CW. Residual, inoperable, or recurrent colorectal cancer: surgical radiotherapy interaction, *Am. J. Surg.*, **139** (1980) 518–25.
9. O'Connell MJ, Childs DS, Moertel CG, et al. A prospective controlled evaluation of combined pelvic radiotherapy and methanol extraction residue of BCG (MER) for locally unresectable or recurrent rectal carcinoma, *Int. J. Radiat. Oncol. Biol. Phys.*, **8** (1982) 1115–1119.
10. Rominger CJ, Gelber R, and Gunderson LL. Radiation therapy alone or in combination with chemotherapy in the treatment of residual or inoperable carcinoma of the rectum and rectosigmoid or pelvic recurrence following colorectal surgery, *Am. J. Clin. Oncol.*, **8** (1985) 118–27.
11. Hindo WA, Soleimani PK, Miller WA, and Henrickson FR. Patterns of recurrent and metastatic carcinoma of colon and rectum treated with radiation, *Dis. Colon. Rectum.*, **15** (1972) 436–40.
12. Rao AR, Kagan AR, Chan PY, Gilbert HA, and Nussbaum H. Effectiveness of local radiotherapy in colorectal carcinoma, Cancer, **42** (1978) 1082–1086.
13. Overgaard M, Overgaard J, and Sell A. Dose-response relationship for radiation therapy of recurrent, residual and primary inoperable colorectal cancer, *Radiother. Oncol.*, **1** (1984) 217–225.
14. Lybert MLM, Martijn H, DeNeve W, Cronmelin MA, and Ribot JG. Radiotherapy for locoregional relapses of rectal carcinoma after initial radical surgery: definite but limited influence of relapse free survival and survival, *Int. J. Radiat. Oncol. Biol. Phys.*, **24** (1992) 241–246.
15. Guiney MJ, Smith JG, Worotniuk V, Ngan S, and Blakey D. Radiotherapy treatment for isolated locoregional recurrence of rectosigmoid cancer following definitive surgery: Peter MacCullum Cancer Institute Experience, 1981–1990, *Int. J. Radiat. Oncol. Biol. Phys.*, **38** (1997) 1019–1025.

16. Gunderson LL, Cohen AM, Dosoretz DE, et al. Residual, unresectable, or recurrent colorectal cancer: external beam irradiation and intraoperative electron beam boost ± resection, *Int. J. Radiat. Oncol. Biol. Phys.,* **9** (1983) 1597–1606.

17. Gunderson LL, Tepper JE, Biggs PJ, et al. Intraoperative ± external beam irradiation, *Current Problems in Cancer,* **7** (1983) 1–69.

18. Gunderson LL, Martin JK, Earle JD, et al. Intraoperative and external beam irradiation ± resection: Mayo pilot experience, *Mayo Clinic Proc.,* **59** (1984) 691–699.

19. Gunderson LL, Martin JK, Beart RW, et al. External beam and intraoperative electron irradiation for locally advanced colorectal cancer, *Ann. Surg.,* **207** (1988) 52–60.

20. Tepper JE, Cohen A, and Wood WC. Treatment of locally advanced rectal cancer with external beam irradiation, surgical resection and intraoperative irradiation, *Int. J. Radiat. Oncol. Biol. Phys.,* **16** (1989) 1437–1444.

21. Willett CG, Shellito PC, Tepper JE, Eliseo R, Convery K, and Wood WC. Intraoperative electron beam radiation therapy for recurrent locally advanced rectal and rectosigmoid carcinoma, *Cancer,* **67** (1991) 1504–1508.

22. Gunderson LL and Dozois RR. Intraoperative irradiation for locally advanced colorectal carcinomas, *Perspect. Colorectal. Surg.,* **5** (1992) 1–23.

23. Wallace HJ, Willett CG, Shellito PC, Coen JJ, and Hoover HC. Intraoperative radiation therapy for locally advanced recurrent rectal or rectosigmoid cancer, *J. Surg. Oncol.,* **60** (1995) 122–7.

24. Gunderson LL, Nelson H, Martenson JA, et al. Intraoperative electron and external beam irradiation with or without 5-Fluorouracil and maximum surgical resection for previously unirradiated locally recurrent colorectal cancer, *Dis. Colon. Rectum.,* **39** (1996) 1379–1395.

25. Haddock MG, Gunderson LL, Nelson H, et al. Intraoperative irradiation for locally recurrent colorectal cancer in previously irradiated patients, *Int. J. Radiat. Oncol. Biol. Phys.,* in press.

26. Gunderson LL and Martenson JA. Gastrointestinal tract radiation tolerance, *Front. Radiat. Ther. Oncol.,* **23** (1989) 277–98.

27. Gunderson LL, Russell AH, Llewellyn HT, Doppke KP, and Tepper J. Treatment planning for colorectal cancer: radiation and surgical techniques and value of small bowel films, *Int. J. Radiat. Oncol. Biol. Phys.,* **11** (1985) 1379–93.

28. Green N, Ira G, and Smith WR. Measures to minimize small intestine injury in the irradiated pelvis, *Cancer,* **35** (1975) 1633–1640.

29. Gallagher MJ, Brereton HD, Rostock RA, et al. A prospective study of treatment techniques to minimize the volume of pelvic small bowel with reduction of acute and late side effects associated with pelvic irradiation, *Int. J. Radiat. Oncol. Biol. Phys.,* **12** (1986) 1565–1573.

30. Gastrointestinal Tumor Study Group. Prolongation of the disease-free interval in surgically resected rectal cancer, *N. Engl. J. Med.,* **312** (1985) 1465–1472.

31. Gastrointestinal Tumor Study Group. Survival after postoperative combination treatment of rectal cancer, *N. Engl. J. Med.,* **315** (1986) 1294–1295.

32. Krook JE, Moertel CG, Gunderson LL, et al. Effective surgical adjuvant therapy for high risk rectal carcinoma, *N. Engl. J. Med.,* **324** (1991) 709–715.

33. O'Connell MJ, Martenson JA, Wieand HS, et al. Improving adjuvant therapy for rectal cancer by combining protracted infusion fluorouracil with radiation therapy after curative surgery, *N. Engl. J. Med.,* **331** (1994) 502–507.

34. Moertel CG, Gunderson LL, Mailliard JA, et al. Early evaluation of combined 5-FU and leucovorin as a radiation enhancer for locally resectable, residual, or recurrent gastrointestinal cancer, *J. Clin. Oncol.,* **12** (1994) 21–27.

35. Duttenhaver JD, Hoskins RB, Gunderson LL, and Tepper JE. Adjuvant postoperative radiation therapy in cancer of the colon, *Cancer,* **57** (1986) 955–63.

36. Nag S, Mills J, Martin E, Bauer C, and Grecula J. IORT using high dose rate brachytherapy or electron beam for colorectal carcinoma. In Vaeth JM (ed.), *Intraoperative Radiation Therapy in the Treatment of Cancer, Frontiers. Radiat. Ther. Oncol.,* **31** (1997) 238–42.

37. Willett CG, Shellito PC, Tepper JE, Eliseo R, Convery K, and Wood WC. Intraoperative electron beam radiation therapy for primary locally advanced rectal and rectosigmoid carcinoma, *J. Clin. Oncol.,* **9** (1991) 843–9.

38. Kramer T, Share R, Kiel K, and Rosman D. Intraoperative radiation therapy of colorectal cancer. In: Abe M, ed. Intraoperative radiation therapy. New York: Pergamon Press 308–10, 1991.

39. Lanciano R, Calkins A, Wolkov H, et al. A phase I, II study of intraoperative radiotherapy in advanced unresectable or recurrent carcinoma of the rectum: a RTOG study. In: Abe M, ed. Intraoperative radiation therapy. New York: Pergamon Press 311–3, 1991.

40. Abuchaibe O, Calvo FA, Azinovic I, Aristu J, Pardo F, and Alvarez-Cienfuegos J. Intraoperative radiotherapy in locally advanced recurrent colorectal cancer, *Int. J. Radiol. Oncol. Biol. Phys.,* **26** (1993) 859–67.

41. Tepper JE, Gunderson LL, Orlow E, et al. Complications of intraoperative radiation therapy, *Int. J. Radiat. Oncol. Biol. Phys.,* **10** (1984) 1831–1839.

42. Shaw EG, Gunderson LL, Martin JK, Beart BW, Nagorney DM, and Podratz KC. Peripheral nerve and ureteral tolerance to intraoperative radiation therapy: clinical and dose response analysis, *Radiother. Oncol.,* **18** (1990) 247–55.

43. Sindelar WF, Tepper J, Travis EL, and Terrill R. Tolerance of retroperitoneal structures to intraoperative irradiation, *Ann. Surg.,* **196** (1982) 601–608.

44. Sindelar WF, Kinsella T, Tepper J, Travis EL, Rosenberg SA, and Glatstein E. Experimental and clinical studies with intraoperative radiotherapy, *Surg. Gyn. Obstet.,* **157** (1983) 205–219.

45. Kinsella TJ, Sindelar WF, Deluca AM, et al. Tolerance of the canine bladder to intraoperative radiation therapy: an experimental study, *Int. J. Radiat. Oncol. Biol. Phys.,* **14** (1988) 939–946.

46. Gillette SL, Gillette EL, Power BE, Park RD, and Winthrow SJ. Ureteral injury following experimental intraoperative irradiation, *Int. J. Radiat. Oncol. Biol. Phys.,* **17** (1989) 791–798.

47. Gillette SM, Gillette EL, Vujaskovic Z, Larva SM, and Park RD. Influence of volume on intraoperatively irradiated canine ureters, *[abstr] Hepato Gastroenterol.,* **41** (1994) 28.

48. Kinsella TJ, Sindelar WF, DeLuca AM, et al. Tolerance of peripheral nerve to intraoperative radiotherapy (IORT): clinical and experimental studies, *Int. J. Radiat. Oncol. Biol. Phys.,* **11** (1985) 1579–1585.

49. Kinsella TJ, DeLuca AM, Barnes M, Anderson W, Terrill R, and Sindelar WF. Threshold dose for peripheral neuropathy following intraoperative radiotherapy (IORT) in a large animal model, *Int. J. Radiat. Oncol. Biol. Phys.,* **20** (1991) 697–701.

50. Le Couteur RA, Gillette EL, Powers EL, Child G, McChesney SL, and Ingram JT. Peripheral neuropathies following experimental intraoperative radiation therapy (IORT), *Int. J. Radiat. Oncol. Biol. Phys.,* **17** (1989) 583–590.

51. Gunderson LL, Nelson H, Martenson JA, et al. Locally advanced primary colorectal cancer: intraoperative electron and external beam irradiation ±5-FU, *Int. J. Radiat. Oncol. Biol. Phys.,* **37** (1997) 601–614.

52. Halberg FE, Cosmatis D, Gunderson LL, et al. RTOG phase I study to evaluate intraoperative radiation therapy and the hypoxic cell sensitizer etanidozole in locally advanced malignancies, *Int. J. Radiat. Oncol. Biol. Phys.,* **28** (1994) 201–206.

53. Peterson IA, Herman RC, Bourland JD, Silbert PL, Dahl RA, and Gunderson LL. Clinical and electrophysiologic changes in canines after intraoperative irradiation (IORT) and intraoperative hyperthermia (IOHT), *[abstr] Hepato. Gastroenterol.,* **41** (1994) 26.

54. Tveit KM, Wiig J, Olsen DR, Storaas A, Poulsen JP, and Giercksky KE. Combined modality treatment including IORT in locally advanced and recurrent rectal cancer: results from a prospective Norwegian study. In Vaeth JM (ed.), *Intraoperative Radiation Therapy in the Treatment of Cancer,* Karger, Basel, *Front. Radiat. Ther. Oncol.,* **31** (1997) 221–23.

55. Bussieres E, Gilly FN, Rouanet P, et al. Recurrences of rectal cancers: results of a multimodal approach with intraoperative radiation therapy, *Int. J. Radiat. Oncol. Biol. Phys.,* **34** (1996) 49–56.

56. Frykholm GJ, Pahlman L, and Glimelius B. Treatment of local recurrences of rectal carcinoma, *Radiother. Oncol.,* **34** (1995) 185–194.

57. Holm T, Cedermark B, and Rutqvist LE. Local recurrence of rectal adenocarcinoma after "curative" surgery with and without preoperative radiotherapy, *Br. J. Surg.,* **81** (1994) 452–455.

58. Merrick HW, Crucitti A, Padgett BJ, and Dobelbower RR Jr. IORT as a surgical adjuvant for pelvic recurrence of rectal cancer. In: Vaeth JM (ed.), *Intraoperative Radiation Therapy in the Treatment of Cancer, Front. Radiat. Ther. Oncol.,* Karger, Basel, **31** (1997) 234–237.

59. O'Connell MJ, Mailliard JA, Kahn MJ, Haller DG, Mayer RJ, and Wieand HS. Controlled trial of fluorouracil and low dose leucovorin given for six months as postoperative adjuvant therapy for colon cancer, *J. Clin. Oncol.,* **15** (1997) 246–250.

60. Wolmark N, Rockette H, Fisher B, et al. The benefit of leucovorin-modulated fluorouracil as postoperative adjuvant therapy for primary colon cancer: results from National Surgical Adjuvant Breast and Bowel Project protocol C-03, *J. Clin. Oncol.,* **11** (1993) 1879–87.

61. International Multicentre Pooled Analysis of Colon Cancer Trials (IMPACT) investigators: efficacy of adjuvant fluorouracil and folinic acid in colon cancer, *Lancet,* **345** (1995) 939–44.

62. Arbuck SG. Overview of clinical trials using 5-FU and Leucovorin for the treatment of colorectal cancer, *Cancer,* **63** (1989) 1036–1044.

63. Doroshow JH, Bertrand M, and Multhauf P. A prospective randomized trial comparing 5-FU vs 5-FU and high-dose folinic acid (HDFA) for treatment of advanced colorectal cancer, *[abstr] Proc. Am. Soc. Clin. Oncol.,* **6** (1987) 96.

64. Erlichman C, Fine S, Wong A, and Elhakeim T. A randomized trial of 5-fluorouracil (5-FU) and folinic acid (FA) in metastatic colorectal carcinoma, *J. Clin. Oncol.,* **6** (1988) 469–75.

65. Petrelli N, Herrera L, Rustan Y, et al. A prospective randomized trial of 5-fluorouracil vs 5-fluorouracil and high-dose Leucovorin vs 5-fluorouracil and methotrexate in previously untreated patients with advanced colorectal carcinoma, *J. Clin. Oncol.,* **5** (1987) 1559–65.

66. Poon MA, O'Connell MJ, Moertel CG, et al. Biochemical modulation of fluorouracil: evidence of significant improvement of survival and quality of life in patients with advanced colorectal carcinoma, *J. Clin. Oncol.,* **7** (1989) 1407–1418.

67. O'Connell M, Poon M, Wieand HS, Krook JE, and Gerstner J. Biochemical modulation of 5-fluorouracil (5-FU) with Leucovorin (LV): confirmatory evidence of improved therapeutic efficacy in the treatment of advanced colorectal cancer, *[abstr] Proc. Am. Soc. Clin. Oncol.,* **9** (1990) 106.

68. Advanced Colorectal Cancer Meta-Analysis Project. Modulation of fluorouracil by leucovorin in patients with advanced colorectal cancer: evidence in terms of response rate, *J. Clin. Oncol.,* **10** (1992) 896–903.

69. Riethmuller G, Schneider-Gadicke E, Schlimok G, et al. Randomized trial of monoclonal antibody for adjuvant therapy of resected Dukes' C colorectal carcinoma, *Lancet,* **343** (1994) 1177–1183.

70. Pacini P, Cionini L, Pirtoli L, Ciatto S, Tucci E, and Sebaste L. Symptomatic recurrences of carcinoma of the rectum and sigmoid, *Dis. Colon Rectum,* **29** (1986) 865–68.

71. Schnabel T, Zamboglou N, Kuhn FP, Kolotos C, and Schmitt G. Intra-arterial 5-FU infusion and simultaneous radiotherapy as palliative treatment of recurrent rectal cancer, *Strahlenther. Onkol.,* **168** (1992) 584–587.

72. Dobrowsky W. Mitomycin-C, 5-fluorouracil and radiation in advanced, locally recurrent rectal cancer, *Br. J. Radiol.,* **65** (1992) 143–147.

73. Mohiuddin M, Marks GM, Lingareddy V, and Marks J. Curative surgical resection following reirradiation for recurrent rectal cancer, *Int. J. Radiat. Oncol. Biol. Phys.,* **39** (1997) 643–649.

74. Pitot HC, Wender DB, O'Connell MJ, et al. Phase 2 trial of irinotecan in patients with metastatic colorectal carcinoma, *J. Clin. Oncol.,* **15** (1997) 2910–2919.

16 HDR-IORT for Colorectal Cancer
Clinical Experience

Louis B. Harrison, Bruce D. Minsky, Carol White,
Alfred M. Cohen, and Warren E. Enker

CONTENTS

1. INTRODUCTION

The clinical experience with high dose rate intraoperative radiation therapy (HDR-IORT) at Memorial Sloan Kettering Cancer Center (MSKCC) for primary unresectable, or locally recurrent colorectal cancer has been previously published in preliminary form *(1,2)*, and has recently been updated *(3,4)*. The updated IORT data will be presented in this chapter (*see* Chapters 14 and 15 for expanded discussion of the natural history in non-IORT patients).

2. PATIENT AND TREATMENT FACTORS

2.1. Patient Group

Between November, 1992 and December, 1996, a total of 112 patients with colorectal cancer were explored in the dedicated HDR-IORT operating room (OR) at MSKCC. Sixty-eight patients were treated with HDR-IORT. All but two of the patients not treated had either unresectable or metastatic disease at exploration. Two patients with minimal resectable disease at surgery were not treated because it was not felt to be indicated: There were 38 males and 30 females with ages ranging from 30–80 yr (median 61). There were 22 patients with primary unresectable disease and 46 who presented with locally recurrent disease. Of the latter 46, 42 are evaluable, and 4 are too recent to report *(6,7)*. There were 64 patients with adenocarcinoma and 4 with squamous-cell cancer. Follow-up time ranged from 1–48 mo, with a median of 17.5 mo.

From: *Current Clinical Oncology: Intraoperative Irradiation: Techniques and Results*
Edited by: L. L. Gunderson et al. © Humana Press, Inc., Totowa, NJ

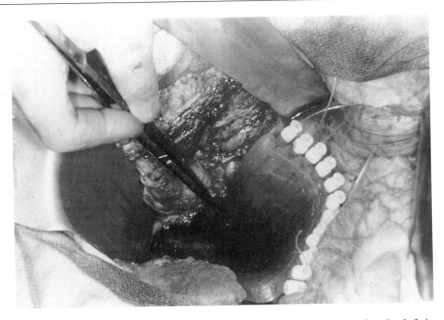

Fig. 1. Harrison-Anderson-Mick (HAM) applicator on a pelvic surface. On the left is a large retractor displacing the bladder anteriorly. The applicator is sitting on the presacral space, and curving to cover the left (inferior of figure) and right (superior of figure) pelvic sidewalls.

2.2. Treatment Factors

An expanded discussion of technical factors for HDR-IORT is found in Chapter 6 and prior publications (1,2). Issues pertinent to the colorectal patients treated at MSKCC will be discussed in this chapter.

This series represents a heterogeneous group of patients. This is reflective of the patient population with primary unresectable and locally recurrent rectal cancer. Therefore, not every patient received the exact same therapy.

In general, patients with primary, unresectable disease received preoperative chemoirradation with concomitant 5-FU (320 mg/m^2/d days 1–5, 29–33) and leucovorin (20 mg/m^2/d days 1–5, 29–33) given during external-beam irradiation (EBRT). Patients received 45 Gy to the whole pelvis, followed by a boost of 5.4 Gy to the primary tumor (total 50.4 Gy) encompassing days 1–38. This regimen has been previously reported (5). Four to six weeks later, the patients underwent surgery and HDR-IORT (10–20 Gy).

Many patients with locally recurrent disease had received prior irradiation. For such patients, further EBRT was not utilized. These patients underwent surgery plus intraoperative irradiation (IORT) alone (10–20 Gy) with the dose prescribed at 5 mm from the surface of the applicator (Figs. 1, 2). There were 13 patients with recurrent disease who had not been previously treated with radiotherapy. They were managed with preoperative combined-modality therapy as described for the primary unresectable group (5). Table 1 outlines the approaches that were used.

Table 2 shows the operative procedures that were performed on each of these patients. Table 3 reveals the summary of the procedure parameters, including procedure times, blood loss, hospital stay, and HDR-IORT dose.

HDR-IORT doses were calculated at a depth of 5 mm in tissue, or 1 cm from the sources in the applicator. The median IORT dose was 12 Gy (range 10–20 Gy). Because

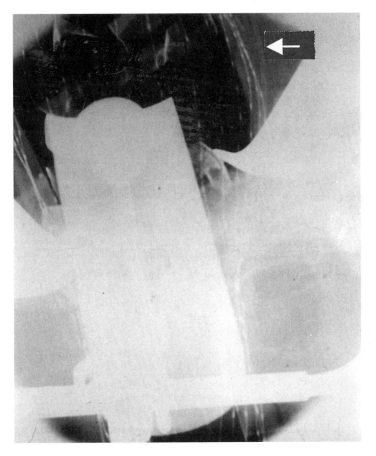

Fig. 2. This is an AP view of the pelvis with dummy wire in the HAM applicator. A large retractor is seen. On the lateral aspects of the pelvis, as the applicator curves anteriorly, the channels appear superimposed. The arrow shows the stent in the ureter, which is displaced from the applicator as much as possible.

of the dose distribution *(1,2)*, there is actually dose escalation within the target area of up to 50%, without dose enhancement to the displaced normal tissue. Thus, the prescribed dose is really a tumor minimum dose. This is clearly different than the doses delivered with electron beam that have only a 10% dose inhomogeneity within the target volume (*see* Chapter 3).

3. CLINICAL RESULTS

3.1. Disease Control and Survival

In primary unresectable cases, the actuarial 2-yr local control rate was 81%. However, margin status was an important factor in the achievement of local control. For patients with negative margins, local control was 92 vs 38% for those with grossly positive margins ($p = 0.002$). Table 4 shows the local control rates by disease presentation and margin status. For locally recurrent disease patients, the 2-yr actuarial local control is 63%. Again, margin status was an important factor. For those with negative margins, local control was 82 vs 19% for those with positive margins ($p = 0.02$). Table 4 shows the local control rates by disease presentation and margin status.

Table 1
Treatment by Disease Presentation, Summary of Management Strategies

Treatment	Primary	Recurrent	Total
Preoperative Chemo/EBRT/Surgery/HDR-IORT	18	13	31
Preoperative EBRT/Surgery/ HDR-IORT	2	3	5
Surgery/HDR-IORT/Chemo	—	1	1
Surgery/HDR-IORT	2	25	27
TOTAL	22	42	64

Chemo = chemotherapy; EBRT = external beam irradiation; HDR-IORT = high-dose-rate brachytherapy.

Table 2
HDR-IORT for Colorectal Cancer:
Operative Procedures Performed at Time of IORT

28 abdominoperineal resection
8 low anterior resection, no colostomy
8 low anterior resection, temporary colostomy
5 resection of pelvic mass
2 low anterior resection with ileostomy
14 pelvic exenteration
3 abdominoperineal resection with subtotal resection

Table 3
HDR-IORT for Colorectal Cancer: Procedure Information

Parameter	Median	Range
Hospital stay	11 days	6–39
Blood loss	1400 cc	200–8500
Anesthesia time	510 min	310–920
OR time	550 min	310–920
Surgical time	490 min	271–870
IORT procedure time	76 min	35–170
IORT delivery time	33.5 min	9–85
IORT dose	12 Gy	10–20

Table 4 also shows the overall disease-free survival rates for both primary unresectable and locally recurrent disease patients as well as these data as a function of the margins of resection. The 2-yr actuarial disease-free survival was 77 vs 38% for negative- vs positive-margin patients ($p = 0.03$) in the primary unresectable cohort. For the locally recurrent disease group, the 2-yr disease-free survival was 71 vs 0% for negative- vs positive-margin patients ($p = 0.04$). These data concerning both survival and local recurrence highlight the importance of resection margins to overall outcome.

The overall survival at 2 yr was 69% for the primary unresectable group, and 47% for the locally recurrent disease group. Whereas the data are early, it is interesting to note the uniformly excellent short-term outcomes for patients with locally recurrent disease who were able to undergo preoperative combined-modality therapy. Table 5 shows outcome

Table 4
HDR-IORT for Colorectal Cancer: Results by Disease Presentation and Margin Status

2 Year Actuarial Data	No. of Patients	Local Control	P Value	DF Survival	P Value
Primary Unresectable	22	81%		69%	
Margin negative	18	92%		77%	
Margin positive	4	38%	.002	38%	.03
Locally Recurrent	42	63%		47%	
Margin negative	26	82%		71%	
Margin positive	16	19%	.02	0%	.04

DF = disease free.

Table 5
HDR-IORT for Colorectal Cancer: Results by Treatment
(Recurrent n = 42)

Data at 2 yr	Chemo n=1	Chemo/EBRT n=13	EBRT n=3	IORT alone n=25
Local Control	1/1 (100%)	13/13 (100%)	2/3 (66%)	16/25 (64%)
Actuarial	100%	100%	0%	51%
Distant Control	1/1 (100%)	13/13 (100%)	2/3 (66%)	14/25 (56%)
Actuarial	100%	100%	50%	52%
DFS	1/1 (100%)	13/13 (100%)	1/3 (33%)	10/25 (40%)
Actuarial	100%	100%	0%	31%

DFS = disease-free survival; Chemo = chemotherapy; EBRT = external beam irradiation; IORT = intraoperative irradiation.

as a function of the treatment program for patients with recurrent disease. All 13 patients in the chemoirradiation group have remained disease free to date. The follow-up is short, however, and more time is needed to manifest the pattern of failure.

3.2. Tolerance

Table 6 reveals the prospectively recorded complications that are all grouped together. These are complex procedures that require extensive resections in a heavily treated patient population. Many patients are also heavily pretreated, and have had extensive prior operations and irradiation. It is often impossible and unfair to characterize a particular complication as a surgical or radiotherapeutic complication. Rather, it is more accurate to consider these events as multifactorial and multidisciplinary, and they are presented as combined morbidity.

4. CONCLUSIONS AND FUTURE DIRECTIONS

The MSKCC group is not the only one investigating HDR-IORT. Simultaneous with the MSKCC development of this procedure, investigators in Germany (6) have also had an interest in this concept, and Ohio State results with either IOERT or HDR-IORT for colorectal cancer (7) are reported in Chapter 15. Huber (6) reported 38 patients treated with HDR-IORT as part of an overall management strategy for T3 (19 patients) and T4

Table 6
Surgery plus HDR-IORT for Colorectal Cancer:
Complications (Grade 3 and higher)

Wound complications	10
Postoperative infection/sepsis	4
Bleeding	4
Neurogenic bladder dysfunction	2
Hydronephrosis	2
Fistula	1
Pain (postop)	3
Compartment syndrome/foot drop	1
Sexual dysfunction	1
Small bowel obstruction or ischemia	2

Note: 26 of 68 patients or 38% had ≥ grade 3 intolerance (some had more than 1 of the above complications).

(19 patients) rectal cancers. The T3 lesions underwent surgery, HDR-IORT (15 Gy) plus postoperative radiation/chemotherapy. The T4 patients received preoperative radiation/chemotherapy followed by resection and IORT (15 Gy). Local recurrence developed in 16% of the T3 group, and 11% of the T4 group, with median follow-up of 25 mo. Total complications, however, were 84%, which was excessive.

In conclusion, the MSKCC approach has shown itself to be feasible, versatile, and consistent with other data using electron beam IORT *(8–16)*. This approach may have certain technical, dosimetric, and logistic advantages, and may offer a cost-effective approach to the majority of world centers that cannot afford IORT with a linear accelerator-based electron program. Whereas this arrangement has worked well at MSKCC, it would have been wiser to have this dedicated OR as part of the main OR facility. This would have allowed more efficient utilization of staff, instruments, and a proximity to the recovery room and the surgical intensive care unit. Groups looking to develop such a facility may wish to weigh the relative merits of the location of the OR, and make the decision based upon the logistics that will work best for their particular program.

Future directions for patients with colorectal cancer should include consideration of further dose escalation for patients with positive margins, and a more uniform strategy of systemic adjuvant therapy. The ultimate goal is to improve both disease control (local and distant) and survival.

REFERENCES

1. Harrison LB, Enker WE, and Anderson L. High dose rate intraoperative radiation therapy for colorectal cancer—Part 1, *Oncology,* **9** (1995) 679–683.
2. Harrison LB, Enker WE, and Anderson L. High dose rate intraoperative radiation therapy for colorectal cancer—Part 2, *Oncology,* **9** (1995) 737–741.
3. Harrison LB, Minsky B, Enker W, et al. High dose rate intraoperative radiation therapy (HDR-IORT) as part of the management strategy for locally advanced primary and recurrent rectal cancer, 1997 ASTRO Abstracts. *Int. J. Radiat. Biol. Phys.,* **39(S)** (1997) 168.
4. Harrison LB, Minsky B, Enker W, et al. High dose rate intraoperative radiation therapy (HDR-IORT) as part of the management strategy for locally advanced primary and recurrent rectal cancer, *Int. J. Radiat. Biol. Phys.,* **42** (1998) 325–330.

5. Grann A, Minsky B, Cohen A, et al. Preliminary results of preoperative 5-fluorouracil low dose leucovorin, and concurrent radiation therapy for clinically resectable T3 rectal cancer, *Dis. Colon Rectum,* **40** (1997) 515–522.
6. Huber FT, Stepan R, Zimmerman F, Fink V, Molls M, and Siewert JR. Locally advanced rectal cancer: resection and intraoperative radiotherapy using the flab method combined with preoperative or postoperative radiochemotherapy, *Dis. Colon Rectum,* **39** (1996) 774–779.
7. Nag S, Mills J, Martin E, Bauer C, and Grecula J. Intraoperative radiation therapy using high dose rate bradytherapy (IOHDR) or electron beam (IOEBRT) for colorectal carcinoma, *Front. Radiat. Ther. Oncol.,* **31** (1997) 238–242.
8. Gunderson LL, Cohen AC, Dosoretz DD, et al. Residual, unresectable, or recurrent colorectal cancer. External beam irradiation and intraoperative electron beam boost ± resection, *Int. J. Radiat. Oncol. Biol. Phys.,* **9** (1983) 1597–1606.
9. Tepper JE, Cohen AM, Wood WC, Hedberg SE, and Orlow E. Intraoperative electron beam radiotherapy in the treatment of unresectable rectal cancer, *Arch. Surg.,* **121** (1986) 421–423.
10. Tepper JE, Wood WC, and Cohen AM. Treatment of locally advanced rectal cancer with external beam radiation, surgical resection, and intraoperative radiation therapy, *Int. J. Radiat. Oncol. Biol. Phys.,* **16** (1988) 1437–1444.
11. Gunderson LL, Martin JK, Beart RW, et al. Intraoperative and external beam irradiation for locally advanced colorectal cancer, *Ann. Surg.,* **207** (1988) 52–60.
12. Gunderson LL and Dozois RR. Intraoperative irradiation for locally advanced colorectal carcinomas. *Persp. Colon Rectal Surg.,* **5** (1992) 1–24.
13. Willett C, Shellito PC, Tepper JE, et al. Interoperative electron beam radiation therapy for primary advanced rectal and rectosigmoid carcinoma, *J. Clin. Oncol.,* **9** (1991) 843–849.
14. Wallace HJ, Willett CG, Shellito PC, et al. Intraoperative radiation therapy for locally advanced recurrent rectal or rectosigmoid cancer, *J. Surg. Onc.,* **60** (1995) 122–127.
15. Gunderson LL, Nelson H, Martenson J, et al. Locally advanced primary colorectal cancer—intraoperative electron and external beam irradiation ± 5-FU, *Int. J. Radiat. Oncol. Biol. Phys.,* **37** (1997) 601–614.
16. Gunderson LL, Nelson H, Martenson J, et al. Intraoperative electron and external beam irradiation ± 5-FU and maximal surgical resection for previously unirradiated locally recurrent colorectal cancer, *Dis. Colon Rectum,* **39** (1996) 1379–1395.

17 Radiation Ablation of Liver Metastases
HDR-IORT With or Without EBRT

Catherine L. Salem and Anatoly Dritschilo

CONTENTS

1. LIVER METASTASES

1.1. The Magnitude of the Problem

Caring for oncology patients has taught physicians much about the strength of the human spirit. Hope bounds eternal for most patients. However, when a diagnosis of liver metastases is shared with patients, it comes as a universally crushing blow. Even those with AIDS-associated malignancies will inquire about their liver status with great trepidation. Further, patients with some of the most aggressive malignancies remain hopeful noting, "Well, at least it hasn't spread to my liver." This indicates that most members of the lay public recognize the grave prognosis of liver metastases.

The presence of liver metastases almost always indicates widespread dissemination that may or may not be detectable. The liver can be involved with metastatic disease from cancer arising in nearly every site in the body. Patients with liver metastases generally belong to one of three prognostic groups: those with colorectal primaries, those with non-gastrointestinal (GI) or upper GI (gastric or pancreas) primaries, and those with neuroendocrine primaries *(1)*. Those with neuroendocrine tumors have a very favorable prognosis, and those with non-GI or upper GI tumor primaries have a very unfavorable prognosis. Most interesting have been patients with colorectal cancers, in whom resection for liver metastases results in impressive survival rates in properly selected patients.

Nearly 131,000 newly diagnosed cases of colorectal cancer in the United States annually result in nearly 55,000 deaths *(2)*. Further, 15–25% of these patients present with liver metastases and another 20–30% develop liver metastases during the course of their illness. For many, the liver lesions will be the cause of death *(1,3,4)*, because surgical resection beneficially affects only 5% of these patients *(5,6)*. Even patients who make it to the operating table for resection of liver metastases can undergo the procedure only

From: *Current Clinical Oncology: Intraoperative Irradiation: Techniques and Results*
Edited by: L. L. Gunderson et al. © Humana Press, Inc., Totowa, NJ

30% of the time, with 31% having unresectable disease confined to the liver, and the remainder having extrahepatic disease *(7)*. This group of patients with unresectable disease confined to the liver at laparotomy has engendered interest from those researching other local modalities of treatment.

1.2. Natural History of Untreated Liver Metastases

Prior to reviewing the results of various therapies it is constructive to review the natural history of colorectal metastases. A prospective study examining prognostic factors in 484 untreated patients provides us with much more insight than the wide range of 3–24 mo, which is commonly reported as median survival time *(1)*. By multivariate analysis, the percentage of the liver replaced by tumor is the most important factor, followed by grade of the primary tumor, presence of extrahepatic disease, mesenteric node involvement, CEA (carcinoembryonic antigen) level, and age *(8)*. Patients with ≤25% of liver volume replaced by tumor, a low-grade primary lesion, no extrahepatic tumor, and no mesenteric nodal involvement do best, with a median survival of 21.3 vs 5.5 mo in those with high-grade primaries, extrahepatic tumor, and nodal metastases, respectively *(8)*. In contrast, for those with more than 25% of the liver replaced by tumor, the prognostic factors described hold less significance. For the entire group of untreated patients less than 1% will survive 5 yr. This information illustrates the power of selection biases and allows a clinician to better determine the effects of a treatment modality on a selected group of patients.

1.3. Surgical Resection

1.3.1. ELIGIBILITY CRITERIA

Resection of metastatic liver disease from colon or rectal carcinoma is an accepted oncologic practice, because surgical resection is the only modality to date that offers patients a chance for 5-yr survival. However, eligibility criteria remain somewhat ill defined. Most surgeons agree that the procedure is indicated only when the liver metastases are completely resectable *(9)*, and is contraindicated when the primary tumor cannot be controlled *(10)*, or in the presence of more than four liver metastases *(3,10,11)*, or extrahepatic metastases, including nodal disease in the porta hepatis *(3,10,12,13)*. In addition, it is not recommended in patients with poor underlying liver function (e.g., hepatitis or cirrhosis) *(1,11)*. Some suggest that the procedure be undertaken with precaution in those with bilobar metastases and those requiring a trisegmentectomy *(10)*, although a prospective randomized study suggests that in a physiologically healthy liver 50–80% of the organ can be removed successfully *(13)*. Many additional prognostic factors have emerged including the primary stage of the tumor, margins of resection, and preoperative CEA level. The importance of disease-free interval has been controversial *(9)*. Still, selection of patients for attempted resection remains rather subjective.

1.3.2. RESULTS

Surgical resection of colorectal liver metastases improves overall and disease-free survival (DFS) with reported 5-yr survivals ranging from 23–40% *(1)*. Table 1 summarizes results with surgical resection. In a review of 800 patients with resected colorectal liver metastases, the overall 5-yr survival was 32% with a 5-yr disease-free survival of 24% *(9)*. The Gastrointestinal Tumor Study Group has shown a doubling of median survival time in those patients for whom resection was completed *(13)*. In a large series

Table 1
Hepatic Resection of Metastatic Colorectal Cancer

Author	No. Patients	Surgical Mortality	5-yr survival	5-yr DFS
Adson (6)	141	2%	25%	—
Hughes (9)	800	—	32%	24%
Lise (4)	39	5%	32%	27%
Nordlinger (5)	1568	2.3%	28%	15%

from France *(5)*, 568 patients underwent resection of liver disease with actuarial survival rates of 88, 64, and 28% at 1, 2, and 5 yr. At 5 yr, the actuarial DFS rate was 15%. Poor prognostic factors include extension of the primary into the serosa, lymphatic spread of the primary, time interval from primary tumor to metastases of less than 2 yr, four or more liver metastases, less than 1 cm margins of resection, and preoperative CEA levels of greater than 30 ug/L. Survival rates at 2 yr vary from 76% in those with 0–2 risk factors to 44% with 5–7 risk factors *(5)*. This information provides a basis for selecting appropriate patients for resection. Mortality rates are less than 3% with significant complications in approx 20%.

1.4. Chemotherapy— IV and Hepatic Arterial Infusion

1.4.1. RATIONALE

Most patients with metastatic colon cancer eventually develop extrahepatic disease, making a systemic chemotherapeutic approach logical as the only treatment or at least as a treatment component. For those with liver-only metastases, treatment with systemic 5-FU results in a 20–30% response rate *(1)*. The addition of leucovorin to 5-FU improves response rates to 30–44% *(1)*. Despite this, no significant survival advantage has been demonstrated, and most of those treated die of progressive disease in the liver.

Because liver metastases are fed preferentially by the hepatic artery, the concept of regional chemotherapy followed. The initial use of external pumps showed improved response rates of 34–83% in the liver, however no survival benefit was demonstrated *(1)*. Eventually, this approach was abandoned, in part because of significant complications with infection, hepatobiliary toxicity, and catheter dislodgment. In order to capitalize on the improved response rates while minimizing complications and taking advantage of diminished systemic side effects, implanted infusion pumps were used. This is less risky in many respects and more economical when four or more courses of therapy are planned *(14)*.

1.4.2. ELIGIBILITY CRITERIA

Multiple randomized trials with arterial chemotherapy delivered via implanted pumps are complete. Whereas somewhat varying criteria for eligibility were used, most patients had unresectable liver disease without evidence of extrahepatic disease. This requires an extensive metastatic evaluation. Patients admitted to these studies have minimally elevated bilirubin levels and a performance status of >70% on the Karnofsky scale *(15)*. Pump placement requires liver arteriogram and laparotomy, suitable anatomy of the arterial system, cholecystectomy, and a highly skilled surgical team *(16)*.

1.4.3. RESULTS

Response rates of over 80% in phase II studies *(15)* and up to 62% in randomized trials *(1,14)*, have been reported. Whereas all of the prospective randomized trials show an improved response rate over systemic chemotherapy, a modest but significant median survival advantage is demonstrated in only two larger studies *(17)*. Furthermore, extra-hepatic progression of disease and toxicity remain drawbacks to the approach. Nonrandomized, single institution trials administering systemic chemotherapy plus intrahepatic chemotherapy show no convincing improvements in survival. To diminish toxicity, many investigators have combined intra-arterial steroids with chemotherapy, and have incorporated delays in the administration of chemotherapy to diminish side effects, but again with no improvement in survival *(15)*.

1.5. External-Beam Irradiation

1.5.1. ELIGIBILITY CRITERIA

The use of external-beam irradiation (EBRT) for liver metastases has been reported. Patients generally have multiple liver metastases, and in some series distant metastases are present. This approach is plagued by the presence of a tumor that requires high doses to eradicate located within radiosensitive liver parenchyma. The accepted total dose to the whole liver with EBRT alone ranges from 21 Gy at 3 Gy per fraction to 30 Gy at 1.8 Gy per fraction *(7)*. When 5-FU-based chemotherapy is combined with EBRT, the whole liver tolerance is reduced to 24–27 Gy in 1.8-Gy fractions.

1.5.2. RESULTS

Series using whole liver EBRT alone, with rather loose acceptance criteria, show an expected median survival of 3–9 mo. A 1-yr actuarial survival of 21% was reported by Sherman *(18)*. Palliation has been achievable in over half of the patients as measured by symptom relief, liver size, and liver function studies. Whereas this approach appears worthwhile for some patients, no long-term survival is achievable by EBRT alone.

1.5.3. RESULTS WITH COMBINED EBRT AND CHEMOTHERAPY

Subsequent studies have used a combination of EBRT plus chemotherapy given systematically or intrahepatically. Although symptom relief was generally good and those with colorectal primaries seemed to fare the best, none of these studies were prospectively randomized, some included patients with distant metastases, and many used large fraction size *(18)*. The results indicate that chemotherapy plus conventional whole-liver EBRT is palliative in the traditional sense.

1.5.4. RESULTS WITH HYPERFRACTIONATION

In an RTOG hyperfractionation study, an attempt was made to capitalize on patients identified to have at least a survival of 6 mo, performance scores of 80–100, colorectal primaries, and no extrahepatic metastases *(19)*. This dose-escalating trial used 1.50 Gy bid to 27, 30, or 33 Gy delivered to the whole liver. Unfortunately the trial was closed early because two patients developed hepatitis at the 33-Gy level. There was no difference in median 4-mo survival among the groups *(20)*. Therefore, this attempt to increase the total dose of radiation delivered to the whole liver failed. A summary of results with EBRT is presented in Table 2 *(20–22)*.

Table 2
External-Beam Irradiation (EBRT) of Liver Metastases

Author	No. Patients	Technique of EBRT	Median Survival[a]
Rotman (21)	23	whole liver + 5 FU	7.5 mos
Leibel (22)	187	whole liver ± misonidazole	4.2 mos
Russell (20)	173	whole liver 1.5 Gy BID	4.2 mos

[a]No long-term survivors are reported in any of these trials.

1.5.5. RESULTS WITH THREE DIMENSIONAL CONFORMAL THERAPY

Building on the use of three-dimensional (3D) conformal therapy in primary hepato-cellular carcinoma, investigators in Michigan have used this modality in patients with unresectable colorectal liver metastases. With the combined use of intraarterial hepatic fluorodeoxyuridine and conformally planned radiotherapy, a 50% response rate was documented in 22 treated patients (23). Total doses delivered to target volumes vary from 48–72.6 Gy depending upon the percentage of normal liver that can be excluded from the high-dose volume. Radiation was delivered bid. The procedure is well tolerated with no patient with partial liver treatment developing hepatitis. The overall median survival was 20 mo; those with extrahepatic disease had a median survival of only 14 mo. As in other modalities, the liver was a primary site of failure with the actuarial freedom from hepatic progression reported as 25% at 1 yr. Investigators suggest that doses attained thus far were inadequate to control liver metastases although the sites of failure within the liver are not specified.

1.6. Rationale for HDR-IORT

The lack of success of whole-liver EBRT has led investigators to attempt to increase the dose of radiation delivered to only a portion of the liver, based on Ingold's observation that limited volumes of the liver can tolerate up to 55 Gy without serious side effects (24). The use of small boost volumes delivered by EBRT is technically limited by continued exposure to larger than necessary volumes of normal liver because of both normal respirations and deeper-seated lesions. Similarly, the use of intraoperative electron irradiation (IOERT) would be limited by technical difficulties of completely encompassing an intrahepatic lesion with an IOERT applicator placed on the surface of the liver.

Capitalizing on the benefits of brachytherapy, investigators at Georgetown University initially used percutaneous interstitial radiotherapy with or without an EBRT boost. This proved feasible (25) and the technique was adapted to the use of intraoperative high dose rate (HDR-IORT) interstitial radiotherapy for patients with hepatic metastases from colorectal carcinoma. This allows the delivery of high doses of radiation to affected portions of the liver while sparing uninvolved parenchyma. Further, tumor-eradicating doses are achievable placing this technique in the potentially curative category. This concept of using HDR-IORT radiotherapy with intention to eradicate all tumor cells in the treated region has been termed radiation ablation. This has obvious implications for nearly one third of patients referred for hepatic resection who have unresectable liver-only metastases (7). This group could potentially enjoy prolonged survival, approaching that of patients with resectable liver lesions, if tumor control is realized. Radiation ablation in this group is an intellectually attractive option that has been explored.

Table 3
HDR-IORT Treatment of Liver Metastases:
Patient Eligibility

Biopsy-proven colorectal carcinoma
Unresectable liver metastases at laparotomy
No significant extrahepatic carcinoma
30–40% of liver remains unirradiated
No age limit
No size or location of lesion limitation

2. TREATMENT FACTORS—RADIATION ABLATION

2.1. Patient Selection

At Georgetown University (26), patients are selected from the group of those with biopsy proven colorectal adenocarcinoma with hepatic involvement by computed tomography (CT) or magnetic resonance imaging (MRI). Only those patients found not suitable for resection at laparotomy go on to receive implants. A greater than 2-mo life expectancy is required. Preoperative evaluation includes a two view chest X-ray, CT, or MRI of the abdomen, hepatic arteriography (as resection was considered), liver function studies, coagulation studies, and CEA. Most have preoperative barium enema and proctosigmoidoscopy. Consent is required prior to participation in this phase I/II study. Extrahepatic disease is largely considered a contraindication to implantation, with approximately two patients ineligible for every one implanted because of unsuspected extrahepatic disease or advanced liver involvement found at laparotomy. Twenty-two patients, including 2 with minimal, isolated, and treatable extrahepatic disease, underwent 24 HDR-IORT procedures as part of this phase I/II study. Eligibility criteria are reviewed in Table 3. None of the patients received EBRT or chemotherapy as a planned component of treatment.

Whereas an unirradiated functioning liver volume of 30–40% is required, the size of an individual lesion and the number of lesions present are not otherwise limiting factors. Age has also not been a limiting factor, with 4 of 22 patients over the age of 73. At laparotomy, patients are considered to either be candidates for surgical resection or implantation with no combination of the two procedures allowable. With mobilization of the liver, location of the lesions did not preclude the procedure.

2.2. Surgical Approach to Radiation Ablation

2.2.1. OPERATING ROOM SHIELDING REQUIREMENTS

Laparotomy with consideration for radiation ablation must be done in a location with adequate shielding available. The use of a specially designed lead-lined operating suite is suggested (27). Portable shields are problematic in that they limit access to the anesthetized patient, are difficult to maneuver, provide incomplete coverage, and pose issues of sterility in the operating room (OR). Shielding criteria based upon nonoccupational exposure rates are used as adjacent ORs and hallways are not controlled with regard to access. The primary OR door must be adequately shielded as most ORs are not spacious enough to allow a maze entry. An alternative access door must be available to assure entry, and the console area must be fitted with anesthesia monitors, closed circuit TVs, and audiointercoms.

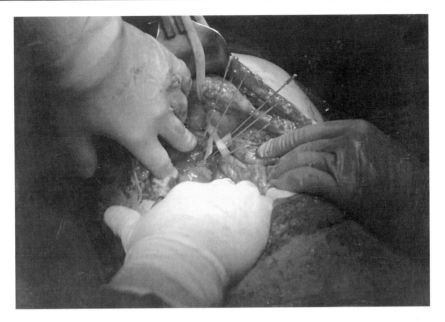

Fig. 1. Placement of applicators into a liver lesion under direct visualization.

2.2.2. MOBILIZATION OF THE LIVER

Patients taken to laparotomy undergo abdominal exploration through a long transverse-subcostal incision or vertical midline incision. If unresectable liver disease is found and the patient was otherwise eligible, the liver is mobilized by division of the lateral peritoneal and diaphragmatic attachments, and dissection of the falciform ligament. If the treated area was to include the gallbladder bed, a cholecystectomy was done to avoid possible complication with biliary fistula *(26,28)*. Retractors above and below the liver allow visualization and adequate distancing from adjacent organs *(29)*.

2.2.3. IDENTIFICATION AND DEFINITION OF THE LESIONS

The liver is carefully examined intraoperatively assessing the number, size, and location of lesions. Preoperative CT or MRI underestimates hepatic disease extent in nearly all patients *(1,26)*. If lesions can not be assessed satisfactorily by palpation, intraoperative ultrasound is used. The irradiator used at Georgetown University, in Washington, DC, is a Gamma Med II allowing remote afterloading with ^{192}Ir. Preplanning based upon CT and MRI volumes is accomplished varying the distance between implant planes, intraplane needle separation, and source location in each needle. Utilizing a catalog of plans, adjustments are made at the time of surgical assessment of treatment volume.

2.2.4. PLACEMENT OF THE NEEDLES

Applicators are closed-ended 14-gage needles with a 45° beveled-end available in lengths of 15, 20, and 25 cm. The applicators are placed under direct visualization (*see* Fig. 1). No area of the liver has proven inaccessible. The deep posterior right lobe was often approached inferiorly. The superior aspect of the left lobe underlies the pericardium directly and care must be taken to avoid needles exiting the hepatic capsule near the heart. The radiation oncologist's hand placed along the liver capsule beneath the left diaphragm assures appropriate needle placement. Up to 12 guide tubes and needle attachments may

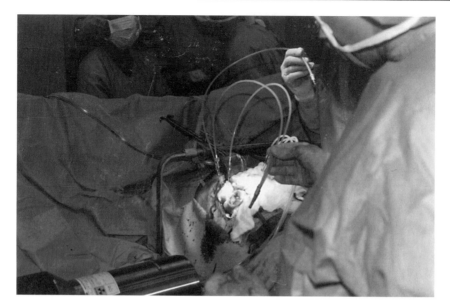

Fig. 2. Applicators are connected to the irradiator by translucent cables.

be placed simultaneously (*see* Fig. 2). Spacing between needles is usually 1–2 cm, and interplane distances of 2–3 cm are used. Along the needle, source stops are 1–2 cm. The needles are placed 0.3 cm beyond the lesions, when feasible, to account for dead space. Gauze packing displaces adjacent radiosensitive structures from the treatment volume.

2.3. Dosimetric Considerations

The patients selected for possible liver implantation are seen in consultation by the radiation oncologists prior to the scheduled surgical procedure. This allows adequate preplanning as outlined above, although some patients will go on to resection. The target volume is modified as necessary after direct tumor palpation or ultrasound evaluation. Up to 30 Gy is delivered to the tumor periphery in a single high-dose fraction. Figure 3 is an example of isodose curves superimposed upon a lesion defined by CT scan. Small volume "hot spots" within the tumor are an unavoidable reality of any brachytherapy procedure but, are minimized with the use of multiple needles and multiple source locations improving homogeneity. Of 24 procedures, dose to the tumor periphery was 20 Gy in 13, 25 Gy in 9, and 30 Gy in 2 procedures *(26)*.

3. RESULTS WITH HDR-IORT

3.1. Radiation Ablation Alone

The use of radiation ablation, or HDR-IORT treatment, for colorectal carcinoma metastatic to the liver has been reported from Georgetown University, using the methods outlined above. Since only small numbers of patients have been reported, the data should be interpreted cautiously. Extrahepatic disease was present in two patients. One had minimal periaortic adenopathy and received postoperative EBRT and one with an adrenal met underwent interstitial irradiation to that site as well.

The median number of lesions treated was 3, with a range of 1–11. In the patient with a solitary liver lesion, cirrhosis was present and precluded resection. The median size of

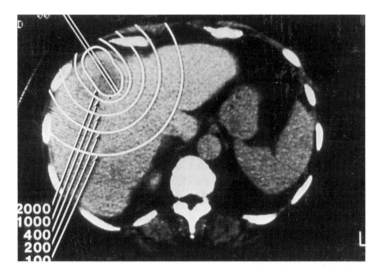

Fig. 3. Preplanned isodose distribution for a 4-cm liver lesion using three source stop positions spaced 1 cm apart.

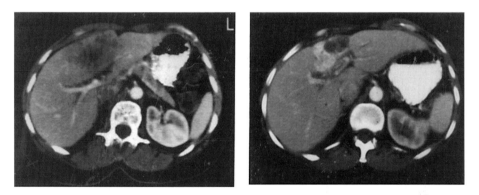

Pre–RT Ablation   **Post RT (1 year)**

Fig. 4. Pre- and postablation CT evaluation showing response of metastatic lesion.

the treated lesions was 5 cm with the largest being 13 cm. The time needed to administer the treatment varied depending upon the number and size of lesions and the strength of the source.

Side effects included bleeding, although significant blood loss requiring transfusion was uncommon. Median hospital stay was 8 d with a maximum of 23 d in a patient with cirrhosis. Two patients developed wound infection and two developed pneumonia, all responding to conservative care. No clinical or laboratory evidence of hepatitis occurred.

CT evaluation both before and after radiation ablation was accomplished showing decreased size of the lesions and improved demarcation of their borders, as revealed in Fig. 4. Biopsies following treatment were accomplished in a few cases allowing pathological confirmation of radiation ablation of liver metastases (*see* Fig. 5).

With a median follow up of 11 mo, and progression defined as a 25% increase in the product of perpendicular dimensions, actuarial local control was 75% at 6 mo and 26%

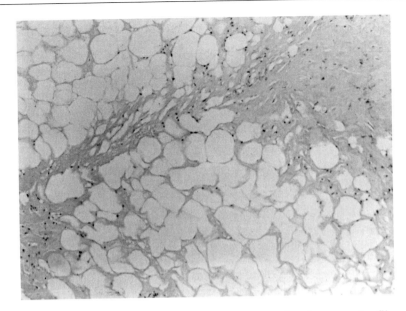

Fig. 5. Postablation biopsy of a metastatic adenocarcinoma showing capsular fibrosis and fat necrosis.

at 26 mo. The median local control was 8 mo. Median survival was 14 mo, with the longest survivor reported at 36 mo.

Even with this relatively short median follow up, 68% of patients had disease recurrence in untreated portions of the liver. Only two patients had re-exploration with biopsy of treated sites. In one no tumor was present at treated sites. In the other, two sites were negative and one was positive at the periphery, suggesting a marginal miss.

3.2. HDR-IORT and Resection

Memorial Sloan-Kettering Cancer Center has used its vast experience in permanent ^{125}I brachytherapy to develop a technique of implantation as an adjunct to surgery. Citing improved survival and local control in patients resected with negative margins as compared to those resected with positive margins (9), investigators use implantation in those in whom gross or microscopic disease was left behind after partial resection of colorectal liver metastases. When gross residual tumor remains after resection, volume implants were done with the use of the Mick applicator, delivering a median 160 Gy to the periphery. When microscopic disease remained, planar implants were done using suture containing ^{125}I seeds, delivering a median 150 Gy to the periphery.

With a total of 17 implants performed in 12 high-risk patients (30,31), the median survival was 18 mo, with 42% of patients surviving 2 yr or more, and 8% surviving 5 yr. Local relapse occurred in 42% of implants with actuarial local control of 44% at 5 yr. The pattern of failure in these patients, with 83% developing distant extrahepatic disease and 25% failing in areas of the liver remote from the site of implantation, underscores the need for more effective systemic and whole-liver treatment. The 42% absolute rate of local failure suggests a need for improved dose delivery at implanted sites as well. No cases of liver toxicity were reported which, combined with reasonable local control results, proves feasibility.

Table 4
HDR-IORT Treatment or Resection of Liver Metastases:
Potential Prognostic Factors

Percentage of liver replaced by tumor	Regional lymph-node involvement
Number and size of metastases	CEA level
Grade of the primary	Age
Stage of the primary	Performance status
Extrahepatic disease	Disease-free interval

The Sloan Kettering investigators suggest that in patients in whom liver-only metastases are not completely resectable because of proximity to vascular structures or to the extent of involved liver parenchyma, an implant should be used as an adjunct to surgery. They also suggest a possible benefit to the combination of ^{125}I implantation and ^{192}Ir implantation with regard to local control. There are no studies reporting on the combination of these techniques.

4. PROGNOSTIC FACTORS IMPACTING RESULTS

The prognostic factors determining outcome in patients undergoing implantation have not been adequately investigated primarily because of the small numbers of patients studied thus far. There is a general assumption that the factors important to the outcome of patients undergoing surgical resection of liver metastases are the same for those undergoing implantation as well. These factors have been outlined previously in this chapter, and are reviewed in Table 4. The best that could be expected for patients undergoing implantation is a survival rate of 5 yr equal to that obtained in patients with surgically resected liver metastases, but this is not currently being accomplished in this group of less highly selected patients. Future studies should investigate the prognostic importance of the percentage of liver involved with tumor, site, grade, and stage of the primary, the presence of extrahepatic disease or mesenteric nodal involvement, CEA level, age (8), underlying medical condition or Karnofsky score, number and size of liver metastases, and disease-free interval following resection of primary colorectal cancer (5). An evaluation of results based upon these presumed prognostic factors would be helpful.

5. DISCUSSION AND FUTURE CONSIDERATIONS

5.1. Role of Radiation Ablation in Liver Metastases

Radiation ablation in patients with liver metastases from colorectal adenocarcinoma, via HDR-IORT, has a potential place in the treatment of patients with no extrahepatic spread of disease, in whom liver disease cannot be resected. Thirty to 40% of healthy remaining parenchyma must remain posttreatment, similar to those undergoing resection. All patients treated with implantation, however, should be entered on prospective phase I or phase II protocols that address the high rate of both liver and distant disease relapse.

5.2. Role of HDR-IORT in Primary Liver Carcinoma

In primary cancer of the liver, the use of HDR-IORT has not yet been reported. Resection remains the only curative modality of treatment with most patients being unresectable at presentation. Even though EBRT has provided palliation, there has been little experience with alternative methods of delivering radiation. For unresectable tumors presenting in patients with adequate hepatic reserve, HDR-IORT treatment combined with tolerable doses of EBRT would be a reasonable experimental avenue to pursue *(32)*.

5.3. HDR-IORT Combined with Other Modalities

5.3.1. EBRT OR CHEMOTHERAPY

A combination of HDR-IORT and EBRT has not been intellectually attractive, primarily because the EBRT doses that can be safely delivered to the entire liver are below those needed to control microscopic disease. Perhaps this is the reason for a lack of investigation in this area. In order for this approach to become more interesting, a systemic agent allowing selective sensitization of liver metastases and/or protection of liver parenchyma would be required. A combination of HDR-IORT and chemotherapy for metastatic disease is theoretically promising but largely awaits a more effective agent. In the interim, it may be of interest to combine HDR-IORT doses of 25 Gy with fractionated whole liver EBRT doses of 24–25 Gy in 1.8- to 2.0-Gy fractions plus a 4-d infusion of concomitant 5-FU and cisplatin, based on results of extended-field EBRT doses of 30 Gy (in 1.8- to 2.0-Gy fractions) plus infusional chemotherapy for anal and esophageal cancers.

5.3.2. 3D CONFORMAL EBRT

Studies of 3D conformal EBRT combined with a more promising radiosensitizer are underway at the University of Michigan. Whereas the use of conformal radiotherapy is attractive in this group of patients as an invasive procedure is avoided, it is important to remember that because of the limitations of imaging studies, in defining both the intrahepatic with or without extrahepatic component of disease, the exact extent of disease is often missed without laparoscopic evaluation. The use of 3D conformal EBRT may be most acceptable in patients who are not considered candidates for HDR-IORT therapy, as a supplement to HDR-IORT or as a substitute for HDR-IORT in institutions without an interest in brachytherapy approaches for liver metastases.

5.3.3. OTHER MODALITIES

The use of ^{90}Yt glass microspheres for liver metastases as well as liver primaries has also been investigated. Selective internal radiotherapy delivered by embolizing microspheres injected into the hepatic artery still result in dose-limiting exposure to normal liver *(33)*. In China, where a large percentage of the world's incidence of hepatocellular carcinoma occurs, studies have been undertaken using intratumoral injection of ^{90}Yt in both primary and metastatic lesions in the liver *(34)*. This method allows delivery of high doses of radiation to the periphery of the lesions although dose calculation is still somewhat uncertain. With an average follow up of 17.6 mo, response rates were excellent, with posttreatment biopsies revealing no tumor in eight of nine patients undergoing the procedure. Dose to surrounding normal tissue is low and allows very high doses to be delivered to the target volume. This promising approach is in the early stages of clinical development. Since patients are being evaluated radiographically without laparoscopy, these investigators are undoubtedly including patients with inadequately defined extrahepatic disease who will not benefit from the procedure.

Another attempt to maximize therapy of colorectal carcinoma metastatic to the liver includes the use of cryotherapy. This modality of treatment does require laparotomy and thus addresses the same population of patients currently considered for HDR-IORT therapy. Whereas this method is shown to control treated lesions well with a median survival of 26 mo in selected patients *(35)*, side effects including severe myoglobinuria and coagulopathy are significant deterrents. Further, the recurring problems of a high rate of failure within the liver and nearly 50% ineligiblity rate at the time of laparotomy, because of the presence of extrahepatic disease or extensive liver disease unappreciated preoperatively, have resulted in limited enthusiasm.

Finally, some investigators have attempted to improve the outcome of patients with liver-only metastases by the use of hyperthermia combined with intra-arterial chemotherapy. Limited single-institution series have shown a modest improvement in partial response and median survival. This remains an area of investigation with continued problems relating to dose delivery.

5.4. Persistent Need for Effective Systemic Therapy

The combination of any of the above methods of local therapy with HDR-IORT therapy is a theoretical possibility, however combined-modality therapies must be undertaken with caution in this group of patients in whom at best 25% are expected to remain disease-free 5 yr after treatment. Quality-of-life issues related to the duration and side effects of therapy, as well as economic issues are major factors and will remain so until significant strides are made in the systemic management of cancers that have metastasized to or originate in the liver.

REFERENCES

1. Niederhuber JE and Ensminger WD. Treatment of metastatic cancer. In DeVita VT, Hellman S, and Rosenberg SA (eds.), *Cancer: Principles and practice of oncology,* Lippincott, Philadelphia, 1993, pp. 2201–2225.
2. Parker SL, Tong T, Bolden S, and Wingo PA. Cancer statistics. *CA: a cancer journal for clinicians.* **47** (1997) 5–27.
3. Lise M, Da Pian PP, Nitti D, and Pilati PL. Colorectal metastases to the liver: present results and future strategies, *J. Surg. Oncol.,* **suppl. 2** (1991) 69–73.
4. Lise M, Da Pian PP, Nitti D, Pilati PPL, and Prevaldi C. Colorectal metastases to the liver: Present status of management, *Dis. Col. & Rect.,* **33** (1990) 688–694.
5. Nordlinger B, Guiguet M, Vaillant J, et al. Surgical resection of colorectal carcinoma metastases to the liver: a prognostic scoring system to improve case selection, based on 1568 patients, *Cancer,* **77** (1996) 1254–1262.
6. Adson MA, van Heerden JA, Adson MH, Wagner JS, and Ilstrup DM. Resection of hepatic metastases from colorectal cancer. *Arch. Surg.,* **119** (1984) 647–651.
7. Daly JM and Kemeny N, Therapy of colorectal hepatic metastases. In, DeVita VT, Hellman S, and Rosenberg SA (eds.), *Important advances in oncology, 1986,* J.B. Lippincott, Philadelphia, 1986, pp. 251–268.
8. Stangl R, Altendorf-Hofmann A, Charnley RM, and Scheele J. Factors influencing the natural history of colorectal liver metastases. *Lancet,* **343** (1994) 1405–1410.
9. Hughes K, Scheele J, and Sugarbaker PH. Surgery for colorectal cancer metastatic to the liver, *Surgical Clin. N. Am.,* **69** (1989) 339–359.
10. Wanebo HJ, Chu QD, Vezeridis MP, and Soderberg C. Patient selection for hepatic resection of colorectal metastases, *Arch. Surg.,* **131** (1996) 322–329.
11. Fegiz G, Ramacciato G, Gennari L, et al. Hepatic resections for colorectal metastases: The Italian multicenter experience. *J. Surg. Oncol.,* **suppl. 2** (1991) 144–154.
12. Saenz NC, Cady B, McDermott Jr WV, and Steele GD. Experience with colorectal carcinoma metastatic to the liver. *Surgical Clin. N. Am.,* **69** (1989) 361–370.
13. Steele Jr G, Bleday R, Mayer RJ, Lindblad A, Petrelli N, and Weaver D. A prospective evaluation of hepatic resection for colorectal carcinoma metastases to the liver: gastrointestinal tumor study group protocol 6584, *J. Clin. Oncol.,* **9** (1991) 1105–1112.

14. Vaughn DJ and Haller DG. Nonsurgical management of recurrent colorectal cancer, *Cancer,* **71** (1993) 4278–4292.
15. Kemeny N, Conti JA, Cohen A, et al. Phase II study of hepatic arterial floxuridine, leucovorin, and dexamethasone for unresectable liver metastases from colorectal carcinoma, *J. Clin. Oncol.,* **12** (1994) 2288–2295.
16. Sugarbaker PH and Steves MA. A cytoreductive approach to treatment of multiple liver metastases, *J. Surg. Oncol.,* **supplement 3** (1993) 161–165.
17. McCall JL, Jorgensen JO, and Morris DL. Hepatic artery chemotherapy for colorectal liver metastases, *Aust. N. Z. J. Surg.,* **65** (1995) 383–389.
18. Minsky BD and Leibel SA. The treatment of hepatic metastases from colorectal cancer with radiation therapy alone or combined with chemotherapy or misonidazole, *Cancer Treat. Rev.,* **16** (1989) 213–219.
19. Leibel SA, Guse C, Order SE, et al. Accelerated fractionation radiation therapy for liver metastases: selection of an optimal patient population for the evaluation of late hepatic injury in RTOG studies, *Int. J. Radiat. Oncol. Biol. Phys.,* **18** (1990) 523–528.
20. Russell AH, Clyde C, and Wasserman TH. Accelerated hyperfractionated hepatic irradiation in the management of patients with liver metastases: results of the RTOG dose escalating protocol, *Int. J. Radiat. Oncol. Biol. Phys.,* **27** (1993) 117–123.
21. Rotman M, Kuruvilla AM, Choi K, et al. Response of colo-rectal hepatic metastases to concomitant radiotherapy and intravenous infusion 5 flourouracil, *Int. J. Radiat. Oncol. Biol. Phys.,* **12** (1986) 2179–2187.
22. Leibel SA, Pajak TF, Massullo V, et al. A comparison of misonidazole sensitized radiation therapy to radiation therapy alone for the palliation of hepatic metastases: results of a radiation therapy oncology group randomized prospective trial, *Int. J. Radiat. Oncol. Biol. Phys.,* **13** (1987) 1057–1064.
23. Robertson JM, Lawrence TS, Walker S, Kessler ML, Andrews JC, and Ensminger WD. The treatment of colorectal liver metastases with conformal radiation therapy and regional chemotherapy, *Int. J. Radiat. Oncol. Biol. Phys.,* **32** (1995) 445–450.
24. Ingold JD, Reed GB, Kaplan HS, and Bagshaw M. Radiation hepatitis. *Am. J. Roentgenol.,* **93** (1965) 200–208.
25. Dritschilo A, Grant EG, Harter KW, Holt RW, Rustgi SN, and Rodgers JE. Interstitial radiation therapy for hepatic metastases: Sonographic guidance for applicator placement, *AJR,* **146** (1986) 275–278.
26. Thomas DS, Nauta RJ, Rodgers JE, et al. Intraoperative high-dose rate interstitial irradiation of hepatic metastases from colorectal carcinoma, *Cancer,* **71** (1993) 1977–1981.
27. Dritschilo A, Harter KW, Thomas DS, et al. Intraoperative radiation therapy of hepatic metastases: technical aspects and report of a pilot study, *Int. J. Radiat. Oncol. Biol. Phys.,* **14** (1988) 1007–1011.
28. Nauta RJ, Heres EK, Thomas DT, et al. Intraoperative single-dose radiotherapy: observations on staging and interstitial treatment of unresectable liver metastases, *Arch. Surg.,* **122** (1987) 1392–1395.
29. Holt RW, Nauta RJ, Lee TC, et al. Intraoperative interstitial radiation therapy for hepatic metastases from colorectal carcinomas, *Am. Surgeon,* **54** (1988) 231–233.
30. Armstrong JG, Anderson LL, and Harrison LB. Treatment of liver metastases from colorectal cancer with radioactive implants, *Cancer,* **73** (1994) 1800–1804.
31. Donath D, Nori D, Turnbull A, Kaufman N, and Fortner JG. Brachytherapy in the treatment of solitary colorectal metastases to the liver, *J. Surg. Oncol.,* **44** (1990) 55–61.
32. Ravoet C, Bleiberg H, and Gerard B. Non-surgical treatment of hepatocarcinoma, *J. Surg. Oncol.,* **suppl. 3** (1993) 104–111.
33. Burton MA, Gray BN, Kelleher DK, and Klepm PF. Selective internal radiation therapy: Validation of intraoperative dosimetry, *Ther. Radiol.,* **175** (1990) 253–255.
34. Tian J, Xu B, Zhang J, Dong B, Liang P, and Wang X. Ultrasound-guided internal radiotherapy using yttrium-90-glass microspheres for liver malignancies, *J. Nuclear Med.,* **37** (1996) 958–964.
35. Weaver ML, Atkinson D, and Zemel R. Hepatic cryosurgery in treating colorectal metastases, *Cancer,* **76** (1995) 210–214.

18 Electron or Orthovoltage IORT for Retroperitoneal Sarcomas

Holger L. Gieschen, Christopher G. Willett,
John Donohue, Ivy A. Petersen, Ira J. Spiro,
Felipe A. Calvo, and Leonard L. Gunderson

CONTENTS

1. INTRODUCTION

Despite impressive advances in surgery and radiation therapy, the management of patients with retroperitoneal sarcoma remains a therapeutic challenge. Published series of surgical resection alone for retroperitoneal sarcoma have shown poor local control and survival rates. Because of the infiltrative nature of these tumors and their anatomic origin, it is frequently difficult to obtain microscopically clear resection margins. The efficacy of postoperative external-beam irradiation (EBRT) after resection is unclear from published reports. Because of the large size of these tumors, significant volumes of normal tissue (liver, small bowel, stomach, kidney, or spinal cord) may be within the EBRT field, and treatment is frequently limited to 45–50 Gy in 1.8- or 2-Gy fractions. It is not surprising that the local failure rate remains unacceptably high after postoperative irradiation because of the dose limitations of normal tissue to EBRT and the likelihood of at least microscopic residual disease after resection. In an effort to improve the local control and survival in patients with retroperitoneal sarcoma, treatment strategies employing intraoperative electron beam irradiation (IOERT) with preoperative or postoperative EBRT and surgery have been explored. This chapter will summarize relevant data on the role of IOERT in the management of patients with retroperitoneal sarcoma.

From: *Current Clinical Oncology: Intraoperative Irradiation: Techniques and Results*
Edited by: L. L. Gunderson et al. © Humana Press, Inc., Totowa, NJ

2. SURGERY WITH AND WITHOUT EBRT

2.1. Surgery Alone or With EBRT

Surgery has been the primary treatment modality of retroperitoneal sarcomas. Therefore, the majority of reports on retroperitoneal sarcoma are surgical series with and without adjuvant EBRT. With advances in surgical techniques, there has been a steady decline in operative mortality, but surgical resection alone is insufficient to control the disease.

Cody et al. analyzed a total of 158 cases of retroperitoneal sarcomas treated at Memorial Sloan Kettering Cancer Center (MSKCC) from 1951 to 1977 with resection with or without EBRT *(1)*. For this analysis the patients were divided into two groups: 78 patients treated from 1951 to 1971, and 80 patients from 1971 to 1977. Over the entire time period the distribution of tumors according to histology type and size remained relatively constant. However, the ability to achieve a gross total resection was 66% in the 1971 to 1977 group as compared to 49% over the entire time period. During the two time periods, overall 5-yr survival in the patients with gross total resection increased only minimally from 37% to 45% despite a marked decline in operative mortality from 21% to 2%. This may be explained by the high 5-yr local recurrence rate of 77% of patients who underwent a complete resection. Histologic grade influenced survival in this series: of the evaluable cases the 5-yr survival for 16 low-grade tumors was 80%, which was superior to 5% for 19 patients with high-grade tumors (values obtained from survival curves in paper). Of interest, the surgeon's intraoperative assessment of the resection margins frequently did not correlate with final margin status. Adjuvant EBRT after gross total resection resulted in an increase in overall survival from 30% to 53%, although this was not statistically significant.

The Mayo Clinic surgical experience with retroperitoneal sarcomas was published in 1989 *(2)*. A total of 116 patients followed for a minimum of 5 yr after operation were included. Total gross resection was possible in 54% of patients; 68% of those with gross resection experienced recurrence with a median time to treatment failure of 1.3 yr. Adjacent organ involvement was the strongest predictor of tumor recurrence. Five- and 10-yr survivals for all patients were 40% and 22%, respectively (54% and 35% 5- and 10-yr survival after complete resection). Survival was significantly improved if gross resection was possible for low-grade sarcomas, for sarcomas not fixed to adjacent organs, and if no metastases were apparent.

A recent series was reported by Karakousis et al. on 90 patients treated for retroperitoneal sarcoma undergoing resection with or without EBRT from 1977 to 1995 *(3)*. Resectability was 100% for 57 patients with primary disease and 88% for 33 patients with recurrent disease. With a median follow-up of 32 mo, the local recurrence rate for the entire group was 30% and varied with the completeness of resection: 56% with local excision and 16% with wide or radical resection. With a minimum follow-up of 5 yr, the overall local failure rates were 50% and 60% at 5 and 10 yr, respectively. Local recurrence was slightly lower with adjuvant radiotherapy (33% vs 22%) but was not statistically significant. Survival was also influenced by the extent of resection: the 5- and 10-yr survival rates were 72% and 61% for patients undergoing wide resection vs 55% and 23%, respectively for local resection.

The importance of complete resection and resection margin status was also reported in the University of Florida experience, by Kilkenney et al. *(4)*. This recent study included patients with primary retroperitoneal sarcoma treated between 1970 and 1994. Patients with complete resection and pathologically negative margins (63% of patients with gross total resection) had a median survival of 68 mo. In cases with positive, uncertain, or close margins, the median survival was 42 mo. In patients with gross residual tumor the median survival was 9 mo; 5 mo in patients who underwent biopsy only. Tumor location within the retroperitoneum did not influence survival. Thirty-seven patients also received EBRT with or without chemotherapy with no apparent survival advantage for these patients, although details on patient selection and dose factors were not specified.

Evidence of improved survival with complete resection is suggested in the Medical College of Virginia series reported by McGrath et al. in 1984 (5). Forty-seven patients with primary retroperitoneal sarcoma were reviewed. Complete resection was defined as surgical removal of all gross disease with microscopically negative margins. Thirty-eight percent of patients had a complete resection by this definition. The disease-free survival for this group was 50% at 5 yr with an overall survival rate of 70%. The local relapse risk at 5 yr was 55% in spite of negative resection margins. The remaining patients undergoing partial resection or biopsy only had a disease-free survival of only 4% at 5 yr.

Storm et al. summarized the results of eight surgical series of patients treated between 1937 and 1987 (6). Of 560 patients who underwent exploratory laparotomy, only half (53%) were able to have a complete resection, as defined by removal of all gross disease. Nineteen percent of the patients had a partial resection, whereas 21% of the patients underwent biopsy only. The survival rates at 2, 5, and 10 yr of 410 resected patients from the combined series were 56%, 34%, and 18%, respectively. The survival was clearly influenced by the completeness of resection. The survival rate at 2, 5, and 10 yr was 81%, 54%, and 46% for completely resected patients. In contrast, these figures were 34%, 17%, and 8%, respectively for patients undergoing partial resection. Even if a complete resection could not be achieved, patients undergoing partial resection fared better than patients who had biopsy only. The rate of local recurrence in patients with gross total resection was high at 72% at 5 yr and ultimately 91% failed locally at 10 yr. This study emphasizes the high local failure rate in patients undergoing resection of retroperitoneal sarcomas.

2.2. Surgery Plus EBRT

The results of adjuvant radiotherapy in the management of patients with retroperitoneal sarcoma treated at the Fox Chase Cancer Center were reviewed by Fein et al. (7). This series also included three patients who received IOERT. Between 1965 and 1992, 21 patients were treated with a follow up ranging from 14–340 mo. Nineteen patients were treated postoperatively and two patients received irradiation preoperatively. EBRT doses ranged from 36.0–61.2 Gy using fractionated treatment with fraction sizes of 1.5–2.0 Gy/d. The three patients who received IOERT were treated with total EBRT doses of 36–61 Gy and IOERT doses of 10 Gy in two patients and 16 Gy in one patient. Two other patients received a brachytherapy boost with [192]Ir. Two out of three patients with IOERT achieved local control, as did the two patients with brachytherapy. For the whole group, the 5-yr actuarial local control and overall survival was 72% and 44%, respectively. Local control rate was influenced by size, stage, grade, or histology of the tumor. A possible dose response was demonstrated in that patients receiving total doses of 55.2 Gy or greater had a lower local failure rate (25%) than that of patients receiving radiation doses of less than 55.2 Gy of irradiation (38%). The only reported complication was a small-bowel obstruction in one patient receiving an external beam dose of 55.2 Gy.

Table 1
Surgical Series With and Without EBRT—Treatment Method and Results

Series/(ref no.)	n	% gross complete resection	EBRT (Gy)	IORT (Gy)	Survival and Local Relapse after Resection		
					DFS 5-yr	OS 5-yr	Local Failure % (yrs)
Surgery ± EBRT							
Cody (1)	158	49	some- no details	No	21[b]	40[b]	77 (5)
Karakousis (3)	90	96	some- no details	No	47	63	50 (5)
Kilkenney (4)	63	87	37 pts-no details	No	—	48	—
McGrath (5)	47	38[a]	60%- no details	No	50[a]	70[a]	55[a] (5)
Storm (6)	560[c]	53	some- no details	No	—	34	72
Surgery + EBRT							
Fein (7)	21	—	36.0 - 61.2	3 pts-10,10,16	—	44	28 (5)
Tepper (8)	17	41	19.3 - 69	No	—	54	54 (5)

[a]Microscopically negative margins.
[b]Patients with complete resection.
[c]Combined results of eight series.

Tepper et al. reviewed 23 patients treated at the Massachusetts General Hospital (MGH) for retroperitoneal sarcoma between 1971 and 1982 (8,9). This series also included six patients who were treated with palliative intent for localized disease. Patients were classified as having a complete resection with histologic negative margins, a partial resection with gross or microscopic residual disease, or no resection. All patients received EBRT with megavoltage radiotherapy except for one palliative case receiving orthovoltage treatment. The stated intent was to deliver at least 50 Gy combined with maximal surgical resection. Doses ranged from 19.28–69 Gy. Seventeen patients were treated with curative intent. Of these, 6 patients received preoperative radiotherapy, 12 patients received postoperative radiotherapy, and one received pre- and postoperative treatment. Complete resection was achieved in seven cases, incomplete resection in seven, and no resection in three. The 5-yr local control and survival rate for patients treated with curative intent was 54%. Analysis suggested that higher doses may increase the likelihood of local control. Four of six patients (67%) who received less than 50 Gy had a local failure, whereas none of the five patients receiving between 50 and 60 Gy, and only one of six receiving more than 60 Gy developed local failure. There was no demonstrable correlation between tumor grade and recurrence rate. The complication rate was not reported.

2.3. Summary

The previously reviewed studies show that surgery remains the single most important treatment modality in the management of patients with retroperitoneal sarcoma (Table 1). Complete resection, i.e., removal of all gross disease, preferably with negative microscopic margins, offers the best chance for survival. Unfortunately, approximately half of all patients undergoing laparotomy are not amenable to a complete resection. Even with a complete resection, local failure remains a substantial problem with 28–91% of these patients ultimately experiencing local disease relapse.

The addition of EBRT to surgical resection is common practice and may be beneficial in patients treated adjuvantly. With documented microscopic residual or in patients with gross residual disease, a benefit for EBRT is less clear, but such treatment may delay the onset of clinical symptoms. However, the above trials and the National Cancer Institute (NCI) randomized trial presented below suggest no benefit of EBRT in patients with gross total but marginal resection. Because of the limitations of normal tissue to EBRT, optimal treatment is hampered with EBRT-only techniques, and IORT has been employed to dose-escalate specific regions in the retroperitoneum at risk for residual disease.

3. IORT TREATMENT FACTORS

3.1. EBRT Factors

The current treatment approach at both MGH and Mayo Clinic for patients with nonmetastatic retroperitoneal sarcoma is to utilize moderate-dose preoperative irradiation (40–50 Gy), surgical resection, and IOERT (if technically feasible). The preoperative EBRT approach is favored for many reasons. First, a high-dose preoperative regimen sterilizes a large percentage of tumor cells and may minimize the risk of tumor implantation in the peritoneal cavity after the marginal resection has been performed. Second, partial regression obtained from EBRT may allow a more complete resection to be performed. Third, these large tumors usually displace abdominal and retroperitoneal viscera to a degree that large volumes of radiosensitive organs such as the stomach and small bowel can be effectively excluded from the preoperative EBRT field. Because of this reduction of normal tissue irradiation by the tumor's displacement of viscera outside the radiation field, it is usually feasible to give daily doses of 1.8 Gy with excellent tolerance, which may not be feasible when done postoperatively.

Anterior-posterior and posterior-anterior fields with 5-cm margins are used when feasible given the limitation of dose-limiting organs (liver, bilateral kidneys, spinal cord) as these tumors frequently extend from the retroperitoneal surface to the anterior abdominal wall. Occasionally, oblique fields are helpful in minimizing the dose to normal structures such as the spinal cord and kidney. Patients with right-sided or left-sided lesions sometimes can receive a portion or all of their treatment in the decubitus position to displace small-bowel loops away from the tumor bed. If irradiation of the tumor or tumor bed requires the inclusion of one kidney to doses beyond tolerance, function of the remaining kidney should be assessed with serum creatinine and blood urea nitrogen levels and a contrast renal study (computerized tomography [CT] scan with iv contrast, renal scan or intravenous pyelogram [IVP]).

3.2. Surgical Factors

The operative management of retroperitoneal sarcomas is hampered by several factors. Chief among these is the frequent large size of these tumors before detection. Because of their substantial bulk, the anatomic confines of the retroperitoneum and the involvement of adjacent viscera, wide excision is the exception rather than the rule for these neoplasms. More commonly a gross total resection of a retroperitoneal sarcoma can be achieved, but some margins are likely to be very close, if not microscopically involved. Whereas incomplete gross resection may alleviate some symptoms related to pressure (i.e., obstruction, pain) or invasion (i.e., hemorrhage, obstruction, pain) of abdominal organs and structures, as well as provide constitutional improvements related to tumor mass, these benefits are often short-lived.

3.2.1. Preoperative Imaging

Preoperative planning is mostly aided by three-dimensional imaging of the abdomen, either with CT or magnetic resonance (MR) scans. The extent of the sarcoma, as well as likely involved normal structures, is readily apparent. Bilateral renal function must be documented because nephrectomy is commonly required to achieve total tumor extirpation. Arteriography, or more commonly venography, may be indicated if major vascular reconstruction is contemplated. A chest radiograph or CT scan is sufficient for evaluation for extra-abdominal metastases. Primary retroperitoneal sarcomas, unlike abdominal visceral sarcomas, are unlikely to form peritoneal metastases; therefore, laparoscopy is not of routine value in these patients. In recurrent disease, this pattern of failure must be considered, especially if ascites are present on the abdominal scan.

3.2.2. Surgical Techniques

Three to six weeks after completion of EBRT, exploratory laparotomy is performed in the dedicated IOERT suite in our respective institutions. At surgery, the abdomen and pelvis are carefully examined for metastases to the liver and/or peritoneal surfaces. If no metastases are found, the patient undergoes resection of the tumor, leaving as little residual sarcoma as possible.

Every effort is made to remove the tumor and involved normal structures *en bloc* without violation or exposure of the tumor surface. Lateral mobilization of the tumor is relatively simple because most vascularity arises from the medial aspect of the tumor. Although normal tissue planes should be used whenever possible, it is easy to get into the sarcoma pseudocapsule, resulting in tumor enucleation and a large amount of microscopic residual disease.

Figures 1A–C demonstrate the removal of a large left-upper quadrant sarcoma along with the distal pancreas, spleen, and left kidney (Fig. 1). With the lateral location of most resectable retroperitoneal sarcomas, the kidney and colon are the most commonly resected organs *(10,11)*. Because the tumor was easily retracted away from the midline vascular structures, the splenic and renal vessels, along with a number of large tumor veins, were ligated early in the procedure, along with division of the pancreatic parenchyma (Fig. 1B). Once the tumor's blood supply was controlled, the lesion could be more safely mobilized with sharp and blunt dissection (Fig. 1C). Bowel anastomoses are usually completed after IOERT has been utilized.

For sarcomas of the iliac fossa and central retroperitoneum, major vascular resections are often necessary if gross total resection is to be achieved. Vascular reconstruction is generally required, usually with prosthetic graft material. If the anastomosis is not overlying a high-risk area for local relapse, it can be excluded from the IOERT field. The graft anastomosis should be shielded from adjacent bowel and, in particular, bowel anastomoses using omentum, peritoneal flaps, or other normal tissues. Figure 1D shows the post resection view of the right abdomen after combined extended right hepatectomy and inferior vena caval resection for a primary leiomyosarcoma.

If no gross tumor remains, frozen section pathologic analysis is carried out on the specimen from areas at greatest risk for residual disease. Biopsy specimens are obtained to examine for the presence of residual sarcoma in the tumor bed. The areas at highest risk for local tumor recurrence are defined by the surgeon and radiation oncologist and outlined with metallic dips and occasionally silk sutures for purpose of visualizing tumor bed through the applicator.

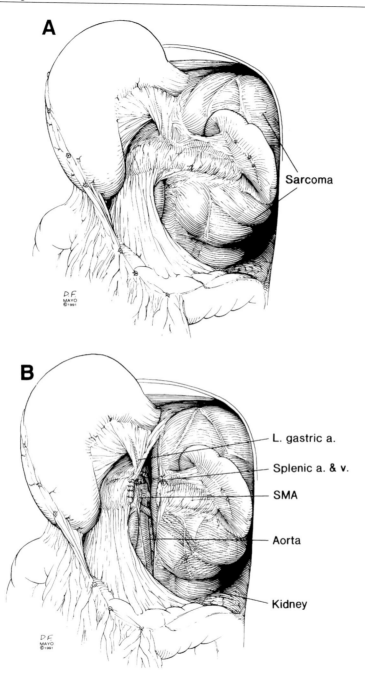

Fig. 1. (A) (32.6): A large left upper quadrant sarcoma is seen posterior to the spleen and distal pancreas. **(B)** (32.7): The medial border of the tumor has been dissected with ligation of the splenic artery and vein and division of the pancreas. The left renal vessels are dissected free in preparation for division, and the aorta has been dissected free with control of tumor vessels. **(C)** (32.9): After posterior and lateral dissection, the tumor and involved structures are removed en bloc. The insert shows the specimen which includes the distal pancreas, spleen, and left kidney. **(D)** (32.14): View of the resection field after removal of a large right upper quadrant sarcoma that involved the retrohepatic inferior vena cava and right liver. A ribbed tube vascular prosthesis has been used to replace the IVC.

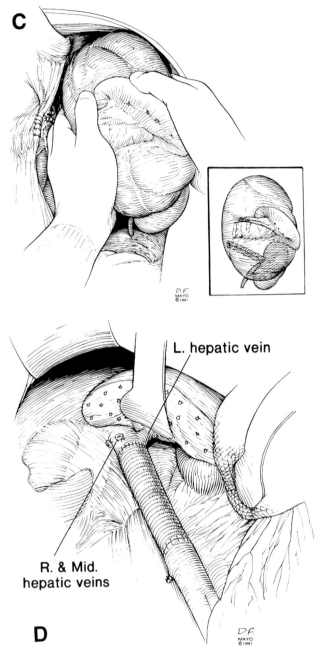

Fig. 1. (*continued*)

3.3. IOERT Factors

To direct the IOERT, applicators (circular, elliptical, or rectangular) are used (Fig. 2). Applicator geometry and size are carefully selected to fully cover the high-risk area. For large sarcomas, abutting fields may be needed to assure that all high-risk areas are included.

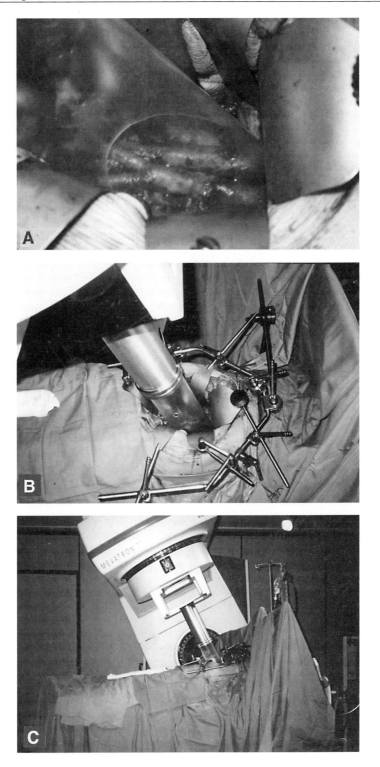

Fig. 2. IOERT treatment sequence after resection of retroperitoneal sarcoma. (**A**) Vena cava, aorta, and iliac bifurcation within IOERT applicator. (**B**) Applicator "docked" with linear accelerator. (**C**) Patient ready for treatment.

The IOERT dose and energy are dependent on amount of residual disease after maximal resection and the volume treated (i.e., length of peripheral nerve in IOERT field, amount of bowel circumference, and so on). For patients with completely resected tumors and negative margins, an IOERT dose of 10 Gy is usually selected, whereas a grossly resected tumor bed with positive microscopic margins will receive 12.5–15 Gy (depending on volume treated). For gross residual disease, doses will range from 15 to 20 Gy depending on the the extent of residual tumor and volume treated. The electron energy is selected according to the desired depth of penetration and ranges typically between 9 and 15 MeV.

4. RESULTS IN SERIES WITH ELECTRON-BEAM IORT

Intraoperative radiotherapy was first used as early as the 1930s with the intent to either overcome the high skin doses that were commonly seen with the available low-energy X-ray machines or as an economical alternative to the costly radium at that time. Modern intraoperative radiotherapy began with clinical studies in Japan in the early 1960s. Initially ^{60}Co was utilized, but soon electron-beam irradiation was used with its more favorable depth-dose distribution. Several pilot studies in the United States and in Europe and Japan, as well as a small randomized study by the NCI evaluated IOERT for retroperitoneal sarcoma.

4.1. NCI Randomized Study—Adjuvant EBRT With or Without IOERT

4.1.1. PATIENT GROUP AND TREATMENT METHOD

Kinsella et al. first reported the preliminary results of a randomized study conducted by the NCI of 35 patients with resectable primary retroperitoneal sarcoma who were randomized to two different adjuvant treatments (12). All patients had a gross total resection, but most had presumed or pathologically positive microscopic residual disease because of marginal resections. Fifteen patients received IOERT of 20 Gy, usually to abutting fields using high-energy electrons of 11–15 MeV, followed by postoperative EBRT of 35–40 Gy (Table 2). Twenty patients received standard postoperative EBRT alone of 50–55 Gy (35–40 Gy to an extended field; 15 Gy within a boost field). All patients receiving IOERT also received misonidazole as a radiosensitizer. In the beginning of the study a second randomization to adjuvant chemotherapy (doxorubicin, cyclophosphamide, and methotrexate) or no chemotherapy was carried out. This randomization was discontinued after the first 13 patients.

4.1.2. RESULTS

4.1.2.1. Disease Control and Survival. In the preliminary analysis by Kinsella et al. with a minimum follow-up of 15 mo, there was no significant difference in the actuarial disease-free survival (DFS) or overall survival (OS) (12). There was a nonsignificant trend towards improved in-field local control for the IOERT group (78 vs 30%).

However, in the follow-up report of this study by Sindelar et al. with a minimum follow-up of 5 yr and a median follow-up of 8 yr, there was a significant difference in local control between the two groups (13). In the IOERT group, only 3 of 15 patients (20%) had an in-field local recurrence, vs 16 of 20 patients (80%) in the EBRT control group ($p < 0.001$) (Table 2). The median survival was similar for both groups: 45 mo for the IOERT group and 52 mo for the control group. Actuarial survival and DFS was correlated

Table 2
Retroperitoneal Sarcoma Resection ± IORT Series—Treatment Method and Results

Series (Author/Institution) (ref. no.)	n	Resection Gross complete No (%)	EBRT (Gy) No., Dose	IORT (Gy) No., Dose	DFS (%) 5-yr	OS (%) 5-yr	In-Field Local Failure % (yrs)
U.S. Series							
Sindelar, NCI	15	15 (100)	35 - 40	20	—	38[b]	20[b]
randomized *(12,13)*	20	20 (100)	50-55	no	—	44[b]	80
Hoekstra, NCI *(16)*	5	5 (100)	1 pt, —	5, 20 - 30	—	—	—
Willett, MGH *(17)*	20	14 (70)	40 - 50	12, 10 - 20	64 (4 yr)	—	19 (4)
Gunderson, Mayo *(18)*	20	—	45 - 52	20, 10 - 20[c]	—	48.5	15
Kiel, RTOG (20)	12	—	45 - 50.4	12, 12.5 - 20	—	—	—
Petersen, Mayo Update *(19)*	87	72 (83)	77, 45-52	87, 10 - 20	—	47	23[d]
European Series							
Pelton *(21)*	41[e]	—	—	41, 10-20	—	—	—
Bussièrs *(22)*	25	11	—	15 - 20	32 (2 yr)	60 (2 yr)	24 (2)
Dubois *(23)*	31[f]	30	28 - 56	31, —	—	64.5	30.7
Willeke *(24)*	25	55	8 - 40.4	11, 18	—	—	—
Calvo *(25,26)*	30	21	39-50	10-20	—	36 (8 yr)	47

[a]Randomized study: 35 patients: 15 with IORT plus EBRT, 20 standard treatment with EBRT.
[b]From graphs $p < 0.05$.
[c]Dependent on amount of residual disease.
[d]Local failure in only 3 of 43 (7%) with primary disease vs 17 of 44 (39%) with recurrent disease.
[e]Includes patients with retroperitoneal sarcoma, colorectal and gastric carcinomas, and other disease sites.
[f]Only 13 of 31 had retroperitoneal sarcomas.

to stage of disease, but not significantly different between the two groups. There was no benefit from chemotherapy in this study.

4.1.2.2. Complications. The overall rate of treatment-related complications was similar in both groups but with marked differences in the types of complications. The treatment mortality rate was 9%, based on one death each in the control and study arm (postoperative pulmonary embolism in the IOERT plus EBRT group and hemorrhage from an aortic mycotic aneurysm in the EBRT-alone control group). Arterial occlusions developed in one IOERT patient and two control patients. Ureteral stenosis occurred in two patients of each group. Both acute and chronic gastrointestinal complications were more common in the EBRT-alone control group. Two IOERT patients (13%) and 10 EBRT-only patients (50%) developed disabling chronic radiation enteritis ($p \leq 0.05$). Peripheral sensory and motor neuropathy were more common in the IOERT group. This was observed in nine IOERT-treated patients (60%) and only one patient (5%) in the EBRT control group. Manifestation of peripheral neuropathy was intermittent pain and motor weakness. The motor weakness resolved in all four affected patients within 6 mo. The high incidence of peripheral neuropathy was likely related to both the 20 Gy IOERT dose (*see* Chapter 10 and refs. *13–15*) and use of abutting IOERT fields in most patients.

4.3. *United States Single Institution and Group Pilot Studies*

4.3.1. NCI

Hoekstra et al. at the NCI reported in 1988 the results of five patients with extensive sarcomas in the pelvic girdle who underwent hemipelvectomy and IOERT with doses of 20–30 Gy *(16)*. The IOERT was directed to the resection margins and surrounding soft tissues using electrons with energies from 11 to 16 MeV. One patient also received postoperative EBRT and one had postoperative chemotherapy. The treatment field sizes for the IOERT were 10×17 cm. Of these five patients, three developed metastatic disease within 3 mo and died. Two were disease free at 43 and 53 mo. Local control was reported in four of five patients. The only reported treatment complication was osteoradionecrosis at 7-mo posttreatment in one patient.

4.3.2. MGH IOERT SERIES

4.3.2.1. Patient Group and Treatment Methods. Willett et al. reported on the MGH experience of IOERT in the management of retroperitoneal sarcoma in a group of 20 patients with either primary ($n = 14$) or recurrent ($n = 6$) disease *(17)* (Table 2). In contrast to other institutions, these patients standardly received preoperative EBRT that was followed by exploratory laparotomy and IOERT. Seventeen of the 20 patients underwent laparotomy and 14 had a complete resection. Three patients had a partial resection and distant metastasis developed during EBRT in three patients. IOERT was given to 12 of the 14 patients. Irradiation doses used were 40–50 Gy EBRT at 1.7- to 2.0-Gy per fraction and 10–20 Gy IOERT with 9–15 MeV electrons. The time interval between EBRT and surgery was 4–6 wk.

4.3.2.2. Results. The 4-year actuarial local control and disease-free survival of the 14 patients undergoing complete resection was 81 and 64%, respectively (Table 2). In this series, five patients developed complications: two with hydronephrosis, two (17%) with sensory neuropathy, and one with a small-bowel obstruction. Based on their experience, the current treatment policy is to limit the IOERT dose to 10–15 Gy for microscopic residual and 17–20 Gy for macroscopic residual disease.

4.3.3. MAYO IOERT SERIES

4.3.3.1. Patient Group and Treatment Methods. In the initial Mayo Clinic experience reported by Gunderson et al., 20 patients received IOERT: 10 with primary tumors and 10 with recurrent disease *(18)* (Table 2). Nineteen of the 20 patients had retroperitoneal tumors. Six patients had planned preoperative irradiation with doses ranging from 45–52 Gy. In all other patients, a partial or gross resection was done prior to any EBRT or IOERT. IOERT was delivered with electrons ranging from 9 to 18 Mev energy. IOERT doses were based on degree of resection: 10–12.5 Gy for microscopic disease, 15 Gy for gross disease less than 2 cm, and 17.5–20 Gy for gross residual disease of 2 cm or greater. IOERT fields include the tumor with a margin of 1 cm, e.g., a 5-cm tumor requires a 7-cm cone. In 15 of 19 patients, treatment was given using only one field. However, in one patient abutting fields were used and two separate fields in the other two patients.

4.3.3.2. Results. The actuarial survival for the initial group of 20 patients was 83% at 2.5 yr and 48.5% at 5 yr with equivalent survival for those with primary or recurrent disease (Table 2). The local failure rate was 15%; only one patient recurred in the IOERT field and three within the EBRT field. Distant metastasis occurred in 25% of all patients but was limited to the group of patients with primary disease. The excellent survival of patients with recurrent disease may be related to the low rate of distant metastasis in this

Table 3
Mayo Clinic IOERT Analysis: Patterns of Local Failure in Patients
with Retroperitoneal and Intrapelvic Sarcomas—Primary vs Recurrent and Low vs High Grade

Pattern of Relapse	Primary n = 43	Recurrent n = 44	Low Grade n = 33	High Grade n = 54	Total n = 87
CF	0	4	2	2	4
LF	2	11	8	5	13
LF and CF	1	2	1	2	3
Total # (%)[a]	3 (7%)[a]	17 (39%)	11 (33%)	9 (17%)	20 (23%)
Prior EBRT excluded[b]	3/41 (7%)	9/31 (29%)	6 (22%)	6 (13%)	12/72 (17%)

CF: central failure in IOERT field; LF: local failure in EBRT field or surgical bed (prior EBRT group)
[a]Patients with prior EBRT included in numerator and denominator.
[b]Patients with prior EBRT excluded from numerator and denominator (primary n = 2, recurrent n = 13).
From ref. 19.

group, which may be explained by a predominance of low-grade lesions. Distant metastasis developed in 13% of patients with low-grade lesions and 42% with high-grade lesions.

Significant complications occurred in 6 of 20 patients (30%), and in 5 patients, IOERT was felt to be a causative factor. Reported complications were: one severe neuropathy (5%) resulting in foot drop, two wound complications, one urologic, and one fibrosis. There were also two cases of small-bowel obstruction that were judged to be related to surgery and EBRT.

An updated Mayo analysis was presented at ASTRO by Petersen et al. in 1996 of 87 patients with retroperitoneal or pelvic sarcomas who had resection plus IOERT at Mayo between March, 1981 and September, 1995 and had ≥ 1 yr of follow-up (median 3.5 yr) (19). More tumors were high grade (62%) and recurrent (52%). At time of operation at Mayo, all gross disease could be removed in 72 patients or 83%. EBRT was given in 77 patients (all 43 with primary lesions and 34 of the 44 patients with recurrent disease).

Forty-nine patients had documented disease relapse with 20 (23%) having local or central failure (central in 7 of 87 or 8%, local in 16 of 87 or 18%) (Table 3). Local or central failure occurred in only 3 of 43 patients with primary lesions (7%) vs 17 of 44 (39%) who presented with recurrent disease. If patients with prior EBRT are deleted from the analysis, the incidence of local or central relapse was 7 and 29% for the primary and recurrent disease patients, respectively.

Five-year OS was 47% with 46 of 87 patients (53%) alive. Five-year OS was unaffected by primary vs recurrent status (52% vs 42%, Fig. 3A) and low- vs high-grade lesions (2-yr 97 vs 75%, 5-yr 45% vs 47%, Fig. 3B). Patients with gross total resection had a trend towards improved survival over those with gross residual disease (median 4.7 vs 3.2 yr, 5-yr 49% vs 36%, p = 0.08, Fig. 3C).

Severe gastrointestinal intolerance was uncommon in primary disease patients (2 of 43 or 5%), but 7 of 44 recurrent disease patients developed grade 3–5 GI fistulae (16%) with one fatality. Grade 3 peripheral neuropathy developed in 4 of 43 patients (9%) with primary disease and 5 of 44 (11%) with recurrent lesions.

The influence of multiple prognostic factors on local and distant disease control and overall survival was analyzed separately for patients who presented with either primary (Table 4) or recurrent disease (Table 5). For patients with primary lesions, both initial lesion size ≤5 cm and the surgeon's ability to achieve a gross total resection prior to

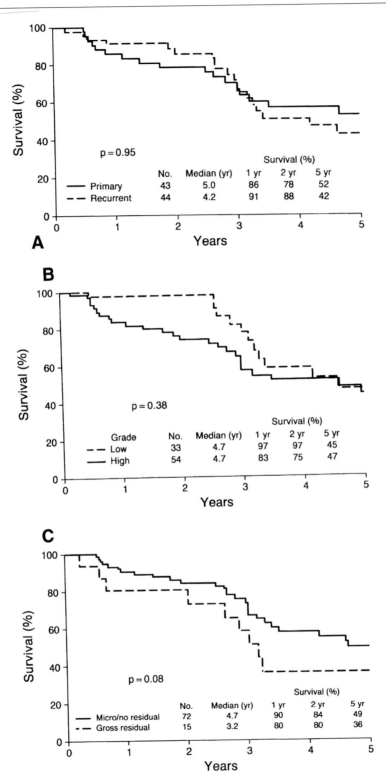

Fig. 3. Overall survival by prognostic factor, Mayo Clinic analysis (*n* = 87). (**A**) Primary (*n* = 43) versus recurrent (*n* = 44). (**B**) Grade—low (grade 1 or 2, *n* = 33) or high (grade 3 or 4, *n* = 54). (**C**) Amount of residual disease after maximal resection—gross (*n* = 15), ≤ microscopic (*n* = 72). (From ref.19.)

Table 4
Primary Retroperitoneal and Pelvic Sarcoma—Influence of Prognostic Factors
on Disease Control and Survival, Mayo Analysis

| | | Overall Survival (%) | | Disease Control | | | |
| | | | | Local (%) | | Distant (%) | |
Prognostic Factor	No.	2 yr	5 yr	2 yr	5 yr	2 yr	5 yr
Residual at IOERT							
≤ Microscopic							
Margin (–)	11	91	62	100	100	71	53
Margin (+)	25	75	54	100	92	65	41
Gross	7	71	29	80	60	43	29
Grade							
Low (1,2)	9	89	42	100	100	88	25
High (3,4)	34	75	54	96	84	55	43
Tumor Size							
≤5	7	100	86	100	83	71	43
>5	35	76	45	96	92	62	46

Mo = months; Yr = year; No = number; Pts = patients; preop = preoperative, postop = postoperative,
EBRT = external beam irradiation.
From ref. *19*.

Table 5
Recurrent Retroperitoneal and Pelvic Sarcoma—Influence
of Prognostic Factors on Disease Control and Survival, Mayo Analysis

| | | Overall Survival (%) | | Disease Control | | | |
| | | | | Local (%) | | Distant (%) | |
Prognostic Factor	No. (%)	2 yr	5 yr	2 yr	5 yr	2 yr	5 yr
Residual at IOERT							
≤ Microscopic							
Margin (–)	5 (11)	80	80	100	100	60	60
Margin (+)	31 (70)	90	44	68	36	65	37
Gross	8 (18)	86	45	100	67	50	33
Grade							
Low (1,2)	24 (55)	100	53	83	28	77	47
High (3,4)	20 (45)	75	35	70	58	42	27
Tumor Size							
≤5 cm	10 (23)	90	58	80	50	60	50
>5 cm	34 (77)	88	40	76	34	61	33

Yr = year; No = number.
From ref. *19*.

IOERT appeared to have a favorable impact on long-term survival (5-yr). Disease control
appeared to be impaired only by the ability to achieve a gross total resection prior to
IOERT. For patients who presented with recurrent disease, the amount of residual disease
at time of IOERT had less apparent impact on disease control or survival. Patients with

low-grade lesions or recurrent tumor size ≤5 cm had more favorable trends for overall survival and disease control.

4.3.4. RTOG IOERT Series

4.3.4.1. Patient Group and Treatment Methods. The Radiation Therapy Oncology Group (RTOG) provided information on their phase II trial of intraoperative radiotherapy (RTOG 85-07). Preliminary results were reported by Kiel et al. at the Third International Symposium of Intraoperative Radiotherapy *(20)* (Table 2). Twenty-eight patients were entered onto RTOG 85-07. Patients with resectable tumors received IOERT at the time of resection followed by postoperative EBRT. Patients with unresectable disease received preoperative EBRT followed by resection and IOERT if possible or IOERT alone. Sixteen patients received no IOERT and were excluded, mainly because of nonsarcoma or benign histology. Twelve patients were treated with IOERT using single doses of 12.5–20 Gy and EBRT with a range of 45–50.4 Gy.

4.3.4.2. Results. With a median follow-up of 18 mo, 6 patients were still alive, one with tumor. Local control was achieved in 10 of 12 patients. This study has not been updated since the original report in 1991 (personal communication with Dr. Kiel).

4.3.5. Fox Chase IOERT Series

4.3.5.1. Patient Group and Treatment Methods. Similar to other series, the importance of resection margins on local control was demonstrated in an IOERT series from Fox Chase Cancer Center, reported by Pelton et al. *(20)* (Table 2). The outcome of 41 consecutive patients who underwent IOERT including patients with retroperitoneal sarcomas, colorectal carcinoma, gastric carcinoma, and other disease sites were reviewed with attention to margin status. Many patients (73%) had failed previous multimodality treatment and 44% had previous EBRT. The median IOERT dose given was 13.75 Gy ranging from 10 to 20 Gy. Patients with prior EBRT had received a median dose of 49.65 Gy. Microscopic margin status was assessed in each case.

4.3.5.2. Results. The 2-yr actuarial OS for the entire group was 72%. The OS in patients with negative resection margin was 100% vs 59% with positive margins. The rate of local control was significantly different for negative and positive margins, 79% vs 48%, respectively. The only predictive prognostic factor in this study was margin status.

4.4. European IORT Data

4.4.1. Institut Bergonie, France— IOERT Series

4.4.1.1. Patient Group and Treatment Methods. A recent study by Bussièrs et al. at the Institut Bergonié, France reviewed 51 patients with either primary ($n = 38$) or recurrent retroperitoneal sarcoma ($n = 13$) referred to their institution *(22)* (Table 2). Of these, 16 patients had already undergone resection without gross residual disease by CT prior to referral and were therefore not included in this study. Five patients were judged unresectable. Of the 26 patients who underwent resection after referral to the Institut Bergonie, 19 received IOERT. Reasons for withholding IOERT were: peritoneal seeding in two, negative frozen section in one, or technically not possible because of either bleeding, tumor size or normal tissue tolerance in three. Of the patients who received IOERT, 14 had primary disease and five had recurrent disease. The median tumor size was 13 cm. Eleven of the 14 patients with primary disease had gross complete resections that required *en block* resection of adjacent organs in seven cases. IOERT was delivered to the tumor bed or residual with a median dose of 17 Gy, range from 15 to 20 Gy. EBRT was delivered postoperatively in 12 patients and preoperatively in one patient. The median dose was 50 Gy, ranging from 40 to 60 Gy at 1.8–2.0 Gy per fraction. EBRT was not added in three cases, because of no residual tumor in one, a second primary discovered at time of surgery in one, and postoperative complication in one.

4.4.1.2. Results. The 2-yr actuarial OS and DFS was 60% and 32%, respectively. In contrast to the Mayo Clinic experience, the five patients with recurrent disease did less well. Three had died of their disease and two patients were alive with disease. Twelve of the 14 patients with primary disease were alive and disease-free. The local control rate at 2 yr was 76%. Similar to other series, the actual failure rate within the field of IOERT was low with only one patient recurring. Distant metastasis occurred in three patients, all were in the group treated for recurrent disease. However, distant recurrence was only recorded as the first site of failure, which underestimates the propensity for distant metastasis.

Postoperative complications were reported in four patients (21%), consisting of one cerebrovascular accident (CVA), one complex pelvic fistula, one anuria caused by hematoma in single kidney patient, and one external pancreatic fistula. Late complications occurred in six patients (32%) resulting in one death (5%). The fatal complication was caused by bleeding secondary to external iliac artery rupture. This patient had received 60 Gy preoperative radiotherapy for a liposarcoma with extension to the iliofemoral area. IOERT consisted of a 15-Gy dose with a field measuring 15×20 cm. This clearly demonstrates the risk of treating large volumes to high doses and in single fractions. Other complications were dehydration, lymphedema in the lower limb, temporary lumbar plexopathy, and two cases of chronic enteritis.

4.4.2. Montpellier Orthovoltage IORT Series

Dubois et al. from Montpellier, France, reported on their experience with intraoperative radiotherapy in 31 patients with soft-tissue sarcomas *(23)* (Table 2). This series included 13 patients with sarcoma located in the retroperitoneum or pelvis. Sixteen patients were treated for primary disease and 15 for recurrent disease; however this information was not separately reported for the group of patients with retroperitoneal tumors. Patients with primary disease also received postoperative EBRT with doses of 28–56 Gy, mean 41.8 Gy. Of the entire group, all but one patient had a gross complete resection. Local recurrence occurred in 4 patients (30.7%), all of whom had had intrapelvic or intra-abdominal disease. A 5-yr survival of 65% was reported for the whole group.

4.4.3. Heidelberg IOERT Series

Willeke et al. published the Heidelberg experience with IOERT in 25 patients with retroperitoneal sarcoma *(24)*. Complete resection with tumor-free margins was achieved in 55% of the patients with 29% of the patients having microscopic and 16% macroscopic residual disease. Only 11 patients received IOERT with a mean dose of 18 Gy. Eight of the 11 patients also received EBRT with a mean dose of 40.4 Gy.

Results were compared to a group of 14 patients treated in the 3 yr prior to IOERT use, who received EBRT alone after resection. In both groups the predominant failure was loco-regional and there was no significant difference between the groups. These investigators concluded that there was no significant difference in the effectiveness of IOERT compared to conventional radiotherapy, although a decrease in toxicity was seen with the use of IOERT.

Table 6
Central Sarcoma IOERT, Pamplona: Disease Relapse vs Prognostic Factors

Prognostic Factor	No. Pts.	Local Relapse		Distant Metastasis	
		No.	(%)	No.	(%)
Disease Status					
Primary	17	3	(18)	6	(35)
Recurrent	13[a]	11[a]	(85)	7	(54)
Size (max diam)					
<10 cm	18	5	(28)	7	(39)
≥10 cm	12	9	(75)	6	(50)
Residual Disease					
≤micro	21	7	(33)	8	(38)
macro (gross)	9	7	(78)	5	(56)

[a]7 had EBRT for primary lesion to site of subsequent recurrence; no further EBRT feasible, Calvo et al. *(25,26).*

4.4.4. PAMPLONA IOERT SERIES

4.4.4.1. Patient Group. Calvo et al. reported the results of the Pamplona Sarcoma series at the International IORT meeting in Lyon in 1994 *(25)* (Table 2). A total of 64 patients with sarcoma had received IOERT—34 with extremity lesions (primary 23, recurrent 11) and 30 with central lesions.

In a recent report, Calvo et al. presented the results of IOERT for the 30 patients with soft-tissue sarcomas of central anatomical sites *(26).* These included tumor locations in the retroperitoneum in eight cases, pelvis in five, trunk in 10, gluteus in four, head and neck in two, and scalp in one. Of the entire group, 13 had recurrent lesions and 17 had primary tumors. Of the 13 retroperitoneal or pelvic tumors, 6 were recurrent, and 7 primaries.

4.4.4.2. Treatment Methods. All patients underwent maximum resection and received IOERT of 10–20 Gy with energies ranging from 6 to 20 MeV. EBRT was given to 23 patients (40–50 Gy at 1.8–2 Gy/fraction) excluding the 7 patients who had received previous EBRT for the primary lesion. Patients with high-grade tumors also received chemotherapy consisting of ifosfamide, dacarbazine, and adriamycin. Chemotherapy was given preoperatively in five patients and as maintenance treatment in 12. A gross total marginal resection was accomplished in 21 patients, and gross residual remained in the other 9 patients.

4.4.4.3. Results. Disease relapse as a function of various prognostic factors is seen in Table 6. Both local recurrence and distant metastases occurred with higher frequency in the 13 patients who presented with local relapse (7 of 13 had received prior EBRT and were treated only with maximal resection and IOERT at time of local relapse). Other factors predicting for an increased risk of local relapse were lesion diameter of >10 vs ≤10 cm and gross (macroscopic) vs microscopic residual after maximal resection. Local control overall was 53% with better local control in patients with microscopic residual disease (67%) vs gross residual (22%). Local control also depended on tumor size: 72% for tumors ≤10 cm and 28% for tumors > 10 cm. For the eight patients with retroperitoneal tumors, the median follow-up was 25 mo. Of these, five developed a local recurrence, two developed distant metastasis in addition to local recurrence, and three are NED at 35, 38, and 63 mo.

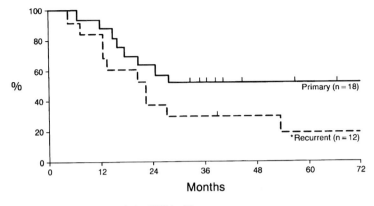

*7 had EBRT for primary lesion; no further EBRT feasible

Fig. 4. Overall survival in primary (n = 18) versus recurrent sarcomas (n = 12) in Pamplona analysis (modified from F. C. Calvo et al. [25]).

With a median follow-up of 25 mo, the OS for the entire group was 36%. Five-year actuarial survival appeared better in the patients who presented with primary vs recurrent lesions at 53% vs 20% (Fig. 4). The difference in survival between the Pamplona and Mayo series in patients with recurrent disease may be related to the fact that a higher percentage of patients in the Pamplona series had received prior EBRT.

Severe toxicity was experienced in 7 of 30 patients. Of the eight retroperitoneal patients, three had severe complications consisting of acute enteritis, chronic enteritis, and neuropathy.

5. CONCLUSIONS AND FUTURE POSSIBILITIES

The natural history of retroperitoneal sarcoma after resection is characterized by a high rate of local recurrence, clearly indicating the need for adjuvant treatment. On the basis of the NCI randomized trial, however, use of adjuvant EBRT without IORT after marginal resection could be questioned, since the rate of tumor-bed relapse with adjuvant EBRT in that trial was 80% (EBRT doses ≤55 Gy) (12,13), which is equivalent to surgery-alone results. In addition, small-bowel tolerance was unacceptable in the EBRT-alone patients in that series. The excellent salvage of patients with recurrent disease in the Mayo IOERT analyses further supports this stance.

A preferable approach for patients with locally advanced primary or locally recurrent disease is to give preoperative EBRT (with or without concomitant chemotherapy) after thin-needle biopsy and perform the resection at an institution that has the capability of giving an IORT supplement with IOERT or HDR-IORT (27,28, and Chapter 19). Treatment programs of EBRT with surgery and IORT have been evaluated at a number of centers in the United States, Europe, and Asia. The data is convincing that local control in the retroperitoneum is improved when IORT is utilized as a component of treatment. Its ultimate benefit in improving overall survival is unknown because of the small numbers of patients treated by this modality and the presence of only one small controlled trial (Table 2).

Local, regional, and distant failures are still common in spite of combination treatment with EBRT, resection, and IORT emphasizing the need for further improvement in local therapy and an effective systemic treatment. For high- and moderate-grade retroperito-

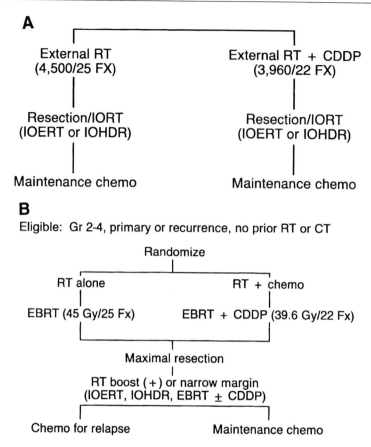

A

External RT
(4,500/25 FX)

External RT + CDDP
(3,960/22 FX)

Resection/IORT
(IOERT or IOHDR)

Resection/IORT
(IOERT or IOHDR)

Maintenance chemo

Maintenance chemo

B

Eligible: Gr 2-4, primary or recurrence, no prior RT or CT

Randomize

RT alone

RT + chemo

EBRT (45 Gy/25 Fx)

EBRT + CDDP (39.6 Gy/22 Fx)

Maximal resection

RT boost (+) or narrow margin
(IOERT, IOHDR, EBRT ± CDDP)

Chemo for relapse

Maintenance chemo

Fig. 5. Potential multi-institutional trials. **(A)** Phase 2 studies testing EBRT with or without con-comitant cisplatin (CDDP) and maintenance postoperative multidrug chemotherapy. **(B)** Potential phase 3 international trial testing the addition of concurrent cisplatin and maintenance multidrug chemotherapy to aggressive local treatment (EBRT, maximal resection, IORT boost with IOERT or HDR-IORT or postoperative supplement with EBRT).

neal sarcomas, it would be reasonable to develop pilot studies which combine chemo-therapy with preoperative EBRT, maximal resection, and IORT. The rationale for this is based on positive survival results in a randomized Italian study testing the addition of multidrug chemotherapy to maximal local treatment for extremity sarcomas (see Chapter 20 and Ref. 30). When regimens with appropriate tolerance are defined in multiinstitu-tional phase 2 studies (Fig. 5A), it would be pertinent to conduct phase 3 studies testing the addition of chemotherapy to EBRT, maximal resection, and IORT (Fig. 5B). This may require an international effort under the aegis of the ISIORT.

REFERENCES

1. Cody HS 3d, Turnbull AD, Fortner JG, and Hajdu SI. The continuing challenge of retroperitoneal sarcomas, *Cancer,* **47** (1981) 2147–52.
2. Dalton RR, Donohue JH, Mucha P Jr, et al. Management of retroperitoneal sarcomas, *Surgery,* **106** (1989) 725–33.
3. Karakousis CP, Gerstenbluth R, Kontzoglou K, and Driscoll DL. Retroperitoneal sarcomas and their management, *Arch. Surg.,* **130** (1995) 1104–1109.

4. Kilkenny JW 3rd, Bland KI, and Copeland EM 3rd. Retroperitoneal sarcoma: the University of Florida experience, *J. Am. Coll. of Surg.,* **182** (1996) 329–39.

5. McGrath PC, Neifeld JP, Lawrence W Jr, et al. Improved survival following complete excision of retroperitoneal sarcomas, *Ann. Surg.,* **200** (1984) 200–204.

6. Storm FK and Mahvi DM. Diagnosis and management of retroperitoneal soft-tissue sarcoma, [*Review*] *Ann. Surg.,* **214** (1991) 2–10.

7. Fein DA, Corn BW, Lanciano RM, et al. Management of retroperitoneal sarcomas: does dose escalation impact on locoregional control?, *Int. J. Radiat. Oncol. Biol. Phys.,* **31** (1995) 129–134.

8. Tepper JE, Suit HD, Wood WC, et al. Radiation therapy of retroperitoneal soft tissue sarcomas, *Int. J. Radiat. Oncol. Biol. Phys.,* **10** (1984) 825–830.

9. Suit HD and Spiro I. Role of radiation in the management of adult patients with sarcoma of soft tissue, *Semin. Surg. Oncol.,* **10** (1994) 347–356.

10. Jaques DP, Coit DG, Hajdu SI, and Brennan MF. Management of primary and recurrent soft tissue sarcoma of the retroperitoneum, *Ann. Surg.,* **212** (1990) 51–59.

11. Alvarenga JC, Ball ABS, Fisher C, et al. Limitations of surgery in the treatment of retroperitoneal sarcoma, *Br. J. Surg.,* **78** (1991) 912–916.

12. Kinsella TJ, Sindelar WF, Lack E, et al. Preliminary results of a randomized study of adjuvant radiation therapy in resectable adult retroperitoneal soft tissue sarcomas., *J. Clin. Oncol.,* **6** (1988) 18–25.

13. Sindelar WF, Kinsella TJ, Chen PW, et al. Intraoperative radiotherapy in retroperitoneal sarcomas. Final results of a prospective, randomized, clinical trial, *Arch. Surg.,* **128** (1993) 402–410.

14. LeCouteur RA, Gillette EL, Powers BE, et al. Peripheral neuropathies following experimental intraoperative radiation therapy (IORT), *Int. J. Radiat. Oncol. Biol. Phys.,* **17** (1989) 583–590.

15. Kinsella TJ, DeLuca AM, Barnes M, et al. Threshold dose for peripheral neuropathy following intraoperative radiotherapy (IORT) in a large animal model, *Int. J. Radiat. Oncol. Biol. Phys.,* **20** (1991) 697–701.

16. Hoekstra HJ, Sindelar WF, and Kinsella TJ. Surgery with intraoperative radiotherapy for sarcomas of the pelvis girdle: a pilot experience, *Int. J. Radiat. Oncol. Biol. Phys.,* **15** (1988) 1013–1016.

17. Willett CG, Suit HD, Tepper JE, et al. Intraoperative electron beam radiation therapy for retroperitoneal soft tissue sarcoma, *Cancer,* **68** (1991) 278–283.

18. Gunderson LL, Nagorney DM, McIlrath DC, et al. External beam and intraoperative electron irradiation for locally advanced soft tissue sarcomas, *Int. J. Radiat. Oncol. Biol. Phys.,* **25** (1993) 647–656.

19. Petersen I, Haddock M, Donohue J, et al. Use of intraoperative electron beam radiation therapy (IOERT) in the management of retroperitoneal and pelvic soft tissue sarcomas, *ASTRO Abst. Int. J. Radiat. Oncol. Biol. Phys.,* **36** (1996) 184.

20. Kiel KD, Won WH, Witt RT, et al. Preliminary results of protocol RTOG 85-07: Phase II of intraoperative radiation for retroperitoneal sarcomas, In Abe M and Takahashi M (eds.), *Intraoperative Radiation Therapy. Proceedings of the Third International Symposium of Intraoperative Radiation Therapy,* Pergamon, New York, 1991, pp. 371–372.

21. Pelton JJ, Lanciano RM, Hoffman JP, et al. The influence of surgical margins in advanced cancer treated with intraoperative radiation therapy (IORT) and surgical resection, *J. Surg. Oncol.,* **53** (1993) 60–65.

22. Bussieres E, Stockle EP, Richaud PM, et al. Retroperitoneal soft tissue sarcomas: a pilot study of intraoperative radiation therapy, *J. Surg. Oncol.,* **62** (1996) 49–56.

23. Dubois JB, Debrigode C, Hay M, et al. Intra-operative radiotherapy in soft tissue sarcomas, *Radiother. Oncol.,* **34** (1995) 160–163.

24. Willeke F, Eble MJ, Lehnert T, et al. [Intraoperative radiotherapy within the treatment concept of retroperitoneal soft tissue sarcomas]. [German] Chirurg, **66(9)** (1995) 899–904.

25. Calvo FA, Azinovic I, Martinez R, et al. IORT in soft tissue sarcomas: 10 years experience, *Hepato-Gastroenterology,* **41** (1994) 4.

26. Calvo FA, Azinovic I, Martinez R, et al. Intraoperative radiotherapy for the treatment of soft tissue sarcomas of central anatomical sites, *Radiat. Oncol. Invest.,* **3** (1995) 90–96.

27. Donath D, Clark B, Evans M, and Brown K. Postoperative adjuvant HDR brachytherapy in the treatment of poor prognosis soft tissue sarcoma (meeting abstract), *Lyon Chirurgical* **89** (1993)151.

28. Nag S, Olson T, Ruymann F, et al. High-dose-rate brachytherapy in childhood sarcomas: a local control strategy preserving bone growth and function, *Med. Pediatr. Oncol.,* **25** (1995) 463–469.

29. Nambisan RN, Karakousis CP, Holyoke ED, and Dougherty TJ. Intraoperative photodynamic therapy for retroperitoneal sarcomas, *Cancer,* **61** (1988) 1248–1252.

30. Pieci P, Frustaci S, DePaoli, et al. (for the Italian Cooperative Group). Localized high grade soft tissue sarcomas of the extremities in adults: preliminary experience of the Italian Cooperative Study Group. Abstract in Proceedings of the Connective Tissue Oncology Society. April 1997.

19 HDR-IORT for Retroperitoneal Sarcomas

Louis B. Harrison, Lowell Anderson, Carol White, and Murray F. Brennan

CONTENTS

INTRODUCTION
MATERIALS AND METHODS
RESULTS
CONCLUSIONS
REFERENCES

1. INTRODUCTION

It has been clearly documented that complete resection plus radiation therapy can locally control the overwhelming majority of soft-tissue sarcomas of the extremity and superficial trunk *(1–18)*. In this regard, the radiation-therapy approach can be either by external beam, brachytherapy, or a combination of both *(1–18)*. The value of adjuvant brachytherapy over surgery alone for high-grade lesions has been demonstrated in a prospective randomized trial at Memorial Sloan Kettering Cancer Center (MSKCC) *(19,20)*. Suit *(2,3,9,12)* has demonstrated excellent local control for low-grade lesions using surgery with external-beam irradiation (EBRT). Other investigators have successfully employed a combination of adjuvant EBRT and brachytherapy *(8,10,11,17,18)*. Local control rates between 80 and 100% have been reported when both surgery and radiotherapy are properly integrated.

Sarcomas arising in the retroperitoneum have been a far different story *(21–25)*. The extent of these lesions has made complete resection difficult, with gross or microscopic disease left behind in a high percentage of cases. In addition, the proximity of normal organs, such as viscera and major vascular structures, has made the delivery of therapeutic doses of postoperative EBRT problematic. To deliver adequate doses of EBRT (>60 Gy) to most patients would result in unacceptable toxicity. The delivery of doses of irradiation that are acceptable to abdominal and retroperitoneal organs are suboptimal for tumor control as discussed in Chapter 1. This therapeutic dilemma is unfortunate, and better strategies are needed.

From: *Current Clinical Oncology: Intraoperative Irradiation: Techniques and Results*
Edited by: L. L. Gunderson et al. © Humana Press, Inc., Totowa, NJ

Table 1
Breakdown of Patients by Histology

Histology	Number of Patients
Liposarcoma	20
Leiomyosarcoma	3
MFH[a]	3
Spindle cell sarcoma	3
Leiomyoblastoma	1
Mesenchymona	1
Myosarcoma	1
TOTAL	32

[a]MFH = malignant fibrous histiocytoma.

For these reasons, a new approach to retroperitoneal sarcomas was developed at MSKCC. In addition to standard surgery, high-dose-rate intraoperative irradiation (HDR-IORT) has been added. This portion of the irradiation is delivered at the time of surgery, with normal organs displaced out of the field. When moderate-dose postoperative EBRT is added, the bowel dose remains within acceptable limits, but the tumor bed receives both the HDR-IORT dose *and* the EBRT portion, bringing this area to a more therapeutic level. Preliminary data using HDR-IORT for colorectal cancers have already been reported *(26–28)*. The purpose of this chapter is to report the initial experience using this approach for retroperitoneal sarcoma, and to use this as a basis for future strategies.

2. MATERIALS AND METHODS

2.1. Patient Group

Between November, 1992 and December, 1996, 32 patients with retroperitoneal sarcoma were treated at MSKCC on a prospective protocol. There were 19 males and 13 females whose ages ranged from 24 to 79 yr (median 58). Twelve patients presented with primary retroperitoneal sarcomas, having never received prior therapy, whereas 20 patients presented with locally recurrent disease, having had prior surgery with or without irradiation. Table 1 shows the distribution of patients by histology. In all, 20 patients had high-grade lesions, whereas 12 had low-grade tumors. Tumor size ranged from $5 \times 5 \times 1$ cm to $49 \times 45 \times 35$ cm, with a median size of $20 \times 12.5 \times 11$ cm. Therefore, by any criteria, this would be considered a challenging group of patients. Follow-up in these patients has ranged from 1–40 mo, with median follow-up of 15 mo.

2.2. Treatment Factors

2.2.1. SURGERY

The treatment program consists of surgery and radiotherapy. The entire operative procedure takes place in a specially designed operating room that is appropriately shielded for the delivery of the HDR-IORT using a high-dose-rate remote afterloading machine. The details of the design of this facility, applicator system, treatment planning algorithms, and so on have been previously reported *(26,27)* and are discussed in Chapters 5 and 6 of this textbook. All patients underwent grossly complete resections, although five

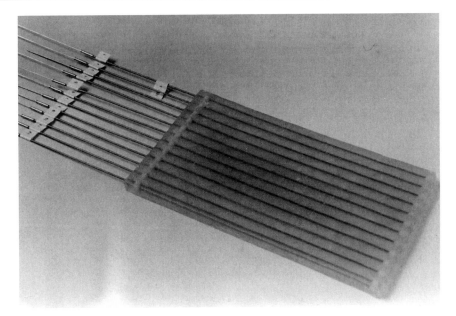

Fig. 1. Harrison-Anderson-Mick (HAM) applicator.

patients were known to have inadequate procedures by virtue of clinically obvious (and pathologically documented) positive microscopic margins.

After the resection is accomplished, normal organs are displaced from the tumor bed, exposing the area to be treated, utilizing appropriate retractors. Metallic clips are placed on the field to demarcate the target region. This generally consists of the resected tumor bed plus a 2–3 cm margin. The extent of margin is sometimes limited by obvious proximity of normal tissue such as spinal cord.

2.2.2. HDR-IORT

With normal tissue maximally retracted, and the target area exposed, an appropriately sized Harrison-Anderson-Mick (HAM) applicator is placed *(26,27)* (Fig. 1) onto the contour of the target area for the delivery of HDR-IORT. With appropriate packing and suturing (when needed), the applicator is assured to be in good position. Because the HAM applicator is transparent, it is easy to make certain that the clipped area is properly covered. Appropriate lead shielding discs can then be strategically interposed between the treated area and nearby normal tissue to enhance their protection. Figures 2–4 show clinical examples.

The set-up procedure for HDR-IORT has also been extensively described *(26,27)*. With the applicator in position, connection tubing is placed to connect the applicator to the HDR remote after-loading machine. A stabilizing bar is often used to maximize the steadiness of the system. When feasible, a fluoroscopy unit is brought into the operating room, and a plain film is taken for documentation purposes. In many cases, this is not feasible, and not performed.

With the system in place, HDR-IORT treatment is ready to proceed. Using a prepared dosimetry atlas that has been described *(26,27)*, the dwell times of the sources are determined. A total dose of 15 Gy at tissue depth of 5–10 mm is delivered, depending upon

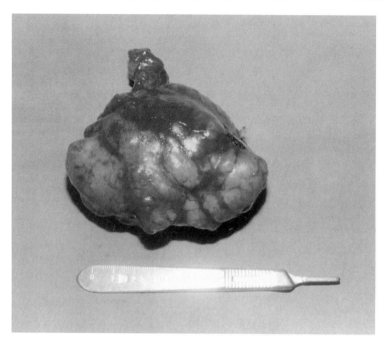

Fig. 2. Resected retroperitoneal sarcoma.

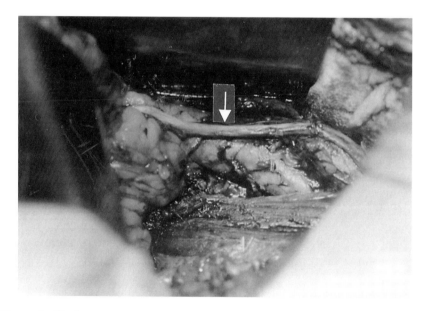

Fig. 3. Tumor bed in the retroperitoneum. The psoas muscle is the tumor bed. The liver and kidney are retracted superiorly (left of figure) and the bowel is moved inferiorly (right of figure). The ureter is seen medially (top of figure, arrow).

the exact anatomical situation. The HAM applicator has a 5-mm thickness on the treatment surface, so the dose is prescribed to 5–15 mm from the sources. Everyone leaves the room, and the treatment is delivered. The patient and the actual treatment delivery are monitored by remote control cameras by the anesthesiologist, radiation oncologist, and

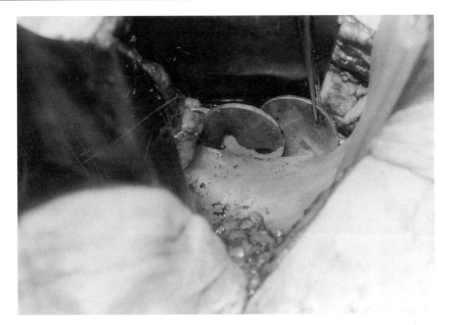

Fig. 4. The same view as Fig. 3, except with the HAM applicator in place, and lead discs protecting the ureter.

surgeon. Once the treatment has been completed, the entire apparatus is dismantled, and the applicator is removed. The surgeon then resumes the case, and closes the patient.

2.2.3. EBRT

After postoperative recovery, usually within 4–6 wks, the patient returns for external beam irradiation (EBRT). A total of 45 Gy in 25 fractions over 5 wks is usually delivered using a linear accelerator of 6 MeV photons or higher. Typically, the patient is turned on his/her side, to help displace bowel away from the target area. Either AP/PA or other planned portal arrangements are used to help minimize dose to normal tissue yet adequately covering the target area. There have been some patients in whom a tissue expander or a special mesh was also placed during the operative procedure, as a further attempt to protect normal organs from the field of irradiation.

3. RESULTS

3.1. Feasibility of Procedure

Table 2 lists the various procedural and treatment-related parameters and times, including HDR-IORT delivery time, IORT procedure time, estimated blood loss from entire surgery/IORT procedure, entire procedure time, hospital stay, and so on. As can be seen, depending upon the size of the region treated, activity of the HDR source, and complexity of the set-up procedure, 30 min to over 4 hr are added to the OR time because of the HDR-IORT procedure, with a median of 110 min. It should be remembered that the entire procedure is done in the same OR, obviating the need for patient transport, which is required with most IOERT programs. There was one case in which an afterloader malfunction made the delivery of HDR-IORT impossible. That patient received a permanent ^{125}I implant instead to three contiguous sites. In all other cases, IORT was delivered

Table 2
HDR-IORT for Retroperitoneal Sarcoma:
Procedural and Treatment Related Parameters

Parameter	Number
Complete resection	27 patients
Incomplete resection	5 patients
Estimated blood loss	1000 cc
	range 150–4700 cc
Hospital stay	9 d
	range 5–50 days
OR time	445 min
	range 205–730 min
IORT procedure	110 min
	range 32–250 min
IORT delivery time	54 min
	range 17–165 min
IORT dose	15 Gy at 0.5 cm.
	from the surface of the HAM applicator

as planned. In no instance did the treatment require interruption for anesthesiology problems or patent monitoring issues. Also, in no instance was the anatomy of the tumor bed unsuitable for treatment using this technique.

3.2. Disease Control and Survival

3.2.1. LOCAL CONTROL

Crude local control has been obtained in 10 of 12 (83%) primary cases, and 15 of 20 (75%) recurrent cases, for an overall crude local control to date of 15 of 32 patients (78%). The actuarial 2-yr local control is 92% for primary cases and 73% for recurrent cases, for an overall 2-yr actuarial local control of 80%.

3.2.2. DISEASE-FREE SURVIVAL

Crude disease-free survival (DFS) is 8 of 12 (67%) for primary cases and 14 of 20 (70%) for recurrent cases with an overall crude DFS of 22 of 32 (69%). The actuarial 2-yr DFS is 66% for primary cases and 69% for recurrent cases, for an overall 2-yr actuarial DFS rate of 66%.

3.2.3. OVERALL SURVIVAL

Crude overall survival (OS) is 10 of 12 (83%) for primary cases and 15 of 20 (75%) for recurrent cases, for an overall crude survival of 25 of 32 (78%). The 2-yr actuarial survival is 81% for primary cases and 67% for recurrent cases, for an overall rate of 72%.

3.2.4. COMPLICATIONS

Table 3 lists the treatment-related complications for the primary cases, whereas Table 4 lists them for the recurrent cases. There were two patients in the recurrent-disease category who died as a result of treatment. Complications from all causes are listed together, as it is frequently impossible to differentiate pure surgical from pure radiotherapeutic

Table 3
HDR-IORT Severe Complications: Primary Presentation

Gastric dysmotility, left flank and abdominal wound cellulitis, pleural effusion, poor bowel function	1 patient
Gastrointestinal fistula/femoral nerve palsy (mild)	1 patient
Ileocolic intussception	1 patient
Total – 3/11 (27%)	

Table 4
HDR-IORT Complications: Recurrent Disease Presentation

Small bowel obstruction	1 patient
Femoral nerve palsy (mild)	1 patient
Renal failure, severe bleeding gastritis, prolonged ileus, bowel necrosis, and death	1 patient
Dehydration, acidosis, stroke	1 patient
Retroperitoneal abscess, sepsis, renal artery bleed, fistula, and death	1 patient
Total – 5/15 (33%)	

complications. Complications are frequently multifactorial in nature, and grouping them together seems most appropriate.

4. CONCLUSIONS

The early local control, disease-free survival, and overall survival in the MSKCC HDR-IORT series for retroperitoneal sarcoma are very encouraging and compare favorably with results obtained in IOERT series from National Cancer Institute *(29)*, Massachusetts General Hospital *(9,30)* and Mayo Clinic *(31,32)* *(see* Chapter 19). Complications are not insignificant with the HDR-IORT approach, but appear acceptable, given the complex and challenging patient population under study. More follow-up is needed to assess the long-term stability of these preliminary data.

REFERENCES

1. Ellis F. Tumor bed implants at the time of surgery, removable interstitial implants with iridium-192, in Hilaris BS (ed). *Afterloading: 20 Years Experience, 1955–1975.* Proceedings of the 2nd International Symposium on Radiation Therapy. New York, NY, Memorial Sloan Kettering Cancer Center, 1975, pp. 125–32.
2. Suit H, Russell W, Martin R. Management of patients with sarcoma of soft tissue in an extremity. *Cancer,* **31** (1973) 1247–1255.
3. Suit H, Russell W, Martin R. Clinical and histopathologic parameters and response to treatment. *Cancer,* **35** (1975) 1478–1483.
4. Lindberg R, Martin R, Romsdahl M, et al. Conservative surgery and radiation therapy for soft tissue sarcomas, in *Management of Primary Bone and Soft Tissue Tumors.* Chicago, IL, Year Book Medical, 1977, pp. 289–298.
5. Rosenberg SA, Kent H, Costa J, et al. Prospective randomized evaluations of the role of limb-sparing surgery, radiation therapy and adjuvant chemoimmunotherapy in the treatment of adult soft tissue sarcomas. *Surgery,* **84** (1978) 62–69.
6. Hilaris B, Shiu M, Nori D, et al. Perioperative brachytherapy and surgery in soft tissue sarcomas, in Hilaris BS (ed), *Brachytherapy Oncology 1982.* New York, NY, Memorial Sloan-Kettering Cancer Center, 1982, pp. 111–117.

7. Shiu M, Turnbull A, Nori D, et al. Control of locally advanced extremity soft tissue sarcomas by function saving resection and brachytherapy, *Cancer*, **53** (1984) 1385–1392.

8. Hilaris B, Shiu M, Nori D, et al. Limb-sparing therapy for locally advanced soft tissue sarcomas, *Endocur. Hypertherm. Oncol.*, **1** (1985) 17–24.

9. Suit H, Mankin H, Wood W, et al. Preoperative, intraoperative, and postoperative radiation in the treatment of primary soft tissue sarcoma, *Cancer*, **55** (1985) 2659–2667.

10. Roy H, Hilaris B, Nori D, et al. Adjuvant endocurietherapy in the management of liposarcomas of the extremities, *Endocur. Hypertherm. Oncol.*, **2** (1986) 29–35.

11. Karakousis C, Emrich L, Rao U, et al. Feasibility of limb salvage and survival in soft tissue sarcomas, *Cancer*, **57** (1986) 484–491.

12. Suit H, Mankin H, Wood W, et al. Treatment of patients with stage M0 soft tissue sarcoma, *J. Clin. Oncol.*, **6** (1988) 854–862.

13. Willett C, and Suit H. Limited surgery and external beam irradiation in soft tissue sarcoma, Adv. Oncol., **5** (1989) 26–29.

14. Shiu M, Hilaris B, Harrison L, et al. Brachytherapy and function saving resection of soft tissue sarcoma arising in the limb, *Int. J. Radiat. Oncol. Biol. Phys.*, **21** (1991) 1485–1492.

15. Zelefsky M, Nori D, Shiu M, et al. Limb salvage and soft tissue sarcomas involving neurovascular structures using combined surgical resection and brachytherapy, *Int. J. Radiat. Oncol. Biol. Phys.*, **19** (1990) 913–918.

16. Zelefsky M, Harrison L, Shiu M, et al. Combined surgical resection and iridium 192 implantation for locally advanced and recurrent desmoid tumors, *Cancer*, **67** (1991) 380–384.

17. Gemer L, Trowbridge D, Neff J, et al. Local recurrence of soft tissue sarcoma following brachytherapy, *Int. J. Radiat. Oncol. Biol. Phys.*, **20** (1991) 587–592.

18. Schray M, Gunderson L, Sim F, et al. Soft tissue sarcoma—integration of brachytherapy, resection and external irradiation, *Cancer*, **66** (1990) 451–456.

19. Pisters PWT, Harrison LB, Leung DH, Woodruff JM, Casper ES, and Brennan MF. Long term results of a prospective randomized trial evaluating the role of adjuvant brachytherapy in soft tissue sarcoma, *J. Clin. Oncol.*, **14** (1996) 859–868.

20. Harrison LB, Franzese F, Gaynor J, and Brennan F. Long-term results of a prospective randomized trial of adjuvant brachytherapy in the management of completely resected soft tissue sarcomas of the extremity and superficial trunk, *Int. J. Radiat. Oncol. Biol. Phys.*, **27** (1993) 259–265.

21. Cody H, Turnbull A, Fortner J, and Hajdu S. The continuing challenge of retroperitoneal sarcomas, *Cancer*, **47** (1981) 2147–2152.

22. Tepper JE, Suit HD, Wood WC, Proppe KH, Harmon D, and McNulty P. Radiation therapy of retroperitoneal sarcoma, *Int. J. Radiat. Oncol. Biol. Phys.*, **10** (1984) 825–830.

23. Harrison LB, Gutierrez E, and Fischer JJ. Retroperitoneal sarcomas: the Yale experience and a review of the literature, *J. Surg. Onc.*, **32** (1986) 159–164.

24. Jacques D, Coit DG, Hajdu S, and Brennan MF. Management of primary and recurrent soft-tissue sarcoma of the retroperitoneum, *Ann. Surg.*, **212** (1990) 51–59.

25. Catton CN, O'Sullivan B, Kotwall C, Cumming B, Hao Y, and Fornasier V. Outcome and prognosis in retroperitoneal soft tissue sarcoma, *Int. J. Radiat. Oncol. Biol. Phys.*, **29** (1994) 1005–1010.

26. Harrison LB, Enker WE, and Anderson L. High dose rate intraoperative radiation therapy for colorectal cancer—part 1, *Oncology*, **9** (1995) 679–683.

27. Harrison LB, Enker WE, and Anderson L. High dose rate intraoperative radiation therapy for colorectal cancer—part 2, *Oncology*, **9** (1995) 737–741.

28. Harrison LB, Minsky B, Enker W, et al. High dose rate intraoperative radiation therapy (HDR-IORT) as part of the management strategy for locally advanced primary and recurrent rectal cancer, *Int. J. Radiat. Biol. Phys.*, **39S** (1997) 168.

29. Sindelar WF, Kinsella TJ, Chen PW, DeLaney TF, Tepper JE, Rosenberg SA, and Glatstein E. Intraoperative radiotherapy in retroperitoneal sarcomas, *Arch. Surg.*, **128** (1993) 402–410.

30. Willett CG, Suit HD, Tepper JE, et al. Intraoperative electron beam radiation therapy for retroperitoneal soft tissue sarcomas, *Cancer*, (1991) 278–283.

31. Gunderson LL, Nagorney DM, McIlrath DC, et al. External beam and intraoperative electron irradiation for locally advanced soft tissue sarcomas, *Int. J. Radiat. Oncol. Biol. Phys.*, **25** (1993) 647–656.

32. Petersen I, Haddock M, Donohue J, et al. Use of intraoperative electron beam radiation therapy (IOERT) in the management of retroperitoneal and pelvic soft tissue sarcomas, ASTRO Abst. *Int. J. Radiat. Oncol. Biol. Phys.*, **36(1)** (1996) 184.

20 Extremity and Trunk Soft Tissue Sarcomas

EBRT With or Without IORT

Ivy A. Petersen, Felipe A. Calvo,
Leonard L. Gunderson, Douglas J. Pritchard,
Ignacio Azinovic, Michael G. Haddock,
and Michael Eble

CONTENTS

1. BACKGROUND

1.1. Extremity Sarcomas

The treatment of extremity soft tissue sarcomas has evolved from amputation or radical compartmental resections to limb-salvage therapy utilizing a combination of wide local excision and radiation therapy. Results from a randomized study done by the National Cancer Institute and multiple retrospective reviews have revealed no significant survival advantage with the more radical surgical procedure *(1–4)*.

Two randomized studies of wide local excision with or without irradiation have been reported recently. The Memorial Sloan Kettering Cancer Center (MSKCC) study was done using brachytherapy alone for high-grade soft tissue sarcomas and revealed a local control advantage for the patients who received the irradiation without any survival compromise *(5)*. The NCI study involved patients with both high- and low-grade sarcomas who were randomized to be observed or treated with postoperative external beam irradiation (EBRT). Local control was significantly improved with the addition of irradiation but no survival difference was observed *(6)*.

From: *Current Clinical Oncology: Intraoperative Irradiation: Techniques and Results*
Edited by: L. L. Gunderson et al. © Humana Press, Inc., Totowa, NJ

Table 1
Outcome of Truncal vs. Extremity Soft Tissue Sarcomas

Study (ref)	No. of Patients	Local Control	
		Trunk	Extremity
Brant (16)	48	83%	92%
Cakir (14)	67	65%	74%
Dinges (15)	83	71%	83%
LeVay (13)	269	71%	84%
Coindre (18)	445	67%	71%

Local control of sarcomas following wide local excision and radiation therapy is high with control rates of greater than 85% at 5 years (2,7,8). In addition functional outcome in patients with the limb-salvage approach has been excellent in the majority of patients (9–12). Despite these results with limb-salvage therapy the foremost issue in the management of these tumors is how to individualize the treatment in order to enhance tumor control in the most challenging tumors and still provide the patient with the best functional outcome.

1.2. Truncal Sarcomas

Truncal soft tissue sarcomas are less common than their extremity counterparts and their management varies considerably. Review of the literature would suggest that overall local control is poorer in this population in comparison to extremity soft tissue sarcomas (Table 1). Local recurrence rates after surgery alone have been reported as low as 27% in one institution, but have been as high as 45% in other series (13–17). Local failure problems in these tumors may be related to several factors such as the difficulty obtaining clear resection margins and the lack of uniform use of adjuvant irradiation. Adjuvant irradiation is often employed only if adequacy of margins or resectability are in question, but may not be as frequently used as in extremity sarcomas (17–20).

2. RATIONALE OF TREATMENT OPTIONS

2.1. Surgical Factors

2.1.1. EXTENT OF RESECTION

With the use of a more conservative limb-sparing surgical approach, investigators have endeavored to define the adequacy of the surgery necessary to obtain good local control. Enneking categorizes the surgical procedures into four types: intracapsular excision, marginal excision, wide excision, and radical amputation (21).

Optimally all patients with soft tissue sarcomas will undergo a wide excision, which entails removal of the tumor with a margin of normal surrounding tissue in continuity. Unfortunately, what constitutes an adequate amount of normal surrounding tissue has not been well established because different investigators use variable definitions of necessary distance from tumor to resection margin and large prospective analyses correlating local control with the amount of radial margin are lacking. Furthermore, a marginal surgical resection, where just the tumor and pseudocapsule are excised, may be the only feasible option when the sarcoma abuts structures such as the neurovascular bundle or bone without resulting in additional significant morbidity. In addition, the necessary

Table 2
Outcome of Extremity Soft Tissue Sarcomas after Limb Salvage Surgery and Radiotherapy

Study (ref)	No. of Patients	Local Control	Disease-free[a] or Overall Survival[b]
NCI (1)	27	80%	71%[a]
MSKCC (25)	1041	75%	76%[b]
Mayo (7)	189	86%	65%[b]
MGH (2)	220	86%	70%[a]
Toronto (53)	62	95%	—
Royal Marsden (54)	175	—	72%[b]

Table 3
Influence of Pathologic Margins on Outcome

Study (ref)	No. of Patients	Local Control		Survival	
		Margin (+)	Margin (−)	Margin (+)	Margin (−)
Pisters (25)	1041	60%	80%[a]	69%	78% (DSS)
Heslin (29)	168	63%	89%[a]	—	—[a] (DSS)
Tanabe (26)	95	62%	91%	70%	65% (OS)
Bell (27)	100	50%	92%[a]	—	—
Sadoski (30)	132	83%	97%[a]	—	—
Sawyer (7)	172	82%	88%	78%	67%
Marcus (33)	76	79%	90[b]	—	—

[a]$p < 0.05$.
[b]$p = 0.076$.

margins for patients receiving adjuvant irradiation is unknown. A wide excision may be unnecessary if adequate irradiation is administered, just as radical excision may eliminate or at least diminish the need for adjuvant irradiation (7,22). Wide excision alone is reported to have local relapses up to 50% and marginal excision results in an even higher local recurrence rate of up to 90% (6,23–25).

The addition of irradiation to either a wide or marginal excision yields excellent local control rates as outlined in Table 2. Despite adjuvant treatment, the type of surgical procedure remains important. Review of the Helinski University experience revealed a 3-yr local control rate of 76% in patients receiving inadequate surgery despite the addition of irradiation as compared to 92% in patients having optimal surgery (26). The advantage of the use of an intraoperative irradiation (IORT) approach for supplemental irradiation to EBRT is the more precise definition of narrow margins at the time of resection, which enables investigators to define and treat the area of highest risk.

2.1.2. Pathologic Margins

Multiple studies in patients with extremity sarcomas have suggested that the surgical pathologic margins are important indicators of local control (7,27–31) (Table 3). Pister reviewed over a thousand patients with primary extremity soft tissue sarcomas who were treated with surgery with or without irradiation or chemotherapy at MSKCC (25). In this population the local control rate at 5 yr was 80% and 60% for negative and positive margins, respectively ($p = 0.0001$). However, this difference in margins status did not influence overall survival.

In a select population of patients from MSKCC treated on a randomized study of resection with or without high dose brachytherapy, local recurrences occurred in 28 of the 135 patients with negative surgical margins *(5)*. Twenty of these occurred in the surgery alone arm (20 of 72 or 28%) as compared to 8 of 63 (13%) in the adjuvant brachytherapy arm ($p = 0.04$). However, among the 29 patients with microscopically positive margins, five each occurred in the brachytherapy and surgery alone population ($p = 0.99$).

A second series from the same institution reviewed the patients who received low-dose brachytherapy with or without additional EBRT *(32)*. Positive margins resulted in a 59% local control rate in the patients who were treated with adjuvant brachytherapy alone as compared to 90% in the group that received EBRT in addition to brachytherapy ($p = 0.08$). In this review negative surgical margins status resulted in a statistically improved local control on both univariate and multivariate analysis.

In a series in which patients had resection with or without irradiation, LeVay found pathologic margins significantly related to local control as well with 7% local failures in patients with wide margins of greater than 4 cm as compared to 17% for those with surgical margins within 1 cm *(13)*. Gross residual resulted in a local failure rate of 77%. The addition of irradiation to resection resulted in a local control rate of 88% after clear margins of greater than 1 cm and 78% in those with microscopically positive margins. In comparison, those who underwent surgery only had local control rates of 84% for clear margins and 54% for microscopically positive margins.

In data from the NCI on low-grade nonretroperitoneal soft tissue sarcomas, the surgical margin was a statistically significant factor of local recurrence in multivariate analysis *(33)*. Furthermore, of the four patients with positive margins who did not receive irradiation, 3 recurred locally compared to 1 of 10 with positive margins who did receive irradiation. This suggests that, although margins are significant factors in local recurrence, they may have a smaller role in the setting of adjuvant irradiation. In conclusion, data would suggest that the status of resection margins are important with or without the addition of irradiation.

Surgical management of truncal sarcomas applies the same principles as for extremity tumors. However, wide excisions are less frequent owing to the approximation of vital organs or structures. Margins have also been important in the management of sarcomas at this site as well *(34)*. As a result, adjuvant radiotherapy should be considered in most soft tissue sarcomas of the trunk. IORT in this population can be technically challenging. Owing to the dose limitations of organs inside the thorax or abdomen, the addition of afterloading brachytherapy, intraoperative high-dose-rate brachytherapy (HDR-IORT), or IOERT as a supplement to EBRT allows for increased flexibility in the delivery of optimal irradiation dose to tumors at these sites.

2.2. Irradiation (EBRT, IORT)

2.2.1. IRRADIATION DOSE VS LOCAL CONTROL

Historically, high doses of irradiation have been used to achieve local control of soft tissue sarcomas. The importance of delivering a minimum radiation dose has recently been recognized as critical to the long-term local control of soft tissue sarcomas *(35,36)*.

Fein evaluated 67 patients with extremity soft tissue sarcomas treated with limb-salvage surgery and postoperative irradiation *(35)*. Improved local control was significantly associated with total doses >62.5 Gy. The 5-yr local control was 96% vs 78% in patients receiving >62.5 Gy and ≤62.5 Gy, respectively ($p = 0.04$). This outcome was seen despite the higher dose patients having larger tumors and a higher percentage having high-grade lesions and positive margins.

Mundt also found a dose response in his review of 64 patients with extremity soft tissue sarcomas. His analysis showed a significantly improved local control with total doses > 60 Gy, but no difference was seen for those receiving 60–63.9 Gy vs 64–68 Gy *(36)*.

In a review of 189 patients at the Mayo Clinic, Sawyer et al. found that the use of an irradiation boost, whether given by EBRT, brachytherapy, or IOERT, resulted in significantly improved survival and local control *(7)*. The 5-yr freedom from local relapse was 88% in the patients receiving a boost as compared to 75% in those who did not ($p = 0.02$). Actuarial 5-yr survival was 69% in the patients receiving an irradiation boost as compared to 45% in those not boosted to a higher dose ($p < 0.001$).

The radiation oncologist must therefore consider the importance of delivering a high dose of irradiation in order to optimally control the sarcoma. Dubois compared the total dose received from EBRT and IORT in patients with extremity, truncal, or retroperitoneal sarcomas and showed a significant difference in the doses for those who failed locally compared to those locally controlled *(37)*.

2.2.2. FUNCTIONAL OUTCOME

Local tumor control is only one factor important in the outcome evaluation of patients with extremity and truncal soft tissue sarcomas. Functional endpoints are also paramount to the outcome after definitive local treatment. Multiple methods of evaluating patient status after limb-salvage therapy have been reported *(9,11,12,21)*. These evaluations in retrospective series have shown that the functional outcome after limb-salvage surgery and irradiation is excellent in 68–86% of patients. In contrast the recent report from the NCI where patients were randomized to surgery with or without the addition of postoperative EBRT suggested a poorer quality-of-life outcome for the patients who underwent adjuvant EBRT *(6)*. In this prospective study joint motion as well as transient decrease in limb strength and edema were found to be statistically worse after EBRT. However, it is important to note that the global quality of life and performance of activities of daily living were not significantly different, suggesting that the long-term toxicity of irradiation is outweighed by the improved local control.

In addition, several authors have noted a correlation between irradiation dose and fibrosis. {13,70} Karasek reported that the volume of tissue that received ≥ 55 Gy more strongly correlated with increased fibrosis and skin changes *(10)*. Robinson reviewed 54 patients and found that in 14 who received doses > 60 Gy the functional outcome was worse. Given this information, the high EBRT dose delivered in the recent NCI report may partly account for the poorer quality of life outcome in this study *(6)*. Further reduction in volume of irradiated tissue may be feasible if the EBRT is delivered preoperatively and there is a measurable response of the tumor prior to resection. This may allow for both a reduced surgery and a smaller irradiation boost field. Tumor regression has been reported in up to 60% of patients receiving preoperative irradiation *(16)*. All of this can theoretically result in improved functional outcome of the patient.

2.3. Chemotherapy

Chemotherapy has been utilized in the treatment of soft tissue sarcomas of the extremity and trunk. Most prospective randomized studies have not shown any benefit from this approach *(38–42)*.

A recent study from the Italian Cooperative Group, however, suggests a benefit for adding chemotherapy to optimal local treatment for high-grade extremity sarcomas in adults *(43)*. High-risk patients were defined as having a grade 3 or 4 sarcoma, spindle or pleomorphic, deeply seated, larger than 5 cm, in an extremity or girdle. After local treatment and stratification for size and presentation (primary or recurrent), patients were randomized to receive or not very intensive adjuvant chemotherapy consisting of five cycles of epirubicin (120 mg/m^2 in 2 d), ifosfamide (9 g/m^2 in 5 d) with mesna, and G-CSF (300 mg/d sc d 8/15), q 3 weeks. On interim analysis of 104 patients (51 control, 53 chemotherapy adjuvant), statistically significant advantages were found for both disease-free and overall survival ($p = 0.001$ and 0.005, respectively).

In recurrent disease situations or when resection possibilities are limited or not feasible, it may be reasonable to consider chemotherapy in conjunction with local irradiation. This approach may facilitate a subsequent resection *(19)*.

Because of the excellent control rates with surgery and irradiation, it is difficult to ascertain whether chemotherapy has added to the local control of soft tissue sarcomas despite the response rates that have been demonstrated. However, the Southeastern Cancer Study Group did report a local control rate of 98.5% at a median of 7-yr follow-up after treatment with preoperative doxorubicin and irradiation *(44)*. These data suggest a benefit from the addition of concurrent chemotherapy and deserves further evaluation.

3. IORT—RATIONALE, TECHNICAL FACTORS

3.1. IORT—Theoretical Benefit

The use of IOERT or brachytherapy as an supplement to EBRT allows the radiation oncologist to achieve high local radiation doses to optimize local control, while reducing the volume of tissue taken to that high dose. In addition there are theoretical reasons for an intraoperative approach. An obvious advantage is the ability to clearly define the surgical bed and high-risk region(s). Radiobiologically, the treatment may be given to a field that may be oxygen deprived after surgery and hence more radioresistant. Intraoperative or perioperative treatment can deliver the additional irradiation dose in a rapid fashion before significant fibrosis can occur. Furthermore, in patients who receive their EBRT component preoperatively with supplemental EBRT postoperatively, the overall treatment time and interval between irradiation segments can be quite long. In comparison the irradiation given at the time of surgery (IOERT) or shortly following (brachytherapy) can significantly shorten the overall treatment time. Overall treatment time has been shown to be significant in long-term outcome in several other malignancies including cervix and head and neck tumors but has not yet been correlated with outcome for soft tissue sarcomas.

The diversity of locations found in soft tissue sarcomas of the extremity and trunk add further technical limitations in delivering optimal irradiation doses. A large number of soft tissue sarcomas are found in the thigh *(45)*. Although the thigh itself is not a difficult site to irradiate, the proximal thigh and limb girdle regions remain a high risk site for local recurrence given the close proximity of the neurovascular bundle. Surgical series have demonstrated the high risk of recurrence at this site because of the difficulty obtaining adequate surgical resection *(23)*. High-dose EBRT to this site puts the patient at risk for neurologic, lymphatic, and/or vascular compromise. When the sarcoma extends into the pelvis, bowel and bladder dose limitations also need to be considered.

3.2. IOERT and HDR-IORT—Technical Aspects

At first glance the use of IOERT in extremity or truncal sites may not seem as challenging as intraabdominal treatment. Often the field may be a relatively flat surface that is readily accessible to the use of an IOERT applicator. However, there are several problems that can arise in these patients. The issues that are utilized to determine the optimal irradiation boost include the size of the field, the anatomical constraints of the treatment site, the area deemed at risk, and the subsequent procedures necessary for closure of the surgical site.

It is not infrequent that the necessary treatment field is large owing to the size of the malignancy. After resection there may be minimal tissue to use for anchoring afterloading tubes for brachytherapy, and this is compounded when muscle transfer flaps are utilized. This may call for large IOERT treatment applicators or abutting treatment fields. In order to accommodate some of these large fields, Mayo Clinic has constructed an 8×20 cm elliptical applicator (Fig. 1). When this size is inadequate to encompass the entire tumor bed, abutting fields have been used. Care must be taken to avoid overlap especially if nerves transverse the two fields. Marking the abutting edges with suture or marking pen may help to ensure that tissues are not overdosed. Further use of lead at the margins of the abutting fields may also be indicated if the clinician feels that the bowing of the electrons at depth may result in unreasonable toxicity.

Anatomical constraints are typical reasons for the use of IOERT instead of afterloading low-dose-rate brachytherapy (Figs. 1–4, pp. 366–371). Tumors that approach the limb girdle are frequently difficult to implant. An example of this situation is a tumor in the proximal medial thigh that would require placement of the brachytherapy tubes into the perineum or into the pelvis in order to cover adequately the high risk site. Another example of technical concern is the trunk, where the curvature of the site may make IOERT less optimal in terms of dose homogeneity. In this situation the use of HDR-IORT may be better suited to contour the trunk and minimize the dose to deep structures within the chest or abdominal cavity.

The ability to evaluate intraoperatively the resected site is a major advantage for the radiation oncologist, allowing for the full definition of any narrow margins. Examination of the gross surgical specimen and the frozen section microscopic evaluation both help to define the area(s) of concern. Sometimes the high risk site is only on one side of the resected tumor specimen and other times there may be multiple narrow margins. If multiple margins are in question, then a brachytherapy or EBRT boost approach may be more appropriate. When only the deep margins are critical, then the IOERT option may be more suitable.

Finally, the radiation oncologist needs to consider the subsequent plans for closure of the incision when determining the best irradiation boost method. Patients who have large tumors or tumors in sites where extra tissue is not available to allow primary closure frequently require either a skin graft or a myocutaneous flap *(46)* (Fig. 5, p. 372). If an afterloading low-dose-rate brachytherapy boost were used, this may make the myocutaneous flap more difficult or impossible to perform. Furthermore, the delivery of the irradiation to the risk site(s) may be jeopardized by the placement of the flap. In this situation an alternative approach would be the use of IOERT or HDR-IORT to deliver the

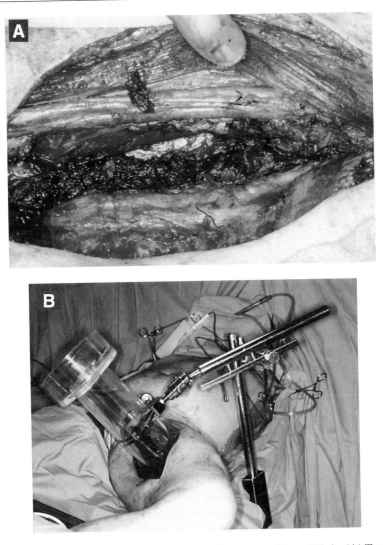

Fig. 1. Use of IOERT for proximal anteriomedial thigh sarcoma, Mayo Clinic. **(A)** Tumor bed after gross total resection. **(B)** 8 × 20 cm lucite applicator in position. **(C)** Applicator docked to linear accelerator. **(D)** Ready for treatment.

irradiation boost and then proceed with the plastic surgery procedure of choice. Use of a postoperative EBRT boost after a myocutaneous transfer or skin graft is probably the least optimal because of the additional time frame needed for adequate healing before postoperative treatment could be initiated.

4. RESULTS WITH IOERT OR HDR-IORT

4.1. Mayo IOERT Series

4.1.1. Patient Group

Between June 1986 and September 1995, 91 patients with limb girdle or extremity soft tissue sarcomas were treated at Mayo Clinic using IOERT as a component of their therapy. The tumor and patient characteristics are outlined in Table 4 (see p. 373) *(47)*.

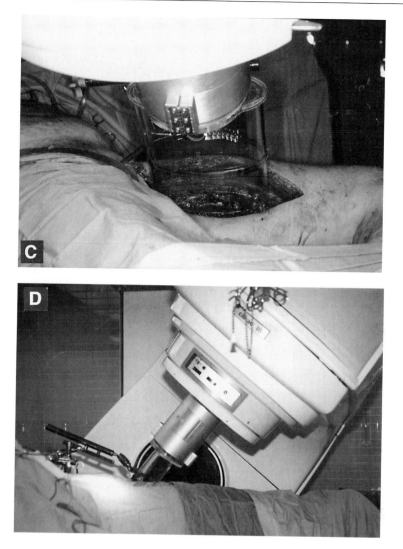

Fig. 1. (*continued*)

4.1.2. SURVIVAL

With a median follow-up of 2.9 yr (range 0.5–10 yr) the 3-yr overall survival was 76%. The survival was better for patients with low-grade lesions with an 87% 3-yr survival compared to 70% for the high-grade lesions (*p* = 0.06). Size of tumor also predicted for outcome with patients with tumors ≤ 5 cm and > 5 cm having a 96% and 65% 3-yr overall survival, respectively (*p* = 0.009).

4.1.3. LOCAL CONTROL

Local control was comparable to other series using EBRT and brachytherapy with a 92% local control at 3 yr. The disease status of the patient impacted local control with a 95% local control in primary lesions vs 81% in recurrent tumors (*p* = 0.014). This local control difference did not translate into a survival difference between these two populations. Although survival was influenced by the grade and size of the sarcoma, the local

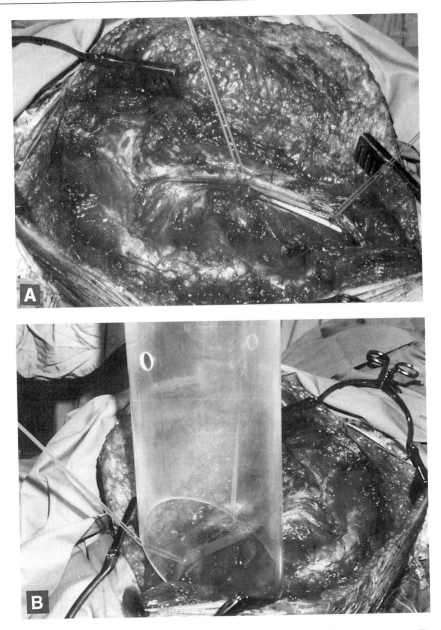

Fig. 2. Tumor bed after resection of a large (8 × 10 × 11 cm) gluteal soft tissue sarcoma, Pamplona. **(A)** Note that the sciatic nerve is in close contact with the surgical resection margin of the sarcoma mass. **(B)** IOERT applicator in position to treat the high risk region (postresected) including the sciatic nerve (12 cm diameter applicator, 30° bevel end).

control was virtually identical. Local and or central (within the IOERT field) failures were seen in six patients. Four of the six had concurrent failures in regional or distant sites.

4.1.4. TOXICITY

Toxicity prospectively charted as nerve tolerance was of particular concern in this population. Only two patients (2%) experienced severe peripheral neuropathy. Moderate neuropathy was seen in an additional nine patients (10%).

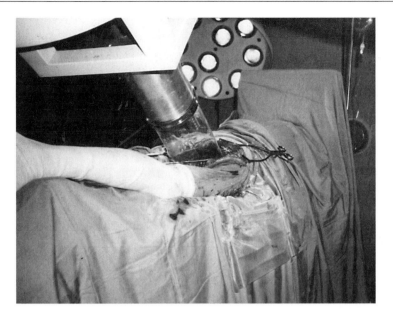

Fig. 3. IOERT procedure after a posterior thigh compartment resection in Pamplona for a large liposarcoma (13 × 10 × 9 cm). The applicator size used is 15 cm diameter with a 45° bevel end.

4.2. Pamplona IOERT Series

4.2.1. PATIENT GROUP

Calvo et al. reported the results of the Pamplona Sarcoma series at the International IORT meeting in Lyon in 1994 *(49)*. Of 64 patients with sarcoma who had received IOERT, 34 had extremity lesions and 30 had central lesions.

Results in 33 evaluable patients with extremity lesions were presented in detail at the ESTRO 94 meeting (personal communication F. Calvo). These included tumor locations in the upper extremity in 6 (arm 2, forearm 4) and lower extremity in 27 (thigh 20, knee-popliteum 4, leg 3). Lesion size was ≤ 5 cm in 5 patients, > 5 cm in 28. Of the 33 evaluable patients, 22 had primary lesions and 11 presented at time of local relapse. Lesion grade was unknown in only 1 patient. In the remaining 32, grade was 1–2 in 19 patients and grade 3 in the remaining 13.

4.2.2. TREATMENT METHODS

All patients underwent maximum resection and received IOERT of 10–20 Gy (10 to 12 Gy, 15 patients; 15 Gy, 21 patients; 20 Gy, 8 patients). A gross total resection was accomplished in all patients with wide margins in 22 patients, close (≤ 5 mm) in 5, and microscopically involved in 2 patients. IOERT energies ranged from 6 to 20 MeV (6–9 MeV, 28 patients; 12–15 MeV, 14 patients; 18–20 MeV, 2 patients). EBRT was given to 30 patients (40–50 Gy at 1.8, 2 Gy/Fx) excluding 3 patients who had received previous EBRT for the primary lesion. Thirteen patients with high-grade tumors received chemotherapy consisting of Ifosfamide, Dacarbazine, and Adriamycin.

4.2.3. RESULTS

Disease relapse was analyzed as a function of primary vs recurrent disease presentation. Distant metastases occurred with equal frequency in both groups of patients (4 of

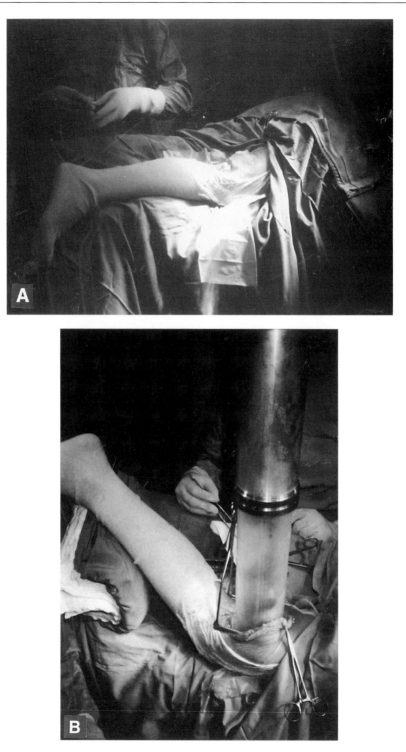

Fig. 4. (A) Pre-IOERT applicator positioning in a patient after resection of a popliteal synovial sarcoma. **(B)** View with the applicator in place to encompass the surgical bed region. Note that the distal leg has been elevated to facilitate exposure of the popliteal fossa. **(C)** Field within a field IOERT technique in which the second treatment component is given after retraction of the peripheral nerve out of the IOERT field (white tissue structure visible in the center of the photo).

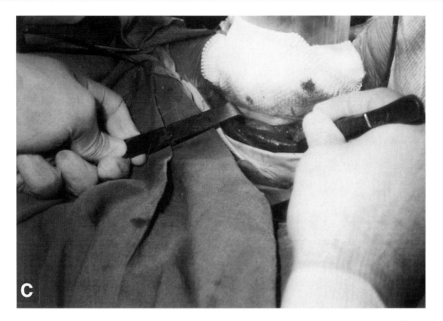

Fig. 4. (*continued*)

22 primary or 18%, 3 of 11 recurrent or 27%). All distant metastases were to the lungs. Local relapse occurred in only 1 of 11 (9%) who presented at time of local relapse vs 3 of 22 (14%) with primary lesions (1-LF alone; 2 LF & DM). Three of 4 local relapses were salvaged with further surgery.

With a median follow-up of 36 months, overall survival for the total group was 76% (25 of 33 alive). Three-year actuarial survival appeared better in the patients who presented with primary vs recurrent lesions at 77% vs 54%.

4.3. Heidelberg IOERT Series

4.3.1. PATIENT GROUP AND TREATMENT METHODS

Twenty-five patients with stage IIB–IIIB extremity sarcoma had IOERT as a component of treatment between 7/91–5/95 (liposarcoma $n = 10$, malignant fibrous histiocytoma $n = 9$; miscellaneous, $n = 6$; recurrent sarcomas $n = 10$; stage IIB, $n = 11$, IIIA, $n = 4$, IIIB $n = 10$) (49). Microscopic residual disease after surgery was found in 4 of the 25. Site was as follows: upper arm, 5; lower arm, 4; thigh, 12; knee, 3; and calf, 1.

The mean IORT dose was 15.3 Gy (range 15–20 Gy), using a mean field size of 11.3 cm (5–26 cm). External beam irradiation was started 3–6 wk postoperatively for a mean dose of 44 ± 5 Gy.

4.3.2. RESULTS

After a mean follow-up of 26.8 months, a 92% local control rate was achieved. The local control rate was independent of the extent of the surgical margin and tumor stage. Lymph node relapse was documented in two patients. Distant failure was observed in five patients, all had stage III disease.

The overall and disease-free actuarial survival were 77% and 58% at 4 yr. For patients with stage III disease, overall and disease-free survival were reduced to 60% and 42%, respectively, because of the rate of distant metastasis.

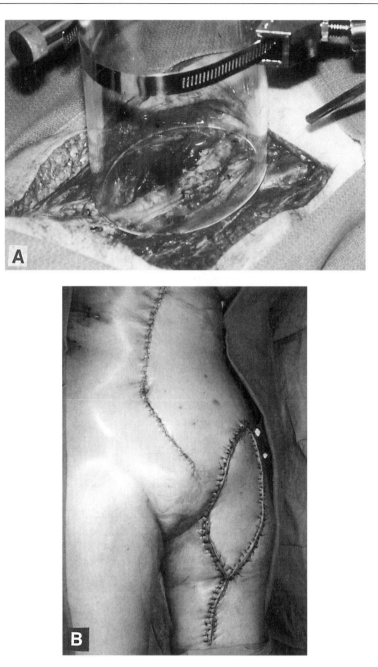

Fig. 5. Use of IOERT when mycocutaneous flap is planned for wound closure after resection of soft tissue sarcoma in left groin, Mayo Clinic. (**A**) Lucite applicator in place over neurovascular bundle. (**B**) Rectus abdominus reconstruction of left groin defect.

Perioperative wound healing problems occurred in three patients requiring additional surgical treatment in one. In six patients a late adverse effect was observed (marked decrease in limb excursion, 2; bone fracture, 2; neuropathy, 1; osteitis and delayed wound healing, 1).

Table 4
Mayo IOERT Patient Characteristics Extremity
and Limb Girdle Soft Tissue Sarcomas

Characteristic (N = 91)	No. (%)
Grade	
Low	29 (32)
High	62 (68)
Median size in cm (range)	9 (0.7–33)
Disease status	
Primary	74 (81)
Recurrent	17 (19)
Site	
Lower extremity limb girdle	17 (19)
Lower extremity	54 (59)
Upper extremity	20 (22)
External beam irradiation	
Preoperative	69 (76)
Postoperative	19 (21)
None	3 (3)
Median dose in Gy (range)	50.4 (19.8–59.4)
IOERT	
Median dose in Gy (range)	10 (7.5–20)

4.4. University of Kansas IOERT Series

4.4.1. PATIENT GROUP AND TREATMENT METHODS

Twenty-eight patients with soft tissue sarcomas diagnosed between June 1987 and December 1989 were treated with wide local excision and IOERT (50). Twenty-one of the 28 patients received additional EBRT. The primary site of tumor was in the extremities in 22 patients.

The dose of IORT delivered ranged from 12.5 to 20 Gy calculated at the 90% isodose line. The energy of electrons ranged from 9 to 16 MeV depending on the thickness of tissue to be treated. EBRT doses ranged from 40 to 50 Gy.

4.4.2. RESULTS

Median follow-up at time of presentation was 21 months. Six patients had failed locally, three patients failed within the IORT field (two despite EBRT), and three patients failed marginally or outside of the IOERT/EBRT fields. Five additional patients developed distant disease primarily in the lung. Nineteen patients were alive without evidence of disease.

4.5. IORT Tolerance

Complications in the patients who have had IOERT as a component of their treatment have indicated that this is a safe modality. Information on the functional status after the use of IOERT is limited and at best suggests no significant difference in outcome, although further evaluation is warranted (7,47,48).

Gemer reported five acute and three long-term complications in the 28 patients treated at University of Kansas Medical Center (50). Four of the five acute complications were

Table 5
Outcome for Different Treatment Approaches of Soft Tissue Sarcomas of the Trunk and Extremity

Study (ref)	No. of Patients	Local Control			DFS		
		Preop RT	Postop RT	Brachy	Preop RT	Postop RT	Brachy
UMN (55)	112	83%	91%	—	56%	67%	—
MGH (2)	220	90%	85%	—	65%	73%	—
MSKCC (5)	164	—	—	82%	—	—	84% (DSS)
Mayo (7)	189	90%	81%	—	—	—	—

* EBRT ± brachytherapy or IOERT

wound related. Two of the chronic complications were neurologic and felt to be directly related to the IOERT with or without surgical resection. The remaining chronic complication was leg edema.

In the Pamplona analysis, neuropathy was reported in 5 of 23 evaluable patients (22%). Neuropathy occurred in 3 of 10 patients with nerve in the IOERT field vs 2 of 13 with nerve excluded (48).

5. SUMMARY AND FUTURE POSSIBILITIES

5.1. Standard Therapeutic Approaches

A variety of approaches are used in the treatment of truncal and extremity soft tissue sarcomas. These include surgery alone, surgery with EBRT done either preoperatively or postoperatively, and surgery combined with brachytherapy with or without EBRT.

5.1.1. SURGERY ALONE RESULTS

Outcome from surgery alone depends significantly on the extent of that surgery. Radical compartment resection or amputation results in excellent local control of greater than 90% in most series. {NCI, Enneking/Simon, Markhede} However, this results in substantial morbidity and diminished quality of life for the patient due to loss of limb or loss of substantial function. In patients in whom a lesser surgery is not feasible due to extent of disease, this may be the only option. Overall survival depends on the size and grade of the primary tumor. Use of surgery alone should be in a very select group of patients with small, low-grade sarcomas. Select cases of small high-grade sarcomas such as those in subcutaneous sites may be amenable to surgery alone without local control compromise (22,51,52).

5.1.2. SURGERY AND ADJUVANT IRRADIATION

Adjuvant irradiation has decreased the need for radical surgical procedures without compromising the longevity of the patient. Local control is not as high as in patients who have more radical surgical procedures but the functional outcome is superior to amputation. Table 5 displays the results of multiple studies with preoperative or postoperative EBRT with or without brachytherapy or IOERT supplements. Most of these series have used EBRT solely in order to deliver doses of greater than 60 Gy to the tumor site. The Scandinavian series have generally used irradiation only in patients who have marginal resections and have not had significant local recurrence problems in their surgery alone

Table 6
IORT as a Supplement to EBRT and Resection in Truncal and Extremity Soft Tissue Sarcomas

Series Author, Inst. (ref)	No. Pts (No. Relapse)	Local Recurrence No (%)	Actuarial LC (%)	Overall Survival
Petersen, Mayo (47)	91 (37)	6 (7)	92% (3 yr)	76% (3 yr)
Primary	74 (31)	3 (4)	95%	76%
Recurrent	17 (6)	3 (17)	81%	72%
Calvo, Pamplona (48)	33 (9)	4 (12)	88% (3 yr)	76% (3 yr)
Primary	22 (5)	3 (14)	—	77%
Recurrent	11 (4)	1 (9)	—	54%
Elbe, Heidelberg (49)	25 (7)	2 (8)	—	77% (4 yr)
Stage II	11	1 (9)	—	100
Stage III	14	1 (7)	—	60
Gemer, U Kansas (50)	28 (8)	4 (14)	not given	68% DFS
Dubois, Montpelier (37)	18	0	—	—
Takahashi (56)	38 (20)	14 (37)	not given	—
Bergman (57)	7	1	not given	—

* 3 of 4 salvaged with further surgery.
Relapse = any tumor progression (local or distant), LC = local control.

patients (52). MSKCC has published substantial experience with the use of brachytherapy as the sole component of irradiation in a randomized study and found results for patients with negative margin high-grade sarcomas to be comparable to the use of EBRT, with or without brachytherapy as a treatment component.

5.1.3. FUNCTIONAL OUTCOME

Functional outcome has been measured by a multitude of devices (7,10–12). Although these methods of evaluation differ significantly, the end results have been favorable throughout. Quality of life evaluation is currently being evaluated in patients receiving treatment on a NCIC study and should be helpful in defining which patients are most compromised with the use of high-dose external beam irradiation.

5.2. Newer Therapeutic Approaches—IOERT or HDR-IORT

In the last decade the use of IORT, delivered primarily as electron beam irradiation (IOERT), or intraoperative high-dose-rate brachytherapy (HDR-IORT) has been used in the treatment of extremity and truncal soft tissue sarcomas. Results that have been published with the use of IOERT indicate that the outcome of patients who have received this treatment are similar to other approaches (7,47–50) (see Table 6).

5.3. Future Possibilities

Further improvements in local control of soft tissue sarcomas are not likely to be great given the high local control rate currently achieved. However, there is sufficient opportunity to optimize the use of all treatment modalities including chemotherapy, radiation therapy, and surgery. In view of the positive survival results in the recently presented Italian trial by Picci et al. (43), more routine use of adjuvant chemotherapy may need to be considered for patients with high-grade lesions.

IOERT allows for other options in the delivery of high dose irradiation to the site of highest risk as determined intraoperatively. Complication rates are low if this modality is used in moderately low doses. The use of HDR-IORT would allow similar flexibility in dose delivery. Further exploration of the use of these modalities is warranted especially in sites where postoperative EBRT would entail significant morbidity because of treating a large volume of tissue.

REFERENCES

1. Rosenberg SA, Tepper J, Glatstein, E, et al. The treatment of soft-tissue sarcomas of the extremities. *Ann. Surg.,* **196** (1982) 305–315.
2. Suit HD, Mankin HJ, Wood WC, et al. Treatment of the patient with stage M0 soft tissue sarcoma, *J. Clin. Oncol.,* **6** (1988) 854–862.
3. Suit HD, Russell WO, and Martin RG. Management of patients with sarcoma of soft tissue in an extremity, *Cancer,* **31** (1973) 1247–1255.
4. Lindberg RD, Martin RG, Romsdahl MM, and Barkley HT. Conservative surgery and postoperative radiotherapy in 300 adults with soft-tissue sarcomas. *Cancer,* **47** (1981) 2391–2397.
5. Pister PWT, Harrison LB, Leung DHY, et al. Long-term results of a prospective randomized trial of adjuvant brachytherapy in soft tissue sarcoma, *J Clin Oncol.,* **14** (1996) 859–868.
6. Yang JC, Chang AE, Baker AR, et al. Randomized prospective study of the benefit of adjuvant radiation therapy in the treatment of soft tissue sarcomas of the extremity, *J. Clin. Oncol.,* **16** (1998) 197–203.
7. Sawyer TE, Petersen IA, Pritchard DJ, et al. External beam sequencing and boost irradiation issues in the treatment of soft tissue sarcomas of the extremities, *Radiology,* **193(P)** (1994) (Abstract) 309.
8. Harrison LB, Franzese F, Gaynor JJ, and Brennan MF. Long-term results of a prospective randomized trial of adjuvant brachytherapy in the management of completely resected soft tissue sarcomas of the extremity and superficial trunk, *Int. J. Radiat. Oncol. Biol. Phys.,* **27** (1993) 259–265.
9. Bell RS, O'Sullivan B, Davis A, Langer F, and Fornasier VL. Functional outcome in patients treated with surgery and irradiation for soft tissue tumours, *J. Surgical Oncol.,* **48** (1991) 224–231.
10. Karasek K, Constine LS, Rosier R. Sarcoma therapy: Functional outcome and relationship to treatment parameters, *Int. J. Radiat. Oncol. Biol. Phys.,* **24** (1992) 651–656.
11. Robinson MH, Spruce L, Eeles R, et al. Limb function following conservative treatment of adult soft tissue sarcoma, *Eur. J. Cancer,* **27** (1991) 1567–1574.
12. Wexler AM, Eilber FR, and Miller TA. Therapeutic and functional results of limb salvage to treat sarcomas of the forearm and hand, *J. Hand. Surg.,* **13** (1988) 292–296.
13. LeVay J, O'Sullivan B, Catton C, et al. Outcome and prognostic factors in soft tissue sarcoma of the adult, *Int. J. Radiat. Oncol. Biol. Phys.,* **27** (1993) 1091–1099.
14. Cakir S, Dincbas FO, Uzel O, Koca SS, Okkan S. Multivariate analysis of prognostic factors in 75 patients with soft tissue sarcoma, *Radiother. and Oncol.,* **37** (1995) 10–16.
15. Dinges S, Budach V, Budach W, Fledmann HJ, Stuschke M, and Sack H. Local recurrence of soft tissue sarcomas in adults: in retrospective analysis of prognostic factors in 102 cases after surgery and radiotherapy, *Eur. J. Cancer,* **30A** (1994) 1636–1642.
16. Brant TA, Parsons JT, Marcus RB, et al. Preoperative irradiation for soft tissue sarcomas of the trunk and extremities in adults, *Int. J. Radiat. Oncol. Biol. Phys.,* **19** (1990) 899–906.
17. Gordon Mark S, Hajdu Steven I, Bains Manjit S, and Burt Michael E. Soft tissue sarcomas of the chest wall, *J. Thorac. Cardiovasc. Surg.,* **101** (1991) 843–854.
18. Coindre J-M, Terrier D, Binh BN, et al. Prognostic factors in adult patients with locally controlled soft tissue sarcomas: a study of 546 patients from the French Federation of Cancer Centers Sarcoma Group, *J. Clin. Oncol.,* **14** (1996) 869–877.
19. Ryan MB, McMurtrey MJ, and Roth JA. Current management of chest-wall tumors, *Surg. Clin. N. Amer.,* **69** (1989) 1061–1080.
20. Wallner KE, Nori D, Burt M, Bains M, and McCormack P. Adjuvant brachytherapy for treatment of chest wall sarcomas, *J. Thorac. Cardiovasc. Surg.,* **101** (1991) 888–894.
21. Enneking WF, Spanier SS, and Malawer MM. The effect of anatomic setting on the results of surgical procedures for soft parts sarcoma of the thigh, *Cancer,* **47** (1981) 1005–1022.
22. Peabody TD, Monson D, Montag A, Schell MJ, Finn H, Simon MA. A comparison of the prognoses for deep and subcutaneous sarcomas of the extremities, *J. Bone Joint Surg.,* **76** (1994) 1167–1173.

23. Simon MA and Enneking WF. The management of soft-tissue sarcomas of the extremities, *J. Bone Joint Surg.,* **58-A** (1976) 317–327.
24. Markhede G, Angervall L, and Stener B. A multivariate analysis of the prognosis after surgical treatment of malignant soft-tissue tumors, *Cancer,* **49** (1982) 1721–1733.
25. Pister PWT, Leung DHY, Woodruff J, Shi W, and Brennan MF. Analysis of prognostic factors in 1,041 patients with localized soft tissue sarcomas of the extremities, *J. Clin. Oncol.,* **14** (1996) 1679–1689.
26. Wiklund T, Huuhtanen R, Blomqvist C, et al. The importance of a multidisciplinary group in the treatment of soft tissue sarcomas, *Eur. J. Cancer,* **32A** (1996) 269–273.
27. Tanabe KK, Pollock RE, Ellis LM, Murphy A, Sherman N, and Romsdahl MM. Influence of surgical margins on outcome in patients with preoperatively irradiated extremity soft tissue sarcoma, *Cancer,* **73** (1994) 1652–1659.
28. Bell RS, O'Sullivan B, Liu FF, et al. The surgical margin in soft-tissue sarcoma, *J. Bone Joint Surg.,* **71** (1989) 370–375.
29. Herbert SH, Corn BW, Solin LJ, et al. Limb-preserving treatment for soft tissue sarcomas of the extremities, *Cancer,* **72** (1993) 1230–1238.
30. Heslin MJ, Woodruff J, and Brennan MF. Prognostic significance of a positive microscopic margin in high-risk extremity soft tissue sarcoma: implications for management, *J. Clin. Oncol.,* **14** (1996) 473–478.
31. Sadoski C, Suit HD, Rosenberg A, Mankin HJ, and Efird J. Preoperative radiation, surgical margins, and local control of extremity sarcomas of soft tissues, *J. Surgical Oncol.,* **52** (1993) 223–230.
32. Alekhteyar KM, Leung DH, Brennan MF, and Harrison LB. The effect of combined external beam radiotherapy and brachytherapy on local control and wound complications in patients with high-grade soft tissue sarcomas of the extremity with positive microscopic margin, *Int. J. Radiat. Oncol. Biol. Phys.,* **36** (1996) 321–324.
33. Marcus SG, Merino MJ, Glatstein E, et al. Long-term outcome in 87 patients with low-grade soft-tissue sarcoma, *Ann. Surg.,* **128** (1993) 1336–1343.
34. Singer S, Corson JM, Demetri GD, Healey EA, Marcus K, and Eberlein TJ. Prognostic factors predictive of survival for truncal and retroperitoneal soft-tissue sarcoma, *Ann. Surg.,* **221** (1995) 185–195.
35. Fein DA, Lee WR, Lanciano RM, et al. Management of extremity soft tissue sarcomas with limb-sparing surgery and postoperative irradiation: Do total dose, overall treatment time, and the surgery-radiotherapy interval impact on local control?, *Int. J. Radiat. Oncol. Biol. Phys.,* **32** (1995) 969–976.
36. Mundt AJ, Awan A, Sibley GS, et al. Conservative surgery and adjuvant radiation therapy in the management of adult soft tissue sarcoma of the extremities: clinical and radiobiological results, *Int. J. Radiat. Oncol. Biol. Phys.,* **32** (1995) 977–985.
37. Dubois JB, Debrigode C, Gely S, Rouanet P, Saint-Aubert B, and Pujol H. Intra-operative radiotherapy in soft tissue sarcomas, *Radiother. and Oncol.,* **34** (1995) 160–163.
38. Bramwell V, Rouesse J, Steward W, et al. Adjuvant CYVADIC chemotherapy for adult soft tissue sarcoma-reduced local recurrence but no improvement in survival: a study of the European Organization for Research an Treatment of Cancer Soft Tissue and Bone Sarcoma Group, *J. Clin. Oncol.,* **12** (1994) 1137–1149.
39. Alvegård TA, Sigurdsson H, Mouridsen H, et al. Adjuvant chemotherapy with doxorubicin in high-grade soft tissue sarcoma: a randomized trial of the Scandinavian Sarcoma Group, *J. Clin. Oncol.,* **7** (1989) 1504–1513.
40. Antman K, Amato D, Lerner H, et al. Adjuvant doxorubicin for sarcoma: data from the Eastern Cooperative Oncology Group and Dana-Farber/Massachusetts General Hospital studies, *Cancer Treat. Symp.,* **3** (1985) 109–115.
41. Antman K, Suit H, Amato D, et al. Preliminary results of a randomized trial of adjuvant doxorubicin for sarcomas: lack of apparent difference between treatment groups, *J. Clin. Oncol.,* **2** (1984) 601–608.
42. Chang AE, Kinsella T, Glatstein E, et al. Adjuvant chemotherapy for patients with high-grade soft-tissue sarcomas of the extremity, *J. Clin. Oncol.,* **6** (1988) 1491–1500.
43. Picci P, Frustaci S, De Paoli A, et al. Localized high grade soft tissue sarcomas of the extremities in adults: preliminary results of the Italian Cooperative Study. Connective Tissue Oncology Society Meeting 1997 (Abstract).
44. Wanebo HJ, Temple WJ, Popp MB, Constable W, Aron B, Cunningham SL. Preoperative regional therapy for extremity sarcoma, *Cancer,* **75** (1995) 2299–2306.
45. Brennan MF. Management of extremity soft-tissue sarcoma, *Am. J. Surg.,* **158** (1989) 71–78.
46. Cordeiro PB, Neves RI, and Hidalgo DA. The role of free tissue transfer following oncologic resection in the lower extremity, *Ann. Plastic Surg.,* **33** (1994) 9–16.

47. Petersen IA, Haddock MG, Pritchard D, and Gunderson LL. IORT in the management of extremity and limb girdle soft tissue sarcomas, *Front Radiat. Ther. Oncol.,* **31** (1997) 151–152.

48. Calvo FA, Azinovic I, Martinez-Monge R, et al. IORT in soft tissue sarcomas: 10 years experience, *Hepato-Gastroenterol.,* **41** (1994) 4 (Abstract).

49. Elbe MJ, Lehnert T, Schwarzbach M, Ewerbeck V, Herfarth C, and Wannenmacher M. IORT for extremity sarcomas, *Front Radiat. Ther. Oncol.,* **31** (1997) 146–150.

50. Gemer L, Neff J, Smalley S, and Huntrakoon M. The use of IORT in the treatment of soft tissue sarcomas, International IORT meeting, Kyoto, 1990 (Abstract), p. 75.

51. Healey E, Corson J, Demetri G, and Singer S. Surgery alone may be adequate treatment for select stage IA-IIIA soft tissue sarcomas, *J. Clin. Oncol.,* **14** (1995) 517.

52. Rydholm A, Gustafson P, Willen H, and Berg NO. Subcutaneous sarcoma, *J. Bone Joint Surg.,* **73** (1991) 662–667.

53. Wilson AN, Davis A, Bell RS, et al. Local control of soft tissue sarcoma of the extremity: the experience of a multidisciplinary sarcoma group with definitive surgery and radiotherapy, *Eur. J. Cancer,* **30A** (1994) 746–751.

54. Stotter AT, A'Hern RP, Fisher C, Mott AF, Fallowfield ME, and Westbury G. The influence of local recurrence of extremity soft tissue sarcoma on metastasis and survival, *Cancer,* **65** (1990) 1119–1129.

55. Cheng EY, Dusenberry KE, Winters MR, and Thompson RC. Soft tissue sarcomas: preoperative versus postoperative radiotherapy, *J. Surgical Oncol.,* **61** (1996) 90–99.

56. Bergman K, Koh WJ, Conrad E, Collins C, Griffin T, and Laramore G. Intraoperative electron beam therapy for soft tissue sarcomas, *Strahlenther Onkol.,* **168** (1992) 479 (Abstract).

57. Takahashi M, Shibamoto Y, Abe M, Kotoura Y, and Yamamuro T. Intraoperative radiation therapy for soft tissue tumors, *Strahlenther Onkol.,* **168** (1992) 480 (Abstract).

21 IORT for Bone Sarcomas

Felipe A. Calvo, Luis Sierrasesumaga,
Norman Willich, Santiago Amillo,
and José Cañadell

CONTENTS

1. INTRODUCTION

Bone sarcomas are rare entities in clinical oncology, in which the histological subtype and site of involvement define the natural history of the disease and in particular the appropriate treatment strategy *(1)*. Ewing sarcoma is a chemo- and radiation-sensitive disease in which combined-modality therapy (more recently including a surgical component) is mandatory for radical management *(2)*. Osteosarcoma survival rates have been significantly improved by adjuvant chemotherapy and extremity preservation rates by neoadjuvant chemotherapy *(3)*. Other uncommon bone sarcomas such as malignant fibrous histiocytoma (MFH) or chondrosarcoma are considered marginally sensitive to chemotherapy or radiotherapy and the primary radical treatment modality is surgery *(4,5)*. A universal feature in the natural history of bone sarcomas is the tendency to involve the extraosseous soft tissue and neurovascular structures once the tumor growth and infiltration acquires a certain size.

In extremity bones, amputation usually achieves a radical surgical margin in the circumferential and distal dimensions, and the only concern is to assure an adequate proximal margin distance *(6)*. Amputation is being replaced by extremity-preservation surgical procedures. In the case of bone sarcomas this requires bone resection and prosthesis replacement of the operated extremity, which is in part related to the feasibility of muscle removal; the circumferential oncology safe margin is compromised by more limited bone and soft-tissue removal.

Intraoperative irradiation (IORT) with electrons or brachytherapy are available technologies to precisely treat the high-risk or involved surgical margins after extremity

From: *Current Clinical Oncology: Intraoperative Irradiation: Techniques and Results*
Edited by: L. L. Gunderson et al. © Humana Press, Inc., Totowa, NJ

bone-sarcoma resection (8). Both radiation modalities have a comparable accuracy in radiation dose-deposit for the treatment of less than 0.5 cm target-volume thickness. Theoretical advantages are the use of a radiation component of treatment at the time of surgery, which after resection, may allow a decrease or deletion of the need for a fractionated external-beam irradiation (EBRT) treatment component that would be given after the prosthesis or graft has been placed (potential detrimental effect on graft viability and/ or dosimetric uncertainty because of the presence of metallic elements in the radiation field). Finally, IORT during sarcoma surgery, and in particular bone-sarcoma resection, is a suitable situation for the use of field-within-a-field radiation technique, in which a larger area is treated with doses able to control microscopic disease (10–12.5 Gy) yet not exceeding the tolerance dose for dose-sensitive structures (peripheral nerve), and a second reduced-field target region can be defined and treated with an additional dose (5–10 Gy) and either excluding or reducing the volume of dose-limiting tissues.

Bone sarcomas arising in central bones generally have less options for radical surgery, and the need to develop new therapeutic alternatives to promote local control is more evident (9). In this situation IORT is again a feasible technique to complement surgical exposure of unresectable bone tumors (protecting normal uninvolved abdominothoracic organs), postdebulked anatomic regions or a postcurettage surgical bed. The ability to locally control these patients will be related to the integral treatment intensity able to be delivered with the available radiation-therapy modalities (EBRT plus IORT) and the chemotherapy programs integrated in chemosensitive tumors (10,11).

An overview of the IORT-relevant experiences reported in the management of bone-sarcoma patients is described, grouping the data by histological subtypes in which the treatment strategy is considered rather uniform, and the peculiarities of IORT technique and contribution to final results in special situations. The data regarding the experience at the University Clinic of Navarra is an update of the previously published Ewing's sarcoma and osteosarcoma results (12).

2. EWING'S SARCOMA

Ewing's sarcoma is a malignant disease that requires multimodal treatment to obtain high cure rates (13). Irradiation is an important component of the treatment of the primary lesion (14). The reported rates of local control attributed to radiation therapy vary widely (15). Tumor volume and the site of the primary tumor have been related to major differences in local tumor control. Thus isolated local recurrences have been reported in 15% of patients with lesions of the extremities, in 47% with rib primaries, and in 69% with pelvic tumors (16). The rate of local persistence/tumor recurrence, as evaluated by clinical and autopsy findings, was reported to be 35, 25, and 7% in patients treated with primary radiation therapy for central, proximal-extremity, and distal-extremity lesions, respectively (17). Overall rates of local tumor control with radiotherapy are in the region of 90% for lesions less than 8 cm in maximum diameter, and 70% for those more than 8 cm in maximum diameter (18).

Surgical resection has attracted increasing interest in the management of Ewing's sarcoma. Several reports have described improvements in local control and survival with the addition of surgery (16,19–21). With reference to the clinical data available, it has to be noted that surgery in Ewing's sarcoma has been used in selected patients with positive prognostic factors such as lesions of the extremities, small tumor volumes, and a good response to chemotherapy. The use of surgery in the management of Ewing's sarcoma

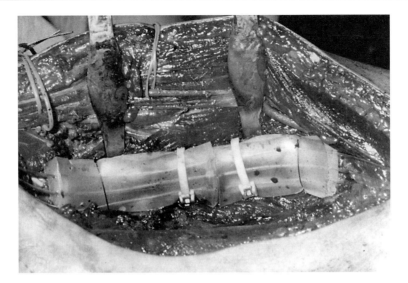

Fig. 1. Flab molded to the high-risk area in HDR-IORT procedure at the University of Münster.

patients simultaneously provides an opportunity to consider the use of IORT as a radiation boost modality in areas of residual disease or at high risk of local recurrence.

The conceptual advantages of the inclusion of IORT in the local treatment of Ewing's sarcoma include the accuracy with which the area at high risk for recurrence can be identified at the time of surgery, the ability to protect normal uninvolved tissues when lesions are located in central anatomic zones (pelvic bones, vertebra, and so on), and the possibility of reducing the total EBRT dose *(22)*.

2.1. HDR-IORT Experience, University of Münster

2.1.1. TREATMENT FACTORS

In cooperation with the Department of Radiotherapy-Radiooncology and the Orthopedic Department of the University of Münster, Germany, the application of high-dose-rate IORT (HDR-IORT) brachytherapy boost after preoperative radiochemotherapy was tested in patients, in whom the surgical margins proved to be close to the tumour. Generally, the brachytherapy applicators were introduced into flab applicators. In a few cases, intraosseous applicators were used. The flab applicator consisted of soft plastic material with a thickness of 1 cm. Parallel longitudinal channels penetrated the material at 1 cm distance from each other. In the channels, tubes were placed and the brachytherapy source could be introduced into these tubes. Different sizes of flab applicators were available depending on the extension of the tumor. Furthermore, the flab could be cut in the operating theater to the necessary size. Because of the flexibility of the material, it was possible to mold the applicator to the *in situ* structures *(23)*. The fitting of the flab was done in the presence of the radiation oncologist and the surgeon (Fig. 1). To avoid an overdose, especially to nerves and vessels, they were distanced by ordinary cloth. No more than 10 Gy was allowed to these critical structures. After the flab had been positioned, the wound was provisionally closed. Perpendicular X-rays of the flab *in situ* were taken with markers in the tubes in order to identify the position of the applicators. The images were digitalized and the isodoses were calculated by the physicist (Fig. 2). For the radiation itself, the anesthetized patient was transported to the radiotherapy department.

Table 1
Tumor and Treatment Characteristics of Ewing's Sarcoma (ES)
Patients Treated with HDR-IORT Brachytherapy at the
University of Münster (July, 1992 to May, 1995)

Characteristics	#	Characteristics	#
Histology		*Tumor volume*	
Ewing's sarcoma	10	<100 mL	4
Atypical ES	5	>100 mL	16
PNET	3		
Extraosseous ES	2	*Dose of brachytherapy*	
Localization		10 Gy	16
Pelvis	9	11 Gy	1
Humerus	4	12 Gy	2
Ulna	1	20 Gy	1
Femur	5		
Fibula	1		

In general, 10 Gy was applied at a distance of 5 mm from the flab surface using an HDR-afterloading device. This was equivalent to a surface dose of approx 20 Gy in unmolded flabs. After the procedure, the patient was brought back to operating theater, the flab applicator was removed, and the wound was closed.

2.1.2. PATIENT GROUP

From July, 1992 to February, 1995, 20 HDR-IORT brachytherapy boosts have been performed. The male to female ratio was 13 to 7. Four patients had tumors smaller than 100 mL, 16 patients had tumors larger than 100 mL. There were 10 Ewing's sarcomas, 5 atypical Ewing's sarcomas, 3 primitive neuroectodermal tumor (PNET) and two extraosseous Ewing's sarcomas. Nine tumors were located in the pelvis, five in the femur, four in the humerus, one in the ulna, and one in the fibula. Six patients had initial metastases, one in the lung, three in the bone, and two with combined pulmonary and osseous manifestations. The tumor characteristics are summarized in Table 1. Eight patients received vincristine, iphosfamide, doxorubicin, actinomycin D (VAIA), 12 patients etoposide plus vincristine, iphosfamide, doxorubicin, actinomycin D (EVAIA) chemotherapy. Two patients had an intralesional resection, 5 patients a marginal resection, and 13 patients a wide resection following the Enneking criteria *(24)*. The radiation doses applied ranged from 10 to 20 Gy with 16 patients receiving 10 Gy measured at 5 mm from the flab surface. The median follow up of the patients was 24 mo (range 14–46 mo). The median operation time including HDR-IORT was 7 h, 45 min (min. 5 h 45 min, max. 10 h, 35 min). On average the brachytherapy procedure took 2 h, 20 min (min. 1 h, 35 min, max. 4 h, 15 min). The median blood loss was 2600 mL (min. 200 mL, max. 10.000 mL).

2.1.3. RESULTS

There have been no intraoperative complications, and postoperative complications have been observed in 40% of the patients. There have been four cases of delayed wound healing and one wound infection, there have been two hematomas, one thrombosis, one paresis of the radial nerve, one hemorrhagic cystitis, one case of edema, and one of proctitis and abscess (Table 2). Postoperative chemotherapy could be continued on

Table 2
Toxicity and Complications Observed with HDR-IORT Brachytherapy in Ewing's
Sarcoma Patients Treated at the University of Münster (July, 1992 to May, 1995)

Observations	#	Observations	#
Delayed wound healing	4	Hemorrhagic cystitis	1
Wound infection	1	Edema	1
Hematoma	2	Abcess and proctitis	1
Thrombosis	1	Paresis of the radial nerve	1

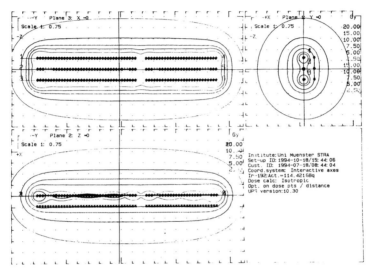

Fig. 2. Isodose distribution with the inserted HDR-IORT brachytherapy applicators in a treatment procedure for a Ewing's sarcoma patient.

average after 19 d (min. 10 d, max. 27 d). There have been three cases of surgical intervention because of complications: In two patients, a wound revision was performed, in one patient, an abscess was removed.

In an August, 1996 analysis, 13 of 20 patients were in complete remission. Six patients had developed metastases and one patient had a combined local and systemic relapse.

2.1.4. Summary

The preliminary results show that an HDR-IORT brachytherapy boost in Ewing's sarcoma using the flab technique is a feasible method. There has been no event of an intraoperative complication caused by the additional radiotherapy. In patients that have mostly large tumors with predominantly pelvic location, the complication rate of 40% is not increased when compared to patients who did not receive brachytherapy (25). The early start of postoperative chemotherapy shows that the perioperative morbidity of the patients was not of major concern. The follow-up is still too short to make definite statements about the local success of the applied boost. So far local control was good with only one local failure combined with a systemic relapse.

Intraoperative high-dose-rate brachytherapy in Ewing's sarcoma is a feasible method with a low perioperative complication rate. Especially in patients, in whom limb-

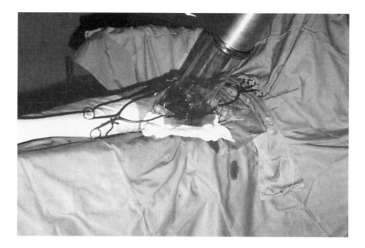

Fig. 3. General view of an IOERT procedure for a femoral Ewing sarcoma at the time of bone resection: 10 cm diameter applicator with a 15° beveled end; 9-MeV electron energy; 1000-cGy total dose; one IOERT field.

preserving surgery is possible only with narrow resection margins, it offers the potential of increased local control. The follow up in the present experience is too short to judge local control and the risks of cumulative late toxicity need to be evaluated in the future.

2.2. NCI IOERT Animal Data And Clinical Experiences

The use of IOERT for bone sarcomas has been reported in only a few series. At the National Cancer Institute (NCI), IOERT was used in some patients with pelvic primary lesions (58), but no conclusions can be drawn from this limited experience. Tolerance studies in normal tissue involving the use of surgery and IOERT alone or in combination with EBRT have suggested that the acceptable tolerated doses in peripheral nerves, muscle, large vessels, and bone are in the range of 15–20 Gy (26–31).

2.3. University Navarra IOERT Clinical Series

2.3.1. PATIENT GROUP AND TREATMENT METHODS

At the University Clinic of Navarra from September, 1984 to February, 1996, 24 pediatric patients with Ewing's sarcoma have been treated with a IOERT component integrated in a multimodal program (Fig. 3). In patients with primary disease, preoperative, concurrent systemic chemotherapy, and EBRT were used. Alternating courses of two regimens were used, containing adriamycin, methotrexate, cyclophosphamide, actinomycin D, vincristine (regimen 2), every 3 wk. External-beam radiotherapy has been delivered to a volume encompassing the entire bone with a 3–5 cm margin beyond the known soft-tissue extension. The total dose administered has been 45–50 Gy, 1.8–2 Gy per fraction, 5 fractions per week. Four to six weeks after completion of preoperative EBRT, patients were considered for surgery and an IOERT boost (10–20 Gy) delivered to the residual tumor or tumor-bed area. After surgery, alternating multiagent chemotherapy was maintained for 1 yr according to the T_{11} protocol (32).

Patients with recurrent disease (four patients with local recurrence) received a reinduction course of systemic chemotherapy followed by maximal surgical resection plus a single IOERT dose of 20 Gy to the tumor bed. All patients had previously received

Table 3
Toxicity and Treatment Characteristics
of Ewing's Sarcoma Pediatric Patients Treated
at the University Clinic of Navarra with IOERT (1984–1996)

Characteristics	#	Characteristics	#
Tumor size (volume)		Electron energy	
<300 cm^3	11	6–9 MeV	18
>300 cm^3	13	12–20 MeV	6
Involved bone		Total dose	
Extremity	20	10 Gy	13
Central	4	15 Gy	9
Postsurgical residue		20 Gy	2
Macroscopic	7	Number of fields	
Microscopic	17	Single	21
IOERT parameters		Multiple	3
Applicator diameter			
6–8 cm	12		
9–12 cm	13		
15 cm	15		

a radical dose of EBRT. Systemic chemotherapy was given as adjuvant therapy for 1 yr or until the development of disease progression.

In the group of patients with primary disease there were three cases of protocol violation that have to be described in order to explain the types of toxicity later found. Two patients with large primary tumors in the lower extremities received a single dose of EBRT of 10 Gy the day before surgery (flash technique); the remaining EBRT was given postoperatively in a conventional program. One additional patient underwent surgical resection after 60 Gy of fractionated radical irradiation. Apart from these protocol violations, the primary disease group was consistently treated with moderate preoperative irradiation and IORT boost (10–15 Gy).

Patient characteristics were: 16 males and 8 females, age range 6–18 yr old (median 12 yr), patients were recurrent to previous therapy. Tumor characteristics are described in Table 3.

2.3.2. RESULTS

The patterns of tumor progression revealed five combined local and systemic failures: one vertebral, one iliac, one rib, and two humerus locations; four cases with a volumetric tumor-size estimation over 300 cm^3—patients with recurrent disease to initial induction therapy. Three additional patients developed distant metastasis alone: one femur and one radius more than 300 cm^3 in size and one clavicle (Table 4). Actuarial survival at 14 yr is 63% for the entire group. There is a statistically significant relationship between risk of disease relapse and initial tumor volumetry (>300 cm^3) ($p = 0.04$).

Selective toxicity analysis for IOERT report of results purposes is focused on the description of local observations in the area of surgery and radiotherapy. Patients had several infectious and aplasic episodes as a result of the adjuvant chemotherapy program. In three patients, delayed wound healing and severe soft-tissue necrosis were seen in the follow-up period. These three cases comprised the two treated with high-dose flash

Table 4
Patterns of Disease Relapse in Pediatric Ewing's Sarcoma Treated
at the University Clinic of Navarra (1984–1996)

Disease Status	#	Local Alone	Local + Distant	Distant Alone
Primary	20	—	1	3
Recurrent	4	—	4	—
Total	24	—	5[a] (20%)	3[b] (12%)

[a] 4 cases with >300 cm^3 tumor volumetry.
[b] 3 cases with >300 cm^3 tumor volumetry.

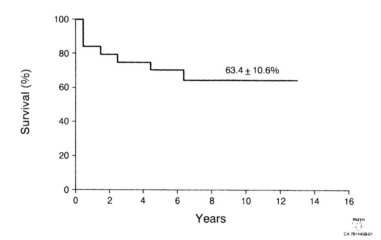

Fig. 4. Actuarial survival of Ewing's pediatric sarcoma patients treated with an IOERT component at the University Clinic of Navarra (1984–1996).

(10 Gy) preoperative radiotherapy and one additional case that was operated on after radical EBRT (60 Gy). Two had repair of their lesions with a myocutaneous flap. Two patients required amputation after failure of conservative management.

In seven patients, a minor-to-moderate degree of soft-tissue fibrosis was evident during the follow-up period. Four developed a shortened extremity and one an articular retraction.

2.3.3. SUMMARY

An up-date of a 13-yr experience exploring IOERT in a pediatric radiosensitive tumor such as Ewing's sarcoma confirms the preliminary observations that the initial local-control rate is encouraging, particularly in primary disease (95%) (Fig. 4). Surgery is now being considered more frequently in the overall management of this disease, and IOERT is an interesting modality that can be included in combined treatment programs. The availability of IORT might decrease the total EBRT dose, and enable a boost dose to be delivered to areas of residual disease or at high risk for local recurrence with an accurate electron-beam field. The complications observed in our initial series have been caused by intensive local treatment. IOERT appears to be very attractive for the treatment of Ewing's sarcoma located in central bone (pelvis, vertebra, ribs, and so on), and it is already a well-tested technique in lesions of the extremities.

3. OSTEOSARCOMA

The treatment of osteosarcoma has changed dramatically in the last decade. Neoadjuvant and adjuvant chemotherapy have significantly increased both survival and tumor resectability rates *(33,34)*, and extremity preservation is an important goal of modern treatment *(35)*. Moreover, whereas osteosarcoma has historically been considered a "radioresistant" tumor type and there has been a lack of interest in exploring radiotherapy in the multidisciplinary approach to bone tumors *(36)*, more recently this treatment modality has been employed in the local treatment of osteosarcoma of the extremities.

In the era prior to adjuvant chemotherapy the only alternative to amputation for the treatment of the primary lesion was local radiotherapy. The so-called Cade technique was an approach that delivered high-dose local EBRT to allow amputation to be delayed for 4–6 mo while patients were observed to see whether pulmonary metastases would develop *(37–40)*. In the modern practice of radiotherapy, the treatment modality has been reserved for lesions located in sites inaccessible to radical surgery *(41,42)*. Several trials have explored the possible role of whole-lung irradiation as an adjuvant treatment for initially localized osteosarcomas *(43,44)*. There have also been studies using high-dose preoperative EBRT and planned surgery *(45)*, and preoperative EBRT with local hyperthermic perfusion *(46)*.

3.1. Kyoto University IOERT Series

3.1.1. PATIENT GROUP AND TREATMENT METHODS

The pionering experience using IORT in osteosarcoma patients has been reported from Kyoto University *(47)*. Between 1978 and 1984, 21 patients with osteosarcoma received IOERT as a part of the treatment designed for their disease. Involved bones were femur—12, tibia—7, humerus—1, and iliac—1. The primary lesion was treated with IOERT alone in 11 cases, and eight patients underwent prosthetic replacement 3 mo after IOERT.

The IOERT technique was described as multifocal bilateral irradiation, using electron beams in the energy range of 6–12 MeV and delivering a total dose of 50–60 Gy to an area of the bone determined according to the computed tomography (CT) findings. Skin and surrounding tissues were retracted to protect them from the radiation beam.

3.1.2. RESULTS

Histologic changes were described in an initial report *(48)*, and clinical results published in a later update showed several findings compatible with treatment efficacy, such as normalization of initially elevated serum alkaline phosphatase, a marked decrease in the uptake of contrast media in bone scintigrams, and complete necrosis of the tumor cells throughout the primary lesions that were resected and analyzed in serial histologic examinations. Two patients developed extensive skin necrosis apparently related to the surgical procedure.

The overall cumulative survival was 32%. This has improved since 1982 with the inclusion of chemotherapy in the treatment program; the estimated 5-yr survival rate in 10 patients treated with the new multidisciplinary program was 60% *(49)*. In the most recent update from this group, 2 out of 23 patients (9%) are reported to have developed a local recurrence, probably caused by a marginal miss of the IORT fields. The most common complication has been fracture of the involved bone. The present recommen-

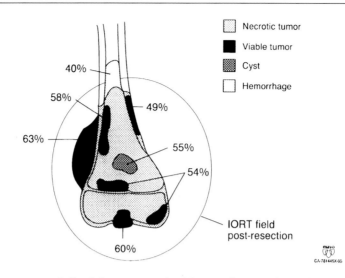

Fig. 5. Osteosarcoma of distal femur treated with neoadjuvant chemotherapy with diagram of pathologic findings following induction chemotherapy and definition of IOERT target volume to include the soft tissues around the tumor.

dation for patients free of distant metastases 8–10 wks after IOERT is reoperation for bone resection and prosthetic replacement *(50).*

In a recent update of the experience generated by Kyoto University *(51),* 17 patients treated with preoperative chemotherapy (cisplatin and doxorubicine) had a 5-yr cumulative survival of 78% and no local recurrences (the IORT dose range delivered to the exposed bone was reported as 50–100 Gy).

3.2. IOERT Experience—University Clinic of Navarra (1985–1997)

3.2.1. Treatment Methods

In the present experience, IOERT is used as a treatment component to boost the tumor-bed area and surrounding tissues following bone resection. Moderate-to-high single doses of electrons were expected to sterilize residual osteosarcoma cells after surgical *en bloc* tumor resection. In addition, neoadjuvant chemotherapy was employed, since this induces even higher tumor-necrosis rates (Fig. 5). On the other hand, it was elected to omit EBRT in those patients in whom metallic prosthetic devices would have been included in the field. This is the only instance in the IOERT program in Pamplona in which IOERT was not complemented by EBRT.

The treatment protocol has been quite uniform in the patients reviewed in this series. Once osteosarcoma was confirmed histogically, patients were entered in a treatment program comprising three major components.

3.2.1.1. Neoadjuvant Chemotherapy. Three preoperative courses of neoadjuvant chemotherapy were given, commencing at 3-wk intervals. Using the transfemoral Seldinger approach, cisplatin 40 mg/m^2 was administered intra-arterially on days 1, 3, and 5 of each cycle. On day 5 of each cycle doxorubicin 60 mg/m^2 iv was added to the program.

3.2.1.2. Surgery. Following the three neoadjuvant courses of chemotherapy, patients were considered for surgical *en bloc* tumor resection. The general aims of surgery were

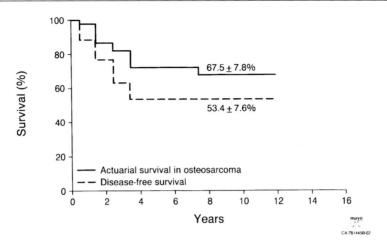

Fig. 6. Overall survival and disease-free survival in Osteosarcoma patients treated with a component of IOERT at the University Clinic of Navarra (1985–1997).

to remove all the involved bone and a margin of normal surrounding tissues if possible. Functional reconstruction of the extremity was done on an individual basis using endoprosthetic devices or bone graft. Before the reconstruction, the patient received IOERT to the tumor-bed area, using a single dose in the range of 10–20 Gy. The electron-beam energy selected was based on the thickness of tumor tissue left after surgery.

3.2.1.3. Systemic Adjuvant Chemotherapy. Three weeks after surgery, intensive adjuvant systemic chemotherapy was initiated using the following regime of cytostatic agents: cisplatin 120 mg/m^2 and doxorubicin 60 mg/m^2 in weeks 1, 5, 15, 25, 33, and 45; high-dose methotrexate 8 g/m^2 with folinic acid rescue in weeks 3, 4, 8, 9, 13, 14, 18, 19, 23, 24, 28, and 29; bleomycin 30 mg/m^2, cyclophosphamide 1200 mg/m^2, vincristine 1.5 mg/m^2, and actinomycin D 1.2 mg/m^2 in weeks 10, 12, 36, 42, and 48.

External-beam radiotherapy was not routinely used in this treatment program. Occasionally, patients with recurrent and/or macroscopic residual after maximal resection received additional fractionated EBRT.

3.2.2. Results

In a 12-yr period, 44 patients with osteosarcoma were treated with an IOERT treatment component (two metastatic patients in complete remission following thoracotomy). Tumor characteristics are described in Table 5. Most frequent histological subtype was osteoblastic (65%) and half of patients had femur locations.

Actuarial survival rate projected to 12 yr is 67% and disease-free survival 53% (Fig. 6). There has been observed 69 local recurrences (4 in condroblastic subtypes, $p = 0.0102$; Table 6).

Toxicity and complications observed in these patients are mainly related to surgical manipulation and adaptation of the anatomy to prosthesic devises. The contribution of IOERT to late normal-tissue sequelae is not well established because of the multifactorial treatment related tissue damage. In the reported experience asymmetry (45%), graft necrosis (4%), graft fracture (15%), local infection (22%), and pseudoathrosis (15%) have been complications observed in the follow-up period. An anecdotical case of skin recall phenomenon during adjuvant high-dose methotrexate is illustrated in Fig. 7.

Table 5
Osteosarcoma Characteristics
in the IOERT Experience at the
University Clinic of Navarra (1985–1997)

Histological Subtype	#	(%)
Osteoblastic	29	(65)
Chondroblastic	9	(20)
Fibroblastic	4	(9)
Telangiectatic	2	(4)
Involved Bone	#	(%)
Femur	22	(50)
Tibia	17	(38)
Fibula	1	(2)
Humerus	3	(6)
Iliac	1	(2)

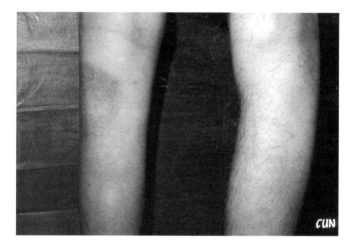

Fig. 7. Recall phenomenon during adjuvant high-dose methotrexate in an osteosarcoma patient. Notice the circular skin erythema in the external region of the left leg, defining the IOERT beam-exit site.

3.2.3. Summary

The goal of osteosarcoma treatment today is not only systemic disease control but also extremity preservation. In this context, the addition of IORT might improve local control rates as it has been achieved in extremity soft-tissue sarcomas with conventional external irradiation (52). External-beam radiotherapy might be more hazardous in osteosarcoma patients who have undergone resection because of the interaction of the radiation with metallic prosthetic reconstructive devices and the intensive chemotherapy programs required to cure these patients. As with soft-tissue sarcomas, the tolerance of peripheral nerves to single high doses of electron irradiation is an important and still open question for radiobiology modulation.

Table 6
Patterns of Osteosarcoma Recurrence at the University Clinic of Navarra (1985–1997)

Histological Subtype	#	Local Alone	Local + Distant	Distant Alone
Chondroblastic	9	—	4 (44%)	3 (33%)
No Chondroblastic	35	—	2 (5%)	7 (20%)
Total	44	—	6 (13%)	10 (22%)

3.3. IOERT Tolerance

The normal tissues at risk of receiving high-to-moderate single doses of IOERT for postresected osteosarcoma of the extremities are muscles, peripheral nerves, ligaments, and skin. Occasionally, structures such as cartilage and bone would be included in the IOERT field. These normal tissues have been extensively investigated to define their tolerance to escalating doses of IOERT alone or in combination with fractionated EBRT. In the case of osteosarcoma patients, the treatment program at the University Clinic of Navarra and Kyoto University did not include the addition of EBRT. The changes in normal tissues described in muscles, peripheral nerves, and bone following a 15–20 Gy single dose of IOERT alone are compatible with acceptable tolerance, although neurologic damage has been observed in a certain proportion of animals after 20 Gy (26,28–31). This dose by extrapolation is considered the upper dose limit in IORT trials in which nerves will be included in the field.

4. MALIGNANT FIBROUS HISTIOCYTOMA

MFH represents 0.7% of all malignant primary bone tumors, of relatively recent description, with a particular tendency to develop extraosseous tumor extension (52). Extremity preserving yet radical surgical approaches have been recommended selectively for cases shown to have oncologic safe tissue margins on the preoperative imaging evaluation (54). Transient remission of lung metastases have been reported with chemotherapy (55) and its role has been suggested to contribute to improve survival both in patients treated with amputation or conservative surgery (56).

4.1. University Navarra IOERT Series

4.1.1. Treatment Methods

The results of the experience at the University Clinic of Navarra with intense multidisciplinary therapy including IOERT after resection is described in Table 7 (Fig. 8) (57). Nine patients with bone MFH were treated with neoadjuvant chemotherapy (CDDP 40 mg/m^2 day 1, 3, and 5 of each induction week; and doxorubicin (10 mg/m^2 iv days 2, 4, and 6 of each induction week; treatment was repeated every 21 d to a total of three cycles), surgical resection (with preservation of the extremity) plus an IOERT boost (10–20 Gy), followed by fractionated EBRT (40–50 Gy) and adjuvant chemotherapy regimen including Cyclophosphamide, Vincristine, Actinomycin D, Dacarbacine (CYVADIC, six cycles). Initial tumor size was >10 cm maximum diameter in four cases. Cortical bone was ruptured in all cases with radiological evidence of soft-tissue involvement. Bone fracture was a presenting sign of disease in four patients. Pathologic positive margins in the resected specimen were identified in two cases.

Table 7
IOERT Experience Description and Results
in MFH of Bone at the University Clinic of Navarra

Case	Site	IOERT dose	EBRT dose	Neuropathy	Status	Follow-up
1	femur	10 Gy	50 Gy	yes	NED	15[c]
2	humerus	20 Gy[a]	50 Gy	yes	DWD	37
3	femur	20 Gy[b]	46 Gy	no	NED	50[c]
4	ischium	15 Gy[a]	45 Gy	no	DWD	8
5	femur	15 Gy[b]	40 Gy	no	NED	43[c]
6	iliac	10 Gy 10 Gy	45 Gy	no	DWD	10
7	femur	10 Gy[b]	46 Gy	no	NED	2[c]
8	femur	15 Gy[b]	60 Gy[c]	no	NED	49[c]
9	femur	15 Gy[b]	38 Gy	yes	NED	18[c]

[a] Neuro-vascular structures protected or mobilized.
[b] Neuro-vascular structures included in the IORT field.
[c] Previous radiotherapy.
NED: alive with no evidence of disease; DWD: dead with disease; follow-up: months since IOERT.

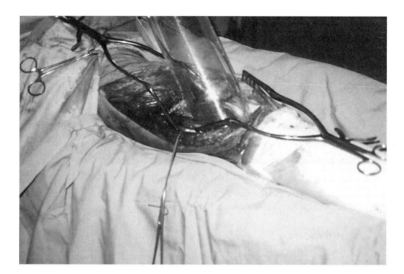

Fig. 8. IOERT for femoral malignant fibrous histiocytoma after resection. Notice that the nerve has been disected and mobilized out of the electron field (7 cm diameter applicator; 30° beveled end; 9-MeV electron energy; 15-Gy total dose).

A single IOERT field was used in eight procedures. The electron energy selected was 12 MeV or less in eight. Applicator size was 6–7 cm in three and 8–10 cm in six.

4.1.2. RESULTS

The median follow-up time at publication was >19 mo (range >20 to >50 mo). One local and systemic progression had been observed in an iliac partially resected patient 8 mo after surgery. Actuarial survival is projected as 63% at 5 yr. Three patients developed symptomatic neuropathy, one of whom has a permanent motor and sensation deficit.

Table 8
IOERT Case Report Description
in Chondrosarcoma Patients Treated at the University Clinic of Navarra

Case	Site	IOERT dose	EBRT dose	Neuropathy	Status	Follow-up
1	sacrum	20 Gy[a]	50 Gy	yes	NED	72c
2	fibula	15 Gy[b]	50 Gy	yes	NED	49c
3	femur	10 Gy 10 Gy	50 Gy	no	NED	20c

[a] Neurovascular structure protected or displaced.
[b] Neurovascular structure included in the IOERT field.
[c] Previous radiotherapy.
NED: alive with no evidence of disease; follow-up: months from IOERT procedures.

5. CHONDROSARCOMA

Chondrosarcoma is considered a radioresistant bone tumor controlled by surgery only if radical margins are possible to be achieved *(1,5,11)*. In the IORT literature there is only one previous limited report of results with this histological subtype.

5.1. Kyoto University

Up to 1991, three chondrosarcoma patients were treated with radical IOERT (50–100 Gy). No local recurrence had been observed at the time of publication *(50)*.

5.2. University Clinic of Navarra

In the experience up to December, 1990, three cases of chondrosarcoma were treated with surgery plus IOERT and EBRT. Table 8 describes characteristics and results. The information should be interpreted as anecdotal, but of relative value for patients with tumor rupture of the bone cortex, candidates with extremity-preserving procedures with close surgical margins or unresectable lesions for cure.

REFERENCES

1. Malawer MM, Link MP, and Donaldson SS. Sarcomas of the bone. In VT De Vita, S Hellman, and SA Rosenberg (eds.) *Principles and Practice of Oncology,* 5th ed. Lippincott-Raven, Philadelphia, 1997, pp. 1789–1816.
2. Rosen G. Primary Ewing's sarcoma: the multidisciplinary lesion, *Int. J. Radiat. Oncol. Biol. Phys.,* **4** (1978) 527–532.
3. Glasser DB, Lane JM, Huvos AG, Marcove RC, and Rosen G. Survival prognosis, and therapeutic response in osteogenic sarcoma. The Memorial Hospital experience, *Cancer,* **69** (1992) 698–708.
4. McCarthy SF, Matsuao F, and Dorfman HD. Malignant fibrous histiocytoma of bone: a study of 35 cases, *Hum. Path.,* **10** (1979) 57–70.
5. Marcove RC. Chondrosarcoma: diagnosis and treatment, *Orthop. Clin. Nort. Am,* **8** (1977) 811–819.
6. Cortes EP, Holland JF, Wang, JJ, et al. Amputation and Adriamicyn in primary osteosarcoma, *N. Engl. J. Med.,* **291** (1974) 998–1000.
7. Eilber FR, Eckhardt J, and Morton DL. Advances in the treatment of sarcomas of the extremity. Current status of limb salvage, *Cancer,* **54** (1984) 2695–2701.
8. Calvo FA, Antos M, and Brady LW. *Intraoperative Radiotherapy. Clinical experiences and results,* Springer Verlag, Heidelberg, 1992.
9. Martínez A, Goffinet DR, Donaldson SS, et al. Intra-arterial infusion of radiosesnitizer (BUdR) combined with hypofractionated irradiation and chemotherapy for primary treatment of osteogenic sarcoma, *Int. J. Radiat. Oncol. Biol. Phys.,* **2** (1980) 123–128.

10. Tefft M, Razek A, Perez C, et al. Local control and survival related to radiation dose and colume and to chemotherapy in non metastatic Ewing's sarcoma of the pelvic bones, *Int. J. Radiat. Oncol. Biol. Phys.*, **4** (1978) 367–372.

11. Krochak R, Harwood AR, Cummings BJ, et al. Results of radical radiation for chondrosarcoma of bone, *Radiother. Oncol.*, **1** (1983) 109–115.

12. Calvo FA, Ortíz De Urbina D, Sierrasesumaga L, Abuchaibe O, Azinovic I, Antillon F, Santos M, and Cañadell J. Intraoperative radiotherapy in the multidisciplinary treatment of bone sarcomas in children and adolescents, *Med. Pediatr. Oncol.*, **19** (1991) 478–485.

13. Barbieri E, Emiliani E, Zini G, Mancini A, Toni A, et al. Combined therapy of localised Ewing's sarcoma of bone: analysis of results in 100 patients, *Int. J. Radiat. Oncol. Biol. Phys.*, **19** (1990) 1165–1170.

14. Dunst J, Jürgens H, Sauer R, Pape H, Paulussen M, Winkelmann W, and Rübe CH. Radiation therapy in Ewing's sarcoma: an update of the CESS 86 trial, *Int. J. Radiat. Oncol. Biol. Phys.*, **32** (1995) 919–930.

15. Halperin EC, Kun LX, Constantine LS, and Tarbell NJ. *Pediatric Radiation Oncology,* Raven Press, New York, 1989.

16. Brown AP, Fixen JA, and Plowman PN. Local control of Ewing's sarcoma: an analysis of 67 patients, *Br. J. Radiol.*, **60** (1987) 261–268.

17. Tepper J, Glaubiguer D, Lichter A, Wackenbut J, and Glatstein E. Local control of Ewing's sarcoma of bone with radiotherapy and combination chemotherapy, *Cancer,* **46** (1980) 1965–1973.

18. Marcus RB, and Million RR. The effect of primary tumor size on the prognosis of Ewing's sarcoma, *Int. J. Radiat. Oncol. Biol. Phys.*, **10 (Suppl 1)** (1994) 88.

19. Bacci G, Picci P, Gitelis S, Borghi A, and Campanacci M. The treatment of localized Ewing's sarcoma. The experience at the Instituo Ortopedico Rizzoli in 163 cases treated with and without adjuvant chemotherapy, *Cancer,* **49** (1982) 1561–1570.

20. Jurgens H, Exner U, Gadner H, et al. Multidisciplinary treatment of primary Ewing's sarcoma of bone. A 6-year experience of a European Cooperative Trial, *Cancer,* **61** (1988) 23–32.

21. Sailder SL, Harmon DC, Mankin HJ, Truman JT, and Suit HD. Ewing's sarcoma: surgical resection as a prognostic factor, *Int. J. Radiat. Oncol. Biol. Phys.*, **15** (1988) 43–52.

22. Evans R, Nesbit M, Gehan E, Garnsey L, et al. Multimodal therapy for the management of localized Ewing's sarcoma of pelvic and sacral bones: a report from the second intergroup study, *J. Clin. Oncol.*, **9** (1991) 1173–1180.

23. Kronholz K, Prott FJ, Anders C, and Willich N. Flabs zur intraoperativen Bestrahlung. Medizinische Physik. Hrsg: H. Leitner, G. Stücklshweiger, S. 1996, pp. 39–40.

24. Enneking WF. A system of staging musculoskeletal neoplasms, *Ballieere's Clinical Oncology,* **1** (1987) 97–110.

25. Brant T, Parsons J, Marcus R, Spanier S, Heare T, et al. Preoperative irradiation for soft tissue sarcomas of the trunk and extremities in adults, *Int. J. Radiat. Oncol. Biol. Phys.*, **19** (1990) 899–906.

26. Kinsella TJ, Sindelar WF, and De Luca AM. Threshold dose for peripheral nerve injury following intraoperative radiotherapy (IORT) in a large animal model, *Int. J. Radiat. Oncol. Biol. Phys.*, **15 (Suppl 1)** 205.

27. Powers BE, Gillette EL, Mcchesney SL, et al. Muscle injury following experimental intraoperative irradiation, *Int. J. Radiat. Oncol. Biol. Phys.*, **17 (Suppl 1)** (1989) 246.

28. Gillete EL, Powers BE, Mcchesney SL, et al. Response of aorta and branch arteries to experimental intraoperative irradiation, *Int. J. Radiat. Oncol. Biol. Phys.*, **15 (suppl 1)** (1988) 202.

28. Powers BE, Gillette EL, Mcchesney SL, et al. Bone necrosis and tumor induction following experimental intraoperative irradiation, *Int. J. Radiat. Oncol. Biol. Phys.*, **17** (1989) 559–567.

29. Le Coteur RA, Gillette EL, Powers BE, et al. Peripheral neuropathies following experimental intraoperative radiation therapy (IORT), *Int. J. Radiat. Oncol. Biol. Phys.*, **11** (1989) 1579–1585.

30. Kinsella TJ, Sindelar WF, De Luca AM, et al. Tolerance of peripheral nerve to intraoperative radiotherapy (IORT): clinical and experimental studies, *Int. J. Radiat. Oncol. Biol. Phys.*, **11** (1985) 1579–1585.

31. Powers BE, Gillette EL, Mcchesney SL, et al. Bone necrosis and tumor induction following experimental intraoperative irradiation, *Int. J. Radiat. Oncol. Biol. Phys.*, **17** (1989) 559–567.

32. Rosen G, Caparros B, Nirenberg A, Marcove RC, Huvos AG, Kosloff C, Lane J, and Murphy ML. Ewing's sarcoma. Ten-years experience with adjuvant chemotherapy, *Cancer,* **47** (1981) 2204–2213.

33. Eilber F, Giuliano A, Edkardt J, Patterson K, Moselev S, and Goonight J. Adjuvant chemotherapy for osteosarcoma: a randomized prospective trial, *J. Clin. Oncol.*, **5** (1987) 21–26.

34. Bacci G, Springfield D, Capnna R, et al. Neoadjuvant chemotherapy for osteosarcoma of the extremity, *Clin. Orthop.,* **224** (1987) 268–276.

35. Wong ACW, Akahoshi Y, Takeuchi S. Limb-salvage procedures of osteosarcoma: an alternative to amputation, *Int. Orthop.,* **10** (1986) 245–251.

36. Sugimoto M, Togochida J, Kotoura Y, Yamamuro T, and Utsumi H. In vitro radiosensitivity of osteosarcoma lines, *Strahlenther. Onkol.,* **165** (1989) 782.

37. Poppe E, Liverud K, and Efskind. Osteosarcoma, *Acta Chir. Scand.,* **134** (1968) 549–556.

38. Allen CF and Stevens KR. Preoperative irradiation for osteogenic sarcoma, *Cancer,* **31** (1973) 1364–1366.

39. Jenkin RDT, Allt WEC, and Fitzpatrik PJ. Osteosarcoma: an assessment of management with particular reference to primary irradiation and selective delayed amputation, *Cancer,* **30** (1972) 393–400.

40. Philips TL and Sheline GE. Radiation therapy of malignant bone tumors, *Radiology,* **92** (1969) 1537–1545.

41. Chambers RG and Mahoney WD. Osteogenic sarcoma of the mandible: current management, *Am. Surg.* **36** (1970) 463–471.

42. Suit HD. Radiotherapy in osteosarcoma, *Clin. Orthop.,* **111** (1975) 71–75.

43. Breur K, Cohen P, Schweisguth O, and Amm H. Irradiation of the lungs or an adjuvant therapy in the treatment of osteosarcoma of the limbs. An EORTC randomized study, *Eur. J. Cancer,* **14** (1978) 461–471.

44. Burgers JM, van Glabbeke M, Bussan A, et al. Osteosarcoma of the limbs. Report of the EORTC-SIOP 03 trial 20781 investigating the value of adjuvant treatment with chemotherapy and/or prophylactic lung irradiation, *Cancer,* **61** (1988) 1024–1031.

45. Farrell C and Raventos A. Experiences in treating osteosarcoma at the hospital of the University of Pennsylvania, *Radiology,* **83** (1964) 1080–1083.

46. Cavaliere R. Hyperthermic treatment of osteogenic sarcoma, *Chemoter. Oncol.,* **2** (1978) 190–196.

47. Abe M, Takahashi M, Shibamoto Y, and Ono K. Application of intraoperative radiation therapy to refractory cancers, *Ann. Radiol.,* **32** (1989) 493–494.

48. Nagashima T, Yamamuro T, Kotoura Y, Takahashi M, and Abe M. Histological studies of the effect of intraoperative irradiation on osteosarcoma, *Nippon Seikeigeka Gakkai Zasshi,* **57** (1983) 1681–1697.

49. Yamamuro T, Kotoura Y, Kasahara K, Tadahashi M, and Abe M. Intraoperative radiotherapy for osteosarcoma, *Strahlecther. Onkol.,* **165** (1989) 783.

50. Abe M, Takahashi M, Shibamoto Y, Ono K, Yabumoto E, and Mori K. Derzeitige Stellung der intraoperativen Strahlentherapie, *Chirurg.,* **59** (1988) 211–217.

51. Kotoura Y, Yamamuro T, Kasahara K, Shibamoto Y, Takahashi M, and Abe M. Intraoperative radiation therapy for malignant bone tumors. In FW Schildberg, N Willich, and HJ Krämling (eds.) *Intraoperative Radiation Therapy,* Die Blane Eule, Essen, 1993, pp. 456–458.

52. Rosenberg SA, Tepper JE, Glastein EJ, et al. The treatment of soft tissue sarcomas of the extremities. Prospective randomized evaluations of (1) limb-sparing surgery plus radiation therapy compared with amputation and (2) the role of adjuvant chemotherapy, *Ann. Surg.* **196** (1982) 305–314.

53. Feldman F and Norman D. Intra and extraosseus malignant histiocytomas (malignant fibrous xanthoma) of bone, *Radiology,* **104** (1972) 97–108.

54. Campana R, Bertoni F, Baccini P, Bacci G, Gerra A, and Camapanacci M. Malignant fibrous histicytoma of bone. The experience at the Rizzoli Institute: report of 90 cases, *Cancer,* **54** (1984) 177–187.

55. Spanier SS, Enneking WF, and Enriquez P. Primary malignant fibrous histiocytoma of bone, *Cancer,* **36** (1975) 2084–2098.

56. Bacci G, Avella M, Picc I et al. The effectiveness of chemotherapy in localized malignant fibrous histiocytoma of bone: the Rizzoli Institute Experience with 66 patients treated with surgery alone or surgery + adjuvant or neoadjuvant chemotherapy, *Chemioterapie,* **7** (1989) 481–494.

57. Castillo I, Calvo FA, Aristu J, et al. Tratamiento intensivo de sarcomas óseos de histología miscelánea: histiocitoma fibroso maligno y condrosarcoma, *Oncología,* **15** (1992) 351–358.

58. Stea et al. 1987.

22 Locally Advanced Primary and Recurrent Gynecologic Malignancies

EBRT With or Without IOERT or HDR-IORT

Michael G. Haddock, Rafael Martinez-Monge, Ivy A. Petersen, and Timothy O. Wilson

CONTENTS

1. INTRODUCTION

The prognosis for women with locally advanced gynecologic tumors with direct tumor extension to pelvic sidewall structures or gross lymphatic spread to pelvic or para-aortic nodes is poor. Although high-dose external-beam radiation (EBRT) with or without brachytherapy is often utilized to treat primary locally advanced malignancies with some success, aggressive local therapy is often not considered in patients with locally advanced recurrent disease in whom standard radiation or surgical therapy has failed. This chapter will summarize the results of standard therapy for locally advanced gynecologic malignancies and present preliminary data from series of patients treated with intraoperative irradiation (IORT)-containing regimens. The future potential of IORT in the management of locally advanced gynecologic malignancies will be discussed.

2. RESULTS WITH NON-IORT TREATMENT APPROACHES

2.1. Primary Gynecologic Malignancies

2.1.1. MANAGEMENT OF THE PRIMARY CERVIX TUMOR

Patients with early cervical cancer which has not spread beyond the cervix (stage I) may be effectively treated with either radical hysterectomy or EBRT plus brachytherapy with 5-yr survival rates > 90% with either approach. Tumor extension into the lateral

From: *Current Clinical Oncology: Intraoperative Irradiation: Techniques and Results*
Edited by: L. L. Gunderson et al. © Humana Press, Inc., Totowa, NJ

Table 1
Survival and Pelvic Control in Stage III Cervical Carcinoma:
External-Beam Radiation with or without Chemotherapy

Series	Ref. No.	No. Pts	Chemotherapy	Survival 5 yr (%)	Disease-Free Survival 5 yr (%)	Pelvic Control 5 yr (%)
Fyles, PMH	(85)	329	none	—	41	—
Komaki, 1978 POC	(86)	115	none	39	33	49
1983 POC		24	none	47	39	69
Petereit, Wisconsin	(87)	61	none	46	—	63
Teshima, Osaka	(88)	82	none	45	—	54
Mitsuhashi, Gunma	(89)	148	none	52	—	86
Ito, Keio U.	(90)	366	none	47	—	68
Patel, India	(91)	114	none	50	—	76
Montana, Duke	(92)	107	none	—	36	55
Perez, Wash. U.	(4)	259	none	—	40	61
Jones, ACS	(93)	630	none in 92%	38	—	—
Horiot, France	(94)	482	none	50	—	57
Souhami, Brazil	(61)	52	none	39	—	46
		39	neoadjuv BOMP	23	—	50
Brunet, Barcelona	(95)	31	neoadjuv BMP	49	47	—
Benedett-Panici, Rome	(96)	70	neoadjuv CDDP, bleo[b]	49	—	—
Pras, Groningen	(97)	18	conc CBDCA, 5-FU	47	—	—
Fields, Einstein	(98)	28	conc CDDP	67[a]	67[a]	77[a]
Stehman, GOG	(99)	53	conc hydroxyurea	47	48	—
Thomas, PMH	(100)	89	conc 5-FU ± mito C	43 (3-yr)	—	52 (3-yr)

CBDCA = carboplatinum; 5-FU = 5-fluorouracil; CDDP = cisplatinum; mito C = mitomycin C; BMP = bleomycin; methotrexate, cisplatinum; BOMP = bleomycin; vincristine, mitomycin, cisplatinum; conc = concurrent.
[a]Crude survival and disease control.
[b]Chemotherapy followed by surgery or radiation therapy.

parametrial tissue precludes a curative attempt with surgical resection alone; standard therapy is EBRT plus brachytherapy. Because of the relatively high normal-tissue radiation tolerances of the upper vagina, cervix, and uterus, very high central tumor doses may be safely delivered with intracavitary brachytherapy. EBRT plus brachytherapy is highly effective for cervical carcinomas that have not spread to the pelvic sidewall with 5-yr tumor control rates > 90% for stage I cancers and 75–90% for stage II cancers (1). However, when the tumor extends beyond the zone of high-dose irradiation achievable with intracavitary brachytherapy, the minimum tumor dose becomes a function of the maximum EBRT dose and tumor-control rates fall (2). Five-year pelvic control rates for patients with involvement of the pelvic sidewall (stage III) treated with EBRT plus brachytherapy range from 50–65% in most series; corresponding 5-yr control rates for those with bladder or rectum invasion (stage IVA) are in the 25–35% range (1).

A number of strategies have been explored to attempt to improve tumor control rates in stage III patients including altered fractionation schemes, concomitant radiation and chemotherapy, hypoxic cell sensitization, and neoadjuvant chemotherapy followed by radiation or surgery. A summary of survival and pelvic control rates in stage III cervical cancer treated with EBRT plus brachytherapy with or without chemotherapy is presented in Table 1. The addition of chemotherapy or hypoxic cell sensitizers has not resulted in significant improvements in survival or disease control when compared to that achievable with radiation therapy alone. However, neoadjuvant chemotherapy followed by concurrent chemotherapy and EBRT has not been investigated.

Retrospective studies have suggested a radiation dose response for pelvic control in patients with stage III cervical cancer. Perez et al. *(3)* reported improved pelvic control rates with point A doses (combined brachytherapy and EBRT) > 60 Gy (38% pelvic recurrence vs 72%, $p \leq 0.01$) and pelvic sidewall doses > 40 Gy (39% pelvic recurrence vs 71%, $p \leq 0.01$). In another Washington University analysis *(4)* the pelvic failure rates were 58% for point A doses ≤ 60 Gy, 43% for 60–75 Gy, and 32% for 75–90 Gy. Pelvic failure rates in this series were also correlated with pelvic sidewall doses: 65% local failure in stage III patients who received ≤ 45 Gy to the sidewall vs 35% for > 45 Gy *(4)*. Other investigators have reported similar results. Chism et al. *(5)* reported pelvic failure rates for stage III cervical cancer of 80% for > 60 Gy, 63% for 60–80 Gy, and 50% for > 80 Gy total point A doses. Hanks *(6)* reported the results of a national practice patterns of care survey (PCS) which showed improved pelvic control rates in patients who received PCS paracentral point doses greater than the PCS lower limit (75 Gy for stage IIIB disease).

The use of higher radiation doses to improve tumor control rates results in an increase in severe complications. Kottmeier and Gray reported improved survival with higher radiation doses in women with locally advanced cervical cancer at a cost of increased severe bladder and rectal complications *(7)*. In the 1973 PCS survey of five major centers, Hanks reported severe complications (required hospitalization) in 15% of all women and 26% of survivors with stage III cervix cancer. An increase in major complications was noted in patients who received > 85 Gy to the PCS paracentral point and > 45 Gy to the pelvic sidewall *(6)*. Other investigators have reported similar results. Perez has reported increased small bowel complications in patients who received > 50 Gy to the pelvic sidewall *(3,8)*.

The likelihood of severe complications has been specifically associated with the EBRT dose in several retrospective reports. Hanks reported that for a given dose, EBRT was more likely to produce complications than brachytherapy *(6)*. Nearly all the severe complications reported in the series of Unal et al. *(9)* occurred in patients who received > 35 Gy EBRT in addition to brachytherapy. In another report from MD Anderson, Hamberger et al. *(10)* analyzed complication rates in patients with loco-regional control of disease as a function of the whole-pelvis EBRT dose: severe complications were seen in 3% with 40 Gy, 11% with 50 Gy, and 20% with 60 Gy.

2.1.1.1. Summary and Future Possibilities. The minimum tumor dose in cervix-cancer patients with pelvic sidewall extension is largely a function of the whole-pelvis or split-pelvis EBRT dose as the radiation dose to the pelvic sidewall from intracavitary brachytherapy is minimal. It is likely that currently utilized EBRT and brachytherapy doses are at or near maximum tolerated levels. Given the sharp increase in complications seen as EBRT doses are escalated above the 45–50 Gy range, increasing the EBRT dose above 45–50 Gy to improve the poor local control rates in stage III patients is not advisable.

Preoperative EBRT (with or without concomitant chemotherapy) followed by surgical resection and pelvic sidewall IORT is a potential management strategy that may result in increased effective pelvic sidewall doses and tumor control without excessive toxicity. This strategy has not yet been fully explored.

2.1.2. MANAGEMENT OF NODAL DISEASE IN PRIMARY CERVIX CANCERS

Standard therapy for patients with metastases to pelvic or para-aortic nodes is EBRT to the pelvis with or without para-aortic node regions. Potish *(11)* reported on the results of surgical staging followed by extended-field EBRT in patients with involved pelvic or para-aortic lymph-node metastases. Relapse-free survival was 57% in women with grossly involved but resectable pelvic nodes and 0% in women with unresectable pelvic nodes. Pelvic failure was noted in 20% of those with resected grossly positive nodes and 56% of those with unresectable pelvic nodes. Because of adjacent bowel, the dose that may be safely delivered to pelvic nodes is in the range of 50–60 Gy *(11)*. Although doses in this range may control microscopic nodal metastases in approx 90% of cases, the control rate for grossly involved nodes would be expected to be less than 50% *(12)*.

In a multivariate analysis of prognostic variables in patients with cervix cancer treated on Gynecologic Oncology Group protocols, nodal status was the most significant variable associated with tumor recurrence; patients with involved para-aortic nodes had the worst prognosis *(13)*. Microscopic or limited-volume macroscopic para-aortic nodal metastases can be controlled with tolerable EBRT doses. Komaki *(14)* treated 15 patients with microscopic or limited-volume macroscopic para-aortic nodal metastases with 40–58 Gy (median 50 Gy) EBRT. Control of para-aortic disease was obtained in 11 of 15 (73%), the small-bowel obstruction rate was 14% and actuarial 3- and 5-yr disease-free survival was 60 and 40%, respectively. Others have reported long-term survival in 25–50% of patients with positive para-aortic nodes (usually microscopic or limited-volume macroscopic disease) using doses of 45–51 Gy *(15–17)*.

Doses necessary to control macroscopic para-aortic nodal metastases exceeds small-bowel tolerance doses. Para-aortic EBRT doses up to 45 Gy are well tolerated in patients who are not surgically staged, but severe small-bowel complications occur in as many as 14% of patients who receive doses of 50–55 Gy without surgical staging and 19% of patients who receive 43–55 Gy with surgical staging *(18)*. Piver et al. *(19)* treated 31 women with para-aortic metastases; intestinal complications were seen in 62% of those who received 60 Gy compared to 10% for those who received 44–50 Gy. A total of 16% of the women in this series died of complications of radiation without evidence of recurrent disease. Wharton *(20)* also reported a fatal intestinal complication rate of 14% in a group of surgically staged patients who received extended-field doses of 55 Gy if they were found to have positive nodes. Despite the relatively high EBRT doses, only 10% were alive without evidence of diseases at 5 yr (all survivors had microscopic nodal disease at the time of EBRT) and on postmortem examination 9 of 14 (64%) had recurrent disease in the para-aortic region *(19)*. When IORT is utilized in conjunction with surgical resection or debulking, increased effective dose may be delivered while limiting EBRT doses to the tolerable 45–50 Gy range.

2.1.3. PRIMARY ENDOMETRIAL CANCER

Although endometrial cancer is commonly confined to the uterus at diagnosis, clinically detectable extension beyond the uterus is present in 5–10% of cases *(21)*. In patients with tumor extension to the pelvic sidewall who are unresectable for cure, survival is poor and EBRT plus intrauterine brachytherapy is associated with a high rate of pelvic failure. Danoff *(21)* treated 19 patients with clinical evidence of extrauterine tumor extension confined to the pelvis with EBRT with or without brachytherapy; the 5-yr survival was 12% and 37% suffered local relapse. There were no 5-yr survivors among the group of patients with extension of tumor to the pelvic sidewall *(21)*. Others have also reported poor results in patients with macroscopic extra-adnexal spread *(22,23)* and/or tumor extension to the pelvic sidewall *(24)*. Pelvic recurrence of persistence of disease has been reported in 90% of women with clinical stage III endometrial cancer after treatment with EBRT plus brachytherapy *(24,25)*. Local failure occurs in 30–40% of patients with clinical stage III endometrial cancer treated with surgical resection and adjuvant radiotherapy *(23,25)*.

As is the case with cervical cancer, microscopic, or limited-volume macroscopic nodal metastases from endometrial adenocarcinoma may be controlled with tolerable doses of EBRT, but the EBRT doses necessary to control gross adenopathy exceed normal tissue tolerance. Komaki *(14)* treated seven patients with para-aortic nodal metastases (microscopic or limited volume) with 40–58 Gy and achieved local control in the para-aortic nodes in six of seven (87%); the 3- and 5-yr DFS was 60%. Several investigators have reported 5-yr survivals in the range of 40–60% after extended-field EBRT for endometrial cancer with para-aortic nodal metastases *(26,27)*. However, most long-term survivors have only microscopic nodal disease and nearly all patients with macroscopic nodal disease suffer disease relapse after doses of 50 Gy EBRT *(26,28)*.

2.2. Recurrent Gynecologic Malignancies

2.2.1. RECURRENT CERVIX CANCER

Salvage therapy for recurrent cervical cancer with surgery or radiation is historically unsuccessful. Early studies of salvage therapy reported 5-yr survivals of 2–4% with the majority of long-term survivors having recurrent disease confined to the central pelvis *(29,30)*. In a group of 39 patients with recurrent cervical cancer who were selected for attempted curative therapy from a group of 193 with recurrent cervix cancer, Calame reported a salvage rate of 21% (8 of 39) *(30)*. Perez reported 5-yr survival in only 5% of stage III patients treated for pelvic recurrence *(4)*. As many as 60% of women who die of cervical or endometrial cancer have local failure as the major cause of death *(31)*.

Successful salvage of patients with pelvic recurrence of cervix cancer following primary radiation therapy is rare with most investigators reporting 5-yr survival rates of ≤ 5% *(4,32)*. Selected patients with locally recurrent disease that is confined to the central pelvis may be cured with exenterative surgery. Fatal complications have been reported in up to 10% of patients with 5-yr survivals in the 25–50% range *(33–36)*. Subsequent pelvic rerecurrence has been reported in approx 30% of patients *(34,35)*. Factors that have been shown to predict for survival include negative margins, small tumor size (< 3 cm), interval from initial radiation therapy to exenteration > 1 yr, and lack of sidewall fixation *(34)*.

Shingleton et al. *(34)* performed pelvic exenterative procedures in 143 women with recurrent cervical cancer; the 5-yr survival was 0% after anterior exenteration with positive margins and 63% after anterior exenteration with negative margins. After total exenteration with positive margins the 5-yr survival was 10 vs 49% with negative margins. In addition, all nine patients who were noted to have some degree of pelvic sidewall fixation preoperatively died. Hatch reported 5-yr survival of 70% after exenteration when the tumor was confined to the cervix vs 24% for patients with any degree of extension beyond the cervix (most commonly to the bladder in this series) *(35)*.

Some patients with recurrent cervix cancer following radiotherapy may be salvaged with radical hysterectomy instead of exenterative surgery, but this approach has been associated with a high rate of complications. In the series of Coleman *(37)* 50 patients with recurrence (32) or persistence (18) of cervical carcinoma following primary radiation therapy were treated with radical hysterectomy. Although the 5-yr survival was 65% in 32 recurrent patients, subsequent loco-regional failure was noted in 42%, and severe complications were noted in 42% including bladder dysfunction in 20%, ureteral injury in 22%, vesicovaginal fistula in 24%, and rectovaginal fistula in 20%. The salvage rate was 22 of 33 (67%) for patients in whom the disease was confined to the cervix, 4 of 11 (36%) for those with vaginal extension, and 0 of 6 for those with parametrial extension.

Successful salvage therapy for patients with locally recurrent cervix cancer may be more likely in patients treated with primary surgery than in patients who recur following radiotherapy. Shingleton reported a 5-yr survival rate of 10% in a series of 67 women with local recurrence; the 3-yr survival was 14% for those who recurred after primary radiation therapy, and 27% for those who recurred after primary surgical therapy (38). Overall 5-yr survival rates with salvage EBRT with or without brachytherapy in previously unirradiated patients ranges from 15 to 50% (38–43).

The likelihood of successful salvage radiotherapy for patients with cervical cancer who have loco-regional recurrence following radical hysterectomy is dependent on the extent of the recurrent disease. Small volume central recurrence limited to the vagina is adequately treated with EBRT plus brachytherapy in many instances and 5-yr salvage rates of 40–80% have been reported (40,42,44,45). Local control and survival are poor in patients with extension of disease beyond the vagina; 5 year survival rates of 4–27% have been reported with local control achieved in only 20–30% of patients (36,39,40,42,44,46). When peripheral relapse is limited in volume with only unilateral sidewall extension, 15–30% may be salvaged with radiotherapy; salvage rates for those with massive peripheral relapse involving both sidewalls are less than 5% (44,46). Patients who recur within 6 mo of surgery have been reported to have a worse prognosis with a median survival of 6 vs 12 mo in patients who were diagnosed with recurrence after a longer interval (39).

Interstitial brachytherapy alone has been used for salvage therapy in patients with recurrent cervix or other gynecologic malignancies. Nori et al. (47) treated 75 patients with recurrent cervix cancer and reported a 10% 5-yr disease-free survival with a median survival of 11 mo; 5-yr survival in women with disease confined to the central pelvis was 31%. The median survival in 21 women with noncervical primaries was also 11 mo with 1 of 21 surviving 5 yr (5%). The majority of patients in this series had been previously irradiated. Better results were reported by Monk et al. (48) who treated 28 locally recurrent patients (18 cervix, 10 corpus) with interstitial brachytherapy with or without EBRT; long-term disease-free survival was reported in 36% and local control in 54%. None of the patients with sidewall involvement were salvaged (48).

Patients with locally advanced recurrent cervix cancer may respond to chemotherapy in as many as 2 of 3 cases, but chemotherapy with currently available drugs has no potential for long-term cure (49). Fifteen patients with locally recurrent cervix cancer were treated with chemotherapy alone in the series of Potter (43) and all died of disease. Chemotherapy given concomitantly with radiation therapy for salvage of local recurrence may improve salvage rates, however. In a preliminary Princess Margaret Hospital study, 17 patients with recurrent cervix cancer were treated with EBRT and concomitant 5-FU with or without mitomycin; 8 of 17 (47%) were rendered disease free and remained alive a median of 34 mo (range 21–58 mo) following salvage therapy (32). The need for effective systemic therapy in patients with recurrence apparently limited to local sites is evidenced by the fact that 50% of patients treated for local recurrence develop distant metastases *(4)*.

2.2.2. RECURRENT ENDOMETRIAL CANCER

The results of salvage therapy for local recurrence of endometrial cancer following primary surgical therapy are similar to those reported for cervical cancer with prognosis dependent upon the extent and location of the recurrence. In women with isolated vaginal recurrences, treatment with EBRT plus brachytherapy results in long-term disease control and survival in 25–60% *(50–55)*. Salvage therapy is less effective if the vaginal recurrence extends into the pelvis; Kuten *(53)* reported 5-yr disease-free survival in 40% and pelvic control in 59% of women with recurrences limited to the vagina vs 20% 5-yr disease-free survival and 17% pelvic control in those with extension of disease into the pelvis. Survival rates for women with pelvic recurrence with or without vaginal recurrence range from 0–20% at 5-yr *(50,52–54)*. Local failure has been reported in 100% of patients with lateral pelvic recurrence treated with EBRT alone *(50)* or EBRT with or without brachytherapy *(53)*.

3. PATIENT SELECTION AND TREATMENT FACTORS FOR IORT

3.1. Patient Selection

Potential candidates for IORT should be jointly evaluated by the radiation oncologist and the gynecologic oncologist. A thorough history should be taken and detailed examination performed; pelvic examination under anesthesia may be required in some cases to accurately determine the extent of pelvic tumor. Staging studies should be directed towards the most common sites of distant metastases; these would include liver function tests, imaging of the abdomen and pelvis with computed tomography (CT), and imaging of the chest (chest X-ray or CT). Magnetic resonance imaging (MRI) may be useful to delineate tumor extent within the pelvis. In patients with known para-aortic adenopathy, consideration should be given to biopsy of scalene lymph nodes prior to proceeding with exploration and IORT.

General criteria for selection of patients with gynecologic malignancies for IORT have been detailed in publications from Mayo Clinic *(56,57)*. Patients should be able to tolerate a major operation and have local or nodal disease that would not be adequately controlled with surgical resection alone; EBRT doses needed for local control should exceed normal tissue tolerances and there should be no evidence of distant metastases. Candidates for IORT would include those with advanced primary or recurrent gynecologic malignancies (most commonly cervix or corpus origin) with direct extension to the pelvic sidewall, or those with gross nodal metastases to pelvic or para-aortic lymph nodes *(58)*. Patients with ovarian cancer are generally not considered for IORT, with the exception of the rare patient with localized recurrent disease, because of the high rate of generalized intraabdominal metastases.

3.2. Sequencing of Treatment Modalities

Patients with primary locally advanced gynecologic malignancies in whom surgery plus IOERT is being considered should receive preoperative EBRT (with or without concomitant chemotherapy) to increase the probability of achieving a gross total resection. Doses in the range of 45–50 Gy in 1.8-Gy fractions can be safely delivered to the pelvis or para-aortic nodal regions. The role of chemotherapy is not defined; studies of neoadjuvant chemotherapy in locally advanced cervical cancer have either been negative or favored irradiation alone (59–62). Concomitant 5-FU plus cisplatinum (CDDP) and EBRT may be safely delivered and this approach is currently being evaluated by the Gynecologic Oncology Group in a randomized clinical trial. Postoperative chemotherapy has not been fully evaluated; one randomized study of postoperative radiotherapy with or without cisplatinum, vinblastine, and bleomycin in node-positive cervix cancer patients following radical hysterectomy showed no benefit to the addition of chemotherapy (63).

Preoperative EBRT with or without chemotherapy is also the preferred sequence in those with locally advanced recurrent disease who have not been previously irradiated. In previously irradiated patients, however, full-dose EBRT is not feasible and the preoperative EBRT dose in these cases depends on the prior radiation dose, the time interval from initial treatment to recurrence, and the location of the recurrence with respect to normal dose-limiting structures such a small bowel. Investigators at Thomas Jefferson University (64) have demonstrated that retreatment doses of 30–36 Gy to the posterior pelvis via lateral fields which exclude small bowel in patients who have previously received 45–50 Gy are tolerable when given in conjunction with low-dose continuous infusion 5-FU for patients with recurrent rectal cancer.

Preoperative chemotherapy should be considered in patients with limited external-beam options to increase the probability of gross total resection. In a phase II study using the MVAC (methotrexate, vinblastine, doxorubicin, cisplatinum) regimen in women with recurrent cervical or vaginal malignancies, an objective response rate of 66% and clinical complete response rate of 21% was reported (65). For those with fixed small-bowel loops in the pelvis that prevent preoperative EBRT, chemotherapy followed by maximal resection plus IOERT and pelvic reconstruction with omentum or mesh to exclude the small bowel from the tumor bed may allow postoperative EBRT to be delivered and is the preferred sequencing of modalities.

3.3. Irradiation Factors

3.3.1. EBRT

In previously unirradiated primary or recurrent patients, EBRT doses of 45–50 Gy (with or without concomitant chemotherapy) should be delivered to the pelvis or para-aortic regions in 1.8-Gy fractions. For pelvic lesions, treatment should be delivered on a linear accelerator with ≥ 10 MeV photons and four shaped-field techniques. In women with cervix or uterine primaries, the external and internal iliac lymph nodes should be included in the treatment field. In patients with involved pelvic lymph nodes, consideration should be given to inclusion of the lower para-aortic nodes in the EBRT field. If there is disease extension to the lower one-third of the vagina, techniques to include the inguinal lymph nodes should be utilized.

External-beam treatment of para-aortic nodal metastases should also be done using a four-field technique and ≥ 10 MeV photons with the patient in the prone position. Use of a false table-top technique for the lateral fields often results in anterior displacement of small bowel and stomach away from nodal regions and may result in better target volume coverage with less small-bowel dose. This has the potential for improving both acute and chronic tolerance. The dose contribution from lateral fields should be limited to 18 Gy so that kidney tolerance is not exceeded. If IOERT to the para-aortic region is contemplated, the spinal-cord dose should be limited to 35–40 Gy as additional spinal-cord dose may be delivered with IOERT.

External-beam treatment of previously irradiated patients must be individualized. The target volume is usually limited to the gross tumor recurrence with a 2-cm margin. If small bowel can be excluded from the target volume, doses of 25–30 Gy preoperatively may be delivered. If small-bowel contrast films obtained at the time of simulation show fixed loops of bowel adjacent to the target volume, EBRT should be delivered postoperatively after surgical exclusion of the small bowel from the tumor bed.

3.3.2. IOERT Treatment Factors

3.3.2.1. Dose and Energy. IOERT is delivered at the time of surgery after maximum surgical resection. At Mayo, a refurbished Clinac 18 is located within a dedicated IORT suite in the operating rooms and electron energies from 6 to 18 MeV are available. The choice of electron energy depends on the depth of the target volume and the location of critical deep structures such as spinal cord. The IOERT dose is calculated at the 90% isodose line; if 6-MeV electrons are used, bolus material may be placed over the IOERT field to compensate for the lower surface dose of low-energy electrons. If abutting fields are indicated, silk sutures should be placed to mark the edge of the initial field (inner portion of the applicator) to facilitate accurate matching of the subsequent field.

The IOERT dose depends on the amount of residual disease and the amount of EBRT that has been delivered preoperatively or is planned postoperatively. If EBRT doses of 45–50 Gy have been delivered or can be delivered postoperatively, 10–12.5 Gy is used for narrow margins or microscopically positive margins, 15–17.5 Gy for gross residual ≤ 2 cm in diameter and 20 Gy for gross residual > 2 cm in diameter. When the EBRT dose is limited to 20–30 Gy because of prior treatment, higher IOERT doses of 15–20 Gy may be used even for microscopically positive margins; however, IOERT doses higher than 20 Gy are rarely given.

3.3.2.2. IOERT Applicators. A variety of shapes and sizes of lucite applicators are necessary to conform to the anatomy of the presacrum, pelvic sidewall, anterior pelvis, and para-aortic lymph-node regions. In the pelvis, circular applicators with 15° or 30° bevels are usually selected. Elliptical or rectangular applicators with flat or 20° bevel ends are often utilized in the para-aortic region (Fig. 1). The availability of a variety of applicator sizes ensures optimal coverage of the resected tumor bed or residual disease while minimizing normal tissue risks. At Mayo Clinic, circular applicators are available in 0.5-cm increments from 5.0 to 9.5 cm. Elliptical applicator sizes include 7 × 12 cm, 9 × 12 cm, 8 × 15 cm, and 8 × 20 cm; rectangular applicator sizes include 8 × 9 cm, 8 × 12 cm, and 8 × 15 cm.

3.3.3. Surgical Considerations

The addition of IORT to the surgical procedure has not resulted in increased acute surgical complications compared to that seen with EBRT plus surgery without IORT *(66–68)*. Tepper reported complications in 35% of patients who received preoperative EBRT without IORT and 32% in patients who received IORT in addition to EBRT and surgical resection *(67)*.

A midline incision is usually necessary to achieve adequate exposure for resection and IORT in the abdomen and pelvis. The incision may need to be more extensive than usual to allow for placement of the IOERT applicator. When both abdominal and perineal incisions are necessary for resection of low-lying pelvic lesions, the tumor bed may be visualized and treated more appropriately through the perineal incision *(66)*.

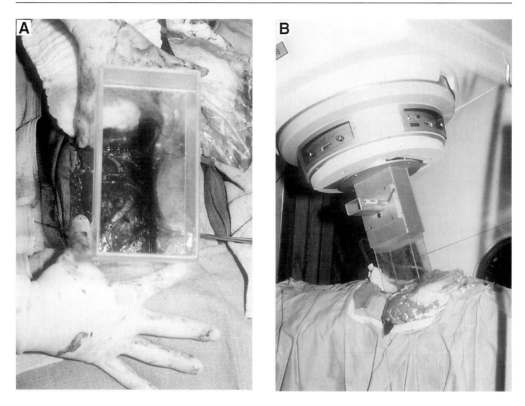

Fig. 1. Treatment of para-aortic region, Mayo Clinic. **(A)** Rectangular applicator 8 × 15 cm with 20° bevel positioned to cover the para-aortic region after mobilization of the small bowel. **(B)** Applicator "docked" with linear accelerator and patient is ready for treatment.

A thorough exploration of the abdomen and pelvis should be performed to detect clinically occult hematogenous distant metastases (i.e., to the liver) or peritoneal spread of disease that would be a contraindication to aggressive local therapy unless the metastasis is solitary in nature and can be resected with negative margins. Patients with locally advanced cervix or endometrial cancer should undergo pelvic lymph-node dissection, and if positive lymph nodes are reported on frozen section analysis, the para-aortic nodes should be dissected. In patients with known para-aortic lymph-node metastases, consideration may be given to scalene lymph-node biopsy prior to laparotomy.

The goal of the surgical procedure is gross total resection if it can be safely accomplished. Maximum resection of the tumor should take place before IORT. The availability of frozen-section pathology analysis is critical to allow for identification of the limits of gross and microscopic tumor extensions. Patients with invasion of the bladder or rectum or those with recurrence in the pelvis after previous irradiation usually require anterior or posterior exenteration. Reconstruction should be done after IORT (i.e., reanastomosis of the rectum) to allow for full exposure of the tumor bed and to avoid irradiating the anastomosis. However, if a vascular reconstruction is required this should be performed prior to IORT *(58)*. Inclusion of large-vessel anastomoses in the IORT field appears to be safe; arterial anastomoses have been shown to heal adequately after IORT doses as high as 45 Gy in dogs *(69)*.

If postoperative EBRT may be indicated, a number of surgical options exist to optimize tumor-volume reconstruction and displacement of dose-limiting organs. Placement

Table 2
Survival Results with IORT-Containing Regimens
for Locally Advanced Gynecologic Malignancies, United States Series

Series, Patient Group	No. Pts.	Median (mo.)	Survival (%)			Disease-Free Survival (%)		
			2 yr	3 yr	5 yr	2 yr	3 yr	5 yr
Mayo, All (70)	63	15	44	30	27	36	27	21
Primary[a]	8	12	14	14	14	14	14	14
Recurrent	55	20	48	32	29	38	29	21
Cervix	36	15	40	25	25	30	24	21
Endometrium	10	56	80	57	38	60	50	17
Other[b]	9	14	44	33	33	44	22	22
U. Washington, recurrent cervix (72)	21	22	—	—	32	—	—	—

[a]4 cervix, 2 vagina, 1 endometrium, 1 uterine sarcoma.
[b]3 vagina, 4 uterine sarcoma, 2 ovary.

of clips to mark the borders of the IORT field is helpful for follow-up evaluation and for design of postoperative EBRT fields, if indicated. When postoperative pelvic EBRT is planned, reconstruction of the pelvic floor and mechanical exclusion of the small bowel from the pelvis (using omentum if available vs tissue expanders or absorbable mesh) may improve EBRT tolerance and decrease the risk of treatment-related small-bowel complications. In patients with a history of prior EBRT in whom aggressive retreatment approaches include additional EBRT, maximal resection, and IORT, pelvis reconstruction with a vascularized rectus abdominus flap may be useful in improving healing and displacing small bowel if an omental flap is not feasible.

4. RESULTS—IOERT WITH OR WITHOUT EBRT

4.1. United States

IOERT has been used at Mayo Clinic (56,57,70) for both locally advanced primary and recurrent gynecologic malignancies and at the University of Washington (71,72) for recurrent cervical cancer. Survival and disease control with IORT containing regimens from these two institutions are summarized in Tables 2 and 3. None of the patients in either series were considered potentially curable with surgery and/or EBRT alone. The 5-yr overall survivals of 27 and 32% and 5-yr local-control figures of 50–55% are encouraging given the historical poor results with standard salvage therapy.

4.1.1. PRIMARY DISEASE

There is very little information in the literature regarding the use of IORT in primary locally advanced malignancies. Patients with primary cervix or uterine malignancies with disease extension to the pelvic sidewall or locally advanced nodal metastases are those with the potential for benefit from the addition of IORT to the treatment program.

Some of the earliest results with IOERT in the treatment of gynecologic nodal metastases in the United States were reported by investigators at Howard University (73). Delgado et al. (74) treated 16 patients with locally advanced cervical cancer with IOERT to the para-aortic region; 11 patients had para-aortic metastases; and 5 were treated

Table 3
Locally Advanced Gynecologic Malignancies, Disease Relapse in United States IORT Series

Series, Patient Group	No. at risk	Local Relapse (%)			Central Relapse (IORT) (%)			Distant Relapse (%)		
		No. (%)	3 yr	5 yr	No. (%)	3 yr	5 yr	No. (%)	3 yr	5 yr
Mayo, All (70)	63	23 (37)	45	45	16 (25)	33	33	25 (40)	43	47
Primary [a]	8	4 (50)	62	62	3 (38)	43	43	2 (25)	36	36
Recurrent	55	19 (35)	43	43	13 (24)	31	31	23 (42)	44	48
Cervix	36	14 (39)	50	50	11 (31)	40	40	17 (47)	52	58
Endometrium	10	2 (20)	22	22	0	0	0	3 (30)	33	33
Other [b]	9	3 (33)	50	50	2 (22)	42	42	3 (33)	33	33
U. Washington, recurrent cervix (71)	22	10 (45)	52	52	—	—	—	6 (27)	—	—

[a]4 cervix, 2 vagina, 1 endometrium, 1 uterine sarcoma.
[b]3 vagina, 4 uterine sarcoma, 2 ovary.
[c]Disease-specific survival.

prophylactically. IOERT doses ranged from 15–20 Gy and only two patients received para-aortic EBRT. Four of 11 patients with nodal metastases were alive 10–36 mo following IOERT, 2 without evidence of disease.

In addition to the Mayo series (Tables 2 and 3) (70) and the Howard University series (74), two other small series patients with primary gynecologic malignancies who have received IOERT have been reported. Yordan reported the results of IOERT in five women with primary gynecological malignancies (two cervix, three corpus) at Rush or Pamplona (75). Four of five were without evidence of disease at the time of publication and there were no local failures. IOERT doses were 10–15 Gy for microscopic disease and 15–26 Gy for macroscopic disease. Konski et al. (76) reported treating eight patients with cervix cancer with IOERT to the para-aortic region. IOERT doses ranged from 10–25 Gy (median 20 Gy) and no patient received EBRT to the para-aortic region. Two patients had bulky para-aortic metastases, five microscopic disease, and one was treated prophylactically. The median survival was 27 mo and the actuarial 2-yr survival was 63%. Para-aortic nodal recurrence was diagnosed in three of eight (38%).

4.1.2. Recurrent Disease

IORT has been more frequently utilized in patients with isolated nodal or locally recurrent gynecologic malignancies than in primary malignancies. Preliminary results from Howard University (74) and Massachusetts General Hospital (MGH) (77) suggested that IOERT was feasible in locally recurrent patients. Orthovoltage IORT without EBRT was utilized in a Roswell park series (78) of 23 recurrent patients; median survival was 7 mo with 2- and 3-yr survivals of 20 and 13%, respectively. Konski et al. (76) treated six patients with para-aortic nodal recurrences of gynecologic malignancies (two endometrial, two cervix, one uterine sarcoma) with IOERT doses of 10–25 Gy following surgical debulking. Four of six received 45 Gy EBRT to the para-aortic region in addition to IOERT. Two of six were alive at the time of publication; one at 11 mo with no evidence of disease and one at 19 mo with para-aortic recurrence.

4.1.2.1. Mayo Clinic and University of Washington Series. The largest United States series of IOERT in recurrent patients are from Mayo Clinic and the University of Washington. Results are summarized in Tables 2 and 3 and Figs. 2 and 3.

In the University of Washington series *(71,72)* of patients with recurrent cervical cancer, IOERT was combined with either preoperative or postoperative EBRT in 13 of 22 (59%) patients. Nine of 15 previously irradiated patients received no additional EBRT, whereas six were reirradiated using conformal fields to doses ranging from 26 to 50 Gy. The median IOERT dose in all patients was 22 Gy at the point of maximum dose.

In the Mayo series *(56,57,70),* IOERT was combined with preoperative or postoperative EBRT in seven of eight (88%) primary patients and 36 of 55 (65%) recurrent patients. Nine of 28 (32%) patients with recurrence in a previously irradiated field were reirradiated with EBRT doses ranging from 9 to 50 Gy. The median IOERT dose in all patients (dose prescribed at 90% isodose line) was 15 Gy for microscopic residual tumor and 20 Gy for gross residual tumor. Eleven of 28 patients with recurrence in a previously irradiated field received preoperative MVAC chemotherapy in an attempt to increase the probability of gross total resection which was achieved in seven (64%) patients.

The reported 5-yr survivals of 29 and 32% in the Mayo series (Fig. 2) and the University of Washington series of patients with recurrence are encouraging as none of the patients in either series were considered potentially curable with surgical resection alone. Local control was reported in 57% in the Mayo series and 48% in the University of Washington series, an apparent improvement compared to historical controls. Despite careful staging to rule out detectable distant metastatic disease, subsequent distant recurrence was a significant problem in both series (Table 3).

4.1.3. OVARIAN CANCER

Limited numbers of patients with recurrent ovarian cancer have been treated with IOERT. Konski et al. *(79)* treated five patients with recurrent ovarian cancer with surgical debulking, IOERT, and postoperative whole-abdomen EBRT. Two of the five patients had gross residual tumor at the time of IOERT; median survival was 14 mo (range 8–46). Two patients in the Mayo series *(70)* had localized ovarian cancer recurrences and were treated with IOERT; one of these patients was alive without evidence of disease > 7 yr following treatment.

4.2. European Results

There have been three major published European series of IOERT for locally advanced gynecologic malignancies *(46,80,81).* Survival and disease-control rates from these series are summarized in Table 4.

4.2.1. LYON SERIES

Gerard et al. *(81)* reported results in 54 patients treated in Lyon for either primary or recurrent disease. Twenty women with locally advanced primary cervix cancer (7 stage IIB, 12 III, 1 IV) were treated with 44 Gy EBRT plus one cycle 5-FU/CDDP plus IOERT. At a median follow-up of 18 mo (range, 12–34 mo), only 4 pelvic relapses (20%) had occurred. Fourteen of 20 (70%) were without evidence of disease, and 15 of 20 (75%) were alive at the time of publication. An additional 34 patients with pelvic recurrence (28 cervix, 6 endometrial; sites of recurrence—central pelvis in 4, sidewall in 25, para-aortic lymph nodes in 5) were treated with IOERT; 16 of 34 received EBRT in addition to

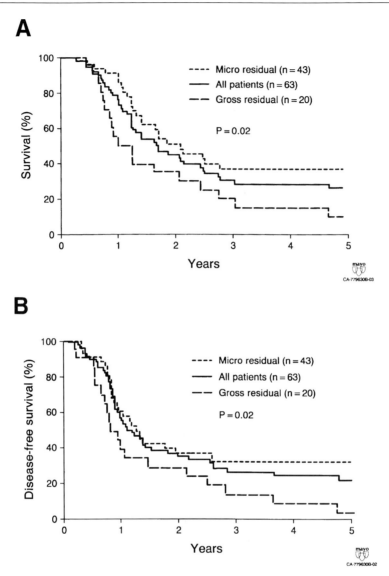

Fig. 2. Actuarial survival as a function of amount of residual disease at the time of IOERT after maximal resection, Mayo analysis. (**A**) Overall survival. (**B**) Disease-free survival.

IOERT. Gross residual tumor was present in the 22 of 34 patients at the time of IOERT. The 4-yr actuarial survival was 32% and central failure occurred in 6 of 34 (18%) patients.

4.2.2. FRENCH IORT GROUP

The largest series of IOERT for recurrent cervix cancer is from the cooperative French Intraoperative Group who reported results of IOERT for 70 recurrent cervix-cancer patients treated in seven French institutions *(46)*. Median survival was 11 mo and 3-yr survival was only 8%. Subsequent local relapse was noted in 75% of patients. Forty of the 70 patients in this series received no EBRT, and some of the 37 patients with gross residual had no resection of tumor.

Table 4
Locally Advanced Gynecologic Malignancies, Survival and Disease Control in European IORT Series

Series	Patient group	No. Pts.	Median Survival	Overall Survival	Local Relapse (%)	Central Relapse (%)	Distant Relapse (%)
U. Navarre (80)	recurrent cervix, prior EBRT	14	7 mo	7% 4 yr	6/10 (60)	2/9 (22)	2/10 (20)
	1° or recurrent cervix, no prior EBRT	24	38 mo	47% 4 yr	3/19 (16)	1/19 (5)	2/19 (11)
	miscellaneous[a] recurrent	10	19 mo	30% 4 yr	4/9 (44)	3/9 (33)	6/9 (67)
France (46)	recurrent cervix	70	11 mo	8% 3 yr	50/67 (75)	—	22/67 (33)
Lyon (81)	primary cervix	20	—	15/20 (75%)[b]	4/20 (20)	—	2/20 (10)
	recurrent cervix/uterus	34	—	32% 4 yr	—	6/34 (18)	—

EBRT = external-beam radiation therapy, 1° = primary, yr = year.
[a]4 endometrium, 4 ovary, 2 vulva.
[b]Crude survival, follow-up 12–34 mo, median 18 mo.

4.2.3. UNIVERSITY OF NAVARRE, PAMPLONA

At the University of Navarre in Pamplona, 48 women with locally advanced gynecologic malignancies have been treated with IOERT (80). Survival results were poor in women with locally recurrent cervix cancer who had been previously irradiated with a 7-mo median and 7% 4-yr survival. Local relapse was reported in 60% of retreatment patients but only 22% relapsed within the IOERT field. Better results were seen in women with primary or recurrent cervix cancer without prior EBRT with a 38-mo median survival and 47% 5-yr survival. The local relapse rate was only 16% and central relapse 5%.

4.3. Prognostic Factors for Disease Control and Survival

4.3.1. AMOUNT OF RESIDUAL DISEASE AFTER MAXIMAL RESECTION AND EXTENT OF RESECTION

Improvements in survival and local control have been reported in both United States and European series when the surgeon is able to perform a gross total resection prior to IOERT. A summary of survival and disease control according to the amount of residual disease is summarized in Table 5. Five-year survivals of 40 and 42% were reported for recurrent patients with microscopic residual tumor in the University of Washington (72) and the Mayo (70) series vs 29 and 11%, respectively, for those with gross residual tumor. In the Mayo series (70), the rate of distant metastases was more than doubled in the group of patients with gross residual vs microscopic residual disease (log rank p value = 0.001) and 5-yr survival was 11 vs 40% ($p = 0.02$) (Fig. 2). Local failure at 5 yr was noted in 49% of patients with microscopic residual and 23% of patients with gross residual disease ($p = 0.44$). The low local-failure rate in Mayo patients with gross residual disease may be partially attributable to the high rate of distant failure and subsequent death before local relapse was clinically evident. In contrast to the Mayo experience, there was no difference in distant metastatic rates in the French series (46). However, the rate of local failure in the group with gross residual was 84% (some of these patients had no resection,

Table 5
Gynecologic IOERT, Locally Recurrent, Survival
and Disease Control by Amount of Residual Disease at IOERT

Series	Residual[a]	No. Pts.	Median survival	Survival 5-yr	Local Failure (%)	Local Failure 5-yr	Distant Mets (%)	Distant Mets 5-yr
U. Washington (72)	micro	10	25 mo	40%	—	45%	—	—
	gross	12	18 mo	29%	—	64%	—	—
Mayo (70)	micro	36	26 mo	42%	14/36 (39)	49%	10/36 (28)	31%
	gross	19	11 mo	11%	5/19 (26)	23%	13/19 (68)	78%
France (46)	micro	30	13 mo	—	19/30 (63)	73% 3 yr	9/30 (30)	—
	gross	37	10 mo	—	31/37 (84)	89% 3 yr	11/37 (30)	—
Spain (101)	micro	7	—	71% crude	—	—	—	—
	gross	19	—	5% crude	—	—	—	—

[a]micro = microscopic residual disease, gross = macroscopic residual disease.

Table 6
Locally Advanced Gynecologic Malignancy IOERT, Survival,
and Local Control by Prior Irradiation Status

Series	Prior EBRT	No. Pts.	Median Survival	Actuarial Survival	Local Relapse
U. Navarre (80)	yes	14	7 mo	7% 4 yr	6/10 (60%) crude
	no[a]	24	38 mo	47% 4 yr	3/19 (16%) crude
Mayo (70)	yes	28	15 mo	25% 5 yr	10/28 (36%) crude, 53% 5 yr
	no[b]	26	20 mo	31% 5 yr	9/26 (35%) crude, 37% 5 yr

[a]Includes primary cervical cancer and those with recurrence following surgery.
[b]Includes eight previously irradiated patients with recurrence outside the radiation field.

only biopsy of disease) and it is likely that many of these patients died of their local disease prior to manifestation of distant metastases. When a gross total resection is not possible, tolerable doses of IORT without EBRT is unlikely to result in local control of tumor. In the Roswell Park series, nine patients with recurrent cervix cancer were treated with 15-Gy orthovoltage IORT without EBRT; all four patients with gross residual disease had central recurrence of disease (78).

The extent of the surgical procedure, pelvic exenteration vs less extensive surgery was evaluated in the University of Washington series. No difference in disease-specific survival was reported (71).

4.3.2. PRIOR EBRT

The prognostic significance of prior EBRT is uncertain; some have reported inferior results in previously irradiated patients, whereas others have found no difference. A summary of results from the Mayo series (70) and the University of Navarre series (80) is presented in Table 6. In the Mayo series there was no significant decrement in survival or disease control in recurrent patients who had previously been irradiated compared to those who recurred after primary surgical treatment or those who recurred outside the prior irradiation field. Similarly, the University of Washington group (71) reported similar disease-specific survivals for previously irradiated and unirradiated patients with recurrent cervical cancer. In contrast, in the University of Navarre experience, survival was only 7% at 4 yr in previously irradiated patients compared to 47% at 4 yr for primary cervix cancer patients or those who recurred following surgical therapy.

4.3.3. IRRADIATION DOSE—EBRT, IOERT

The dose of EBRT or IOERT has not been consistently associated with outcome. In the Mayo series (70), there was no association of EBRT dose or IOERT dose with survival, local control, or distant control. In a small combined Rush Presbyterian/Pamplona series of 10 recurrent gynecologic malignancy patients, the EBRT dose did not correlate with local control using a dividing point of 40 Gy. However, they did note improved local control for those in whom the sum of the EBRT dose and twice the IOERT dose (effective IOERT dose is 2–3 times fractionated EBRT dose) was > 70 Gy with four of seven patients controlled locally vs none of three with effective doses < 70 Gy (75).

4.4. Distant Control

Distant failure is a significant problem, especially in the group of patients with gross residual disease at the time of IOERT. In the Mayo series (70), the 5-yr distant recurrence rate was 47% for all patients and 78% for recurrent patients with gross residual disease.

Improvements in survival in patients with locally advanced gynecologic malignancies will require effective systemic therapy. The most effective single agent for the treatment of squamous-cell carcinoma of the cervix is cisplatinum with an objective response rate of approx 30% (49). The duration of response in patients with recurrence following radiation or surgery is on the order of 4–6 mo, and few patients survive longer than a year (49). Salvage chemotherapy with currently available agents is largely ineffective (49).

Patients with unresectable recurrent disease after previous irradiation may be considered for combination chemotherapy to increase the likelihood of a gross total resection and decrease the distant metastasis rate. The MVAC regimen has been shown to have significant activity in advanced cervical cancer with a response rate of 66% (21% complete response, 45% partial response) (65). There was a trend towards a reduction in distant metastases in the Mayo series with the use of chemotherapy (largely MVAC) with 5-yr distant recurrence rates of 54 vs 27% ($p = 0.09$) (Fig. 3), but the administration of chemotherapy did not appear to impact on survival.

4.5. Tolerance of IOERT

Peripheral nerve is the dose-limiting structure for IORT in the pelvis and para-aortic lymph-node region. Painful neuropathy has been reported in 5–30% of patients who receive IORT (57,71,80,82). In the University of Washington series (71), 9 of 22 (41%) women developed painful peripheral neuropathy (minor motor deficits in addition to pain in two patients) following IOERT doses ranging from 14 to 27.8 Gy (median 22 Gy) calculated at the depth of maximum dose. In two cases the neuropathy was caused by recurrent tumor rather than IOERT. The risk of neuropathy was not related to IOERT field size or dose. There was an association noted with cumulative EBRT dose; neuropathy developed in 4 of 4 with cumulative EBRT doses > 75 Gy and 3 of 18 with < 75 Gy. Reirradiation with EBRT doses of 26–50 Gy (median 30.6 Gy) was done in 6 of 15 previously irradiated patients. Four patients had resolution of neuropathy after 6–18 mo; the remaining three patients had neuropathy that persisted until death.

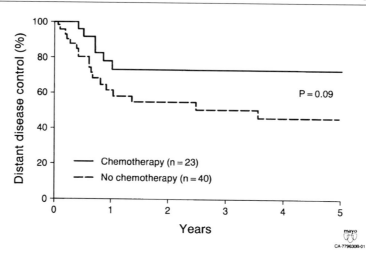

Fig. 3. Distant disease control in patients who received or did not receive chemotherapy as a component of treatment, Mayo Analysis

The risk of peripheral neuropathy has been associated with IOERT dose in patients with recurrent colorectal cancer. In the Mayo analysis, the risk of grade 2 or 3 neuropathy was 7% with IOERT doses ≤ 12.5 Gy vs 19% with higher doses *(83)*. In the Mayo series of primary or recurrent gynecologic malignancy patients, only 2 of 63 (3%) have developed grade 3 neuropathy *(70)*.

Grade 3 or higher toxicities of any nature related to IOERT were diagnosed in 11 of 63 (17%) of patients in the Mayo gynecologic series *(70)*. Toxicities other than neuropathy included intestinal fistula or obstruction in 8%, soft-tissue injury in 3%, and ureteral obstruction in 3%. If tumor is adherent to the ureter prior to resection, the ureter should be included in the IORT field with a stent placed either prophylactically or if subsequent obstruction develops to prevent loss of renal function.

5. SURGERY PLUS HDR-IORT WITH OR WITHOUT EBRT

Intraoperative irradiation may be delivered with a high-dose-rate brachytherapy source (HDR-IORT) after placement of temporary catheters along the tumor bed. German investigators have reported preliminary results of postoperative high-dose-rate brachytherapy using catheters placed at the time of operation for women with recurrent gynecologic malignancies that involve the pelvic sidewall *(84)*. Whereas this approach has the advantage of allowing for fractionation of the radiation dose, normal tissues such as small bowel cannot not be displaced to the same degree achievable with true HDR-IORT.

6. CONCLUSIONS AND FUTURE POSSIBILITIES

Survival and disease-control rates in patients with locally recurrent surgically inoperable gynecologic malignancies who are treated with aggressive local therapy that includes IOERT compare favorably to historical controls. Research efforts should concentrate on efforts to improve the likelihood of gross total resection given the poor results seen in patients with gross residual disease. Preoperative concomitant chemoradiotherapy should be explored where feasible. For patients in whom gross total resection cannot be accomplished, use of intraoperative irradiation dose modifiers needs to be evaluated (sensitizers, hyperthermia, and so on). Evaluation of IORT in unresectable locally advanced primary malignancies deserves further exploration. Given the unacceptably high rate of distant metastases, more effective systemic strategies need to be developed.

Long-term control of locally advanced gynecologic malignancies is possible in a significant number of carefully selected patients with aggressive multimodality local therapy that includes IORT. Further evaluation of IORT by those centers with demonstrated expertise seems warranted.

REFERENCES

1. Marcial VA and Marcial LV. Radiation therapy of cervical cancer, *Cancer,* **71** (1993) 1438–1445.
2. Jampolis S, Andras EJ, and Fletcher GH. Analysis of sites and causes of failures of irradiation in invasive squamous cell carcinoma of the intact uterine cervix, *Radiology,* **115** (1975) 681–685.
3. Perez CA, Fox S, Lockett MA, et al. Impact of dose in outcome of irradiation alone in carcinoma of the uterine cervix: analysis of two different methods, *Int. J. Radiat. Oncol. Biol. Phys.,* **21** (1991) 885–898.
4. Perez CA, Kuske RR, Camel HM, et al. Analysis of pelvic tumor control and impact on survival in carcinoma of the uterine cervix treated with radiation therapy alone, *Int. J. Radiat. Oncol. Biol. Phys.,* **14** (1988) 613–621.
5. Chism SE, Keys HM, and Gillin MT. Carcinoma of the cervix: a time-dose analysis of control and complication, *Am. J. Roentgenol.,* **123** (1975) 84–90.
6. Hanks GE, Herring DF, and Kramer S. Patterns of care outcome studies—results of National Practice in Cancer of the Cervix, *Cancer,* **51** (1983) 959–967.
7. Kottmeier HL and Gray MJ. Rectal and bladder injuries in relation to radiation dosage in carcinoma of cervix, *Am. J. Obstet. Gynecol.,* **82** (1961) 74–82.
8. Perez CA, Breaux S, Bedwinek JM, et al. Radiation therapy alone in the treatment of carcinoma of the uterine cervix II: analysis of complications, *Cancer,* **54** (1984) 235–246.
9. Unal A, Hamberger AD, Seski JC, and Fletcher GH. An analysis of the severe complications of irradiation of carcinoma of the uterine cervix: treatment with intracavitary radium and parametrial irradiation, *Int. J. Radiat. Oncol. Biol. Phys.,* **7** (1981) 999–1004.
10. Hamberger AD, Unal A, Gershenson DM, and Fletcher GH. Analysis of the severe complications of irradiation of carcinoma of the cervix: whole pelvis irradiation and intracavitary radium, *Int. J. Radiat. Oncol. Biol. Phys.,* **9** (1983) 367–371.
11. Potish RA, Downey GO, Adcock LL, Prem KA, and Twiggs LB. The role of surgical debulking in cancer of the uterine cervix, *Int. J. Radiat. Oncol. Biol. Phys.,* **17** (1989) 979–984.
12. Fletcher GH. Subclinical disease, *Cancer,* **55** (1984) 1274–1284.
13. Stehman FB, Bundy BN, DiSaia PJ, Keys HM, Larson JE, and Fowler WC. Carcinoma of the cervix treated with radiation therapy I: a multivariate analysis of prognostic variables in the Gynecologic Oncology Group, *Cancer,* **67** (1991) 2776–2785.
14. Komaki R, Mattingly RF, Hoffman RG, Barber SW, Satre R, and Greenberg M. Irradiation of para-aortic lymph node metastases from carcinoma of the cervix or endometrium, *Radiology,* **147** (1983) 245–248.
15. Berman ML, Keys H, Creasman W, DiSaia P, Bundy B, and Blessing J. Survival and patterns of recurrence in cervical cancer metastatic to periaortic lymph nodes, *Gynecol. Oncol.,* **19** (1984) 8–16.
16. Lovecchio JL, Averette HE, Donato D, and Bell J. 5-year survival of patients with periaortic nodal metastases in clinical stage IB and IIA cervical carcinoma, *Gynecol. Oncol.,* **34** (1989) 43–45.
17. Hughes RR, Brewington KC, Hanjani P, et al. Extended field irradiation for cervical cancer based on surgical staging, *Gynecol. Oncol.,* **9** (1980) 153–161.
18. Potish R, Adcock L, Jones T Jr, et al. The morbidity and utility of periaortic radiotherapy in cervical carcinoma, *Gynecol. Oncol.,* **15** (1983) 1–9.
19. Piver MS, Barlow MD, and Krishnamsetty R. Five-year survival (with no evidence of disease) in patients with biopsy-confirmed aortic node metastasis from cervical carcinoma, *Am. J. Obstet. Gynecol.,* **139** (1981) 575–578.
20. Wharton JT, Jones HW III, Day TD Jr, Rutledge FN, and Fletcher GH. Preirradiation celiotomy and extended field irradiation for invasive carcinoma of the cervix, *Obstet. Gynecol.,* **49** (1977) 333–338.

21. Danoff BF, McDay J, Louka M, Lewis GC, Lee J, and Kramer S. Stage III endometrial carcinoma: analysis of patterns of failure and therapeutic implications, *Int. J. Radiat. Oncol. Biol. Phys.*, **6** (1980) 1491–1495.

22. Potish RA, Twiggs LB, Adcock LL, and Prem KA. Role of whole abdominal radiation therapy in the management of endometrial cancer; prognostic importance of factors indicating peritoneal metastases, *Gynecol. Oncol.*, **21** (1985) 80–86.

23. Bruckman JE, Bloomer WD, Marck A, Ehrmann RL, and Knapp RC. Stage III adenocarcinom of the endometrium: two prognostic groups, *Gynecol. Oncol.*, **9** (1980) 12–17.

24. Antoniades J, Brady LW, and Lewis GC. The management of stage III carcinoma of the endometrium, *Cancer*, **38** (1976) 1838–1842.

25. Greven KM, Curran WJ Jr, Whitington R, et al. Analysis of failure patterns in stage III endometrial carcinoma and therapeutic implications, *Int. J. Radiat. Oncol. Biol. Phys.*, **17** (1989) 35–39.

26. Feuer GA and Calanog A. Endometrial carcinoma: treatment of positive paraaortic nodes, *Gynecol. Oncol.*, **27** (1987) 194–109.

27. Eifel PJ. Can patients with regional metastases from carcinoma of the endometrium be cured with radiation therapy? In Meyer JL (ed.), *The Lymphatic System and Cancer*, Karger, Basel, 1994, pp. 196–203.

28. Hicks ML, Piver MS, Puretz JL, et al. Survival in patients with paraaortic lymph node metastases from endometrial adenocarcinoma clinically limited to the uterus, *Int. J. Radiat. Oncol. Biol. Phys.*, **26** (1993) 607–611.

29. Munnell EW and Bonney WA Jr. Critical points of failure in the therapy of cancer of the cervix, *Am. J. Obstet. Gynecol.*, **81** (1961) 521–532.

30. Calame RJ. Recurrent carcinoma of the cervix, *Am. J. Obstet. Gynecol.*, **105** (1969) 380–385.

31. Brady LW, Perez CA, and Bedwinek JM. Failure patterns in gynecologic cancer, *Int. J. Radiat. Oncol. Biol. Phys.*, **12** (1986) 549–557.

32. Thomas GM, Dembo AJ, Black B, et al. Concurrent radiation and chemotherapy for carcinoma of the cervix recurrent after radical surgery, *Gynecol. Oncol.*, **27** (1987) 254–260.

33. Lawhead RA Jr, Clark DGC, Smith DH, Pierce VK, and Lewis JL Jr. Pelvic exenteration for recurrent or persistent gynecologic malignancies: a 10 year review of the Memorial Sloan-Kettering Cancer Center experience, *Gynecol. Oncol.*, **33** (1989) 279–282.

34. Shingleton HM, Soong SJ, Gelder MS, Hatch KD, Baker VV, and Austin JM Jr. Clinical and histo-pathological factors predicting recurrence and survival after pelvic exenteration for cancer of the cervix, *Obstet. Gynecol.*, **73** (1989) 1027–1034.

35. Hatch KD, Shingleton HM, Soong SJ, Baker VV, and Gelder MS. Anterior pelvic exenteration, *Gynecol. Oncol.*, **31** (1988) 205–213.

36. Prasasvinichai S, Glassburn JR, and Lewis GC. Treatment of recurrent carcinoma of the cervix, *Int. J. Radiat. Oncol. Biol. Phys.*, **4** (1978) 957–961.

37. Coleman RL, Keeney ED, Freedman RS, Burke TW, Eifel PJ, and Rutledge FN. Radical hysterectomy for recurrent carcinoma of the uterine cervix after radiotherapy, *Gynecol. Oncol.*, **55** (1994) 29–35.

38. Shingleton HM, Gore H, Soong SJ, et al. Tumor recurrence and survival in stage IB cancer of the cervix, *Am. J. Clin. Oncol.*, **6** (1983) 265–272.

39. Krebs HB, Helmkamp F, Sevin BU, Poliakiff SR, Nadji M, and Averette HE. Recurrent cancer of the cervix following radical hysterectomy and pelvic node dissection, *Obstet. Gynecol.*, **59** (1982) 422–427.

40. Deutsch M and Parsons JA. Radiotherapy for carcinoma of the cervix recurrent after surgery, *Cancer*, **34** (1974) 2051–2055.

41. Jobsen JJ, Leer JWH, Cleton FJ, and Hermans J. Treatment of locoregional recurrence of carcinoma of the cervix by radiotherapy after primary surgery, *Gynecol. Oncol.*, **33** (1989) 368–371.

42. Friedman M and Pearlman AW. Carcinoma of the cervix: radiation salvage of surgical failures, *Radiology*, **84** (1965) 801–811.

43. Potter ME, Alvarez RD, Gay FL, Shingleton HM, Soong SJ, and Hatch KD. Optimal therapy for pelvic recurrence after radical hysterectomy for early-stage cervical cancer, *Gynecol. Oncol.*, **37** (1990) 74–77.

44. Ciatto S, Pirtoli L, and Cionini L. Radiotherapy for postoperative failures of carcinoma of the cervix uteri, *Surg. Gynecol. Obstet.*, **151** (1980) 621–624.

45. Tan R, Chung CH, Liu MT, Lai YL, and Chang KH. Radiotherapy for postoperative recurrent uterine cervical carcinoma, *Acta. Oncol.*, **30** (1991) 353–356.

46. Mahe MA, Gerard JP, Dubois JB, et al. Intraoperative radiation therapy in recurrent carcinoma of the uterine cervix: report of the French Intraoperative Group on 70 patients, *Int. J. Radiat. Oncol. Biol. Phys.,* **34** (1995) 21–26.

47. Nori D, Hilaris BS, Kim HS, et al. Interstitial irradiation in recurrent gynecological cancer, *Int. J. Radiat. Oncol. Biol. Phys.,* **7** (1981) 1513–1517.

48. Monk BJ, Walker JL, Tewari K, Ramsinghani NS, Syed AMN, and DiSaia PJ. Open interstitial brachytherapy for the treatment of local-regional recurrences of uterine corpus and cervix cancer after primary surgery, *Gynecol. Oncol.,* **52** (1994) 222–228.

49. Alberts DS and Garcia DJ. Salvage chemotherapy in recurrent or refractory squamous cell cancer of the uterine cervix, *Seminars in Oncology,* **21** (1994) 37–46.

50. Pirtoli L, Ciatto S, Taddei G, and Colafrancheschi M. Salvage with radiotherapy of postsurgical relapses of endometrial cancer, *Tumori,* **66** (1980) 475–480.

51. Phillips GL, Prem KA, Adcock LL, and Twiggs LB. Vaginal recurrence of adenocarcinoma of the endometrium, *Gynecol. Oncol.,* **13** (1982) 323–328.

52. Aalders JC, Abeler V, and Kolstad P. Recurrent adenocarcinoma of the endometrium: a clinical and histopathological study of 379 patients, *Gynecol. Oncol.,* **17** (1984) 85–103.

53. Kuten A, Grigsby PW, Perez C, Fineberg B, Garcia DM, and Simpson JR. Results of radiotherapy in recurrent endometrial carcinoma: a retrospective analysis of 51 patients, *Int. J. Radiat. Oncol. Biol. Phys.,* **17** (1989) 29–34.

54. Vavra N, Denison U, Kucera H, et al. Prognostic factors related to recurrent endometrial carcinoma following initial surgery, *Acta. Obstet. Gynecol. Scand.,* **72** (1993) 205–209.

55. Morgan JD III, Reddy S, Sarin P, Yordan E, DeGeest K, and Hendrickson FR. Isolated vaginal recurrences of endometrial carcinoma, *Radiology,* **189** (1993) 609–613.

56. Garton GR, Gunderson LL, Webb MJ, et al. Intraoperative radiation therapy in gynecologic cancer: The Mayo Clinic experience, *Gynecol. Oncol.,* **48** (1993) 328–332.

57. Garton GR, Gunderson LL, Webb MJ, Wilson TO, Cha SS, and Podratz KC. Intraoperative radiation therapy in gynecologic cancer: update of the experience at a single institution, *Int. J. Radiat. Oncol. Biol. Phys.,* **37** (1997) 839–843.

58. Sindelar WF, Hoekstra HJ, and Kinsella TJ. Surgical approaches and techniques in intraoperative radiotherapy for intra-abdominal, retroperitoneal, and pelvic neoplasms, *Surgery,* **103** (1988) 247–256.

59. Tettersall MHN, Lorvidhaya V, Vootiprux V, et al. Randomized trial of epirubicin and cisplatin chemotherapy followed by pelvic radiation in locally advanced cervical cancer, *J. Clin. Oncol.,* **13** (1995) 444–451.

60. Kumar L, Kaushal R, Nandy M, et al. Chemotherapy followed by radiotherapy versus radiotherapy alone in locally advanced cervical cancer: a randomized study, *Gynecol. Oncol.,* **54** (1994) 307–315.

61. Souhami L, Gil RA, Allan SE, et al. A randomized trial of chemotherapy followed by pelvic radiation therapy in stage IIIB carcinoma of the cervix, *J. Clin. Oncol.,* **9** (1991) 970–977.

62. Chiara S, Bruzzone M, Merlini L, et al. Randomized study comparing chemotherapy plus radiotherapy versus radiotherapy alone in FIGO stage IIB-III cervical carcinoma, *Am. J. Clin. Oncol.,* **17** (1994) 294–297.

63. Tattersall MHN, Ramirez C, and Coppleson M. A randomized trial of adjuvant chemotherapy after radical hysterectomy in stage IB-IIA cervical cancer patients with pelvic lymph node metastases, *Gynecol. Oncol.,* **46** (1992) 176–181.

64. Mohiuddin M, Lingareddy V, Rakinic J, and Marks G. Reirradiation for rectal cancer and surgical resection after ultra high doses, *Int. J. Radiat. Oncol. Biol. Phys.,* **27** (1993) 1159–1163.

65. Long HJ III, Cross WG, Wieand HS, et al. Phase II trial of methotrexate, vinblastine, doxorubicin, and cisplatin in advanced /recurrent carcinoma of the uterine cervix and vagina, *Gynecol. Oncol.,* **57** (1995) 235–239.

66. Merrick HW III. Surgical aspects of intraoperative radiation therapy. In Vaeth JM and Meyer JL (eds.), *The role of high energy electrons in the treatment of cancer,* Karger, Basel, 1991, pp. 209–223.

67. Tepper JE, Gunderson LL, Orlow E, et al. Complications of intraoperative radiation therapy, *Int. J. Radiat. Oncol. Biol. Phys.,* **10** (1984) 1831–1839.

68. Avizonis VN, Sause WT, and Noyes DR. Morbidity and mortality associated with intraoperative radiotherapy, *J. Surg. Oncol.,* **41** (1989) 240–245.

69. Kinsella TJ and Sindelar WF. Normal tissue tolerance to intraoperative radiation therapy. Experimental and clinical studies. In Vaeth JM and Meyer JL (eds.), *Radiation tolerance of normal tissues,* Karger, Basel, 1989, pp. 202–214.

70. Haddock MG, Petersen IA, Webb MJ, Wilson TO, Podratz KC, and Gunderson LL. Intraoperative radiotherapy for locally advanced gynecological malignancies, *Front. Radiat. Ther. Oncol.,* **31** (1997) 256–259.

71. Stelzer KJ, Koh WJ, Greer BE, et al. The use of intraoperative radiation therapy in radical salvage for recurrent cervical cancer: outcome and toxicity, *Am. J. Obstet. Gynecol.,* **172** (1995) 1881–1888.

72. Stelzer KJ, Koh W, Greer B, et al. Intraoperative electron beam (IOEBT) as an adjunct to radical salvage for recurrent cancer of the cervix, In Schildberg FW, Willich N, and Essen HJ (eds.), *Intraoperative radiation therapy,* Verlag Die Blaue Eule, Germany, 1993, p. 411.

73. Goldson AL, Delgado G, and Hill LT. Intraoperative radiation of the paraaortic nodes in cancer of the uterine cervix, *Obstet. Gynecol.,* **52** (1978) 713–717.

74. Delgado G, Goldson AL, Ashayeri E, Hill LT, Petrilli ES, and Hatch KD. Intraoperative radiation in the treatment of advanced cervical cancer, *Obstet. Gynecol.,* **63** (1984) 246–252.

75. Yordan EL, Jurado M, Kiel K, et al. Intra-operative radiation therapy in the treatment of pelvic malignancies: a preliminary report. *Bailliere's Clin. Obstet. Gynaecol.,* **2** (1988) 1023–1034.

76. Konski A, Neisler J, Phibbs G, Bronn D, and Dobelbower RR Jr. The use of intraoperative electron beam radiation therapy in the treatment of para-aortic metastases from gynecologic tumors: a pilot study, *Am. J. Clin. Oncol.,* **16** (1993) 67–71.

77. Dosoretz DE, Tepper JE, Shim DS, et al. Intraoperative electron-beam irradiation in gynecologic malignant disease, *Appl. Radiol.,* **13** (1984) 61–63.

78. Hicks ML, Piver S, Mas E, Hemplinig RE, McAuley M, and Walsh DL. Intraoperative orthovoltage radiation therapy in the treatment of recurrent gynecologic malignancies, *Am. J. Clin. Oncol.,* **16** (1993) 497–500.

79. Konski AA, Neisler J, Phibbs G, Brown DG, and Dobelbower RR Jr. A pilot study investigating intraoperative electron beam irradiation in the treatment of ovarian malignancies, *Gynecol. Oncol.,* **38** (1990) 121–124.

80. Martinez-Monge, R. IORT in the management of locally advanced or recurrent gynecologic cancer at high risk for loco-regional relapse. Doctoral Thesis, University of Navarre, Spain, 1994.

81. Gerard JP, Dargent D, Raudrant D, et al. Place de la radiotherapie peroperatoire dans le traitement des cancer de l'uterus. Experience lyonnaise preliminaire, *Bull. Cancer/Radiother.,* **81** (1994) 186–195.

82. Barber HRK and O'Neil WH. Recurrent cervical cancer after treatment by a primary surgical program, *Obstet. Gynecol.,* **37** (1971) 165–172.

83. Gunderson LL, Nelson H, Martenson JA, et al. Intraoperative electron and external beam irradiation with or without 5-fluorouracil and maximum surgical resection for previously unirradiated locally recurrent colorectal cancer, *Dis. Colon. Rectum.,* **39** (1996) 1379–1395.

84. Hockel M, and Knapstein PG. The combined operative and radiotherapeutic treatment (CORT) of recurrent tumors infiltrating the pelvic wall: first experience with 18 patients, *Gynecol. Oncol.,* **46** (1992) 20–28.

85. Fyles AW, Pintilie M, Kirkbride P, Levin W, Manchul LA, and Rawlings GA. Prognostic factors in patients with cervix cancer treated by radiation therapy: results of a multiple regression analysis, *Green,* **35** (1995) 107–117.

86. Komaki R, Brickner TJ, Hanlon AL, Owen JB, and Hanks GE. Long-term results of treatment of cervical carcinoma in the United States in 1973, 1978, and 1983: patterns of Care Study (PCS), *Int. J. Radiat. Oncol. Biol. Phys.,* **31** (1995) 973–982.

87. Petereit DG, Sarkaria JN, Chappell R, et al. The adverse effect of treatment prolongation in cervical carcinoma, *Int. J. Radiat. Oncol. Biol. Phys.,* **32** (1995) 1301–1307.

88. Teshima T, Inoue T, Ikeda H, et al. High-dose rate and low-dose rate intracavitary therapy for carcinoma of the uterine cervix, *Cancer,* **72** (1993) 2409–2414.

89. Mitsuhashi N, Takahashi M, Nozaki M, et al. Evaluation of external beam therapy and three brachytherapy fractions for carcinoma of the uterine cervix, *Int. J. Radiat. Oncol. Biol. Phys.,* **29** (1994) 975–982.

90. Ito H, Kutuki S, Nishiguchi I, et al. Radiotherapy for cervical cancer with high-dose rate brachytherapy—correlation between tumor size, dose and failure, *Green,* **31** (1994) 240–247.

91. Patel FD, Sharma SC, Negi PS, Ghoshal S, and Gupta BD. Low dose rate vs. high dose rate brachytherapy in the treatment of carcinoma of the uterine cervix: a clinical trial, *Int. J. Radiat. Oncol. Biol. Phys.,* **28** (1993) 335–341.

92. Montana GS, Fowler WC, Varia MA, Walton LA, Mack Y, and Shemanski L. Carcinoma of the cervix, stage III: results of radiation therapy, *Cancer,* **57** (1986) 148–154.

93. Jones WB, Shingleton HM, Russell A, et al. Patterns of care for invasive cervical cancer: results of a national survey of 1984 and 1990, *Cancer,* **76** (1995) 1934–1947.

94. Horiot JC, Pigneux J, Pourquier H, et al. Radiotherapy alone in carcinoma of the intact uterine cervix according to GH Fletcher guidelines: a French cooperative study of 1383 cases, *Int. J. Radiat. Oncol. Biol. Phys.,* **14** (1988) 605–611.

95. Brunet J, Alonso C, Llanos M, et al. Chemotherapy and radiotherapy in locally advanced cervical cancer, *Acta. Oncol.,* **34(7)** (1995) 941–944.

96. Benedett-Pacini P, Maneschi F, Cutillo G, et al. Modified type IV-V radical hysterectomy with systematic pelvic and aortic lymphadenectomy in the treatment of patients with stage III cervical carcinoma, *Cancer,* **78** (1996) 2359–2365.

97. Pas E, Willemse PHB, Boonstra H, et al. Concurrent chemo- and radiotherapy in patients with locally advanced carcinoma of the cervix, *Ann. Oncol.,* **7** (1996) 511–516.

98. Fields AL, Anderson PS, Goldberg GL, et al. Mature results of a phase II trial of concomitant Cisplatin/pelvic radiotherapy for locally advanced squamous cell carcinoma of the cervix, *Gynecol. Oncol.,* **61** (1996) 416–422.

99. Stehman FB, Bundy BN, Thomas G, et al. Hydroxyurea versus misonidazole with radiation in cervical carcinoma: long-term follow-up of a Gynecologic Oncology Group trial, *J. Clin. Oncol.,* **11** (1993) 1523–1528.

100. Thomas G, Dembo A, Fyles A, et al. Concurrent chemoradiation in advanced cervical cancer, *Gynecol. Oncol.,* **38** (1990) 446–451.

101. Martinez-Monge R, Jurado M, Azinovic I, et al. Intraoperative radiotherapy in recurrent gynecologic cancer, *Green,* **28** (1993) 127–133.

23 Genitourinary IORT

Felipe A. Calvo, Horst Zincke,
Leonard L. Gunderson, Javier Aristu,
Jean P. Gerard and Jose M. Berian

CONTENTS

BLADDER CANCER IORT
RENAL CANCER IORT—UNITED STATES AND EUROPEAN TRIALS
TOLERANCE ISSUES
FUTURE POSSIBILITIES
REFERENCES

1. BLADDER CANCER IORT

1.1. Introduction

When conventional external-beam irradiation (EBRT) alone was given in an attempt for preservation of bladder and potential cure in operable or inoperable patients, the local bladder cancer was permanently eradicated in <50% of patients *(1–3)*. Radical cystectomy, when combined with preoperative EBRT, eradicated pelvic tumor permanently in 75–90% of patients with invasive cancer *(1,4–6)*.

In reports from Europe and Japan in the 1980s, EBRT plus intraoperative irradiation (IORT) by either removable radium or iridium implant *(7–9)* or IORT with electrons (IOERT) *(10–14)* was shown to be tolerable and preserved bladder function in ≥75% of patients with solitary tumors that invaded into but not beyond bladder muscle (Table 1). Success with combined EBRT plus IORT regimens was related to the ability of open surgery to provide excellent exposure for the selected delivery of more irradiation to the tumor and less to uninvolved bladder.

1.2. General Considerations

In an era of both systemic and local treatment intensification, the issue of organ preservation in bladder-cancer patients continues to be a major theme *(15–18)*. Although EBRT alone produced only a modest rate of bladder preservation and long-term survival in patients with invasive bladder cancer, many cases were referred for EBRT because of poor general status or other conditions that contraindicated radical surgery *(2,19)*. How-

From: *Current Clinical Oncology: Intraoperative Irradiation: Techniques and Results*
Edited by: L. L. Gunderson et al. © Humana Press, Inc., Totowa, NJ

Table 1
Intraoperative Irradiation: Clinical T2 Bladder Cancer

Authors	Ref. #	# Patient	Treatment	5 Year Local Control	5 Year Survival
van der Werf-Messing et al.	7	328	EBRT, Ra-226	77%	56%
Batterman et al.	8	85	EBRT, Ra-226	74%	55%
Mazeron et al.	9	24	Resection, ^{192}Ir, EBRT	92%	58%
Matsumoto et al.	10	28	IOERT, EBRT	82%	62%

EBRT: External beam irradiation; Ra-226: brachytherapy, radium needles; ^{192}Ir: brachytherapy, afterloading iridium; IOERT: intraoperative electrons.

ever, some excellent results in terms of organ preservation have been achieved using sophisticated radiotherapy techniques such as brachytherapy or IOERT in combination with EBRT *(7–14)*.

The modern approach to organ preservation trials including radiotherapy is based upon strict selection criteria: only those patients who exhibit a complete tumor response after initial chemotherapy induction therapy are candidates for high-dose EBRT plus cisplatin in an effort to preserve the bladder *(20)*. Within this frame work, IOERT is an attractive boost modality, as it can accurately treat tumors located in the lateral and posterior bladder walls while avoiding irradiation of the small bowel and rectum *(21,22)*.

1.3. Technical Factors for IOERT

1.3.1. SURGICAL

A baseline pretreatment cystoscopy should be performed prior to treatment with neoadjuvant chemotherapy or chemoirradiation to determine lesion factors (size, location, exophytic vs ulcerative). Three to five weeks following completion of neoadjuvant chemotherapy (MCV vs other), patients should be re-evaluated cystoscopically for the assessment of the primary tumor response to chemotherapy. Both the re-evaluation cystoscopy and the open surgical procedure for IORT should be at least 2 and no more than 5 wk following the completion of the chemotherapy.

1.3.1.1. Surgical Staging and Open Cystotomy. Patients should undergo a limited pelvic lymph-node sampling by an extraperitoneal approach, if possible. The intent is to sample any palpably abnormal pelvic lymph nodes and to excise some inferior external iliac (obturator) and internal iliac lymph nodes on the ipsilateral side, and possibly on the contralateral side for histologic evaluation. The bladder should be opened with an incision that is not directly adjacent to the original tumor site and that is judged to give good exposure for IOERT through a lucite applicator. The extravesical tissue deep to the primary tumor should be palpated and biopsied to assist determination of electron-energy selection. Following IOERT, bladder closure and bladder catheter drainage will be managed conservatively with an anticipation that the healing of the cystotomy may be compromised by prior chemotherapy and EBRT.

1.3.1.2. Cystoscopic Follow-Up. Patients should be evaluated cystoscopically every 3–4 mo following the completion of radiation therapy and chemotherapy for 1 yr, every 6 mo for 2 yr, then annually. Cystectomy for salvage should be done as indicated.

A

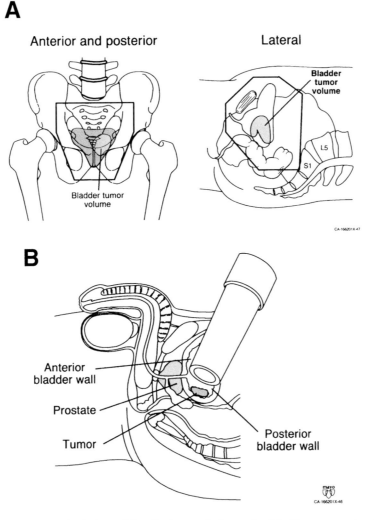

Fig. 1. Idealized artists depiction of irradiation techniques for bladder cancer (modified from Shipley, WU *[21,22]*). (**A**) EBRT four-field technique. (**B**) IOERT treatment.

1.3.2. EBRT

External-beam irradiation fields should be designed on a treatment simulator during which time the bladder is localized by instillation of contrast media and air (only 50 cc total since patients should be treated immediately following voiding; 30–35 cc contrast, 15–20 cc air).

Treatment fields should include the entire bladder, the bladder tumor volume with any extravesical components, the prostate and prostatic urethra, and the lymph nodes immediately adjacent to the bladder (Fig. 1A). The field should extend inferiorly to at least the superior aspect of the obturator foramena (≥ 2.5 cm beyond bladder mucosa) and superiorly to just below the sacral promontory. These fields will include the perivesical, obturator, and external and internal iliac nodes, but not the common iliac lymph nodes. Field width should extend 1.5 cm lateral to the bony pelvis. For lateral fields, the anterior boundary of the fields should be 2 cm anterior to the most anterior portion of bladder mucosa as demonstrated by air-contrast cystogram. Posteriorly the fields should extend at least 2.5 cm posterior to the most posterior portion of the bladder mucosa seen on cystogram, or 2.5 cm posterior to the tumor mass, if palpable or evaluable by pelvic computed tomography (CT) scan. The superior and inferior extents of the lateral fields are identical to those used for the anteroposterior/posteroanterior (AP/PA) fields. The lateral fields should be shaped with corner blocks inferiorly to shield the tissues outside the symphysis and the anal canal. Wedges (usually 15°) should be considered for lateral fields if the transverse contour has a significant slope anteriorly.

1.3.2.1. Concomitant Administration of Cisplatin with EBRT. Cisplatin should be administered during the course of EBRT on days 1 and 21. The usual daily dose is 100 mg/m^2 given as a 30–40-min infusion two or more hours after EBRT.

1.3.3. IOERT

The IOERT applicator size, bevel angle, and beam energy will be chosen so that the total target volume (the pretreatment tumor volume) is enclosed within the 90% isodose lines. The lucite applicators will most likely be between 5 and 7 cm in internal diameter and should allow a 1.0–1.5-cm margin around the entire initial tumor volume (in responders, the margin will be larger with regard to the residual mucosal lesion). Electron-beam energies will likely range between 9 and 18 MeV, but should be adequate to assure coverage at the appropriate depth. There should be protection of the rectum and/or rectosigmoid by angulation of the treatment beam and/or by packing posterior to the target volume with either lead or laparotomy pads to prevent penetration behind the tumor target volume into the structures. Bolus material may be needed to improve surface-dose dependent on the chosen electron energy. A suction catheter should be used to assure that excess urine does not collect over the surface of the tumor during treatment. If the peritoneal cavity has been opened for exposure, the use of omentum to cover either the perivesicle biopsied site and/or the irradiated site should be considered.

A sagittal schematic of IOERT applicator placement for the treatment of a MGH patient with locally advanced—stage T3b—bladder cancer is seen in Fig. 1B. The bladder has been opened superiorly and the treatment applicator is angled laterally to avoid irradiating the right ureteral orifice and the rectum.

1.4. Clinical Results with IORT Electrons

1.4.1. JAPAN SERIES

1.4.1.1. Technical Factors. The largest reported series using IORT in bladder cancer patients has been from Japan (10,23). The characteristics of the treatment program tested were preservation of the bladder in combination with a high-dose IORT boost of 25–30 Gy and fractionated EBRT, starting 3–4 wk postoperatively, to moderate total does of 30–40 Gy in 15–20 fractions over 3–4 wk. Other technical aspects of interest were the use of low-energy electron beams (4–6 MeV) and the size of the applicators (4, 5, and 6 cm in diameter).

1.4.1.2. Patient Group. In a 13-yr period from period from 1965 to 1978, 116 patients were treated. Tumors were generally located at the ureteral orifice (36 patients - 44%), the posterior wall (18 patients - 22%), or the lateral walls (15 patients - 19%). Tumor diameter was less than 3 cm in most cases.

Pathologic tumor stage was Ta, T1, and T2 in 94 cases, and the cumulative total-relapse rate in these early tumor stages was 29% within 6 yr of follow-up. There was a

Table 2
Pamplona and Lyon IOERT Results: Bladder Cancer

Author	#	Stage/Downstage		Local Relapse	Survival
Gerard (Lyon)	25	21 T_2	20 (80%)	3 (12%)[a]	55% (4 yr)
		4 T_3	CCR		
Aristu (Pamplona)	40	7 T_2	27 (67%)	3 (7%)[b]	46% (7 yr)
		17 T_3	pT_0		
		11 T_4			

[a] bladder preserved.
[b] bladder removed.
CCR: clinical complete response.

significant difference in recurrence rate between the group with solitary tumors (8%) and the group with multiple tumors (27%). Cystectomy was performed in five cases as rescue treatment of recurrences. Thirteen local tumor recurrences have been documented in the period evaluated.

1.4.1.3. Results. The survival rate for patients with Ta, T1, and T2 tumors is 72%. No long-term survivors have been seen among T4 patients, but there are some long-term survivors among T3 patients. This information is not available in the published report.

The complications related to the treatment program included three cases of flank pain for several days after irradiation, presumably caused by acute obstruction of the ureteral orifice, which was included in the irradiation field. No serious late complications were observed except in one patient who had a contracted bladder after 30-Gy IOERT and 21.5-Gy EBRT, requiring urinary diversion 12 yr later because of progressive bilateral hydronephrosis. Radiation proctitis or other bowel damage was not experienced. Obstruction of the bladder neck or ureteral orifice did not occur.

1.4.2. WESTERN RESULTS

In Western countries, occasional long-term survivors have been described with a functional bladder following IOERT *(22,24)*. Radiation Therapy Oncology Group (RTOG) attempted, without success, to accrue patients to a phase II trial integrating IOERT as a component of treatment following preoperative MCV and EBRT plus cisplatin.

1.4.3. LYON SERIES

A recent report from the Centre Hospitalier Lyon Sud *(13,14)* has analyzed the results obtained with an IOERT boost in the combined conservative bladder-preservation treatment of muscle-invasive bladder carcinoma (Table 2). In a 4-yr period (April, 1990 to April, 1994), 25 patients (median age 63, male 21) were treated with IOERT and bladder-preservation treatment modalities with the restriction criteria of having a solitary tumor lesion, located in the fixed portion of the bladder and size of less than 6 cm in maximum diameter. Tumor histology was transitional cell in 23 and squamous cell in 2 cases. Clinicopathological stages were T2 (n = 21) or T3 (n = 4) N0M0. Following lymphadenectomy, 5 patients pN1 were detected.

The treatment program included in all patients the administration of preoperative chemoradiation (small pelvis four-field technique, 18 MV photons, 48 Gy/24 fractions/35 d and two concomitant courses of cisplatinum 30 mg/m^2/days 1–3 and 28–30 continu-

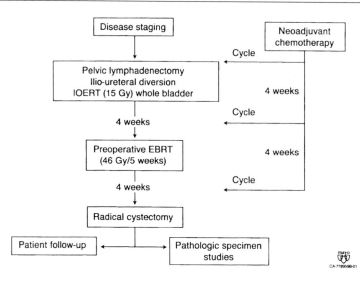

Fig. 2. Multidisciplinary treatment protocol for bladder cancer which integrates IOERT, University Clinic of Navarra (Pamplona, Spain).

ous iv infusion). In 14 patients two cycles of MCV chemotherapy were given before irradiation and one patient pN1 received two adjuvant MCV courses. IOERT was performed with a 6- to 7-cm diameter applicator, selecting in all procedures 9 MeV electron energy and a total single dose of 15 Gy. A limited iliac lymphadenectomy was performed in 20 patients.

Cystoscopic evaluation following the preoperative chemoradiation treatment segment (3 wk after completion of EBRT plus cisplatin) showed 20 patients (80%) in complete clinical response. Local recurrences were proven in three patients (two treated by salvage cystectomy) and distant metastasis were observed in five patients. Four-year survival is 55% for the entire group.

The tissue-tolerance analysis described four cases of asymptomatic superficial bladder radiation necroses and one pubic-bone necrosis. There was no operative mortality.

1.4.4. University of Navarra Series

The University Clinic of Navarra (Pamplona, Spain) explored the integration of IOERT in a multidisciplinary treatment program for locally advanced bladder cancer using preoperative EBRT and more recently a combination of neoadjuvant chemotherapy and preoperative EBRT *(11)*. An important aspect of that experience has been the possibility that it has afforded to analyze the cystectomy specimen and to correlate the pathologic findings with the previous treatment program. This information is of particular value for the development of clinical trials using IOERT as a boost modality in organ-preservation protocols *(12)*. The treatment protocol is outlined in Fig. 2.

1.4.4.1. Technical Factors. The surgical procedure consisted of a midline longitudinal incision to expose the bladder. Both ureters were dissected free over the distal third of their length to ensure that they were excluded from the IOERT field. The IOERT applicator was introduced through the anterior laparotomy incision and the whole collapsed bladder was included in it. The small bowel was mobilized out of the pelvis with fixed retractors. The gantry of the linear accelerator was angulated and the cones were usually beveled (15° or 30°). The rectum was protected with a lead shield in most cases.

Table 3
Pathologic Downstaging (Primary and Nodal) and
Patterns of Relapse, Pamplona Bladder IORT Update 1996

Stage	#	Local	Mixed	Distant	Unknown
pT_0N_0	18	0	1	3	1
$pT + N_0$	7	0	0	3	1
$pT_0N +$	9	0	0	4	0
$pT + N +$	6	1	1	1	0
Total	40	1 (2%)	2 (5%)	11 (27%)	2 (5%)

A dose of 15 Gy was delivered in most patients (range 10–20 Gy) with electron energies of 9–12 MeV.

External-beam irradiation started 4 wk after the first surgical procedure. The treatment consisted of a four-field box technique, including in the target volume the bladder and the pelvic nodal areas. A CT treatment-planning system was available in all cases. The daily dose was 2 Gy, and the total dose delivered to the volume was 46 Gy in 5 wk.

Radical cystectomy was performed 4–6 wk after EBRT. Surgical techniques were uniform for all patients. Male patients underwent radical cystoprostatectomy. An anterior exenteration was carried out in the female patients.

Patients were subsequently pathologically staged. Multiple sections were cut (average: eight) from each cystectomy specimen in order to study the possible presence of tumor cells and other histopathologic features.

Chemotherapy administered in the neoadjuvant group consisted of cisplatin 15 mg/m^2, 24-hr iv infusion days 1–3; 5-FU 1000 mg/m^2 (maximum 1500 mg per 24 h), iv infusion days 1–3; doxorubicin 35 mg/m^2, iv day 1; and hexamethylmelamine 150 mg/m^2, po (maximum dose 200 mg/d) on days 8–17. Three courses of the above-described chemotherapy were given, commencing every 4 wk. The initial cycle started just after the transurethral resection and the confirmation of invasive bladder cancer. The second chemotherapy course was given after the laparotomy for ureteral diversion, IOERT, and lymphadenectomy. The third course started upon the completion of preoperative EBRT, 4 wk before the second surgical intervention for cystectomy.

1.4.4.2. Pamplona Results. The most recent unpublished analysis of these data (study period November, 1987 to October, 1993; analysis performed in December, 1995) showed 40 patients treated with the complete program: median age 60 yr (range 44–74), 35 males; 34 patients with Karnofsky index >70%. Clinicopathologic tumor stages were: 7 T2, 17 T3, 11 T4, 5 N+. Posttreatment pathology showed 27 pT0 (67%) and 15 pN+ (37%). The follow-up period for the entire group ranges from 2–96 mo (median 35 mo).

Patterns of tumor relapse show 24 patients with no evidence of disease (NED), 1 local recurrence alone, 11 patients with distant sites of progression, 2 patients with mixed local and distant failure, and 2 with unknown relapse status. Local recurrences have been observed in 2 of 22 pT + or N+ patients (33%) and 1 of 18 pT0N0 (5%) (Table 3).

Cause-specific survival at 7 yr is projected at 46% for the entire group. Actuarial survival is 52% in pT0N0 vs 38% for any pathology-positive patients. Survival at 7 yr by initial tumor stage is 85% T2, 48% T3, and 10% T4.

1.4.4.3. Summary. The integration of an IOERT boost to the whole bladder in a multidisciplinary protocol combining neoadjuvant systemic chemotherapy, preoperative radiotherapy, and planned cystectomy has proven to be feasible and well tolerated. The sterilization rate of invasive bladder cancer, confirmed in pathologic studies of the cystectomy specimens, is high (in the range of 65%) and seems to be increased by the addition of neoadjuvant chemotherapy to the treatment program *(25–27)*. These findings are of importance with respect to the development of new protocols with the aim of bladder preservation. IORT is a very attractive radiotherapy boost modality to be considered in the future in this cancer site.

2. RENAL CANCER IORT—UNITED STATES AND EUROPEAN TRIALS

2.1. Patient Evaluation; Technical Factors

2.1.1. PRETREATMENT EVALUATION

At the time of an initial multispecialty consultation involving a surgeon, medical oncologist, and radiation oncologist, the extent of pretreatment evaluation and sequencing of treatment modalities should be determined. In addition to a history and physical examination, routine baseline studies should include a complete blood count, serum chemistries including creatinine, chest film, bone scan, and CT abdomen/pelvis. A baseline chest CT study should also usually be obtained.

2.1.2. SURGICAL COMPONENT

The surgical approach to cytoreductive surgery with IORT has to reconcile the two goals of this treatment program; namely, the right approach to the tumor mass to be resected and a similar satisfactory approach for the placement of the applicator for the use of IOERT. If all presurgical criteria are satisfied (namely that of no dissemination in the interim) the patient is usually approached through a subcostal incision transversing the midline in order to approach upper quadrant masses in the retroperitoneum or parallel to the large vascular structures. If the tumor extends distally beyond the renal vessels, a midline approach is used that usually is extended below the umbilicus to the pubic bone to gain satisfactory exposure to the entire retroperitoneum. For this purpose, the retroperitoneum is incised extending from the hepatic flexure of the right colon transversing just below the cecum and extending the retroperitoneal incision towards the ligament of Treitz. This enables the surgeon to exenterate the right colon, transverse colon, and small bowel temporarily onto the chest of the patient to be held in a Lakey pack.

For the left periaortic area, the peritoneum along Toldt's line lateral to the left colon is incised from the splenic flexure to the mesocolon and the large bowel mobilized medially. Usually, the inferior mesenteric artery will be sacrificed to provide excellent exposure to this area.

On secondary exposures, a modified incisional approach might be utilized. For instance, for the pelvic area, a modified Gibson incision has proved quite beneficial.

In all the preparations around the arterial vessels, great emphasis is given to avoid performing an exarterectomy (removing the adventice tissue). This is done to avoid a spontaneous perforation following the EBRT, resection, and IOERT.

All efforts are made to remove all of the visible cancer. This is sometimes facilitated, particularly in renal-cell cancer, through the use of preoperative EBRT which seems to involve the cancer in a capsule that is then easily dissected out from the retroperitoneal area, particularly around the large vasculature of the vena cava and aorta. In cases in which the vena cava is partially occluded by thrombus, the vena cava can be resected with impunity because collateral circulation has developed and is satisfactorily draining the blood from the iliac veins. Lacerations, which occur frequently, particularly in the venous system, are repaired with the appropriate suture material ranging from 4-0 to 7-0 Prolene. Rarely is it necessary to replace vascular structures with a Dacron or Gore-Tex graft.

Closure of the abdomen is achieved with running double-stranded No. 1 Maxon sutures in the anterior fascia, including the posterior fascia for the upper abdomen. Appropriate drains are placed in the retroperitoneum and the subcutaneous tissue, and the skin edges are usually approximated with skin clips.

Patients may suffer from prolonged ileus following the surgical treatment program plus IOERT. Nasogastric suction is usually necessary for a more prolonged period of time.

2.1.3. EBRT

Preoperative EBRT should be delivered with multiple-field techniques for previously unirradiated patients. Field design options include AP/PA plus lateral or obliqued fields to include tumor bed and nodal sites yet sparing the spinal cord. Extended fields are commonly treated to 45 Gy and boost fields to 50.4 Gy in 1.8-Gy fractions. Low-dose preoperative irradiation of 19.6–25.2 cGy in 11–14 fractions can be considered in previously irradiated patients.

Patients who receive moderate-dose preoperative irradiation undergo a restaging evaluation 3–4 wk following completion of irradiation. This includes a history, physical examination, a repeat of baseline laboratory tests, and radiographs including CT of the chest, abdomen, pelvis (Fig. 3), and a bone scan. Patients with systemic metastases do not proceed to exploratory laparotomy or IOERT except for the situation of a solitary resectable lung metastasis.

2.1.4. IOERT

Intraoperative irradiation with 6–12 MeV electrons can usually be delivered to the para-aortic or caval region and/or renal fossa (tumor bed). The dose of IOERT, as calculated at the 90% isodose curve, varies from 10 to 20 Gy depending on amount of residual disease remaining after maximal resection and the dose of EBRT that has been given preoperatively or is feasible postoperatively. Small vascular or titanium clips should be placed around areas of adherence or residual disease, before wound closure, for purpose of follow-up studies and postoperative EBRT, if indicated.

2.1.5. FOLLOW-UP

After completion of treatment, patients should usually be followed at 3- to 4-mo intervals for 1 yr, every 6 mo to 3 yr, then yearly. Studies should include complete blood count, creatinine, chest X-ray, CT abdomen and pelvis, and full physical examination. Bone scans and other studies can be done as indicated. At the time of each evaluation, data should be prospectively collected and computerized with regard to disease status and normal tissue tolerance to treatment.

2.2. Clinical Results with IORT

2.2.1. MAYO RESULTS

IOERT has been used as a supplement to EBRT with or without resection at Mayo in 28 patients with genitourinary (GU) malignancies (bladder - 4, prostate - 4, ureter - 2, renal - 18 including 4 with bone metastases) *(28,29)*. In the 14 patients with locally advanced primary (2 patients) or recurrent (12 patients) renal cancers, histologic cell type was renal cancer in 10, transitional or squamous-cell cancer in 3, and Wilms' in 1.

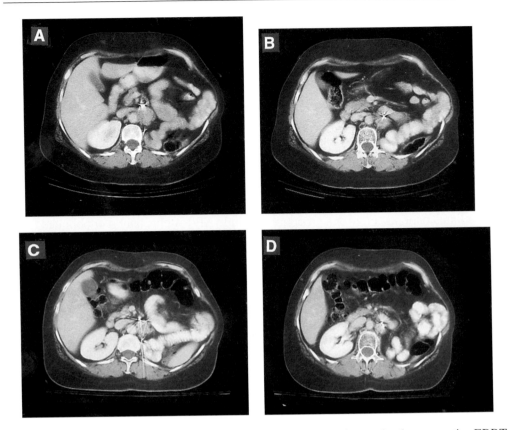

Fig. 3. Tumor regression in a patient with recurrent renal cancer who received preoperative EBRT before resection and IOERT at Mayo Clinic. **(A,B)** Preirradiation CT scan with bulky left para-aortic adenopathy and lack of fat plane adjacent to aorta. **(C,D)** Post-irradiation scan 4 wk following completion of 45 Gy/25 fractions/5 wk and 2.5 mo after initial scan; note shrinkage of mass with improved fat planes relative to aorta. An IOERT dose of 12.5 Gy was given after a marginal gross total resection.

Preoperative EBRT was given in 11 of the 14 patients (dose ≥ 44 Gy in 8) *(62)*. The IOERT dose was 10–20 Gy in 12 of 14 patients (dose of 25 Gy given to 2 patients who had received high-dose EBRT prior to referral to Mayo with disease progression).

In the renal-cell cancer group of patients, 5 of 10 patients were alive at the time data was updated for presentation in Lyon in 1994 *(29)*. Three of 10 or 30% were free of disease at 37, 59, and 56 mo from initiation of treatment. Two other patients died free of disease at 10.5 and 19 mo (5 of 10 or 50% relapse free). Two patients were alive with disease at 22 and 44 mo and 3 patients died of disease at 16, 19, and 31 mo. Of the 4 patients with other cell types, 1 died free of disease at 28.5 mo and 3 died of disease at 5, 8, and 12 mo (Table 4).

Patterns of relapse in the Mayo renal patients are seen in Tables 4 and 5. Local or central relapse occurred in only one patient in each category. The distant metastasis rate was high at 57% (8 of 14 patients).

2.2.2. PAMPLONA SERIES

Feasibility and early clinical results using IOERT at the time of surgical management of recurrent or locally advanced renal cancer has been reported at the University Clinic

Table 4
Renal IORT: Mayo (9/94 analysis)
Survival and Disease Status versus Disease Category

Disease Category/Status	No. (n = 14)	Survival in months (Failure Pattern)
Primary RCC	2	
Alive - NED	1	56
Dead - with disease	1	31 (DM - liver, lung)
Recurrent RCC	8	
Alive - NED	2	37,55
- with disease	2	21.5 (LF, DM - LN)
		44 (DM lung, bone)
Dead - NED	2	10.5 (Cvasc) 19 (Graft sepsis)
- with disease	2	16 (DM lung) 19 (RF, DM - CNS)
Recurrent TCC/SCC	3	
Dead - NED	1	28.5 (postop)
- with disease	2	5 (DM liver) 12 (CF)
Wilms' - Dead with disease	1	8 (PS, DM - liver, LN)

DM = distant metastasis; CF = central failure; LF = local failure; RF = regional failure; LN = lymph node; CNS = central nervous system; Cvasc = cardiovascular; TCC = transitional cell cancer; RCC = renal cell cancer; SCC = squamous cell cancer; NED = no evidence of disease.

Table 5
Renal IORT: Mayo (9/94), Heidelberg (9/96), Pamplona (12/89)
Incidence and Patterns of Failure by Disease Category

Disease Category	Ref. No.	Any Relapse No. %	Central No. %	Local No. %	Regional No. %	Distant No. %
Mayo Series (n = 14)	27,28					
Primary RCC		1/2 (50)	0 —	0 —	0 —	1 (50)
Recurrent RCC		4/8 (50)	0 —	1 (13)	1 (13)	5 (63)
Recurrent TCC/SCC		2/3 (67)	1 (33)	0 —	0 —	1 (33)
Wilms'		1/1 (100)	0 —	0 —	0 —	1 (100)
Mayo Totals		8/14 (57)	1 (7)	1 (7)	1 (7)	8 (57)
Pamplona	29	3/11 (27)	1 (9)	1 (9)	—	3 (27)
Heidelberg	30	5/11 (45)	0 —	0 —	0 —	5 (45)

RCC = renal cell cancer
TCC = transitional cell cancer
SCC = squamous cell cancer

of Navarra (30). In a 20-mo period, 11 consecutive patients with stage III (5 patients), IV (3 patients), or lumbar fossae recurrence (3 patients) were treated with a combination of surgical tumor resection, IOERT to the tumor or tumor-bed region, and postoperative EBRT (not given in 4 patients). Histology was confirmed as clear-cell adenocarcinoma in all surgical samples, except for one recurrent patient in which histology was consistent with transitional-cell carcinoma. Age ranged from 40–70 yr old (median 60). Macroscopic postsurgical residual disease was evident in four cases; close margins or micro residue was assumed in the remaining seven cases.

The IOERT target volume was encompassed by an applicator size of 10 cm diameter in four procedures, 7 cm in three, 8 cm in two, 9 cm and 12 cm in one each. The electron energy selected for treatment was 9 MeV - six, 12 MeV - one, 15 MeV - two, 18 MeV - one, and 20 MeV - one. Total single IOERT dose was 15 Gy - eight, 10 Gy - two, and 20 Gy - one. External-beam fractionated irradiation was added in seven patients, ranging from 30 to 45 Gy (five patients).

With a follow-up period at the time of publication of 2–33 mo (median 8 mo), patterns of tumor progression showed three patients with a distant relapse (three lung metastases together with two liver metastases). One of the three had a local relapse at 7 mo follow-up from IOERT (no EBRT was administered in this particular case, IOERT dose was 20 Gy, residual disease was microscopic and the applicator size and electron energy were 7 cm and 9 MeV, respectively). An interval analysis of the reported group of patients has identified long-term survivors without evidence of recurrent disease (three patients NED with more than 3 yr follow-up).

No early or late relevant toxicity related to the local components of treatment was detected. Therefore, this appears to be an anatomic region that can be reasonably treated by IOERT techniques following tumor with or without lymph-node resection. The introduction of an IOERT radiation-boost component might facilitate the ability to decrease the dose of the EBRT component of treatment needed to control disease in this abdominal region in which radiotherapy management is controversial because of the presence of dose-limiting structures.

2.2.3. Heidelberg Results

At the 6th International IORT meeting in San Francisco, Elbe et al. *(31)* reported results in a series of 11 patients with renal cancer (primary - three, locally recurrent - eight) treated at the University of Heidelberg *(31)* with maximal resection, IOERT (12–20 Gy), and postoperative EBRT (40 Gy in 2-Gy fractions, 5 d/wk). With mean follow-up of 24 mo, all patients were controlled locally, but distant metastases had occurred in 5 of 11 (lung - three, bone - two). Overall and disease-free survival at 3 yr were 47 and 34%, respectively.

3. TOLERANCE ISSUES

IOERT tolerance for intact or surgically manipulated genitourinary organs or structures in animals is seen in Table 6. Bladder and ureteral tolerance will be discussed as a function of both animal and clinical data.

3.1. Bladder

Both clinical and laboratory data indicate that single doses of 20–25 Gy to a portion of the bladder (less than one-third) is very well tolerated with infrequent compromise of lower urinary-tract function *(10,32)*. In the 116 patients treated by Matsumoto et al. there were only four complications related to IOERT, even though a ureteral orifice was included in 44% of patients, and the bladder neck, or trigone, in 11 patients *(10,23)*. Three patients had transient ureteral-vesical junction obstruction, felt caused by edema. In one patient, bilateral hydronephrosis developed requiring urinary diversion. Only one of the 57 patients followed more than 5 yr developed a clinically significant bladder contracture.

An NCI study of IOERT bladder tolerance in foxhounds showed relatively few acute or late harmful effects *(32)*. After cystostomy, IOERT was delivered using a 5-cm circu-

Table 6
Normal Genitourinary Tissue Tolerance to IOERT in Animals (Usually Dogs)

Tissue	Maximum tolerated dose (Gy)	Tissue effect	Dose (Gy)
Intact Structure			
Bladder	30	Contraction and ureterovesical narrowing	≥25
Ureter	30	Fibrosis and stenosis	≥30
Kidney	<15	Atrophy and fibrosis	≥20
Surgically Manipulated			
Bladder	30	Healing but contraction	≥30

lar applicator and a 12-MeV electron beam to an area including the trigone, one ureteral orifice, and proximal urethra, with escalating single doses of 0, 20, 25, 30, 35, and 40 Gy. No fractionated EBRT was delivered. Dogs were electively sacrificed at 1 and 2 yr.

With follow-up to 24 mo, all dogs given ≤ 25 Gy to the bladder neck and to one ureteral orifice in the NCI study had normal renal function, no abnormalities shown by serial intravenous pyelogram (IVP) and no major loss of bladder volume or contractility by serial cystometrics. Obstruction of a ureteral orifice and renal failure secondary to bilateral hydronephrosis was seen in 3 out of 15 dogs that received 25, 35, and 40 Gy. At autopsy, histologic changes comprising mucosa thinning and telangiectasia with submucosal fibrosis were confined to the IORT field and appeared to be dose related. The bladder epithelium remained intact at all doses. The ureterovesical junction in animals receiving 20 Gy showed mild fibrosis of the lamina propria and moderate chronic inflammation. Above 20 Gy the histologic changes at the ureterovesical junction were pronounced, with gross stenosis in three animals. The authors concluded that the bladder trigone will tolerate 20 Gy IORT without major clinical sequelae.

In a recent report *(33)* an interesting and new observation has been described in one of four dogs kept for long-term evaluation. This animal developed a bladder tumor 3 yr after an IORT dose of 30 Gy. This was observed as a filling defect on intravenous pyelography. Microscopic study of the tissue after resection showed a hemangiosarcoma of the bladder within the IORT field.

3.2. Ureter

Dose-sensitive structures identified in early IOERT analyses included ureter and bile duct. Neither structure is dose limiting, however, since stents can be inserted as indicated to overcome obstruction and preserve renal or liver function. In an early Mayo analysis of 51 IOERT patients with pelvic malignancy, 44% of previously unobstructed ureters became partially or totally obstructed when included in the IOERT field *(34)*.

Ureteral tolerance was reanalyzed in two recent Mayo publications utilizing IOERT as a component of treatment in patients with either locally advanced primary colorectal cancer *(35)* (n = 56) or previously unirradiated locally recurrent colorectal cancer *(36)* (n = 123). For the primary disease patients, 3 of 56 patients (5%) developed partial ureteral obstruction, and 6 developed obstruction requiring a stent (11%). Pelvic relapse was the probable cause of total obstruction (grade 3) in one patient and IOERT was a potential contributing factor to obstruction in 8 of the 9 vs 11 patients with ureter in the

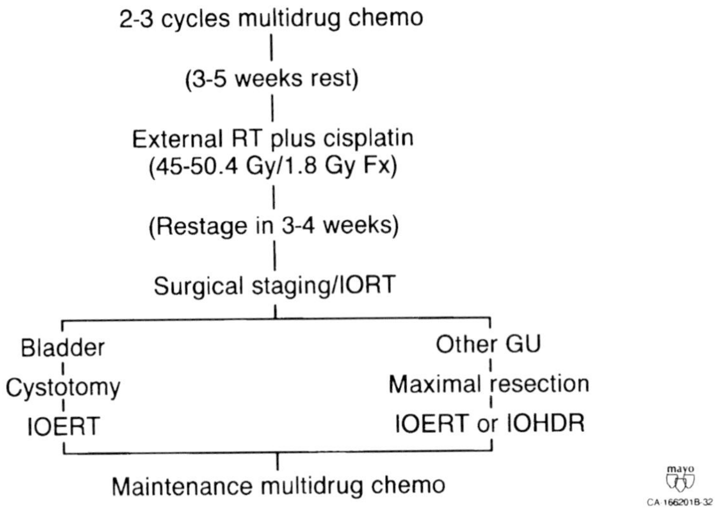

2-3 cycles multidrug chemo
|
(3-5 weeks rest)
|
External RT plus cisplatin
(45-50.4 Gy/1.8 Gy Fx)
|
(Restage in 3-4 weeks)
|
Surgical staging/IORT

Bladder   Other GU
Cystotomy   Maximal resection
IOERT   IOERT or IOHDR

Maintenance multidrug chemo

Fig. 4. Potential multimodality treatment schema for locally advanced genitourinary transitional or squamous cell malignancies.

IOERT field (45% vs 56% incidence). In the locally recurrent patients, 7 of 123 patients (6%) developed partial ureteral obstruction, and 12 (10%) developed an obstruction requiring stents. Of the 33 patients with ureter in an IOERT field, 12 patients (36%) developed some degree of obstruction, either partial or total.

Because stents can be inserted to overcome ureteral obstruction and preserve renal function as indicated, when tumor is adherent to ureter, it should be included in the IOERT boost. At Mayo, ureteral stents are placed only if subsequent obstruction develops because stent-related problems are not infrequent. Although animal studies from CSU suggest that the incidence of IOERT-related ureteral changes is related to length of ureter within the field *(37)*, data concerning length of ureter within IOERT field was not collected prospectively in patients in the Mayo colorectal IOERT series of patients *(35,36)*.

4. FUTURE POSSIBILITIES

4.1. Renal Cell Cancers

Aggressive IOERT containing approaches appear reasonable for locally advanced renal cancers on the basis of small series from Mayo Clinic, Pamplona, and the University of Heidelberg *(28–31)*. The best candidates are previously untreated patients (4 of 6 Mayo patients with progression after IOERT had received EBRT [3 patients] or chemotherapy [2 patients] before referral for IOERT). Good systemic treatment options do not exist at present with regard to chemotherapy. It is hoped that ongoing efforts with immunotherapy or gene therapy will provide some leads.

4.2. Transitional Cell or Squamous Cancers (Bladder, Ureter, or Kidney)

For patients with high-grade transitional-cell or squamous-cell cancers of the bladder, kidney, or ureter, multidrug chemotherapy should be combined with locally aggressive approaches because of increased systemic risks and the availability of effective systemic therapy *(25–27)* (Fig. 4). At the present time, patients are often referred for consideration of EBRT or IORT only after local or regional disease progression while receiving multidrug chemotherapy. It would be preferable to incorporate the systemic therapy in planned sequential fashion by delivering two to three cycles of chemotherapy before proceeding to EBRT ± CDDP. Patients would be restaged to rule out metastases 3–4 wk after EBRT and could then proceed to maximal resection plus IORT. Maintenance multidrug chemotherapy could be considered starting approx 1 mo postoperatively.

REFERENCES

1. Miller LS and Johnson DE. Megavoltage radiation for bladder carcinoma: alone, postoperative, *Seventh National Cancer Conference Proceedings,* (1973) 771–782.
2. Shipley WU, Rose MA, Perrone TL, et al. Full-dose irradiation for patients with invasive bladder carcinoma: clinical and histological factors prognostic of improved survival, *J. Urol.,* **134** (1985) 679–683.
3. Quilty PM and Duncan W. Primary radical radiotherapy for T3 transitional cell cancer of the bladder: an analysis of survival and control, *Int. J. Radiat. Oncol. Biol. Phys.,* **12** (1986) 853–860.
4. Batata MA, Chu FC, Hilaris BC, et al. Preoperative whole pelvis versus true pelvis irradiation and/or cystectomy for bladder cancer, *Int. J. Radiat. Oncol. Biol. Phys.,* **7** (1981) 1349–1355.
5. Van Der Werf-Messing B. Carcinoma of the urinary bladder T3 NXMO treated by preoperative radiation followed by simple cystectomy, *Int. J. Radiat. Oncol. Biol. Phys.,* **8** (1982) 1849–1855.
6. Shipley WU, Coombs LJ, and Prout GR Jr. Preoperative irradiation and radical cystectomy for invasive cancer—patterns of failure and prognostic factors associated with patient survival and disease progression, *J. Urol.,* **135** (1986) 222.
7. Van Der Werf-Messing B, Menon RS, and Hop WL. Cancer of the urinary bladder T2, T3, (NXMO) treated by interstitial radium implant: second report, *Int. J. Radiat. Oncol. Biol. Phys.,* **7** (1983) 481–485.
8. Batterman JJ and Tierie AH. Results of implantation for T1 and T2 bladder tumors, *Radiother. Oncol.,* **5** (1986) 85–90.
9. Mazeron JJ, Marinello G, Pierquin B, et al. Treatment of bladder tumors by iridium-192 implantation: the Creteil technique, *Radiother. Oncol.,* **4** (1985) 111–119.
10. Matsumoto L, Kazizoe T, Mikuriya S, et al. Clinical evaluation of intraoperative radiotherapy for carcinoma of the urinary bladder, *Cancer,* **47** (1981) 509–513.
11. Calvo FA, Henriquez I, Santos M, et al. Intraoperative and external beam radiotherapy in invasive bladder cancer: pathological findings following cystectomy, *Am. J. Clin. Oncol.,* **13** (1990) 101–106.
12. Calvo FA, Aristu J, Abuchaibe O, et al. Intraoperative and external preoperative radiotherapy in invasive bladder cancer: effect of neoadjuvant chemotherapy in tumor downstaging, *Am. J. Clin. Oncol.,* **16** (1993) 61–66.
13. Gerard JP, Hulewicz G, Saleh M, et al. Pilot study of IORT for bladder carcinoma, *Front. Radiat. Ther. Oncol.,* **31** (1997) 250–252.
14. Hulewicz G, Roy P, Coquard C, et al. La radiotherapie per-operatoire dans le traitement conservateur des cancers infiltrants de la vessie, *Progrés en Urol.,* **7** (1997) 229–234.
15. Housset M, Maulard C, Chretien VC, et al. Combined radiation and chemotherapy for invasive transitional-cell cancer of the bladder: a prospective study, *J. Clin. Oncol.,* **11** (1993) 2150–2157.
16. Kaufman DS, Shipley WU, Griffin PP, et al. Selective bladder preservation by combination treatment of invasive bladder cancer, *New Engl. J. Med.,* **329** (1993) 1377–1382.
17. Scher HI, Geller NL, Curley T, et al. Effect of relative cumulative dose-intensity on survival of patients with urothelial cancer treated with M-VAC, *J. Clin. Oncol.,* **11** (1993) 400–407.
18. Logothetis C, Swanson D, Amato R, et al. Optimal delivery of preoperative chemotherapy: preliminary results of a randomized, prospective comparative trial of preoperative and postoperative chemotherapy for invasive bladder carcinoma, *J. Urol.,* **155** (1996) 1241–1245.
19. Mamghan H, Fisher R, Mameghan J, et al. Analysis of failure following definitive radiotherapy for invasive transitional cell carcinoma of the bladder, *Int. J. Radiat. Oncol. Biol. Phys.,* **31** (1995) 247–254.
20. Kachnic LA, Kaufman DS, Heney NM, et al. Bladder preservation by combined modality therapy for invasive bladder cancer, *J. Clin. Oncol.,* **15** (1997) 1022–1029.
21. Shipley WU, Kaufman DS, and Prout GR. Intraoperative radiation therapy in patients with bladder cancer. A review of techniques allowing improved tumor doses and providing high cure rates without loss of the bladder function, *Cancer,* **60** (1987) 1485–1488.
22. Shipley, WU. Intraoperative radiation therapy for bladder cancer: a review of techniques allowing improved tumor doses and providing high cure rates without the loss of bladder function, In Dobelbower

RR and Abe M (eds.), *Intraoperative radiation therapy*. CRC, Boca Raton, FL, (1989) pp. 227–233.

23. Matsumoto K. Intraoperative radiation therapy for bladder cancer, In Dobelbower RR and Abe M (eds.), *Intraoperative radiation therapy*. CRC, Boca Raton, FL, (1989) pp. 217–226.

24. Martinez A and Gunderson LL. Intraoperative radiation therapy for bladder cancer, *Urol. Clin. North. Am.,* **11** (1984) 643–648.

25. Dunst J, Sauer R, Schrott KM, et al. An organ-sparing treatment of advanced bladder cancer: a 10-year experience, *Int. J. Radiat. Oncol. Biol. Phys.,* **30** (1994) 261–266.

26. Schultz TK, Herr HW, Zhang ZF, et al. Neoadjuvant chemotherapy for invasive bladder cancer: prognostic factors for survival in patients treated with MVAC with 5-year follow-up, *J. Clin. Oncol.,* **12** (1994) 1394–1401.

27. Tester W, Caplan R, Heaney J, et al. Neoadjuvant combined modality program with selective organ preservation for invasive bladder cancer: results of Radiation Therapy Oncology Group phase II trial 8802, *J. Clin. Oncol.,* **14** (1996) 119–126.

28. Frydenberg M, Gunderson LL, Hahn G, et al. Preoperative external beam radiotherapy followed by cytoreductive surgery and intraoperative radiotherapy for locally advanced primary or recurrent renal malignancies, *J. Urol.,* **152** (1995) 15–21.

29. Gunderson LL, Zincke H, Robinow J, et al. IORT containing regimens for GU cancer. 5th International IORT Symposium Abstracts, Lyon, *Hepatogastroenterology,* **41** (1994) 5.

30. Santos M, Ucar A, Ramos H, et al. Radioterapia intraoperatoria en el carcinoma renal localmente avanzado: experiencia inicial., *Actas. Urol. Esp.,* **13** (1989) 36–40.

31. Elbe MJ, Stähler G, and Wannenmacher M. IORT for locally advanced or recurrent renal carcinoma, *Front. Radiat. Ther. Oncol.,* **31** (1997) 253–255.

32. Kinsella TJ, Sindelar WF, DeLuca Am, et al. Tolerance of the canine bladder to intraoperative radiation therapy: an experimental study, *Int. J. Radiat. Oncol. Biol. Phys.,* **14** (1988) 939–946.

33. Hoekstra HJ, Sindelar WF, Kinsella TJ, et al. Intraoperative radiation therapy-induced sarcomas in dogs, *Radiat. Res.,* **120** (1989) 508–515.

34. Shaw EG, Gunderson LL, Martin JK, Beart RW, Nagorney DM, and Podratz KC. Peripheral nerve and ureteral tolerance to intraoperative radiation therapy: clinical and dose response analysis, *Radiother. Oncol.,* **18** (1990) 247–255.

35. Gunderson LL, Nelson H, Martenson JA, et al. Locally advanced primary colorectal cancer: intraoperative electron and external beam irradiation ± 5-FU, *Int. J. Radiat. Oncol. Biol. Phys.,* **37** (1997) 601–614.

36. Gunderson LL, Nelson H, Martenson JA, et al. Intraoperative electron and external beam irradiation with or without 5-fluorouracil and maximum surgical resection for previously unirradiated locally recurrent colorectal cancer, *Dis. Colon. Rectum.,* **39** (1996) 1379–1395.

37. Gillette EL, Gillette SM, Vujaskovic Z, et al. Influence of volume on canine ureters and peripheral nerves irradiated intraoperatively, In Schildberg FW, Willich N, and Krämling H (eds.), *Radiation Therapy—Proceedings 4th International IORT Symposium,* Munich, 1992, Essen. Verlag Die Blaue Eule, (1993) 61–63.

24 Lung Cancer
EBRT With or Without IORT

Javier Aristu, Felipe A. Calvo, Rafael Martínez, Jean Bernard Dubois, Manuel Santos, Scott Fisher, and Ignacio Azinovic

CONTENTS

1. RESULTS OF STANDARD TREATMENT—RATIONALE FOR IOERT

1.1. Small Cell Lung Cancer

Small-cell lung cancer (SCLC) is considered at high risk for metastatic disease at time of diagnosis, and combined-modality therapy with chemotherapy and thoracic external beam irradiation (EBRT) is the treatment of choice. Surgery for patients with SCLC could probably be reserved for stage I disease. Patients with more advanced SCLC are not considered to be surgical candidates, and early EBRT obtains acceptable thoracic control rates. Intraoperative electron irradiation (IOERT) has not been reported in this tumor histology.

1.2. Non-Small-Cell Lung Cancer

Radiation therapy has been the standard treatment in stage III disease. However, few patients can be actually cured, local control rates in the long term are modest, and reported 5-year survival rates are only about 5% (1,2). In selected patients with a good performance status and without weight loss, the 5-year survival was only 7% (3).

The rationale to intensify the loco-regional treatment for non-small-cell lung cancer (NSCLC) is based on the observation that 30–40% of patients die with active loco-regional disease (1,4), and it is likely that the incidence of local failure is underestimated because most published series did not utilize computed tomography (CT) or bronchos-

From: *Current Clinical Oncology: Intraoperative Irradiation: Techniques and Results*
Edited by: L. L. Gunderson et al. © Humana Press, Inc., Totowa, NJ

copy for treatment planning and/or restaging following EBRT. Histologic examination of bronchoscopic biopsy specimens in patients treated with irradiation or combined chemoirradiation documented a local failure rate of almost 80% (5). Another reason for the underestimated local failure rate in patients with NSCLC is the development of distant metastases in the early follow-up period; local control is uncertain when assessed in patients surviving less than 1 year.

Several radiotherapy trials suggest that thoracic control in lung cancer is dose related (6,7), but radiosensitive organs such as the lung, spinal cord, and heart often limit the dose of EBRT to ≤ 60 Gy, a dose usually inadequate to sterilize large NSCLC. In an effort to improve local control and survival, new treatment strategies have seen explored, such as hyperfractionated irradiation (8,9), accelerated fractionation irradiation (10), chemoradiotherapy (11), radiation dose escalation using three-dimensional planning and conformal irradiation (12,13), or IOERT. IOERT is a technique developed to improve the therapeutic index of the combination of surgery and irradiation by increasing the maximum dose to the target volume while sparing adjacent uninvolved or radiosensitive structures (14).

Thoracic tumor control rates might benefit from the combination of surgery and radiotherapy, but only approximately 10% of patients with stage III NSCLC are usually considered operable. Despite this dismal picture, surgical resection rates may be increased by using neoadjuvant chemotherapy and preoperative EBRT (15–17). IOERT permits the delivery of a high single dose of radiation during lung cancer surgery to high-risk areas of residual or marginally resected tumor in the mediastinum, chest wall, and hilum while normal tissues can be displaced or protected from the irradiation beam (18) (Fig. 1).

2. CLINICAL EXPERIENCES: TECHNICAL CONSIDERATIONS FOR IOERT

In properly selected patients for thoracic surgery, the only relative or absolute contraindication to IOERT procedures using a high-energy electron beam is in the anterior chest wall region. A lateral thoracotomy incision is usually preferred for IOERT exposure (Fig. 2). This approach permits the introduction of cylindric and beveled IOERT applicators into the thoracic cavity to obtain the maximum inclusion of one side of the mediastinum or hilium after lobectomy, atypical resection, or pneumonectomy.

At the University Clinic of Navarra, investigation have been using custom-made cylindric, straight and beveled, IOERT applicators with a fixed docking mechanism in a nondedicated accelerator to deliver an IOERT boost with electrons ranging from 6 to 20 MeV to selected regions including the hilum (Fig. 3), mediastinum (Fig. 4), chest wall, or thoracic apex (Fig. 5). If anatomically feasible and appropriate from the cancer treatment view, radiosensitive organs such as the esophagus, spinal cord, and heart were protected with lead blocks. The bronchial stump is recommended to be protected with a vacularized flap to prevent suture dehiscence, after IOERT treatment.

The IOERT methodology used has been reported in detail in previously published articles (19,20). Macroscopic residual surgical masses, especially in Pancoast's tumors treated with preoperative chemoradiation, may not contain a viable tumor at the definitive pathology report. To properly select IOERT doses and electron energies, a biopsy of the surgical bed is informative. An IOERT boost to the medial aspect of the thoracic cavity

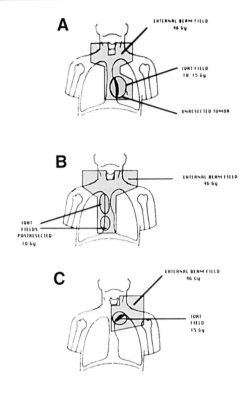

Fig. 1. Integration of external and intraoperative irradiation in lung cancer patients: (**A**) unresected left hiliar tumor; (**B**) right postlobectomy situation (two fields, nonoverlaping including bronchial stump and mediastinum); (**C**) Pancoast lesion.

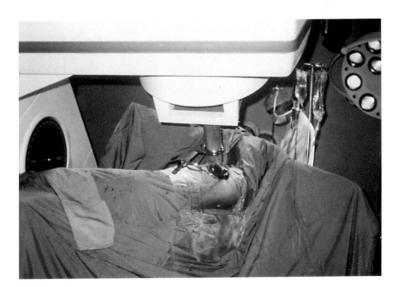

Fig. 2. General view of thoracic IORT with electrons through left lateral thoracotomy.

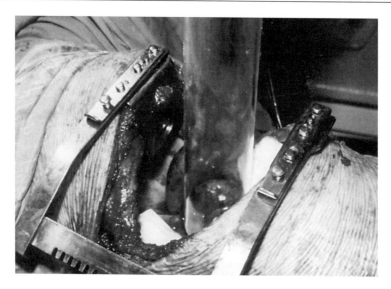

Fig. 3. IOERT applicator positioning during exploratory thoracotomy for an unresectable right-lobe NSCLC. Note that the tumor has been introduced in a 6-cm (0°) applicator, including normal lung parenchyma just around the tumor.

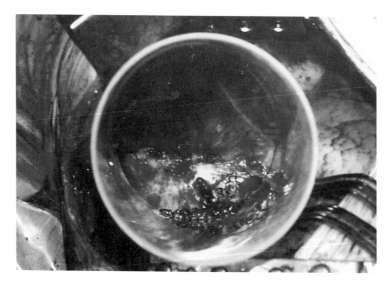

Fig. 4. Simulation for applicator selection (size, beveled angle, positioning, and maneuvers for normal tissue protection) after right superior lobectomy. The IOERT target volume includes right mediastinum and bronchial stump; the remaining normal lung is mobilized out of the electron field.

apex in superior pulmonary sulcus tumors is frequently difficult to access, but through a Trendelenberg position of the surgical coach, IOERT can usually be accomplished.

3. INTERNATIONAL IOERT CLINICAL EXPERIENCES AND RESULTS

The clinical experience of IOERT in lung cancer is still limited and the available data regarding treatment of NSCLC were obtained in phase I–II trials in a small series of

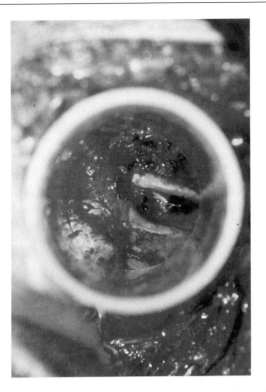

Fig. 5. Postresection simulation for a Pancoast tumor. The target volume includes the tumor bed region (posterior and superior chest wall and paravertebral space), and the remaining normal lung is mobilized out of the intraoperative field.

patients. Abe and collegues in the initial Japanese experience did not use IOERT in lung neoplasms because of the early systemic dissemination of disease *(21)*.

3.1. NCI Series

Based on a previous canine experimental model involving the use of pneumonectomy and IOERT doses of 0, 20, 30, and 40 Gy, a limited phase I National Cancer Institute (NCI) clinical trial demonstrated considerable toxicity with 25 Gy of IOERT to two separate fields encompassing the superior and inferior mediastinum following pneumonectomy *(22)*. Early complications were described in three out of four patients: one case of bronchial stump dehiscence, one bronchopleural fistula, and one case of reversible esophagitis. Three patients with late complications showed one case of irreversible radiation esophagitis, one contralateral esophagobronchial fistula, and one case of reversible esophagitis. Only one long-term survivor is free from disease (more than 3 years). The retrospective analysis of toxic events detected overlapping of the fields in one toxic case. This study recognized the feasibility of IOERT during lung cancer surgery and recommended a decrease in the IOERT dose to 15–20 Gy.

3.2. Graz University Experience

3.2.1. Patient Group

More recently, combined IOERT (10–20 Gy) and postoperative EBRT (46–56 Gy) were used in 21 inoperable tumors at the University Medical School of Graz (Austria)

(23). The analysis included 12 patients with N0 disease. The radiosensitive mediastinal structures such as the heart, spinal cord, esophagus, and large vessels could be mobilized or protected from the IOERT beam by shielding maneuvers.

3.2.2. RESULTS

The response rates in 14 evaluable patients 18 weeks after they completed IOERT and EBRT was excellent with three complete responses (21%) and 10 partial responses (71%). Ten patients are alive and well at a range of 5–20 months (median 12 months).

The same institution updated the results of this program in two consecutive studies *(24,25)*. The IOERT procedure was generally well tolerated, but fatal intrabronchial hemorrhage related to IOERT occurred in two cases with tumor involvement of the pulmonary artery. Local failure was seen in three patients and the 5-year overall and recurrence-free survival rates were 15% and 53%, respectively.

3.3. Montpellier Series

3.3.1. PATIENT GROUP

The Centre Regional De Lutte Contre Le Cancer in Montpellier (France) reported results in 17 patients: 3 stage I, 7 stage II, and 7 stage IIIA (personal communication). The treatment protocol involved the use of IOERT with doses in the range of 10–20 Gy and 45 Gy EBRT in 20–25 fractions with or without a 3-week rest period following a complete surgical excision. Microscopic residual disease in the mediastinal nodes or pleura-chest wall was seen in 12 and 5 patients, respectively. The median follow-up time for the entire group of patients alive was 59 months, with follow-up ranging from 40+ to 120+ months.

3.3.2. RESULTS

Disease control and survival results were as follows. Local control was obtained in 13 out of 17 patients (76%) and central recurrence in the IOERT field has been demonstrated in 4 patients. Three patients are alive without disease at 5.5, 8, and 11 years. Fourteen patients are dead: 7 from distant metastases, 4 from loco-regional recurrence, 1 patient developed a second cancer, and 2 patients had a local recurrence in the EBRT field. The median survival time for the entire group was 36 months and the actuarial survival rate is 18% projected at 11 years.

3.4. University of Navarra, Pamplona Experience

3.4.1. PATIENT GROUP

The largest clinical experience on the use of IOERT in NSCLC is from the University Clinic of Navarra in Pamplona (Spain) *(18–20,26,27)*. The most recent revision of the institutional experience with IOERT in NSCLC is available for communication. Between the period November 1984 and November 1993, 104 patients with histologically confirmed stage III NSCLC were treated with IOERT as a treatment component of multidisciplinary management. The retrospective analysis of the treatment programs in this period of time allows grouping of the patients into four categories. Between 1984 and 1989, 22 patients were treated with surgery, IOERT, and postoperative EBRT. From 1989 to 1993, 82 patients received neoadjuvant chemotherapy. Responders or resectable patients after neoadjuvant chemotherapy (46 patients) were managed with surgery, IOERT, and postoperative EBRT. Nonresponders, unresectable disease (17 patients), or Pancoast's tumors (19 patients) received preoperative chemoradiotherapy, surgery, and an IOERT boost.

3.4.2. TREATMENT TECHNIQUES

3.4.2.1. Neoadjuvant Chemotherapy. Neoadjuvant cisplatin (CDDP)-based chemotherapy consisted of two different protocols. The initial one (1985–1990) included 120 mg/m^2 CDDP 6-h iv infusion on day 1, 8 mg/m^2 mitomycin C (MMC) 1-h iv infusion on day 1, and 3 mg/m^2 (maximum 5 mg) vindesine (VDS) 3-h iv infusion on days 1 and 14 (MVP regimen). In 1990, a new chemotherapy regimen was evaluated in which CDDP and VDS were maintained, MMC was omitted, and intrarterial carboplatin 150 mg/m^2 was added (MCP regimen). Chemotherapy was repeated every 4 weeks (MVP regimen) or 5 weeks (MCP regimen).

3.4.2.2. Surgery. Patients with an objective clinical response or stable disease considered resectable underwent surgical resection, including the primary tumor and mediastinal lymphadenectomy 4–5 weeks after the last cycle of induction chemotherapy.

3.4.2.3. IOERT. IOERT dose and energy were dependent on the amount of residual disease. Total single doses ranged from 10 to 15 Gy. IOERT boosted a single anatomic site of residual disease in 79 procedures and 2 nonoverlapping fields were used in 25 procedures. The most common applicator diameters employed were 7, 8, and 9 cm (66%). The IOERT dose was 10 Gy (62%), 12.5 Gy (5%), 15 Gy (16%), and 18–20 Gy (17%) (generally administered for unresected tumors). Electron energies most frequently selected were 9 and 12 MeV.

3.4.2.4. EBRT. Thoracic EBRT was started 4–5 weeks after surgery. Treatment was delivered with a 15-MV linear accelerator employing the anteroposterior-posteroanterior (AP–PA) technique to encompass the treatment volume which included the bronchial stump, ipsilateral hilium, the bilateral mediastinal, and supraclavicular lymph nodes. Patients were treated with daily fractions of 2 Gy, 5 times per week, reaching a cumulative dose of 46 Gy in 23 fractions. A similar approach was used for preoperative irradiation.

3.4.3. PATIENT AND TREATMENT CHARACTERISTICS, SUMMARY OF PAMPLONA IOERT SERIES

3.4.3.1. Patients Characteristics. Among the 104 treated patients, there were 101 males and 3 females, with a median age of 61 years (range 27–79 years). The median performance status was 80%. Squamous cell carcinoma was the predominant tumor type (63%) followed by adenocarcinoma, large-cell carcinoma, mixed histology, and undifferentiated carcinoma. Forty-eight patients (46%) were classified as stage IIIA (60% N2 disease) and 56 (54%) patients as stage IIIB.

3.4.3.2. Treatment Characteristics. A median of three cycles of chemotherapy were administered. Objective response to chemotherapy or chemotherapy plus preoperative EBRT was identified in 60 out of 82 patients (73%). In the early part of this program, a large proportion of tumors were considered unresectable and tumor resection was not attempted. Poor prognostic patients were classified as nonresponders to neoadjuvant chemotherapy or considered unresectable.

Tumor resection was performed in 90 patients and the type of resection included 73 (70%) lobectomies, 8 atypical resections, 8 segmentectomies, and 1 pneumonectomy. Complete gross resection with microscopically clear margins was achieved in 73% of stage IIIA patients and 37% of stage IIIB patients. Differences between these parameters were statistically significant ($p = 0.0007$).

3.4.4. TREATMENT RESULTS, PAMPLONA IOERT SERIES

3.4.4.1. Local Control. Regarding the quality of resection, the local control rates observed in patients with microscopic residual disease were 18/24 (75%), 4/14 (29%) and

Table 1
Patterns of Failure According
to Disease Stage and Surgical Residue, Pamplona IOERT Analysis

Surgical Residue	Local Control[a]	Distant[b]
Micro/absent		
IIIA	18/24 (75%)	7/24 (29%)
IIIB	4/14 (29%)	4/14 (29%)
Pancoast tumors	11/12 (92%)	2/12 (17%)
Macroscopic/Unresected		
IIIA	3/7 (43%)	6/7 (86%)
IIIB	7/30 (23%)	12/30 (40%)
Pancoast tumors	5/5 (100%)	1/5 (20%)

[a]Local control = no local failure with or without distant metastases.
[b]Distant failure = distant failure alone or distant and local failure.

11/12 (92%) for stages IIIA and IIIB and Pancoast's tumors, respectively. Local control in patients with macroscopic residual disease were 3/7 (43%), 7/30 (23%), and 5/5 (100%) for stages IIIA and IIIB and Pancoast's tumors, respectively (Table 1).

3.4.4.2. Survival. At the time of this analysis, 16 patients (15%) remain alive and free of disease. Five-year overall survival rates for the entire group are 40% for stage IIIA and 18% for stage IIIB patients ($p = 0.01$). Five-year local disease-free survival regarding residual disease is as follows: 69% and 42% for microscopic or no residual disease for stages IIIA and IIIB, respectively, and 58% and 41% for macroscopic (gross) residual disease for stages IIIA and IIIB, respectively. Anecdotally, 19 patients survived more than 5 years after IOERT, with a follow-up range from 64+ to 107+ months. Among patients surviving more than 5 years, there were three second tumors (colon, esophagus, and head and neck) and one cancer unrelated death.

3.4.4.3. Treatment-Related Toxicities. Treatment toxicity and complications are outlined in Table 2. Four patients died in the postoperative period due to possible IOERT-related toxicity: two bronchopleural fistula and two pulmonary hemorrhage. The first bronchopleural fistula occurred in a lobectomized patient, in whom the bronchial stump was not included into the IOERT field. Another patient died 3 months after surgery due to a bronchopleural fistula in a microscopically tumor-involved bronchial stump. One patient developed fatal massive hemoptysis at 2 months following IOERT because of pulmonary artery rupture. This latter patient had prior hemoptysis and a left hiliar unresected tumor treated by tumor exposure and 15 Gy (20 MeV) IOERT plus 46 Gy postoperative EBRT. The autopsy study showed a necrotic cavity in the primary tumor with no viable residual tumor cells and a fistulous tract communicating between the pulmonary artery and the bronchial tree. A nonresected patient treated with three cycles of MVP regimen, preoperative EBRT (44 Gy), and IOERT (15 Gy) died early in the postoperative period from pulmonary hemorrhage.

Esophagitis grade III-IV was noted in 26 (25%) patients and esophageal damage with ulcerated or necrotic tissue was observed in 2 patients (Fig. 6). One out of two patients who developed esophageal ulcer died 8 months after surgery from fatal hemorrhage. This patient had a T4 tumor infiltrating the descending portion of the aorta and the esophagus. He was treated with three cycles of MVP chemotherapy regimen, preoperative EBRT (46 Gy), surgery (atypical resection plus chest wall resection), and 10 Gy IOERT boost

Table 2
Toxicity and Complications for the Entire Group
(104 patients) Treated with Combined Modality
Therapy and an IOERT Component, Pamplona Analysis

Toxicity and Complications	No. of Episodes
Postoperative period	
Pneumonia	4
Abscess–empyema	4
Pulmonary embolism	1
Peritonitis	1
Hemomediastinum	1
Pulmonary hemorrhage	2
Bronchopleural fistula	2
Acute vena cava syndrome	1
Short term	
Esophagitis grade III–IV	26
Symtomatic pneumonitis	6
Bronchopleural fistula	1
Pulmonary embolism	1
Pneumonia	2
Long term	
Transient neuropathy	6
Lung fibrosis	7
Bronchopleural fistula	1
Esophageal ulcer	2
Esophageal stricture	1
Instability of chest wall	1

(12 MeV). No viable microscopic tumor was encountered in the resected specimen and the necropsy findings revealed a connection between the esophagus and the aorta without histologic evidence of tumor cells.

Symptomatic radiation acute pneumonitis was observed in six patients (Fig. 7). Seven patients were diagnosed of severe long-term fibrosis who require chronic corticotherapy administration.

Neurologic toxicity was noted only in patients treated with IOERT which included the thoracic apex or chest wall. Six patients developed transient neuropathy (four Pancoast's tumors) with pain and paresthesia in the superior ipsilateral extremity or chest wall.

Severe infectious complications were seen in 11 patients. Six of these patients were diagnosed with simultaneous thoracic tumor progression coexisting with an abcess. IOERT-related major toxicities according to treatment characteristics are summarized in Table 3.

3.5. The Allegheny University Hospital: Graduate Hospital of Philadelphia Experience

This unique experience in the United States was preliminarily reported in 1994 (28). The present update includes 21 patients treated from 6/92 to 9/97 as part of a pilot feasibility experience for stage I ($N = 1$), II ($N = 2$), and III ($N = 18$) NSCLC patients managed by surgical resection, IOERT (10 Gy), and EBRT (45.0–59.4 Gy, 16 preoperatively and 5 postoperatively). Chemotherapy was administered to all patients. The median

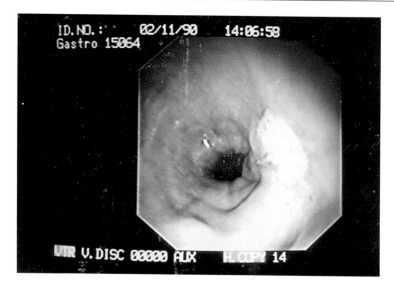

Fig. 6. Endoscopic view of an esophageal ulcer located in the internal portion of an IOERT field after lobectomy and treatment of the ipsilateral mediastinum. Symptoms were increased during the administration of adjuvant chemotherapy with radiopotentiating agents.

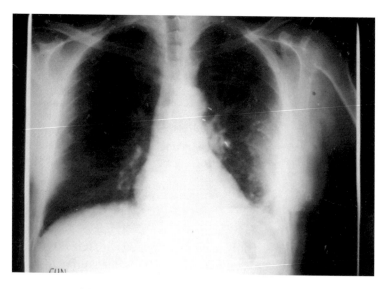

Fig. 7. An acute pneumonitis was identified in a patient treated with IOERT for an unresectable left hiliar NSCLC on a 7-days' postoperative chest x-ray showing a linear distribution of parenchymal increase density; the resolution of pneumonitic changes was demonstrated after 15 days of steroid therapy.

survival time for the alive patients is 33 months. Patterns of relapse have shown 3 (14%) thoracic and 12 (55%) systemic. Actuarial 5-year survival is 33%.

3.6. Instituto Madrileño de Oncología (Madrid, Spain)

From February 1992 to July 1997, 18 patients with stage III non-small-cell lung cancer (11 Pancoast tumors) received IOERT as a part of a multidisciplinary program including

Table 3

Tumor Treatment and IOERT Technical Characteristics in Patients with Possible Intrathoracic IOERT-Related Major Toxicities, Pamplona Analysis

Toxicity	Stage	Type of Surgery	IOERT Dose/energy/residue	IOERT Volume (Applicator diameter)	Bronchial stump	EBRT	Surgery interval (days)
Bronchopleural fistula	IIIA	Lobectomy	11 Gy/9 MeV/microscopic	Pulmonary apex + mediastinum (8 cm)	Suture	—	30
Bronchopleural fistula	IIIB	Lobectomy	10 Gy/12 MeV/microscopic	Hilium[a] (9 cm + 7 cm)	Flap	Preop (32 Gy)[b]	45
Bronchopleural fistula	IIIA	Lobectomy	10 Gy/9 MeV/microscopic	Hilium[a] (9 cm + 7 cm)	Suture	Postop (44 Gy)	270
Bronchopleural fistula	IIIB	Lobectomy	10 Gy/12 MeV/macroscopic	Hilium + mediastinum (9 cm)	Flap	Postop (6 Gy)[b]	60
Pulmonary hemorrhage	IIIB	Tumor exposure	15 Gy/20 MeV/macroscopic	Mediastinum (9 cm)	—	Postop (50 Gy)	60
Pulmonary hemorrhage	IIIA	Tumor exposure	15 Gy/18 MeV/macroscopic	Hilium (8 cm)	—	Preop (44 Gy)	8
Esophageal ulcer	IIIA	Lobectomy	10 Gy/9 MeV/microscopic	Hilium (6 cm)	Flap	Postop (46 Gy)	146
Esophageal ulcer	IIIB	Atypical R.	10 Gy/12 MeV/microscopic	Mediastinum (10 cm)	—	Postop (46 Gy)	215
Esophageal stricture	IIIB	Lobectomy	15 Gy/12 MeV/microscopic	Chest wall + mediastinum (9 cm)	Flap	Preop (46 Gy)	310

[a]IOERT multiple (N=2) fields. [b]EBRT was stopped for toxicity

447

surgical resection in all cases, chemotherapy in 13, preoperative EBRT in 7, and postoperative EBRT in 7. Tumor residue at the time of surgery was macroscopic (gross) in eight cases. The median survival time for the entire series is 14 months. Intrathoracic recurrence has been identified in two patients. Five-year actuarial survival is projected as 22% (cause-specific 33%). Long-term toxicity observed included neuropathy (two cases) and esophageal stricture (one case).

4. TISSUE TOLERANCE STUDIES—MEDIASTINAL IOERT

The tolerance of mediastinal structures to IOERT has been prospectively analyzed in experimental animal studies. In a dose-escalation study (29) delivering 20, 30, and 40 Gy to two separate intrathoracic IOERT fields which included collapsed right upper lobe, esophagus, trachea, phrenic nerve, right atrium, and blood vessels, pathologic changes were observed at 30 Gy in the trachea and esophagus, with severe ulceration and peribronchial and perivascular chronic inflammation in the normal lung. A dose of 20 Gy produced minimal changes in the esophagus, trachea, and phrenic nerve, but major vessels and the atrium showed medial and adventitial fibrosis, obliterative endarteritis of the vasa vasorum, and severe coagulative necrosis. Acute pneumonitis was seen at all doses, and changes in the contralateral lung were detected using 12-MeV electrons.

De Boer et al. (30) studied the effects of 20, 25, and 30 Gy in mediastinal structures. The bronchial stump healed in all dogs. Severe tissue damage was seen at all doses and included bronchovascular and esophagoaortic fistulas and esophageal stenosis.

At the National Cancer Institute (22), an experimental program evaluated the tolerance of surgically manipulated mediastinal structures to IOERT in 49 adult foxhounds and a limited phase I clinical trial (four patients with stage II or III NSCLC). Normal healing of the bronchial stump was found after pneumonectomy and IOERT doses of 20, 30, and 40 Gy, but there were late changes with tracheobronchial irradiation damage at all doses (5–10 months after treatment). Two out of four receiving 20 Gy developed esophageal ulceration at 6 months without late stricture. In dogs given 30 and 40 Gy, esophageal damage was severe (esophagoaortic fistula and stenosis) and one dog developed carinal necrosis. The same institution reported the results of five dogs reserved for long-term studies and one stage II NSCLC patient alive at 5 years. They conclude that IOERT in the mediastinum may be safe at dose levels that do not exceed 20 Gy (31).

Additional experimental analysis of canine esophagus tolerance to IOERT has been reported by the NCI investigators (32). After right thoracotomy with mobilization of the intrathoracic esophagus, IOERT was delivered to include a 6-cm esophageal segment using a 9-MeV electron beam with escalating single doses of 0, 20, and 30 Gy. Dogs were followed clinically with endoscopic and radiologic studies and were electively sacrificed at 6 weeks or 3, 12, or 60 months after treatment. Transient mild dysphagia and mild esophagitis was observed in all dogs receiving 20 Gy, without major clinical or pathological sequelae except in one dog that developed achalasia requiring a liquid diet. At a dose of 30 Gy, changes in the esophagus were pronounced with ulcerative esophagitis and chronic ulcerative esophagitis inducing gross stenosis after 9 months.

Zhou et al. (33) analyzed the acute responses of the mediastinal and thoracic viscera in nine canines sacrificed after they received single IOERT doses of 25, 35, and 45 Gy. No pathological changes were found in the spinal cord and vertebra. Microscopic examination of trachea, esophagus, and lung showed mild or severe histological changes at 30

Table 4
Clinical and Pathologic Findings Observed in Animal Experimental Models

IORT doses	Bronchial Stump	Esophageal Damage	Lung Damage	Pathologic Changes in Heart and Vessels
20 Gy	Normal healing	Transient mild disphagia	Mild	Moderate
30 Gy	Normal healing	Chronic ulcerative esophagitis	Moderate	Moderate–severe
40 Gy	Normal healing	Esophageal perforation, esophageal stricture	Severe	Severe

Source: Data from refs. 29–33.

days at the level of 25 Gy versus 35–45 Gy, respectively. Severe and unrepaired histologic changes were found in the heart and aorta receiving 35–45 Gy.

Based on these data, active clinical programs using thoracic IOERT agree that 20 Gy is the upper single-dose limit that can be safely tolerated by mediastinal and thoracic viscera (Table 4) with IOERT alone. There are no reported experimental normal-tissue tolerance studies of IORT used in combination with EBRT.

5. SUMMARY

The modern developments in the treatment of localized NSCLC confirm the oncology tendency to intensify systemic and local treatment to promote disease control. Although a large number of patients with stage III NSCLC die of systemic disease, local failure remains a substantial problem. The Cancer and Leukemia Group B Protocol has recently reported patterns of disease failure in stage IIIA patients treated with induction chemotherapy, surgery, and thoracic irradiation (34). The study found that of 52 out of 74 patients had failures and the thorax was the first site of isolated or combined local failure in 36 patients (69%). Similarly, Le Chevalier et al. (5) reported that local control at 1 year documented by bronchoscopy was poor (15%) in the chemotherapy plus radiotherapy arm.

Unfortunately, approximately less than 20% of stage III patients have resectable disease for cure at diagnosis and the optimal management of patients with unresectable disease remains controversial. In spite of improvement in resectability rates with neoadjuvant approaches, stage III NSCLC patients have a high incidence of local recurrence. Based on these observations, higher tumor doses may result in improved local control, and several trials have emerged in an attempt to promote thoracic control by escalating total radiation doses exploring altered fractionation or three-dimensional radiation planning (8,9,35,36).

Intraoperative irradiation has been integrated into the multidisciplinary management of NSCLC in several small prospective single institution pilot trials as a sophisticated electron boost of radiation, confirming the feasibility of IOERT procedure during surgical exploration of NSCLC patients. IOERT doses between 10 and 15 Gy combined with EBRT (46–50 Gy) induces acute and late toxic events at a clinically acceptable level. Table 5 is a summary of international IOERT clinical trials regarding local control and survival data in NSCLC.

Definitive conclusions based on the available IORT experiences discussed in this chapter cannot be established, but thoracic control and survival seems to be related to

Table 5
IOERT International Clinical Experiences in NSCLC

Authors	No. of patients	Stage	Treatment Protocol	Local Control	5-Year Survival
Smolle-Jeuttner[a] (ref. 30)	24	12 I 1 II 10 IIIA	IOERT 10–20 Gy + EBRT 46–56 Gy	19/23 (83%)	15%
Dubois (personal communication)	17	3 I 7 II 7 IIIA	S[b] + IOERT (10–20 Gy) + EBRT 45 Gy	13/17 (76%)	18%
Pamplona experience (present report)	104	19 IIIA (N0) 29 IIIA (N2) 56 IIIB	Multidisciplinary treatment (see text) with IOERT 10–20 Gy + EBRT (46 Gy) with and without CT	48/92 (52%)	40% (IIIA) 18% (IIIB)
Philadelphia experience (ref. 33 plus present report)	21	1 I 2 II 15 IIIA 3 IIIB	Neoadjuvant CT with and without preop EBRT + S[b]+IOERT with and without postop EBRT	18/21 (86%)	33%
Madrid experience (present report)	18	11 IIIA 6 IIIB 1 IV	Neoadjuvant CT with and without preop EBRT + S[b]+IOERT with and without postop EBRT	16/18 (90%)	22%

[a]Inoperable patients; CT: chemotherapy
[b] Surgery

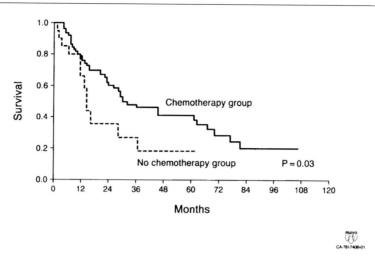

Fig. 8. Actuarial survival in patients treated with an IOERT component at the University of Navarra: chemotherapy contributed to survival prolongation ($p = 0.03$).

tumor stage and location, surgical residue, and neoadjuvant chemotherapy (Fig. 8). Remarkable local control rates in Pancoast and stage IIIA tumors with microscopic residual disease have been detected.

The effect of IOERT on the group of patients presenting with stage IIIB appear to be favorable. This point is illustrated by the fact that patients with macroscopic residual disease or unresected disease achieved modest rates of local control (23%), but a few long-term survivors are identified.

Further confirmatory trials will be necessary to define the implication of IOERT in thoracic control and survival of patients with NSCLC. IOERT as a component of treatment can be integrated in phase III trials with treatment strategies that may include surgical thoracic exploration. This effort will require international cooperation among expert IOERT institutions.

REFERENCES

1. Perez CA, Pajak TF, Rubin P, et al. Long-term observations of the patterns of failure in patients with unresectable non-oat cell carcinoma of the lung treated with definitive radiotherapy. Report by the Radiation Therapy Oncology Group, *Cancer,* **59** (1987) 1874–1881.
2. Johnson DH, Einhorn LH, Bartolucci A, et al. Thoracic radiotherapy does not prolong survival in patients with locally advanced, unresectable non-small cell lung cancer, *Ann. Intern. Med.,* **113** (1990) 33–38.
3. Dillman RO, Herndon J, Seagren SL, et al. Improved survival in stage III non-small cell lung cancer: seven year follow-up of cancer and leukemia Group B (CALGB) 8433 trial, *J. Nat. Cancer Inst.,* **88** (1996) 1210–1215.
4. Cox JD. Failure Analysis of of inoperable carcinoma of the lung of all histopathologic types and squamous cell carcinoma of the esophagus, *Cancer Treat. Symp.,* **2** (1983) 77–86.
5. Le Chevalier T, Arriagada R, Quoix E, Ruffie P, Martin M, and Tarayre M. Radiotherapy alone versus combined chemotherapy and radiotherapy in nonresectable non-small-cell lung cancer: first analysis of a randomized trial in 353 patients, *J. Nat. Cancer Inst.,* **83** (1991) 417–423.
6. Emami B and Perez CA. Carcinoma of the lung. In Perez CA and Brady LW (eds.), *Principles and practice of radiation oncology,* Philadelphia, PA, (1987) Lippincott pp. 650–683.
7. Perez CA, Bauer M, Eldestein BS, Guillispe BD, and Birch R. Impact of tumor control on survival in carcinoma of the lung treated with irradiation, *Int. J. Radiat. Oncol. Biol. Phys.,* **12** (1986) 539–547.

8. Cox JD, Azarnia N, Byhardt RW, Shin KH, Emami B, and Pajak TF. A randomized phase I/II trial of hyperfractionated radiation therapy with total dose of 60.0 to 79.2 Gy. Possible survival benefit with >69.6 Gy in favorable patients with RTOG stage III non-small cell lung carcinoma. Report of Radiation Therapy Oncology Group 83-11, *J. Clin. Oncol.,* **8** (1990) 1543–1555.

9. Cox JD, Pajak TF, Herskovic A, et al. Five year Survival after hyperfractionated radiation therapy for non-small cell lung carcinoma of the lung (NSCLC): results of RTOG protocol 81-08, *Am. J. Clin. Oncol.,* **12** (1991) 280–284.

10. Byhardt RW, Pajak TF, Emami B, Herskovic A, Dogget RS, and Olsen LA. A phase I/II study to evaluate accelerated fractionation via concomitant boost for squamous, adeno, and large cell carcinoma of the lumg: report of Radiation Therapy Oncology Group 84-07, *Int. J. Radiat. Oncol. Biol. Phys.,* **26** (1993) 459–468.

11. Sause WT, Scott C, Taylor S, et al. Radiation Therapy Oncology Group (RTOG) 88-08 and Eastern Cooperative Oncology Group (ECOG) 4588: preliminary results of a phase III trial in regionally advanced, unresectable non-small-cell lung cancer, *J. Nat. Cancer Inst.,* **87(3)** (1995) 198–205.

12. Emami B, Purdy JA, Manolis J, et al. Three-Dimensional Treatment Planning for Lung Cancer, *Int. J. Radiat. Oncol. Biol. Phys.,* **21** (1991) 217–227.

13. Armstrong JG, Burman C, Leibel S, et al. Three-dimensional conformal radiation therapy may improve the therapeutic ratio of high dose radiation therapy for lung cancer, *Int. J. Radiat. Oncol. Biol. Phys.,* **26** (1993) 685–689.

14. Gunderson LL. Rationale for and results of intraoperative radiation therapy, *Cancer,* **74** (1994) 537–540.

15. Pass HI, Progebniak HW, Steinberg SM, Mulshine J, and Minna JD. Randomized trial of neoadjuvant therapy for lung cancer: interim analysis, *Ann. Thorac. Surg.,* **53** (1992) 992–998.

16. Rosell R, Gomez-Codina J, Camps C, et al. A randomized trial comparing preoperative chemotherapy plus surgery with surgery alone in patients with non-small cell lung cancer, *N. Engl. J. Med.,* **330** (1994) 153.

17. Roth JA, Fossella F, Komaki R, et al. A randomized trial comparing perioperative chemotherapy and surgery with surgery alone in resectable stage III non-small cell lung cancer, *J. Nat. Cancer Inst.,* **86** (1994) 673–680.

18. Calvo FA, Santos M, and Ortíz de Urbina D. Intraoperative radiotherapy in thoracic tumors, *Front. Radiat. Ther. Oncol.,* **25** (1991) 307–316.

19. Calvo FA, Ortiz de Urbina D, Abuchaibe O, et al. Intraoperative radiotherapy during lung cancer surgery: technical description and early clinical results, *Int. J. Radiat. Oncol. Biol. Phys.,* **19** (1990) 103–109.

20. Aristu J, Martínez-Monge R, Aramendía JM, et al. Cisplatin, mitomycin, and vindesine followed by intraoperative and postoperative radiotherapy for stage III non-small cell lung cancer: final results of a phase II study, *Am. J. Clin. Oncol.,* **20** (1997) 276–281.

21. Abe M and Takahashi M. Intraoperative radiotherapy: the Japanese experience, *Int. J. Radiat. Oncol. Biol. Phys.,* **7(7)** (1981) 863–868.

22. Pass HI, Sindelar WF, Kinsella TJ, et al. Delivery of intraoperative radiation therapy after pneumonectomy: experimental observations and early clinical results, *Ann. Thorac. Surg.,* **44** (1987) 14–20.

23. Jeuttner FM, Arian-Schad K, Porsch G, et al. Intraoperative radiation therapy combined with external irradiation in nonresectable non-small-cell lung cancer: preliminary report, *Int. J. Radiat. Oncol. Biol. Phys.,* **18** (1990) 1143–1150.

24. Arian-Schad, Juellner FM, Ratzenhofer B, et al. Intraoperative plus external beam irradiation in nonresectable lung cancer: assessment of local response and therapy-related side effects, *Radiother. Oncol.,* **119** (1990) 137–144.

25. Smolle Juettner, Geyer E, Kapp KS, et al. Evaluating intraoperative radiation therapy (IORT) and external beam radiation therapy (EBRT) in non-small cell lung cancer (NSCLC), *Eur. J. Cardio-thorac. Surg.,* **8** (1994) 511–516.

26. Calvo FA, Ortiz de Urbina D, Herreros J, and Llorens R. Lung Cancer, In Calvo FA, Santos M, and Brady LW (eds.), *Intraoperative Radiotherapy. Clinical Experiences and Results,* Springer-Verlag Berlin Heidelberg 1992, pp. 43–50.

27. Martinez-Monge R, Herreros J, Aristu JJ, Aramendia JM, and Azinovic I. Combined treatment in superior sulcus tumor, *Am. J. Clin. Oncol.,* **17** (1994) 317–322.

28. Fisher S, Fallahnejad M, Lisker S, et al. Role of intraoperative radiation therapy (IORT) for stage III non small cell lung cancer, *Hepato-gastroenterol.,* **41** (1994) 15.

29. Barnes M, Pass H, De Luca A, et al. Response of mediastinal and thoracic viscera of the dog to intra-operative radiation therapy (IORT), *Int. J. Radiat. Oncol. Biol. Phys.,* **13** (1987) 371–378.

30. De Boer WJ, Mehta DM, Oosterhius JW, et al. Tolerance of mediastinal structures to intraoperative radiotherapy after pneumonectomy in dogs, *Strahlenther. Oncol.,* **165** (1989) 768.

31. Tochner ZA, Pass HI, Sindelar WF, et al. Long term tolerance of thoracic organs to intraoperative radiotherapy, *Int. J. Radiat. Oncol. Biol. Phys.,* **22(1)** (1992) 65–69.

32. Sindelar WF, Hoekstra HJ, Kinsella TJ, et al. Response of the canine esophagus to intraoperative electron beam radiotherapy, *Int. J. Radiat. Oncol. Biol. Phys.,* **15** (1992) 663–669.

33. Zhou GX, Zeng DW, and Li WH. Acute responses of the mediastinal and thoracic viscera of canine to intraoperative irradiation. In Schildberg FW, Wilich N, and Krämling HJ (eds.), *Intraoperative Radiation Therapy,* Proceedings 4th International Symposium, Munich 1992, pp. 50–52.

34. Kumar P, Herndon II J, Langer M, et al. Patterns of disease failure after trimodality therapy of nonsmall cell lung carcinoma pathologic stage IIIA (N2). Analysis of Cancer and Leukemia Group B Protocol 8935, *Cancer,* **77** (1996) 2393–2399.

35. Hazuka MB, Turrisi AT, Martel MK, et al. Dose-escalation in non-small cell lung cancer (NSCLC) using conformal 3-dimensional radiation treatment planning (3DRTP): preliminary results of a phase I study, *(Abstract) Proc. Am. Soc. Clin. Oncol.,* **13** (1994) 337.

36. Choi NC, Carey RW, Daly W, et al. Potential impact on survival of improved tumor downstaging and resection rate by preoperatively twice-daily radiation and concurrent chemotherapy in stage IIIA non-small-cell lung cancer, *J. Clin. Oncol.,* **15** (1997) 712–722.

25 Pediatric Malignancies
IORT Alone or With EBRT

Paula J. Schomberg, Thomas E. Merchant, Gerald Haase, and Javier Aristu

1. IORT RATIONALE—STANDARD TREATMENT RESULTS

In pediatric tumors, local control when combined with intensive adjuvant systemic therapy often leads to long-term survival. In other words, because of greater sensitivity of systemic disease to chemotherapy, local control becomes of greater importance than in many adult malignancies. For example, in adult pancreatic cancer, improved local control does not translate into improved survival due to the high rate of systemic failure because of inadequate chemotherapy whereas an approximately 30% 5-year survival is seen in pediatric group IV rhabdomyosarcoma patients *(1)* and in metastatic Ewing's sarcoma patients *(2)*.

The problem of achieving local control with a suitable therapeutic ratio is especially difficult in the pediatric population. The morbidity of high-dose irradiation in growing bones and soft tissues adds to the challenge of radiosensitive organs such as the kidney, liver, spinal cord, stomach, and bowel in both adults and children. Neuhauser et al. *(3)* were the first to describe the relationship among growth compromise, radiation dose, and age in children. A significantly greater tendency toward vertebral body deformation with doses in excess of 20 Gy and age under 2 years was identified. A recent review of radiation growth effects in children stated that the challenge was to modify or eliminate treatment likely to produce irreparable damage without compromising the chance for cure *(4)*. Adequate local control with acceptable treatment morbidity remains a problem in the treatment of malignancies of the abdomen, pelvis, and retroperitoneum in children as well as adults.

From: *Current Clinical Oncology: Intraoperative Irradiation: Techniques and Results*
Edited by: L. L. Gunderson et al. © Humana Press, Inc., Totowa, NJ

Possible situations for the use of intraoperative irradiation (IORT) in pediatric malignancies include those in which surgery and/or chemotherapy would not be expected to result in local control or in which external beam irradiation (EBRT) doses in excess of 50 Gy would be necessary. In addition, there are cases in which the substitution of IORT for a part of the EBRT dose would decrease the dose to normal structures and, therefore, minimize damage to these tissues. Consideration should be given to the use of IORT as a component of treatment in the primary management of rhabdomyosarcoma. Ewing's sarcoma, epithelial tumors and other soft tissue sarcomas, and in select cases of Wilms' tumor, neuroblastoma, and hepatoblastoma.

The most common pediatric malignancies are leukemia, lymphoma, and primary brain tumors (5). These tumors comprise a group of patients for whom, with relatively few exceptions, IORT may be impractical in the primary setting. Excluding these most common pediatric malignancies, other childhood cancers differ substantially from adult malignancies in histogenesis, clinical presentation (axial vs peripheral), and response to combined modality therapy. It is easy to be optimistic and consider that all pediatric solid tumors may be amenable to IORT. However, if one considers that for many of these tumors, (1) survival is relatively high, (2) morbidity of standard therapy is small, (3) local control may not be a substantial problem, or (4) the role of radiation therapy is being limited or reduced, it would seem that treatment at the time of recurrence, especially in the setting of prior irradiation, would be the ideal way for IORT to find a niche in the treatment of the pediatric patient. Local disease may be an important component of management problems in these patients.

1.1. Soft Tissue Sarcoma

Complete surgical resection with pathologically negative margins is accomplished in a minority of patients with pelvic and retroperitoneal sarcomas, and despite such aggressive surgical approaches, the local recurrence rate may exceed 50% (6). Crist et al. (6) reported on the 101 patients entered on the first and second Intergroup Rhabdomyosarcoma studies (IRS-I and -II) with a retroperitoneal space primary site (excluding genitourinary and hepatobiliary primary sites). Significantly more of these patients (87%) were of advanced group (III or IV) at diagnosis as compared to the IRS-I and -II studies as a whole (66%), and tumor volumes were larger than primaries occurring in other locations. In 39% of the patients, there were major difficulties in the delivery of the specified irradiation related to the large tumor volume, an inability to adequately define margins, and the frequent presence of normal structures in the field. In 13 patients, the radiation dose was too low, in 11 others no radiation was administered, in 5 patients the EBRT volume was too small to encompass the tumor, in 9 patients both the dose and volume were too small, and in 1 patient improper timing of EBRT was used. In one-half of these patients, the EBRT violations were of such a magnitude that the patient was deemed inevaluable. Of the 70 evaluable patients, 40 (57%) relapsed. Sixty percent of the relapses were local or regional with or without a distant metastatic component. Of patients experiencing relapse, 98% died of their disease.

1.2. Neuroblastoma

There is a potential role for IORT in the management of neuroblastoma due to the young age of the patients and EBRT dose restrictions. Most children are less than 4 years old and the median age at diagnosis is 21 months. Thirty percent of cases occur in infants less than 1 year of age (7). In addition, older children with neuroblastoma require higher radiation doses for tumor control. There is a high incidence of spinal deformities in long-term survivors of neuroblastoma. These include kyphosis and/or scoliosis and have been reported to develop in more than 75% of 5-year survivors *(7)*. Garaventa et al. *(8)* reviewed the experience with localized but unresectable neuroblastoma in 21 Italian institutions. They concluded that risk categories can be defined by age and primary site with children aged 1–15 years with intra-abdominal primaries faring worse than those with extra-abdominal sites or those less than 1 year of age (progression-free survival at 5 years of 30% vs 64% vs 72%, $p < 0.01$ and $p < 0.001$, respectively). They could not prove a role for irradiation, at least in the doses and schedules used in their patients. Castleberry et al. *(9)* demonstrated the benefit of irradiation in neuroblastoma. They conducted a randomized comparison of chemotherapy with and without irradiation in a high-risk patient group (older than 1 year with Pediatric Oncology Group Stage C disease). Differences in complete remission rate, event-free and overall survival in favor of the group receiving irradiation were significant ($p = 0.013$, 0.009, and 0.008). IORT is a potential way to administer all or part of the irradiation.

1.3. Wilms' Tumor

In Wilms' tumor, the standard flank dose of 10.8 Gy has acceptable morbidity. However, patients with residual disease after maximal resection who require a boost could receive IORT in place of EBRT in an attempt to minimize treatment morbidity. Patients with bilateral Wilm's tumors not suitable for partial nephrectomy or with local recurrence pose a difficult problem. One is faced with the possibility of bilateral nephrectomies followed by hemodialysis and/or renal transplantation and a poor survival rate. DeMaria et al. *(10)* reported a 29% survival in bilateral Wilms' tumor patients undergoing transplantation. The excess death rate was related to a higher incidence of sepsis thought to be due to the use of radiotherapy, chemotherapy and the resulting immunosuppression in these patients. The use of IORT in combination with nephron-sparing surgery may permit obliteration of both gross and microscopic tumor while preserving maximum residual renal function.

1.4. Hepatoblastoma

The only long-term survivors of hepatoblastoma are those in whom complete surgical excision is accomplished. In a series compiled by Exelby et al. *(11)*, 67% of patients with hepatoblastoma underwent resection and 58% of those who had a complete resection survived. None of their patients with unresectable tumors survived. Normal liver tolerance is not compatible with curative radiation doses when large treatment volumes are necessary to encompass tumor. Radiation therapy can be utilized in an attempt to make an unresectable tumor resectable or in cases with a marginal resection. The use of IORT to deliver a part of the dose may limit the radiation dose to normal liver. Shafer and Selinkoff *(12)* reported three cases of initially unresectable hepatoblastoma which became operable following chemotherapy and EBRT. Focal irradiation combined with chemotherapy was utilized by Habrand et al. *(13)* in the management of patients with hepatoblastoma who had residual disease following resection. Tolerance to irradiation was good and 75% have remained free of disease at 4–83 months (median 32 months).

1.5. Bone Sarcoma

Local control is an essential component of the successful management of bone sarcoma patients. The addition of neoadjuvant chemotherapy to conservative surgery (combined with EBRT and possibly IORT) may facilitate en bloc tumor resection, with functional reconstruction sparing the patient amputation or other debilitating surgery.

2. TREATMENT FACTORS FOR IORT

Children are small relative to adults. The issue of size challenges the tenets of IORT because of the close proximity of critical structures, internal organs, and the need to treat physically small (or occasionally relatively large) areas in these patients. High dose rate brachytherapy IORT (HDR–IORT) has an applicator or delivery system designed to treat confined spaces which may restrict or prevent the introduction of a rigid intraoperative electron irradiation (IOERT) applicator.

The use of this modality in children requires extraordinary communication and planning among the pediatric oncologist, the surgeon, and the radiation oncologist. Each operation is planned with the intent to completely excise the tumor. However, the extent of resection attained is determined at operation and is not necessarily predictable by tumor biology, histologic subtype, response to therapy, or preoperative imaging. For most pediatric tumors, the strategy involving IORT considers two points in time: an immediate surgical procedure at diagnosis and a subsequent secondary operation or delayed primary resection after biopsy of the tumor and chemotherapy +/– EBRT.

The primary objective of an immediate operation is to confirm the histologic diagnosis, provide adequate tissue for prognostic and biologic specimens, and evaluate the site and extent of disease. The safest procedure necessary to accomplish this is generally recommended. However, if the tumor is localized, more extensive operative exposure may be carried out to determine resectability and accomplish a complete resection, if feasible. If the tumor location, friability, invasion of adjacent organs, or other factors suggest excessive risk of resection, the procedure should be abandoned and no consideration of the use of IORT is made at the initial operation. A definitive secondary procedure will be delayed until chemotherapy response (alone or in combination with EBRT) allows for more effective local tumor control at a subsequent time. IORT may be employed during the initial operation after complete gross tumor resection, but where a high suspicion of microscopic residual disease exists such as with an inflammatory pseudocapsule containing viable tumor cells or in cases of a difficult marginal surgical dissection. If a nearly complete resection is attained and minimal gross disease is left in surgically inaccessible areas, IORT is a reasonable adjunctive measure to utilize during initial operation but would need to be supplemented by postoperative EBRT +/– simultaneous chemotherapy.

The most common utilization of IORT in children occurs during the delayed primary or second-look procedure after initial chemotherapy (14). The delayed operation is carefully planned based on imaging studies and is appropriately timed within the patient's overall treatment regimen, as this approach generally provides the best opportunity for complete local tumor resection. Patients with initially unresectable disease, residual tumors, or local recurrences who have demonstrated any response to chemotherapy are reasonable candidates for IORT. Extensive tumor progression is a contraindication except in the most extraordinary circumstances. Because of the limited experience with these techniques in children, the use of hemodilution, regional hyperthermia, and circulatory arrest with cardiopulmonary bypass would currently also eliminate the possibility of IORT.

Because of the potential magnitude of this procedure, preoperative monitoring of the patient's hematologic coagulation status is mandatory. Adequate red blood cell and platelet transfusion is accomplished before operation and all blood components including fresh frozen plasma must be available for intraoperative infusion *(15)*. The anesthetic management requires invasive monitoring or arterial pressures, urine output and central venous pressures in anticipation of sudden hemorrhage, fluid sequestration, ventilatory restriction, or major vascular compression. Obviously, adequate large-bore peripheral venous access may be critical depending on which body cavity is being operated upon.

Fortunately, in pediatric patients, most uninvolved structures can be adequately mobilized so that IOERT applicators from 3 to 7 cm (or larger) in diameter or in length along outside edges can be comfortably placed even in the deepest body cavities without cumbersome lead shielding. In the Mayo pediatric patient series, applicator sizes used varied from 4.5 to 9 cm for circular applicators and from 6×11 cm to 8×15 cm for rectangular or elliptical applicators. If necessary, the use of multiple but nonoverlapping fields may be planned in the operating room before patient transport. In one $3\,^{1}/_{2}$-year-old Mayo patient with marginal resection of a $17 \times 10 \times 8$-cm retroperitoneal ganglio-neuroblastoma, five IOERT fields were required to cover the areas at risk (two abutting fields for the under surface of the liver and three abutting fields to cover the right retroperitoneum).

Bench surgery for renal tumors such as bilateral Wilms' tumors offers the advantages of careful palpation and dissection of the tumor, avoids tumor spillage into the field, and permits extensive renal resection. For the management of recurrent bilateral Wilm's tumors, the substitution of ex vivo irradiation for ex vivo surgical excision in appropriately selected patients may offer the advantage of delivering a large radiation dose to a precisely localized tumor while avoiding damage to uninvolved renal structures and leaving neighboring structures unirradiated. This is especially beneficial for patients who have small renal lesions unsuitable for resection or who have had previous abdominal irradiation.

Logistical considerations aside *(16,17)*, HDR-IORT may be more advantageous than IOERT when treating certain pediatric patients. The size of the patient and the geometry of the site may allow flexible HDR-IORT applicators to be more functional than rigid Lucite or metal IOERT applicators. Solid tumors most likely to benefit from HDR-IORT are the same as for IOERT, as previously discussed. Specific locations that may benefit from the more flexible HDR-IORT applicators include anterior or lateral chest wall and anterior or anterolateral abdomen or pelvis.

The potential advantage of HDR-IORT over conventional brachytherapy is not specifically related to the radiobiologic or invasive characteristics of HDR-IORT (the subject of a far more reaching debate and of Chapters 6 and 7 in this book). It is related to the rapidity of treatment while normal dose-limiting organs are surgically displaced and logistical considerations that make the use of indwelling catheters for conventional brachytherapy difficult. Indwelling catheters and sources are problematic for the pediatric patient, their parents, and caregivers. Small patients require prolonged immobilization or specialized care when afterloading catheters and high-photon-energy sources such as iridium are used.

3. IOERT RESULTS

3.1. Denver Children's—General Results

Limited data exists in the literature to assess the role of IOERT in the management of pediatric malignancies. The largest single institution series from the Children's Hospital

Table 1
IOERT General Results

Author/Institution (ref.)	No. of Patients	Local Control (%)	Survival (%)	Follow-up (Months)
Haase—Denver Children's (14)				
Benign	11	91	100	51 mean
Malignant	48	75	63	51 mean
Schomberg—Mayo Clinic (18)	11	91	73	99 median

of Denver (Table 1) suggests efficacy of IOERT in children (14). They reported 59 pediatric patients with a variety of tumor types treated since 1984. IOERT doses of 10–17 Gy were delivered with 5- to 11-MeV electrons to 84 fields in 64 procedures. Some patients also received EBRT. The local control rate in 11 patients with histologically benign, but locally aggressive lesions was 91%. In the 48 patients with malignant tumors, local control was reported in 75%, and survival was 63% at a mean of 51 months after diagnosis (range 14–104 months). Results in the 25 patients with neuroblastoma and 6 patients with osteosarcoma will be reported in the subsequent results sections dealing with those pediatric disease sites.

3.2. Mayo Clinic Series

3.2.1. Patient Group and Treatment Method

A smaller series of 11 patients with locally advanced primary or recurrent abdominal–pelvic tumors was reported by Schomberg et al. from the Mayo Clinic (Table 1) (18). Tumor histologies included four neuroblastomas, two desmoids, and one each of the following: embryonal rhabdomyosarcoma, synovial cell sarcoma, neurofibrosarcoma, malignant fibrous histiocytoma, and paraganglioma. Maximum tumor dimension at the initiation of treatment ranged from 5 to 20 cm with a median of 10 cm. All patients received EBRT and six also received multiagent systemic chemotherapy. Intraoperative irradiation with 6- to 15-MeV electrons was delivered to the tumor or tumor bed utilizing 1–5 treatment fields (19 total fields treated). Ten patients received doses between 10 and 20 Gy and the remaining patient received 25 Gy.

3.2.2. Results

Eight of 11 patients (73%) are alive and continuously disease free at 37–126 months. Two died of distant progression at 2 and 18 months from IOERT. The patient dying at 2 months had an autopsy which confirmed local control. The second patient had distant metastases at the time of IOERT, was treated palliatively, and failed at a distant site outside the radiation fields. An additional patient died at 6 months after IOERT with local, central, and distant disease. This patient was treated for a large (8 × 15 cm) retroperitoneal mass which enlarged after initial treatment with external irradiation and chemotherapy. Three months after completion of that initial therapy, salvage treatment was attempted with maximal surgical resection and IOERT. In view of dose-limiting structures, the IOERT field could not encompass the entire surgical bed but was limited to gross residual plus 1-cm margins (cone size 5.5 cm).

Table 2
IOERT Neuroblastoma Results

Author (ref.)	No. of Patients	Local Control (%)	Survival (%)	Follow-up (Years)
Haase (14)	25	72	60	4.25
Ohmuna (20)	17	82	47	>2
Matsuura (21)	6	75	17	NS[a]
Maeno (22)	7	100	71	1.8–4.7
Masaki (23)	13	100	38	>2
Mugishima (25)	18	100	78	3

[a]NS = Not specified.

3.3. Disease-Specific Pediatric IOERT Results

3.3.1. WILMS' TUMOR

Experience with the use of IOERT in the management of Wilms' tumors has been published by several authors. Halberg et al. (19) utilized IOERT either *in situ* or ex vivo in the management of two patients with recurrent bilateral Wilms' tumor. This use of IOERT produced tumor control and maximized preservation of residual renal function in these patients with a traditionally poor prognosis with commonly available treatment methods. Ohmuna et al. (20) reported four cases of Wilms' tumor treated with multimodal therapy combined with IOERT (usually 15 Gy) to the tumor bed and lymph node regions at Chiba University between 1979 and 1990. Three are alive and disease-free at more than 9 years following treatment. The fourth patient had bilateral Wilms' tumor and underwent nephrectomy on one side and partial tumor resection on the other. Surgery was followed by IOERT and chemotherapy, but the patient succumbed to metastatic disease. Matsuura et al. (21) treated one case of stage II Wilms tumor and that patient remained alive and without evidence of recurrence for more than 2 years.

3.3.2. NEUROBLASTOMA

A number of series have reported IOERT results in the treatment of neuroblastoma (Table 2). Results will be reported for seven separate series, including the large Denver experience.

The Denver series (14) includes 25 neuroblastoma patients, 15 (60%) of whom were long-term survivors from 14 to 104 months (mean 51 months) after IOERT. Six of seven stage III (86%) and 9 of 18 stage IV patients (50%) survived. Seven patients (70% of patients failing, 28% of total patient group) died with both local progression and disseminated disease and three (30% of patients failing, 12% of total patient group) had only disseminated disease with autopsy proof of local control.

Ohmuna et al. (20) treated 17 cases of neuroblastoma utilizing multimodal therapy (surgery and chemotherapy) which included IOERT to the tumor bed and regional lymph nodes. Eight of the patients (47%) are alive at longer than 2 years; five (27%) are disease free, and the other three have metastatic disease for which they continue to receive chemotherapy. The other nine patients have died of their disease, primarily metastatic, with six patients having autopsy confirmation of tumor control within the irradiated fields.

Maeno et al. (22) reported seven cases of stage IVA and IVB neuroblastoma, all of whom received multimodality therapy including chemotherapy, maximal resection of residual tumor seen on imaging studies after the initial chemotherapy, and IOERT (7–15 Gy); four of the seven patients also received total body irradiation and autologous bone marrow transplantation. One patient who received bone marrow transplantation without total body irradiation remains alive but with bone metastases. A second patient who received neither the total body irradiation nor the bone marrow transplant died with liver and bone metastases. The five remaining patients (71%) remain alive and disease-free at 1.8–4.7 years.

Matsuura et al. *(21)* reported their experience using surgery, IOERT, multidrug chemotherapy (preoperatively in five of six and postoperatively in all six) +/– bone marrow transplantation (two patients) in six cases of advanced abdominal neuroblastoma. The IOERT field encompassed the tumor bed and the paraaortic lymph nodes and 12–15 Gy was administered. No EBRT was administered. One patient remains alive and without evidence of abdominal recurrence at more than 2 years. Two patients died of complications of bone marrow transplantation at 19 and 23 months. Autopsies revealed no intraabdominal disease. Two patients died of systemic metastases 1 and 2 years after IOERT; the authors did not comment on whether there was confirmation of local control. The last patient, the only one that did not undergo complete resection of nodal disease, progressed in this area despite chemotherapy after an initial response.

Masaki et al. *(23)* reported their experience with 13 patients with advanced neuroblastoma treated with IOERT. All patients achieved local control and 38% are alive and disease-free at greater than 2 years.

Aitken et al. *(24)* reported preliminarily on eight patients with advanced-stage neuroblastoma who received IOERT as part of their multimodality therapy. They concluded that IOERT did not unduly extend operative time or increase complications and that it enhanced local tumor control when combined with maximal tumor resection, EBRT, and chemotherapy.

Mugishima et al. *(25)* utilized either IOERT or EBRT as a component of a multimodality treatment approach for advanced stage neuroblastoma. Thirty-six patients were treated with high-dose chemotherapy, surgery, and an autologous bone marrow transplant followed by 13-*cis*-retinoic acid. Local irradiation was administered in 27 of the patients (IOERT [$n = 18$] or EBRT [$n = 10$]). IOERT was utilized except when it was prohibited by technical factors. No local failures were observed in the 27 patients who received local irradiation. One-third of the patients who did not receive some form of local irradiation failed locally as at least a component of their failure. However, the nonirradiated patient group were of a lower age and therefore, perhaps, were not a strictly comparable patient group. The 65% 3-year disease-free survival in this series compares favorably with other autotransplant series [30–40% *(26–28)*]. However, the small patient numbers do not exclude possible selection bias, and the inclusion of several new modalities simultaneously do not allow one to determine the relative contributions of each. No increase in toxicity was reported in those patients receiving IOERT.

3.3.3. Bone Sarcoma

Yamamuro and Kotoura *(29)* reported their experience with IOERT for osteosarcoma. Since 1978, they have used IOERT in combination with chemotherapy for treating primary and metastatic malignant bone tumors in 32 patients in an attempt to preserve the affected limb. Doses of 50–60 Gy are given to osteosarcomas and 100 Gy to the more radioresistant juxtacortical osteosarcomas. Ten patients later underwent resection of the primary (eight for prosthetic replacement and two for treatment complications), and in

8 complete tumor necrosis was observed. In the remaining two cases, treated with unilateral IOERT, instead of medial and lateral, scattered viable tumor cells were noted in the superficial layers. Three patients experienced local recurrence. Two were in nonirradiated areas; one from tumor implantation in the muscle during the biopsy procedure and the other was due to inadequate tumor volume coverage. The third local recurrence occurred within the irradiated volume in a patient with juxtacortical osteosarcoma. Survival rates for these patients were comparable to patients undergoing resection.

In the Denver series *(14)*, six patients with Ewing's or osteogenic sarcoma were treated with IOERT. Three were long-term survivors. One patient died of infection with no evidence of local disease at autopsy and another died of disseminated disease without detection of local recurrence. Therefore, only one of six patients with bone tumors in their series died with evidence of local failure.

3.4. IOERT Toxicity

Three patients in the Mayo series required surgical intervention for treatment-related complications *(30)*. All are alive and free of disease at intervals of 112, 112, and 113 months after IOERT. Two patients developed bilateral hydronephrosis. One was managed with the creation of bilateral ileal ureters and the second with a left to right transureteroureterostomy with excision of a distal right ureteral stricture and a ureteroureterostomy. Both ureters were within the IOERT field in only one of the patients. These patients had surgical mobilization of their ureters before IOERT, and the ureters were included within the EBRT fields. Both of these factors may have contributed to the development of subsequent ureteral fibrosis. In follow-up, both patients have maintained acceptable renal function. These two patients also developed small-bowel obstruction requiring a single surgical intervention. The third patient developed severe renovascular hypertension secondary to left renal artery, superior mesenteric artery, and aortic stenosis and underwent a spleno-left renal artery anastomosis. She remains on antihypertensive medication with well-controlled blood pressure. The ureteral problems occurred early in the Mayo experience and efforts were subsequently made to minimize ureteral manipulation, which potentially will reduce the urologic complications. An additional two patients developed neuropathies; one consisted of transient leg pain and weakness and the other was persistent leg weakness requiring physical therapy. The latter patient had a hemipelvectomy before any irradiation for an aggressive desmoid. He subsequently had a massive pelvic and left lower abdominal relapse and proceeded to preoperative EBRT, maximal resection (but gross residual), and IOERT. He is alive and disease-free 60 months from initiation of irradiation.

In the Japanese series, complications were not described in detail but were deemed acceptable. Ohnuma et al. *(20)* reported scoliosis at an angle of 15°–29° in four of five long-term survivors, which improved gradually with casting. Masaki et al. *(23)* described one patient who experienced limitation of movement of one lower extremity at 4 months after IOERT for advanced neuroblastoma. Computed tomography (CT) scan revealed swelling of the psoas muscle and symptoms reportedly improved with palliative therapy.

Haase et al. *(14)* reported no increase in operative morbidity or mortality in their IOERT patients and no problems with intracavitary infections related to the patient transport or treatment applications. One of their 64 patients did develop a superficial wound complication and this was easily treated with local care and antibiotics and did not adversely impact the patient's overall treatment or outcome. There were no manifestations of acute intestinal injury. There were no differences in operative morbidity or

Table 3
HDR–IORT Results

Author/Institution (Ref.)	No. of Patients	Local Control (%)	Survival (%)	Follow-up (Months)
Nag/Ohio State (31)	11	NS[a]	41 mos. median	NS
Merchant/MSKCC[b] (32,33)	16	61	54	18
Schuck/Munster (34)	20	95	NS	NS

[a]NS = Not specified.
[b]MSKCC = Memorial Sloan-Kettering Cancer Center.

mortality in patients where IOERT was employed compared to a matched group who underwent tumor resection alone.

Despite the use of high doses of IOERT in osteosarcoma patients, Yamamuro and Kotoura (29) noted good preservation of joint function when active and passive exercise was initiated 7–10 days after IOERT. Full extension and 70–90% flexion of the joint was preserved. However, 58% of patients who underwent neither limb amputation nor prosthetic replacement and survived longer than 1 year sustained a pathologic fracture through the lesion. All attempts at osteosynthesis failed to fuse the fracture site. Fracture was more common in osteolytic than in osteoblastic tumors and, therefore, the authors currently recommend prosthetic replacement 3 months after IOERT for all osteolytic tumors. At this time, the tumor necrosis is complete, and marginal or even intralesional resection is safe. They believe that the bone segment undergoing prosthetic replacement can be made much smaller after IOERT than would otherwise be possible, as irradiated but nonosteolytic parts of the bone do not need to be removed. They recommend intramedullary nailing with special rods after IOERT for osteoblastic or less osteolytic tumors to prevent pathologic fracture and preserve good joint function.

4. HDR–IORT EXPERIENCE—UNITED STATES AND EUROPE

4.1. Ohio State

The pediatric experiences (Table 3) to date include that of the group at Ohio State University (31), where fractionated high dose-rate brachytherapy was used alone in the primary treatment of 11 patients with rhabdomyosarcoma (RMS) and non-RMS soft tissue sarcoma. In that study, catheters were implanted at the time of surgery and left in place for 8–14 days. Fractions of 3 Gy were delivered twice a day to a total dose of 36 Gy. The median disease-free survival was 41 months. Although the Ohio State experience does not match specifically the Memorial Sloan-Kettering definition of HDR–IORT, it does show how function-preserving therapy is applied to the pediatric patient and how logistical considerations make conventional forms of brachytherapy difficult in the pediatric patient.

4.2. Memorial Sloan-Kettering

4.2.1. PATIENT GROUP AND TREATMENT METHODS

In the most recent report of the Memorial Sloan-Kettering pediatric series (32,33), 16 patients with solid tumors were treated with HDR–IORT brachytherapy via a remote afterloader. The study included patients with Ewing's sarcoma, rhabdomyosarcoma, synovial cell sarcoma, Wilms' tumor, and other rare pediatric tumors, including osteo-sarcoma and immature teratoma. HDR–IORT was used in the initial management of nine patients and at the time of recurrence in the remaining seven patients. The indication for treatment after maximal resection included gross residual disease in 5 and suspected microscopic disease in 11. All of the treatment sites were axial. They included thoraco-abdominal ($n = 10$) and pelvic ($n = 6$) sites. In this series, all patients were pretreated with chemotherapy. Only nine patients had prior surgery and five had prior EBRT. HDR–IORT consisted of a 12-Gy single-fraction treatment that was prescribed to a depth of 0.5 cm from the surface of a multichannel tissue-equivalent applicator.

4.2.2. RESULTS

With a median follow-up of 18 months, the actuarial rates of local control, metastasis-free, and overall survival were 61%, 51%, and 54%, respectively. One patient failed locally and one failed with both local and distant disease. The low incidence of distant control was due to both the progression and development of metastatic disease. At the time of HDR–IORT, three patients had disseminated disease within the pleural cavity and one had pulmonary metastases. With a limited number of patients, the Memorial authors were able to conclude that the ability to confine treatment to the primary site and decrease the dose to normal tissues was beneficial and safe.

4.3. University of Munster/Germany

Schuck and colleagues performed an intraoperative brachytherapy boost after pre-operative radiochemotherapy in patients with Ewing's sarcoma as part of a European Intergroup Cooperative Ewing's Sarcoma study *(34)*. The intraoperative brachytherapy boost was administered in 20 patients in whom the surgical margins were close to tumor. In general, 10 Gy was administered at a distance of 5 mm from the flab surface using a HDR-afterloading device.

Preliminary results show the technique to be feasible and only one patient (5%) has experienced a local recurrence (this patient also had systemic relapse). There have been no intraoperative complications due to the additional radiotherapy and the overall com-plication did not differ from that in patients treated without brachytherapy.

4.4. HDR–IORT Toxicity

In the Memorial HDR–IORT series *(32)*, the rate of complications potentially related to HDR–IORT (alone or combined with other treatment components) was 19%. A single patient experienced delayed wound healing. He underwent resection of a synovial cell sarcoma of the ischiorectal fossa following intensive alkylator-based chemotherapy that included cyclophosphamide, doxorubicin, vincristine, ifosfamide, and etoposide. Fol-lowing surgery and IOHDR, he received EBRT (50.4 Gy) and additional chemotherapy with the same agents. The delayed healing was predictable.

One patient experienced an abscess at the HDR–IORT site. This patient had an imma-ture teratoma of the presacral region. She had been treated previously with a subtotal resection and suffered a similar complication. She progressed at the primary site and was treated with chemotherapy followed by resection and HDR–IORT. An abscess formed following the resection and HDR–IORT. This delayed the timely delivery of postopera-tive EBRT and limited the total EBRT dose to 25.2 Gy. She was the only patient with an isolated local recurrence.

One potential problem identified for HDR–IORT and the pediatric patient is the threat of cytopenia introduced by the source. As the source dwells in the patient for the lengthy treatment time that often characterizes HDR–IORT, radiosensitive circulating cells are exposed to radiation. This exposure may lead to postoperative leukopenia, a condition which compromises healing and promotes complications. This situation is relevant for the pediatric patient who is likely to be cytopenic at the time of surgery from prior chemotherapy and who may be receiving treatment with granulocyte or granulocyte–macrophage colony-stimulating factors (G-CSF and GM-CSF, respectively). Recent studies have demonstrated greater sensitivity for mobilized progenitor cells as compared to bone marrow progenitor cells and that may explain source-induced cytopenia resulting from HDR–IORT (35). Although this problem has not been previously described, to our knowledge, Memorial authors have reported the possible occurrence of source-induced leukopenia in one patient. She was treated for desmoplastic small-cell tumor of the mediastinum. Her HDR–IORT site measured 91 cm², covered multiple vertebral bodies, and approximated the great vessels. She also received intensive alkylator-based chemotherapy before and after HDR–IORT and died of pulmonary fungemia presumably due to refractory cytopenia. The cytopenia was seen only after HDR–IORT.

4.5. Future Possibilities for HDR–IORT

There is a single experience with a high-dose-rate intraoperative source that might be amenable to the treatment of children with primary brain tumors. The source, tested in adults with brain metastases, should be mentioned because of its potential for future applications. The photon radiosurgery system is a battery-operated high-voltage X-ray generator which is placed stereotactically in a manner analogous to CT-guided biopsy. It has been used to irradiate small intracranial targets because of its rapid gradient in dose. A feasibility study, previously published to describe the treatment of 14 patients (36), showed the unique ability of this probe to provide interstitial, intraoperative, high-dose rate, single-fraction (10–20 Gy) irradiation following histologic confirmation of malignancy. Its potential applications are intriguing.

5. PROGNOSTIC FACTORS

In the Denver series by Haase et al. (14), three of five patients who had gross residual disease at the time of IOERT failed with local and disseminated disease, suggesting prognostic significance for the amount of residual disease after maximal surgical resection. In the Mayo series by Schomberg et al. (18), all eight patients who underwent gross total resection have been locally controlled, as were two of the three patients with gross residual disease at the time of the IOERT for an overall local control rate of 91%. All the patients in the Mayo series, unlike those in the Haase series, received EBRT in addition to the IOERT. The only patient not locally controlled had unresectable disease at the time of IOERT. The local control rate in the three patients treated at the time of recurrence was 100%.

6. DISCUSSION AND FUTURE POSSIBILITIES

6.1. Discussion

The somatic sequelae of radiation therapy are well documented and are the primary concern when treating pediatric patients. To more accurately irradiate the tumor volume, spare normal tissues from high doses of irradiation, and reduce the possibility of late effects, advanced techniques have been developed to conform the prescription dose to well-defined targets. IOERT and HDR–IORT are two such techniques.

Despite the potential for these techniques to enhance the therapeutic index, they are being adopted without objective evidence that they achieve equivalent or better disease control or reduce radiation-related toxicity. This problem stems from the lack of prospective assessment of these techniques, well-defined endpoints such as disease control or toxicity, and the difficulties associated with organizing collaborative cooperative group studies. Conformal radiation therapy, brachytherapy, IOERT, and HDR–IORT can substantially reduce the volume that receives the prescription dose. In the study of late effects, however, the benefit of localized irradiation using IOERT or HDR–IORT might be offset by the increased likelihood of a late effect from high-dose per fraction treatment.

Another problem associated with IOERT and HDR–IORT is the general lack of understanding of high-dose single-fraction radiation therapy and the inability to classify this treatment in the radiation therapy armamentarium. Understanding the mechanisms of action of high-dose single-fraction irradiation, the relationship of high-dose single-fraction irradiation to fractionated radiation therapy, and the role of this treatment when performed in conjunction with fractionated therapy remains elusive.

At the present time, IOERT and HDR–IORT are not specifically identified with the treatment of a particular pediatric tumor. The limited experience of this technique with pediatric patients makes it difficult to suggest IOERT or HDR–IORT as a treatment option to the pediatric oncologist. This situation is perpetuated by the small role that radiation therapy currently plays in the treatment of pediatric patients.

For the present time, single-fraction IOERT or HDR–IORT is more likely to be an adjunct to rather than a substitute for fractionated EBRT. Thus, IOERT or HDR–IORT should be used in an institutional or cooperative group protocol as a local boost treatment in conjunction with fractionated EBRT and maximal resection. Fractionated preoperative EBRT may facilitate resection by causing tumor shrinkage and induce tumor cell damage to decrease the risk of implantability at the time of surgery. Limited experience exists to suggest that IORT in combination with maximal debulking surgery in pediatric patients with locally advanced or recurrent abdominal, retroperitoneal or pelvic malignancies results in excellent local tumor control and overall survival. Toxicity appeared acceptable considering the poor prognosis of this group of patients with standard approaches and the high risk of tumor-associated morbidity and mortality.

6.2. Future Possibilities

Pediatric cancer management during the past three decades has been characterized by substantial gains in overall disease control and survival. These gains have been achieved primarily for leukemia and lymphomas and early-stage bone and soft tissue sarcomas.

For patients with more advanced solid tumors, the gains in disease control and survival have been less substantial. In fact, for most of these tumors, local control remains an important problem. Such is the catalyst for the current Intergroup Rhabdomyosarcoma Study pilot for stage II patients (groups II and III) (37) for whom local control and overall disease control is known to be poor and for whom new strategies are being sought. In the current pilot study, the interaction of EBRT (41.1–50.4 Gy without dose escalation) and escalating doses of cyclophosphamide are being evaluated. Stage II (group II and III patients) have a poor event-free survival and comprise the majority of patients with this disease entity (1,38). Similar chemoirradiation pilot studies should be considered with irradiation-dose escalation using newer techniques of radiation therapy treatment planning and delivery such as conformal EBRT and IOERT or HDR–IORT.

Unfortunately, the issues of local control are secondary for many high-risk pediatric patients because their overall survival is often influenced by the development of metastases and the lack of data suggesting that local control impacts survival. Investigators are reluctant to rely on EBRT or brachytherapy to solve some of the local control problems because of the late effects that are attributable to these modalities. Indeed, with the advent of more effective chemotherapy and aggressive surgical approaches, investigators are attempting to limit the role of EBRT or its use in terms of dose and volume. These efforts continue despite the knowledge that high doses of radiation offer higher rates of local control and new methods are available to deliver the treatment. In general, the availability of several internal irradiation boost options (IOERT, HDR–IORT) may decrease the dose of the EBRT component of treatment required without compromising the efficacy of the integral radiation dose (the total irradiation dose can be divided between EBRT and IORT). In the pediatric population, the toxicity of concern is expected to be most closely linked to the EBRT component, if IOERT doses are limited to 10–15 Gy.

IOERT or HDR–IORT should be considered as a component of retreatment in a majority of patients with locally recurrent disease in whom re-resection is being considered. For this to occur, patients may need to be referred to major institutions with IORT capability in HDR–IORT brachytherapy, IOERT, or both. These recommendations are independent of a history of prior EBRT in view of preliminary results in adult IORT series for recurrent cervical *(39,40)* and rectal cancer *(41,42)* and retroperitoneal sarcoma *(43–45)*. In those situations, limited-dose HDR–IORT (20–30 Gy in 1.8- to 2.0-Gy fractions) plus chemotherapy precede the surgical attempt of maximal resection and IORT.

IOERT or HDR-IORT should also be considered as an adjunct to surgical resection and preoperative or postoperative EBRT when the preoperative imaging studies or findings at the time of surgery are likely to indicate that high-dose radiation therapy is necessary to prevent local relapse. In this setting, the dose of EBRT can be decreased with substitution of IORT for a part of the EBRT dose, thereby decreasing the dose to normal structures and, therefore, minimizing damage to these tissues.

To clarify the role of IORT in the management of pediatric malignancies, it will be important to collect prospective data on disease control, survival, and tolerance in both single institution and cooperative group settings. High-dose EBRT should be compared to EBRT combined with IORT, in terms of local control and tolerance. It may not be possible to randomly compare results because of limited patient numbers and the small number of institutions with IORT capability. However, protocols can be developed which allow for the option of an IORT boost (IOERT or HDR–IORT) versus EBRT boost (utilizing standard or three-dimensional treatment planning).

REFERENCES

1. Crist W, Gehan EA, Ragab AH, et al. The third intergroup rhabdomyosarcoma study, *J. Clin. Oncol.,* **13** (1995) 610–630.
2. Cangir A, Vietti TJ, Gehan EA, et al. Ewing's sarcoma metastatic at diagnosis, *Cancer,* **66** (1990) 887–893.
3. Neuhauser EDB, Wittenborg MH, Berman LZ, and Cohen J. Irradiation effects of roentgen therapy on the growing spine, *Radiology,* **59** (1952) 637–650.
4. Goldwein JW and Meadows AT. Influence of radiation on growth in pediatric patients, *Clinics in Plastic Surgery,* **20** (1993) 455–464.

5. Gurney JG, Davis S, Severson RK, Fang JY, Ross JA, and Robison LL. Trends in cancer incidence among children in the U.S., *Cancer,* **78** (1996) 532–541.
6. Crist WM, Raney RB, Tefft M, et al. Soft tissue sarcomas arising in the retroperitoneal space in children, *Cancer,* **56** (1985) 2125–2132.
7. Halperin EC, Kun LE, Constine LS, and Tarbell NJ. *Neuroblastoma in Pediatric Radiation Oncology,* Raven, New York, pp. 134–60.
8. Garaventa A, DeBernardi B, Pianca C, et al. Localized but unresectable neuroblastoma: Treatment and outcome of 145 cases, *J. Clin. Oncol.,* **11** (1993) 1770–1779.
9. Castleberry RP, Kun LE, Shuster JJ, et al. Radiotherapy improves the outlook for patients older than 1 year with Pediatric Oncology Group stage C neuroblastoma, *J. Clin. Oncol.,* **9** (1991) 789–795.
10. DeMaria JE, Hardy BE, Brezinski A, and Churchill BM. Renal transplantation in patients with bilateral Wilms' tumor, *J. of Ped. Surg.,* **14** (1979) 577–579.
11. Exelby PR, Filler RM, and Grosfeld JL. Liver tumors in children in the particular reference to hepatoblastoma and heptocellular carcinoma: American Academy of pediatrics surgical section survey, 1974, *J. Ped. Surg.,* **10** (1975) 329–337.
12. Shafer AD and Selinkoff PM. Preoperative irradiation and chemotherapy for initially unresectable hepatoblastoma, *J. Ped. Surg.,* **12** (1997) 1001–1007.
13. Habrand JL, Nehme D, Kalifa C, et al. Is there a place for radiation therapy in the management of hepatoblastomas and hepatocellular carcinomas in children?, *Int. J. Radiat. Onc. Biol. Phys.,* **23** (1992) 525–531.
14. Haase GM, Meagher Jr DP, McNeely LK, et al. Electron beam intraoperative radiation therapy for pediatric neoplasms, *Cancer,* **74** (1994) 740–747.
15. Friesen RH, Morrison Jr JE, Verbrugge JJ, et al. Anesthesia for intraoperative radiation therapy in children, *J. Surg. Oncol.,* **35** (1987) 96–98.
16. Harrison LB, Enker WE, and Anderson LL. Part 1: High-dose-rate intraoperative radiation therapy for colorectal cancer; Part 1, *Oncology,* **9** (1995) 679–683.
17. Harrison LB, Enker WE, and Anderson LL. High-dose-rate intraoperative radiation therapy for colorectal cancer. In: Part 2, technical aspects of brachytherapy/remote afterloader, *Oncology,* **9** (1995) 737–740.
18. Schomberg PJ, Gunderson LL, Moir CR, Gilchrist GS, and Smithson WA. Intraoperative electron irradiation in the management of pediatric malignancies, *Cancer,* **79** (1997) 2251–2256.
19. Halberg FE, Harrison MR, Salvatierra O, Longaker MT, Wara WM, and Phillips Tl. Intraoperative radiation therapy for Wilms' tumor in situ or ex vivo, *Cancer,* **67** (1991) 2839–2843.
20. Ohnuma N, Takahashi H, Tanabe M, Yoshida H, Iwai J, and Iwakawa M. Multimodal therapy combined with intraoperative radiation therapy for malignant abdominal tumor in children. Proceedings of 3rd International Symposium on IORT Kyoto Nov 1990.
21. Matsuura K, Ogata T, Araki K, Inomata T, and Nishioka A. Intraoperative radiation therapy for advanced abdominal neuroblastoma and Wilms' tumor. International Congress of Radiation Oncology 1993. Kyoto, Japan p. 360.
22. Maeno T, Kamata R, Sanuke E, et al. IORT for advanced neuroblastoma. Proceedings of 3rd International Symposium on IORT Kyoto Nov. 1990.
23. Masaki H, Saeki M, Tsuchida Y, et al. Intraoperative radiation therapy for advanced neuroblastoma. Proceedings of 3rd International Symposium on IORT Kyoto Nov 1990.
24. Aitken DR, Hopkins A, Archambeau JO, et al. Intraoperative radiotherapy in the treatment of neuroblastoma: report of a pilot study, *Annals. of Surg. Oncol.,* **2** (1995) 343–350.
25. Mugishima H, Harada K, Suzuke T, et al. Comprehensive treatment of advanced neuroblastoma involving autologous bone marrow transplant, *Acta. Paediatrica. Japonica.,* **37** (1995) 493–494.
26. August CS, Serota FT, Kock PA, et al. Treatment of advanced neuroblastoma with supralethal chemotherapy, radiation, and allogeneic or autologous marrow re constitution, *J. Clin. Oncol.,* **2** (1984) 609–616.
27. Philip T, Bernard JL, Aucher JM, et al. High dose chemoradiotherapy with bone marrow transplantation as consolidation treatment in neuroblastoma: an unselected group of stage IV patients over one year of age, *J. Clin. Oncol.,* **5** (1987) 266–271.
28. Seeger RC, Moss TJ, Feig SA, et al. Bone marrow transplantation for poor prognosis neuroblastoma. In Evans AE, D'Angio GJ, and Seeger RC (eds.), *Advances in neuroblastoma research.* New York, Liss, (1988) pp. 203–213.
29. Yamamuro T and Kotoura Y. Intraoperative radiation therapy for osteosarcoma. In Humphrey GB, Koops HS, Molenaar WM, and Postma A (eds.), *Osteosarcoma in adolescents and young adults: new developments and controversies,* Boston (1993) Kluwer Academic Publishers, pp. 177–183.

30. Ritchey ML, Gunderson LL, Smithson WA, et al. Pediatric urological complications with intraoperative radiation therapy, *J. of Urol.,* **143** (1990) 89–91.

31. Nag S, Olson T, Ruymann F, Teich S, and Pieters R. High-dose-rate brachytherapy in childhood sarcomas: a local control strategy preserving bone growth and function, *Med. Pediatr. Oncol.,* **25** (1995) 463–469.

32. Merchant TE, Zelefsky MJ, Sheldon JM, LaQuaglia MB, and Harrison LB. High-dose rate intraoperative radiation therapy for pediatric solid tumors, *Med. Pediatr. Oncol.,* **30** (1998) 34–39.

33. Merchant TE, Zelefsky MJ, Sheldon JM, LaQuaglia MB, and Harrison LB. High-dose rate intraoperative radiation therapy for pediatric solid tumors, *Radiother. Oncol.,* **39(SI)** (1996) 17.

34. Schuck A, Rube Ch, Hillmann A, Paulussen M, et al. Intraoperative high dose rate brachytherapy after preoperative radiochemotherapy in the treatment of Ewing's sarcoma, personal communication.

35. Scheding S, Media JE, KuKuruga MA, and Nakeff A. In situ radiation sensitivity of recombinant human granulocyte colony stimulating factor recruited murine circulating blood and bone marrow progenitors: evidence for possible biologic differences between mobilized blood and bone marrow, *Blood,* **88** (1996) 472–478.

36. Douglas RM, Beatty J, Gall K, Valenzuela RF, et al. Dosimetric results from a feasibility study of a novel radiosurgical source for irradiation of intracranial metastases, *Int. J. Radiat. Oncol. Biol. Phys.,* **36** (1996) 443–450.

37. Maurer HM. Intergroup rhabdomyosarcoma study V: A pilot study of vincristine (VCR), actinomycind-D (AMD), and escalating dose cyclophosphamide (CTX) therapy for children with localized rhabdomyosarcoma in increased risk of relapse and metastatic rhabdomyosarcoma with a parameningeal site. Protocol activation date: January 24, 1997.

38. Maurer HM, Gehan EA, Beltangady M, et al. The intergroup rhabdomyosarcoma study-II, *Cancer,* **71** (1993) 1904–1922.

39. Garton GR, Gunderson LL, Webb MJ, et al. Intraoperative irradiation in gynecologic cancer: the Mayo Clinic experience, *Gynecol. Oncol.,* **48** (1993) 328–332.

40. Stelzer K, Koh W, Greer B, et al. Intraoperative electron beam therapy (IOERT) as an adjunct to radical surgery for recurrent cancer of the cervix. In Schieldberg GW, Willich N, and Kramling H (eds.), *Intraoperative radiation therapy,* Essen: Verlag Die Blaue (1993), 411–414.

41. Willett CG, Shellito PC, Tepper JE, et al. Intraoperative electron beam radiation therapy for recurrent locally advanced rectal and rectosigmoid carcinoma, *Cancer,* **67** (1991) 1504–1508.

42. Gunderson LL, Nelson H, Martenson JA, et al. Intraoperative electron and external beam irradiation ± 5FU and maximal surgical resection for previously unirradiated locally recurrent colorectal cancer, *Dis. Col. Rect.,* **39** (1996) 1379–1395.

43. Willett CG, Suit HD, Tepper JE, et al. Intraoperative electron beam radiation therapy for retroperitoneal soft tissue sarcoma, *Cancer,* **68** (1991) 278–283.

44. Gunderson LL, Nagorney DM, McIlrath DC, et al. External beam and intraoperative electron irradiation for locally advanced soft tissue sarcomas, *Int. J. Radiat. Oncol. Biol. Phys.,* **25** (1993) 647–656.

45. Petersen IP, Haddock MG, Donohue JH, et al. Use of intraoperative electron beam radiation therapy (IOERT) in the management of retroperitoneal and pelvic soft tissue sarcomas, ASTRO abstracts, *Int. J. Radiat. Oncol. Biol. Phys.,* **36(Suppl 1)** (1996) 185.

26 IORT for Head and Neck Cancer

*Robert L. Foote, Peter Garrett, William Rate,
Subir Nag, Rafael Martinez-Monge,
Thierry Schmitt, and Thomas V. McCaffrey*

CONTENTS

1. STANDARD TREATMENT FOR ADVANCED RESECTABLE OR INCOMPLETELY RESECTED HEAD AND NECK CANCER

Current standard treatment for locally advanced but resectable (stages III and IV and selected stage II) head and neck cancer includes surgery combined with preoperative or postoperative radiation therapy or radiation therapy alone or combined with a neck dissection with surgery reserved for salvage. Chemotherapy may be added. However, other than a neoadjuvant role for organ preservation in advanced larynx or pyriform sinus cancer and a concomitant and maintenance role in advanced nasopharyngeal cancer, the role for chemotherapy remains to be defined *(1–3)*. Despite advances made in recent years with combined modality therapy, local and regional recurrence rates remain unacceptably high (20–60%), and 5-year survival rates remain disappointingly low (30–60%).

Local-regional control and overall survival from representative large retrospective and prospective studies are summarized in Table 1. In the RTOG 73-03 study comparing primary irradiation, with surgery reserved for salvage treatment, to surgery combined with preoperative or postoperative irradiation, 30–44% of the patients died of uncontrolled primary tumor *(4,6)*. Peters et al. found no improvement in local–regional control with higher doses of conventionally fractionated postoperative radiation therapy with doses above 57.6 Gy in patients with negative or microscopically positive margins, except perhaps in the subset of patients with extracapsular nodal extension *(5)*. However, higher doses of conventionally fractionated radiation therapy were associated with

From: *Current Clinical Oncology: Intraoperative Irradiation: Techniques and Results*
Edited by: L. L. Gunderson et al. © Humana Press, Inc., Totowa, NJ

Table 1
Local–Regional Control and Overall Survival
in Locally Advanced Resectable Head and Neck Cancer by Non-IORT Treatment Modality

Treatment Modality and Sequence (ref.)	No. of Patients	Local–Regional Recurrences No.	Local–Regional Recurrences (%)	5-Year Local–Regional Control	p-Value	5-Year Overall Survival	p-Value
RTOG (4)							
RT	43	25	(58)	38%	0.42	30%	0.81
RT + S	43	20	(47)	43%		27%	
S + RT	43	19	(44)	52%		36%	
MDACC (5)							
S + RT	240	61	(25)	70%		30%	
RTOG (6)							
RT + S	136	57	(42)	48%	0.04	29%	0.15
S + RT	141	44	(31)	65%		40%	
MDACC, USF, Mayo (7)							
S + RT (CF)	70	—	—	66%	0.11	38%[b]	0.34
S + RT (AF)	64	—	—	88%		60%[b]	
Intergroup Study 0034 (8)							
S + RT	225	53	(24)	71%	N.S.[a]	44%	N.S.[a]
S + C + RT	223	43	(19)	74%		48%	
Head and Neck Contracts Program (9)							
S + RT	152	—	—	72%	0.89	35%	0.86
CT + S + RT	140	—	—	68%		37%	
CT + S + RT + CT	151	—	—	73%		45%	
SWOG (10)							
S + RT	76	—	—	—		28%	0.27
CT + S + RT	82	—	—	—		28%	
Medical College of Wisconsin (11)							
RT + S	40	16	(40)	—		41%[c]	0.93
CT + RT + S + CT	43	24	(56)	—		35%[c]	

Abbreviations: RT = radiation therapy, S = surgery, CF = conventionally fractionated adjuvant radiation therapy, AF = accelerated fractionated adjuvant radiation therapy, CT = chemotherapy.
[a]N.S. = not significant, 4-year data.
[b]3-Year data.
[c]2-Year data.

higher complication rates (≤57.6 Gy, 1 of 36, 2.8%; 63 Gy, 9 of 117, 7.7%; 68.4 Gy, 7 of 87, 8%) (5).

Significant predictors of local–regional recurrence in completely resected head and neck cancer include close surgical margins, lymph node metastases >3 cm in size, lymph node metastases in two or more lymph nodes or lymph node levels, extracapsular lymph node extension, vascular or lymphatic space invasion, soft tissue invasion, jugular vein invasion, adherence to or invasion of nerve, desmoplastic lymph node pattern, oral cavity primary site, Zubrod performance study ≥2, and delay in the onset of postoperative radiation therapy >6 weeks (5,12).

Incompletely resected head and neck cancer carries an even worse prognosis. The main pattern of treatment failure is uncontrolled disease above the clavicles with relatively few distant metastases. Death results from uncontrolled cancer in the head and neck region in most cases (13–16). Table 2 summarizes local–regional control and survival from representative series of patients treated with surgery alone or combined with irradiation and/or chemotherapy for incompletely resected head and neck cancer. Local and regional recurrence rates are high at 21–100% with long-term survival rates of 5–60%. Zelesfsky et al. from Memorial Sloan-Kettering Cancer Center found improved local–regional tumor control with the use of higher doses of postoperative external beam irradiation (EBRT) in patients with close (≤5 mm) or positive margins: 92% with ≥60 Gy and 44% with >60 Gy, $p = 0.007$. Oral tongue cancers were excluded from the analysis (20). More effective, less toxic treatment is needed for locally advanced but resectable and incompletely resected head and neck cancer.

1.1. Paranasal Sinus Cancers

Cancers arising from or extending into the paranasal sinuses present challenging obstacles to successful treatment for head and neck surgeons and radiation oncologists. Because of their location adjacent to critical structures, complete surgical resection and high-dose EBRT are difficult to accomplish with acceptable morbidity. Local recurrence is the main pattern of treatment failure and a major cause of death (21–24). Five-year local control and survival rates are 53–68% and 39–64%, respectively, with combined surgery and radiation therapy (22,25–35). The total dose of irradiation that can be delivered is limited by the tolerance of adjacent critical normal tissues, including the eye, optic nerve, chiasm, brain, and brain stem.

1.2. Salvage Treatment for Local–Regional Relapse

Local and regional recurrence after curative treatment for locally advanced head and neck cancer is a significant problem. With the exception of larynx cancer, local recurrences following combined modality therapy are rarely salvaged. Once a recurrence develops, 50–60% of patients will die as a direct consequence of uncontrolled local or regional disease (36). Surgical salvage for recurrence following surgery with or without adjuvant irradiation is rarely successful and frequently not feasible due to the size, extent, and/or location of the recurrent disease or involvement of critical structures (5,12). In the clinical trial reported by Peters et al. from the M.D. Anderson Cancer Center, 61 patients (61/240, 25%) developed a local–regional recurrence following surgery and postoperative radiation therapy. Only 36 were eligible for attempts at salvage treatment, with only one patient successfully salvaged (5). Similarly, irradiation as salvage treatment for surgical failures is rarely successful (37,38).

Reirradiation using EBRT (35–65 Gy) with or without chemotherapy has been attempted in patients with local or regional recurrence or a second primary cancer following initial treatment with radiation therapy with some success. Local control rates have been reported as high as 50% with a 5-year survival of 20% (39–42). However, normal tissue tolerance is a dose-limiting concern with an incidence of tissue necrosis following reirradiation varying from 0% to 40% (40–46). Early results from pilot studies evaluating reirradiation and chemotherapy for recurrent head and neck cancer revealed promising response rates (43% complete response, 31% partial response) but significant severe toxicity (11% treatment-related mortality, 11% severe toxicity, 11% severe life-threatening hematologic toxicity) (47–50).

Table 2
Local–Regional Control and Overall Survival
in Incompletely Resected Head and Neck Cancer by Non-IORT Treatment Modality

Treatment Modality and Sequence (ref.)	No. of Patients	Local–Regional Recurrences No.	(%)	5-Year Local–Regional Control	p-Value	5-Year Overall Survival	p-Value
Medical College of Virginia (17)							
S	49	28	(57)	21%	0.0003	34%	0.01
S + RT	35	9	(26)	61%		50%	
MSKCC (15)							
S ± RT (Preop) Total	62	45	(73)	—		31%[b]	
Margins[a]:							
Close (≤5 mm)	19	14	(74)	—		21%	
Premalignant	5	4	(80)	—		60%	
CIS	13	11	(85)	—		23%	
Invasive	25	16	(64)	—		28%	
Roswell Park Memorial Inst. (13)							
S ± RT ± CT							0.001[c]
Margins:							
Close (≤5 mm)	10	4	(40)	—		39%[c]	
CIS	2	1	(55)	—		—	
Invasive	22	12	(55)	—		7%[c]	
Gross	1	1	(100)	—		—	
MDACC (18)							
S (2-year data)							
Margins:							
Negative	146	21	(14)	86%		67%	
Initially positive,							
rendered negative	50	10	(20)	80%		62%	
Positive	20	16	(80)	20%		5%	
RTOG and Intergroup Study 0034 (19)							
S + RT ± CT							
(4-year data)	109	53	(49)	44%		29%	
MSKCC (20)							
S + RT (7-yr data)					0.39		N.S.
Margins:							
Negative	36	5	(14)	79%		46%	
Close (≤5 mm)	41	11	(27)	71%		61%	
Positive	25	4	(16)	79%		56%	

Abbreviations: RT = radiation therapy, S = surgery, CT = chemotherapy.

[a]Positive margins included gross residual cancer or microscopically positive margins involved with invasive cancer, carcinoma *in situ,* or premalignant disease (dysplasia).

[b]Crude results.

[c]Disease-free survival, not overall survival.

Interstitial implantation has been utilized to enhance tumor control in unresectable cancer adherent to deep, bony, or neurovascular structures as a component of primary treatment and as a component of salvage treatment for recurrent head and neck cancer. Placement of afterloading tubes or permanent radioactive seeds can occur intraoperatively. Local control rates of 40–60% and 5-year survival rates of 14% have been reported *(40,51–57)*. However, serious complications can occur in 11–71% of cases. Additional disadvantages of interstitial brachytherapy include increased risk of nosocomial infections during prolonged hospitalization, possible increased risk of exposure of hospital staff to radiation, higher cost and inconvenience of longer hospital stay and operating room time, and technical challenges in areas of difficult geometry.

Hyperthermia has been added to interstitial implants or EBRT with reported complete response rates of 40–70% *(58–60)*. Unfortunately, the size and location of most recurrences limit the optimal use of interstitial implantation or hyperthermia to a small select group of patients.

Chemotherapy has been used for palliation of patients with advanced and/or recurrent head and neck cancer. Response rates of 50% or less and a median survival of 5–6 months are typical *(61)*.

Table 3 summarizes the results of reirradiation for recurrent head and neck cancer, 5-year local–regional control rates are 0–69% with overall survival of 13–45%. Severe complication rates are 6–37%. Outcomes may be improved with use of a higher dose (>50–60 Gy), use of brachytherapy, and in patients with a second primary cancer.

1.3. Summary

The need exists to improve local-regional tumor control and survival in locally advanced primary head and neck cancers with close surgical margins, positive margins, involvement of paranasal sinuses, and in local-regional recurrences or second primary cancers within a previously irradiated field. Intraoperative irradiation, whether by intraoperative electron beam radiation therapy (IOERT) or high-dose rate-intraoperative radiation therapy (HDR-IORT), has great potential for assisting these goals without adding significant treatment-related morbidity or mortality.

2. IORT—TECHNICAL FACTORS FOR HEAD AND NECK CANCERS

2.1. Electron Beam (IOERT) Technical Factors

The anatomy and function of the head and neck region present unique challenges to the head and neck cancer surgeon and radiation oncologist who are involved in intraoperative electron beam irradiation (IOERT). Although surgical exposure, electron beam applicator size determination, and application and docking are typically straightforward when treating cancer in the neck or parotid region, critical normal structures such as the larynx, vascular anastomoses, vertebral bodies, and spinal cord require careful treatment planning. The larynx and its associated cartilages, if present and not at risk, can be shielded by strips of malleable sterilized lead, the thickness of which is determined by the energy of the electron beam utilized. When indicated, lead can also be used to shield bone (usually mandible) and skin edges (Fig. 1). If the jugular vein and carotid artery have not been resected and are at risk, they can tolerate doses of up to 20 Gy even if previously irradiated. However, if a microvascular-free tissue transfer is planned for reconstruction, the vessels identified for microscopic anastomosis to the tissue transfer should be ex-

Table 3
Local–Regional Control and Overall Survival Following
Non-IORT Reirradiation for Recurrent or Second Primary Head and Neck Cancer

Institution (ref.)	No. of Patients	Moderate to Severe Complications	5-Year Local–Regional Control	5-Year Overall Survival
Mallinckrodt Institute of Radiology[a] (39)	99	25%	<50 Gy: 11% >50 Gy: 25%	13%
Oregon Health Sciences University[b] (43)	100	9% (4 fatal)	Recurrent: 27% Second primary: 60%	Recurrent: 17% Second Primary: 37%
Institut Gustave Roussy[c] (40)	35	37% (3 fatal)	<60 Gy: 8% >60 Gy: 55%	19%[j]
M.D. Anderson Cancer Center[d] (62)	53	15% (5 fatal)	EBRT: 27% EBRT + IC: 67% All: 35%	RT: 21% RT + IC: 60%
Centre Claudius Regan[e] (63)	19	11%	S + EBRT: 36% CT + EBRT: 0%	36%*
Massachusetts General Hospital[d] (64)	51	6%	—	≤60 Gy: 45% <60 Gy: 0%
Hong Kong[d] (65)	706	7%	32%	23%
Rotterdam[f] (66)	73	28%	EBRT + B: 50% EBRT: 29%	20%
Fermilab[g] (67)	40	23%	44%	20%[j]
Univ. of Alabama[h] (49)	20	15%	—	56%
Henri Monder Hospital[i] (52)	70	27%	69%	14%
Hopital Necker[i] (68)	23	37%	57%	13%[j]
Centre Alexis Vautrin[i] (69)	123	23%	59%	24%

Abbreviations: EBRT = external beam radiation therapy, IC = intracavitary brachytherapy, B = brachytherapy.
[a] Surgery and EBRT: n = 48; surgery alone: n = 11; EBRT alone: n = 40.
[b] EBRT ± brachytherapy, 85 recurrent cancers, 15 second primaries.
[c] EBRT ± surgery.
[d] Recurrent nasopharynx cancers. EBRT and/or brachytherapy.
[e] Hyperfractionated EBRT postoperatively or combined with chemotherapy.
[f] Recurrent or second primary cancer. EBRT ± brachytherapy. 3-year local control rate.
[g] External fast neutrons. Includes sarcomas. 2-year local control and survival.
[h] EBRT and 5-FU/hydroxyurea, 1-year survival.
[i] Brachytherapy.
[j] 2-Year survival.

cluded from the IOERT field if at all possible. Reconstruction is performed following surgical tumor ablation and IOERT.

Following a complete neck dissection, the soft tissue remaining between the tumor bed and vertebral bodies or skull base (5–10 mm), or spinal cord and brain/brain stem (5–10 mm of soft tissue and approximately 15 mm of bone) can be relatively thin. In the case of recurrence after prior EBRT or planned preoperative or postoperative EBRT, the spinal cord dose needs to be kept to a minimum during IOERT. Because of the limited thickness of the soft tissue at risk in the neck, low-energy electrons are most frequently

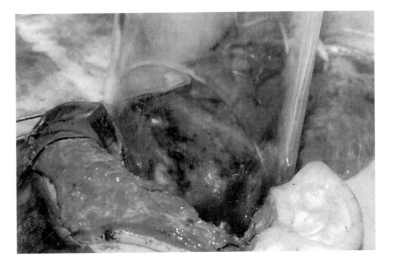

Fig. 1. Malleable sterilized lead shielding skin edge and mandible.

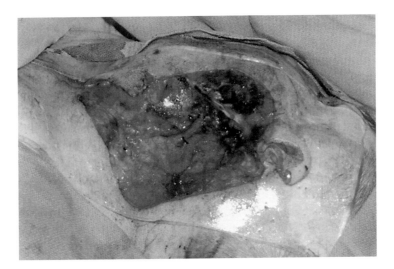

Fig. 2. Elasto-gel bolus material placed over the entire surgical and IOERT field. The transparent nature of the material allows clear identification of underlying anatomy, including vessels, bone, nerves, and metallic clips or suture material outlining the treatment field. The gelatinous pliability fills in air cavities and gaps.

used (4–9 MeV). In most cases, this requires the use of bolus to increase the tumor bed surface dose. Typically, 5 mm of bolus is adequate to encompass the volume at risk within the 90% isodose line when using 6-MeV electrons. If the soft tissue is thicker, higher-energy electrons without bolus may be utilized. If critical structures are deep to the target volume, bolus of 5–15 mm thickness or more can be utilized to reduce the dose at depth. At Mayo, we have found it most efficient to cover the entire surgical bed with bolus material rather than trying to pack bolus deep into a recess or within the end of the treatment applicator (Fig. 2). Elasto-gel (Southwest Technologies, Inc., Kansas City, MO) can be used for bolus material. Studies at the Mayo Clinic and the C. Griffith Cancer Center have documented that high-dose IOERT with various electron energies has no

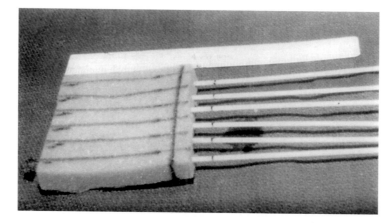

Fig. 3. The foam applicator is 1 cm thick and is custom-made in the operating room. It has parallel catheters placed 1 cm apart within it. (Reprinted from ref. *73,* with kind permission from Elsevier Science Ireland Ltd., Bay 15K, Shannon Industrial Estate, Co Clare, Ireland).

effect on the appearance and property of the Elasto-gel pads. The radiation attenuation and buildup effects of the Elasto-gel pads are very similar to polystyrene or other tissue-equivalent materials. Elasto-gel comes packed in a sterilized envelope, is made of non-toxic material, and is transparent so that the underlying tumor bed, anatomy, and surgical markers (metallic clips or suture material) can be seen during cone placement and docking. The adhesive nature of the material can be removed by moistening it with water. Because of the gel nature, the thickness can be variable, and each pad should be measured in thickness individually. Pads come in approximately 5- and 10-mm thicknesses *(70,71).* Alternatively, wet gauze of the required thickness may be used. At UCSF, the applicators have been modified to incorporate bolus material into the distal end.

Treatment of the skull base, nasopharynx, oropharynx, and paranasal sinuses is more challenging. Even the smallest, 4.0-cm circular applicators, can be difficult to place and dock due to limited surgical exposure. A midline mandibulotomy and mandibular swing can greatly aid tumor resection and access to the skull base and oropharynx. Skin edges should be retracted outside of the treatment cone. Mucosal edges to be used for closing can be safely treated if indicated.

2.2. HDR–IORT Technical Factors

One limitation of IOERT is that it can only be used in areas accessible to the applicator. Because narrow cavities, steeply sloping surfaces, or areas where treatment delivery requires turning a corner are not readily or easily accessible to the applicator, IOERT may be less feasible in some anatomic sites, such as periorbital areas, skull base, and within the sinuses.

At the Ohio State University, a new technique for delivering radiation therapy intra-operatively with high-dose rate brachytherapy was developed to treat tumors in these inaccessible locations *(72).* Various-sized foam or silicone surface template applicators 1.0 cm thick have been developed to fit different sized tumor beds (Fig. 3). Silicone HDR–IORT applicators, having limited flexibility, are used on flat or gently sloping surfaces, and very flexible foam HDR–IORT applicators are used for irregular or curved surfaces, especially in the sinuses and at the base of the skull. One to six (median 3)

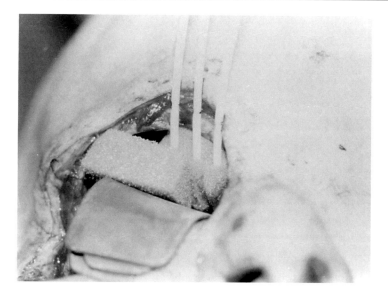

Fig. 4. An area in the superior orbit and base of skull being treated with a foam-based applicator. Pliable lead foils are used to shield normal tissues in the inferior orbit. (Reprinted from ref. *73,* with kind permission from Elsevier Science Ireland Ltd., Bay 15K, Shannon Industrial Estate, Co Clare, Ireland.)

hollow plastic catheters are inserted parallel and 1 cm apart in the selected applicator. The applicator is then placed over the tumor bed and secured by gauze packing or suturing to the underlying tissues. In unusual circumstances, the catheters are individually sutured to the tumor bed. Adjacent normal tissue is retracted with a retractor and/or by packing with gauze. In some instances, bone (maxilla) is temporarily resected to gain access to the tumor site. After treatment, it is regrafted. Nontumorous normal tissues that cannot be retracted (eye or orbit) are shielded by pliable lead shields whenever possible (Fig. 4).

With dummy sources in the catheter, a radiograph is obtained to verify catheter position within the tumor site and to document the site of HDR-IORT dose delivery (Fig. 5). Various preplanned treatment programs corresponding to each applicator and prescribed dose are available. Equal dwell times rather than an optimizing program are used because it is thought that the higher central dose achieved with equal dwell times would be an advantage. Furthermore, errors are less likely using equal dwell times. An appropriate treatment program is then retrieved from the planning computer and transferred to the treatment control panel. The catheters are connected to a mobile high-dose-rate remote afterloading machine that is brought to the shielded operating room from the Radiation Oncology Department. Treatments proceed without delay, as new dosimetry is not required. Because of the rapid fall off in dose for brachytherapy, stating doses to normal tissues is not very meaningful because these were variable.

3. IOERT RESULTS

3.1. Methodist Hospital of Indiana Experience

The Methodist Hospital of Indiana (Indianapolis) began a treatment program for locally advanced primary or locally recurrent head and neck cancer using surgical resection and IOERT in 1982 *(74–81).* Indications for IOERT included close surgical margins, micro-

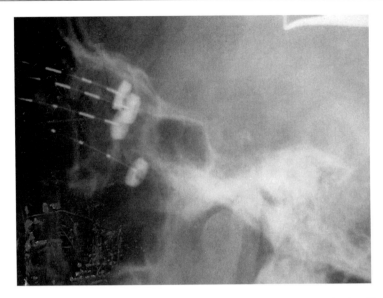

Fig. 5. A lateral radiograph confirms the location of the applicator (with indwelling "dummy" sources) in the base of the brain. (Reprinted from ref. *73,* with kind permission from Elsevier Science Ireland Ltd., Bay 15K, Shannon Industrial Estate, Co Clare, Ireland).

scopically positive margins, or gross residual disease. A total of 355 patients had received IOERT as of September 1996. Their experience is summarized below by site, including salivary gland malignancies, tongue base cancers, and locally advanced cervical nodal disease.

3.1.1. SALIVARY GLAND MALIGNANCIES

Surgical resection is the treatment of choice for both primary and locally recurrent salivary gland malignancies. Locally advanced cancers may infiltrate the facial nerve. Resection often requires the sacrifice of the facial nerve with resulting paralysis.

3.1.1.1. Patient Group. Thirty patients with T3 or T4 cancers with a minimum follow-up of 2-years have been treated with maximal resection plus IOERT at Methodist Hospital. The majority of cancers originated in the major salivary glands including 20 parotid cancers and three submandibular cancers. Minor salivary gland cancers were treated at a variety of sites, including the oral cavity and oropharynx (three cases), nasopharynx, and maxilla (four cases). Tumor histologies included mucoepidermoid carcinoma (13), adenoid cystic carcinoma (10), adenocarcinoma (3), malignant mixed cancers (2), and acinar cell carcinomas (2). Prior radiation therapy had been given to eight patients (27%) with a dose range of 50–72 Gy. The planned IOERT dose was not altered routinely based on prior EBRT.

3.1.1.2. Technical Factors. Attempts were made to preserve the facial nerve, when possible, at the time of resection. If the nerve was involved with gross disease, it was sacrificed. Close surgical margins were obtained in 20 cases, 8 had microscopically positive margins, and 2 had gross residual cancer.

IOERT was utilized in 30 patients (5-MeV electrons were used in 27 patients and 9-MeV electrons in 3). Single fractions of 15 Gy were given to 26 patients, 20 Gy to 3, and 10 Gy to 1. Circular Lucite applicators ranging in size from 5 to 9 cm in diameter defined the treatment fields. The applicators are transparent and offered easy visualiza-

Table 4
Methodist Hospital of Indiana (Indianapolis) Head and Neck IOERT Experience

Site	No. of Patients	Local–Regional Control	5-Year Overall Survival	Complications (See Text)	Treatment Mortality
Salivary gland	30	74% (5-year)	57%	0	2 (7%)
Prior EBRT[a]: No	22	95%	—		
Yes	8	25%	—		
Margins:					
Close	20	80%	66%		
Microscopic	8	57%	38%		
Gross	2	0%	0%		
Tongue base	34	—	30%[b] (3-year)	4 (12%)	2 (6%)
Prior EBRT[a]: No	11	75% (3-year)	68%[b]		
Yes	23	42%	20%[b]		
Neck	82	78% (3-year)	42% (3-year)	8 (10%)	5 (6%)
Margins:					
Close/microscopic	76	85%			
Gross	6	20%			

[a]EBRT: external beam radiation therapy.
[b]Disease-specific survival.

tion of the treatment field. Lead shielding of critical normal structures was individualized. The most common shielded areas were skin edges and pharynx.

Eighteen patients received postoperative EBRT ranging from 40 to 70 Gy. No adjuvant chemotherapy was administered.

3.1.1.3. Results. All patients were transported from the operating suite to the radiation therapy suite without difficulty and with no increased infectious complications or wound breakdown. However, there were two early deaths (<3 months) from other causes. These cases were included in the survival data but not the local control data. There was one death from respiratory failure attributed to pulmonary fibrosis from prior treatment with bleomycin. The second patient died as a result of a carotid artery hemorrhage. The treatment field included the carotid artery which was involved with gross residual disease. Three weeks after surgery and IOERT, tumor necrosis in the radiation field resulted in death from hemorrhage.

Table 4 summarizes the outcome including local-regional control, survival, and complications. Local–regional tumor control was significantly affected by margin status and prior irradiation ($p < 0.001$). Survival was also adversely affected by margin status. Eight intact nerves, most commonly facial nerves, were within the IOERT field. No clinical dysfunction has developed with IOERT doses ranging from 10 to 20 Gy.

3.1.1.4. Summary. IOERT can be safely administered in advanced salivary gland cancers. Local–regional tumor control and survival were adversely affected by margin status and prior radiation therapy. Although the present policy at Methodist Hospital is not to treat patients with gross residual disease because neither patient in this group obtained local control or long-term survival, only two patients had gross residual and results are inconclusive. If the carotid artery is involved with gross disease, IOERT should probably not be given unless the artery is removed or bypassed surgically.

3.1.2. Tongue Base Cancer

The tongue base may be a primary source of cancer or it can be involved by direct extension from tonsil, floor of mouth, oral tongue, or larynx cancers. Standard treatment strategies for cancer invading the tongue base involve either resection or EBRT with or without a brachytherapy boost.

Patients with locally advanced primary or recurrent cancers with tongue base involvement have been treated with surgical resection plus IOERT at the Methodist Hospital of Indiana. The goal of combining IOERT with marginal gross total resection was to preserve as much tongue base as possible and treat microscopic residual disease. In doing so, both speech and swallowing function can be preserved.

3.1.2.1. Patient Group. Thirty-four patients with tongue base involvement have been treated with maximal surgical resection and IOERT with or without EBRT at Methodist Hospital. The minimum follow-up has been 2 years. The tongue base was the most common primary site with 11 patients, followed by floor of mouth with 8 patients, mobile tongue with 6 patients, larynx with 4 patients, tonsil with 3 patients, and retromolar trigone and vallecula with 1 patient each. All cancers were squamous cell carcinoma. Thirty were moderately or poorly differentiated. The 23 patients treated for recurrent cancer had all failed prior EBRT (45–75 Gy with a median of 63 Gy). Eight of the 11 patients treated for primary disease had T3 or T4 cancers and 9 of 11 had at least N2B nodal metastases.

3.1.2.2. Technical Factors. Close surgical margins were obtained in 23 patients and microscopically positive margins in 11 patients. Two patients received IOERT doses of 10 Gy, and the remainder were treated with 15 or 20 Gy. Electron energies of 4–6 MeV were used. Electron applicator size ranged from 4 to 10 cm, with the majority treated with a 5- or 6-cm applicator. Lead shielding was individualized. Nine previously unirradiated patients received postoperative EBRT with a median dose of 58 Gy (45–64 Gy).

3.1.2.3. Results. Table 4 summarizes the treatment results. There were two early deaths (<3 months). One patient died of pneumonia while still in the hospital, and another died of cardiac arrest. These cases were included in the survival data but not the local control analysis. Patients who had received prior EBRT were less likely to achieve local control. Patterns of failure analysis revealed that failures predominantly occurred outside the IORT field in the neck or beyond. There were four complications, including aspiration pneumonia, fistula, wound breakdown, and osteonecrosis. There were no difficulties associated with transferring the patient between the operative suite and radiation therapy suite.

3.1.2.4. Summary. In this series, IOERT as a component of treatment in patients with tongue base involvement produced a high rate of local control and disease-specific survival for primary disease with no apparent additional morbidity.

3.1.3. Cervical Node Metastases

Advanced cervical lymph node metastases may occur at initial presentation or as a regional recurrence. As the size of the cervical lymph node increases, so does the probability of extracapsular extension, resulting in difficulty obtaining complete surgical resection. Combined surgery and irradiation offers the optimal chance for nodal control in such high-risk patients.

IOERT can be used in conjunction with resection and EBRT to enhance nodal control without increasing morbidity or mortality. In the unirradiated neck, IOERT can be used as a boost prior to postoperative EBRT or as the sole radiation treatment in a previously irradiated neck when additional EBRT cannot be given.

3.1.3.1. Patient Group. Eighty-two patients with N2 or N3 nodal disease have been treated at Methodist Hospital and followed for a minimum of 3 years. The cervical lymph node metastases which received IOERT were all clinically >3 cm in size and 80% were fixed to underlying structures. Forty-nine patients were treated for recurrent nodal disease while 33 were treated at the time of primary disease presentation.

3.1.3.2. Technical Factors. Complete surgical resection of nodal and extranodal disease was attempted in all patients in conjunction with IOERT with or without EBRT. Six patients had gross residual disease, 30 microscopically positive margins, and 46 close margins.

IORT was delivered by electron beam utilizing low-energy electrons (4 or 5 MeV) in most cases. A single fraction of 15 Gy (31 patients) or 20 Gy (49 patients) was delivered via a hard docking Lucite applicator system. Neurovascular and skin edge shielding, as well as bolus, were used as appropriate. Treatment was delivered with electron applicators ranging from 4 to 10 cm in diameter.

EBRT was given in 77 of the 82 patients either as prior primary treatment ($n = 14$) or in conjunction with resection with IOERT ($n = 63$). Forty-two patients were treated with preoperative EBRT with a median dose of 60 Gy. Postoperative EBRT was given to 21 patients following IOERT, with median dose 50 Gy. Fourteen patients were treated with IOERT alone following recurrence after primary EBRT, with median dose 65 Gy.

3.1.3.3. Results. Table 4 summarizes the treatment results. Nodal control was significantly affected by margin status ($p < 0.05$). Factors significantly associated with better survival included control at the IORT site, local–regional control, primary disease presentation, minimal disease after surgery, and freedom from distant metastases (all $p < 0.05$). Operative and perioperative mortality (30 days) was 6%. Posttreatment morbidity, consisting of fistula formation, flap necrosis, or osteoradionecrosis developed in eight patients.

3.1.3.4. Summary. In this series, IOERT as a component of treatment in patients with advanced cervical nodal disease produced a high rate of nodal control with no apparent additional morbidity.

Six additional institutions have reported their experience using IORT for advanced primary or recurrent head and neck cancer. These experiences are summarized below.

3.2. Mayo Clinic Experience

3.2.1. PATIENT GROUP

Between January 1992 and April 1994, 31 patients with locally advanced primary or locally/regionally recurrent head and neck cancer were treated with IOERT at the Mayo Clinic in Rochester, Minnesota *(82)*. Eighteen patients had received prior radiation therapy with a median dose of 64 Gy (50–72.4 Gy). The median follow-up at the time of the analysis was 15.1 months. There were 22 patients with squamous cell carcinoma and 2 patients had chondroblastic osteogenic sarcoma. One patient each had the following histologies: adenosquamous carcinoma, basosquamous cell carcinoma, adenocarcinoma, adenoid cystic carcinoma, spindle cell carcinoma, rhabdomyosarcoma, and desmoid.

3.2.2. TECHNICAL FACTORS

Gross total resection was attempted prior to IOERT. This was achieved in 28 of the 31 patients (Table 5). All patients had both resection and IOERT in a dedicated IOERT suite located within the Rochester Methodist Hospital operating rooms.

Table 5

Head and Neck IORT—Local–Regional Control and Overall Survival by Series and Prognostic Factor

Institution (ref.)	No. of Patients	Local– Regional Control	2-Year Overall Survival	Complications (See Text)	Treatment Mortality
Mayo (82)	31	52%	31%	1 (3%)	3 (10%)
Primary	10	70%	38%		
Recurrent	21	43%	28%		
Margins after maximal resection:					
Gross residual	3	67%	35%		
Microscopic	20	50%	30%		
Close	8	50% (2-year)	25%		
S + IOERT	17	41%	25%		
S + IOERT + EBRT	14	64%	39%		
Squamous cell	24	50%	20%		
Non-squamous cell	7	57%	67%		
UCSF (83)	30	60%	70% (3-year)	5 (16%)	0
Primary	5	100%			
Recurrent	25	60%			
Margins after maximal resection:					
Positive	21	67% (3-year)			
Close	9	67%			
Squamous cell	23	70%			
Non-squamous cell	7	57%			

continued

Table 5
(continued)

Institution (ref.)	No. of Patients	Local–Regional Control	2-Year Overall Survival	Complications (See Text)	Treatment Mortality
University of Navarre, Pamplona (84)		33.3%	32%	2 (10%)	—
Primary	8	42.8%	57%		
Recurrence	23	26.2%	31%		
Margins after maximal resection:					
Gross residual	16	25.7%	15.6%		
Microscopic	15	39.2%	26.3%		
Prior EBRT: No	16	46.4%	28.1%		
Yes	15	19%	8.6%		
University of the Ryukyus (85)	25	54.1%[a]	45.1%	32.8%	2 (8%)
Margins after maximal resection:					
Gross residual	7	0%	0%		
Microscopic	12	54.5%	33%		
Close	11	81.8%	70%		
University Hospital Bellevue (86)	43	51%[b]	30%[b]	2 (5%)	0
Primary					
Margins after maximal resection:					
Negative	15	68%[b]	—		
Close or positive	28	44%[b]	—		
Recurrent	10	50%	—	0	0
Ohio State University (72)	40	70%	72%	6 (15%)	1 (3%)
Combined with EBRT: Yes	28	79%	88%		
No	12	50%	33%		

Abbreviations: S = surgery, IOERT = intraoperative electron beam radiation therapy, EBRT = external beam radiation therapy.
[a] Failure within IOERT field.
[b] 5-Year results.
[c] 7 Year results.

485

There were 37 IOERT fields treated in the 31 patients. The applicator size varied from a 4.0-cm circular applicator to a 9 × 12-cm rectangular applicator with a median applicator size of 5.0 cm. The skull base was treated in 16 patients, neck in 11, tongue in 3, skull base and neck in 2, nasopharynx, skull base, and neck in 1, nasopharynx and skull base in 1, prevertebral area in 1, parapharyngeal area in 1, and parotid bed in 1.

A majority of patients received IOERT with low-energy electrons (34 fields were treated with 6-MeV electrons and 2 with 9-MeV electrons). The remaining field was treated with 15-MeV electrons.

A strict IOERT dose protocol was followed which included 20 Gy for gross residual disease >2.0 cm in diameter or prior EBRT, 15 Gy for gross residual disease ≤2.0 cm, and 12.5 Gy for microscopically positive or close margins. The median dose delivered was 15.0 Gy. The dose was prescribed to the 90% isodose line which encompassed the area at risk with a 1–1.5-cm margin.

One patient received 50.4 Gy preoperative EBRT. Twelve patients received postoperative EBRT with a median dose of 63 Gy (30.6–72 Gy). Two patients were to receive planned postoperative EBRT but one died postoperatively and the other developed distant metastases and a local recurrence prior to starting EBRT. No patient received chemotherapy.

3.2.3. Results

Table 5 summarizes the overall treatment results with regard to both local control and survival. Pattern of failure analysis revealed 10 (32%) failures within the IOERT field. There were 15 (48%) failures above the clavicles either within the IOERT field, adjacent to it, or within regional lymph nodes. The 2-year overall survival of the total group of patients was 31%.

A prognostic factor analysis was conducted. Local–regional control at 2 years was best in patients treated with primary cancer (70%) or when preoperative or postoperative EBRT could be added (64%). Two-year overall survival was significantly improved in those patients with nonsquamous versus squamous cell carcinoma histologies (67% vs 20%, $p = 0.03$). The main pattern of treatment failure for patients with squamous cell carcinoma histologies was within the IOERT field [33%] or adjacent to the IOERT field [38%]. The main pattern of treatment failure for patients with nonsquamous cell carcinoma histology was distant metastases (43%), but failure within or adjacent to the IOERT field was still common (29%). There was no difference in the recurrence rates within the IOERT field, adjacent to it, or within regional lymph nodes when analyzed by the amount of residual tumor at the time of IOERT. There was a lower incidence of distant metastases in patients with no residual cancer (0%) versus those with microscopically positive margins (35%), or gross residual tumor (33%).

Treatment tolerance was evaluated by severity and causation at each follow-up interval. Grade 3 or greater toxicity related to IOERT occurred in only one patient (subcutaneous/soft tissue). There has been no bone necrosis, one grade 1 peripheral neuropathy related to IOERT, one fatal hemorrhage due to recurrent cancer, and one fistula secondary to EBRT and surgery.

3.3. University of California, San Francisco Experience

3.3.1. Patient Group

Between March 1991 and December 1994, 30 patients with head and neck cancer were treated with IOERT and maximal resection with or without EBRT (83). Patients included were identified as having high-risk factors for recurrence based on previous history of recurrence, site of disease, extent of disease, and perineural, bony, or vascular invasion. All had either stage III or IV disease. All 25 patients who were treated for recurrent disease had been treated previously with full-course EBRT. There were 23 patients with squamous cell carcinoma, 3 with mucoepidermoid carcinoma, 2 with adenoid cystic carcinoma, 1 with adenocarcinoma, and 1 with anaplastic thyroid carcinoma.

3.3.2. TECHNICAL FACTORS

After maximal resection was accomplished, all patients were transported from the operating suite to the radiation therapy suite. If tumor was noted to invade the carotid arterial system, the vessel was resected along with the tumor.

The IOERT electron energy ranged from 6 to 9 MeV. The median applicator size was 5.7 cm, with the largest applicator size 7 cm. The mandible and cranial nerves were generally shielded. A dose of 15 Gy was delivered to the 90% isodose line which encompassed the tumor volume. A dose rate of 5 Gy/min was originally used, but more recently, the dose rate was increased to 10 Gy/min to deliver the treatment more quickly, without any apparent increase in complications. Ten patients, including four patients with primary disease, received EBRT after IOERT.

3.3.3. RESULTS

Table 5 summarizes the treatment results. The patients have been followed a median of 30 months. Three-year actuarial local control and survival were excellent at 60% and 70%, respectively.

Overall, 10 patients (30%) had some type of local recurrence. There has been only one failure within the IOERT field. However, there have been nine local–regional failures outside the IOERT field. One patient was lost to follow-up 12 months following IOERT. At the time of last follow-up, the patient was free of disease. There have been no local–regional recurrences in any of the five patients treated for primary disease with IOERT with or without EBRT, regardless of the margin status after resection. In the 25 patients with recurrent disease, 43% of those with positive margins developed local–regional recurrence, and 30% with close or negative margins had local–regional recurrence. Of the six patients with recurrent disease who were treated with EBRT after surgery, three developed local–regional recurrences.

Complications possibly attributable to IOERT and/or surgery were one seroma, one abscess, a 1-cm wound dehiscence, one supraglottic edema, and one mucositis. These complications were transient and left no permanent sequelae. One patient developed "carotid syndrome" with vasovagal symptoms, and another patient developed a stroke; both of these were felt to be more likely related to the surgery than to the IOERT. No patient developed necrosis, fistulae, or sensorineural problems related to IOERT.

3.4. University of Navarre Experience

3.4.1. PATIENT GROUP

Between November 1984 and June 1995, 31 patients with locally advanced head and neck cancer were treated with surgery and IOERT with or without EBRT (84). Full-dose preoperative or postoperative EBRT was given to previously unirradiated patients. There were 26 patients with squamous cell carcinoma, 1 patient had a basal cell carcinoma, 1 had a mixed squamous and basal cell carcinoma, 2 had adenoid cystic carcinoma, and had 1 mucoepidermoid carcinoma.

3.4.2. TECHNICAL FACTORS

All patients had maximal resection prior to IOERT. Gross residual disease persisted in 16 patients and microscopic residual in 15.

Thirty IOERT fields were treated with a beam energy of 6–9 MeV, and 10 were treated with beam energies of 12–15 MeV. Lucite applicator sizes varied from 5 to 12 cm. The median applicator size was 7–8 cm. Fourteen patients received 10 Gy, 8 received 12.5 Gy, and 18 received 15 Gy. Twenty-four patients had one field treated, five had two fields treated, and two had three fields treated. A primary tumor site was treated in 17 and the neck in 23.

There were 14 previously unirradiated patients who received EBRT (median dose 50 Gy). Six previously irradiated patients were reirradiated postoperatively (median dose 30 Gy).

3.4.3. RESULTS

Table 5 summarizes the treatment results. Predictors of local–regional recurrence included gross residual disease after maximal resection ($p = 0.1$) and inability to deliver full-dose adjuvant EBRT because of prior radiation therapy ($p = 0.004$). A subset of five patients with primary N3 neck disease treated with preoperative chemoradiation followed by radical neck dissection of the involved nodal areas and IOERT achieved a 3-year actuarial control of 50%. Toxicity attributable to IOERT included one case of long-term pharyngeal fistula and one case of ipsilateral vocal cord paralysis. Four patients developed pharyngeal fistula, and one a failure of heterotopic bone engraftment. Survival was largely influenced by the inability to deliver full-dose adjuvant EBRT because of prior radiation therapy ($p = 0.04$) and by the presence of gross residual tumor ($p = 0.029$).

3.5. University of the Ryukyus Experience

3.5.1. PATIENT GROUP

Between April 1988 and January 1992, 25 patients with locally advanced primary or locally/regionally recurrent head and neck cancers were treated with surgery and IOERT *(85)*. Of the 25 patients, 22 had squamous cell carcinoma. Seventeen patients had recurrent cancer that had been previously treated by surgery and/or radiation therapy. Ten patients had received previous EBRT (26–70 Gy). Eight patients had no prior treatment.

3.5.2. TECHNICAL FACTORS

IORT was delivered to 9 primary tumor sites and 21 metastatic lymph node sites. Adenopathy fixed to the carotid artery was the most common indication. Intraoperative irradiation was given with a 6–18-MeV (median 9 MeV) electron beam. Circular applicators with internal diameters from 2.5 to 12 cm (median 6 cm) were used. A single dose of 10–30 Gy (median 20 Gy), prescribed to the 90% isodose line, was delivered. Bolus was used in two cases.

Preoperative or postoperative EBRT was combined with IORT for 20 sites. A total dose of 10–70 Gy (mean 41.2 Gy) was delivered by means of EBRT.

3.5.3. RESULTS

Table 5 summarizes the treatment results. Two patients were lost to follow-up. The median follow-up period for all patients was 19 months.

Local–regional tumor control data in this series are reported only in relation to within the IOERT field. Intraoperative radiation therapy with or without EBRT was not successful in controlling gross residual disease. Significant differences were observed in the local control rate between gross residual and microscopic residual disease ($p < 0.05$), and between gross residual disease and close margins ($p < 0.01$). The local control rates within the IOERT field were 83.3% in patients with no prior therapy, 75% for recurrences after prior surgery, and 60% for recurrences after prior radiation therapy and surgery. Patterns of treatment failure revealed that only one case, with gross residual tumor, recurred within the IOERT field alone. Other cases tended to recur both inside and outside the field. Four of five patients developing distant metastases had gross residual disease.

Two-year overall survival for the entire patient group was 45%. Survival was significantly better for patients with microscopic residual disease at 33% ($p < 0.05$) and close margins at 70% ($p < 0.01$) when compared to patients with gross residual disease (0% 2-year survival).

Five patients developed late complications. Four patients developed osteoradionecrosis. Three patients with osteoradionecrosis were free from recurrence for 28, 48, and 57 months. One patient who developed cervical vertebral bone necrosis required surgical stabilization. Another with hard palate necrosis was sequestrated and re-epithelialized at 52 months after the onset of necrosis. The third skull base necrosis received conservative follow-up. Three patients, including one with osteoradionecrosis, developed carotid artery hemorrhage. Two of these were fatal. Complication rates were 0% in the patients who had received no prior therapy, 37.5% for recurrence after prior surgery, and 40% for recurrence after prior radiation therapy and surgery. The incidence of complications also increased with IOERT doses > 20 Gy.

3.6. University Hospital Bellevue Experience

3.6.1. PATIENT GROUP

Since 1986, IOERT has been utilized in the treatment of locally advanced (T3, T4) oropharyngeal carcinomas with extension into the tongue base (86). This technique was used as a boost for primary treatment in 43 cases and as a part of salvage treatment in 10 cases.

3.6.2. TECHNICAL FACTORS

All patients underwent gross total tumor resection prior to IOERT. Circular applicators of 4 or 5 cm inner diameter and electron beam energies of 6, 9, or 13 MeV were utilized for IOERT. The IOERT applicators were sutured to the underlying tissues of the tongue base to ensure the best dosimetric conditions for the electron beam (fixed and plane treatment portal, Fig. 6). The 10 patients with recurrent cancers received 20 Gy IOERT at the 90% isodose line encompassing the tumor bed with margin and no further EBRT. Forty-three previously untreated patients with T2, T3, or T4 oropharyngeal cancers have been treated with IOERT as of 1995. Forty-one patients received 20 Gy IOERT and two patients received 25 Gy. All 43 patients received postoperative EBRT to doses of 50–65 Gy.

3.6.3. RESULTS

Table 5 summarizes the treatment results with median follow-up of >24 months. This is the only series mature enough to report 5-year results. Local control was equal in the primary disease and locally recurrent patients. Only one relapse occurred within the IOERT field in the prior EBRT group of 10 patients. Five-year survival was 30% in primary disease patients.

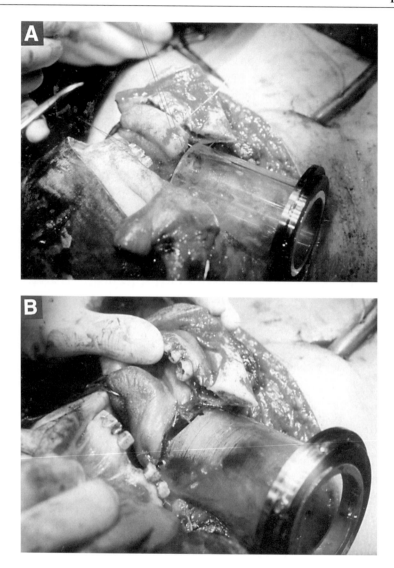

Fig. 6. (A) The IOERT applicator being sutured to the tongue base tumor bed. **(B)** This results in the applicator being fixed in a perpendicular position to the treatment field.

Postoperative complications included an orocutaneous fistula, a flap dehiscence, three flap necroses, one flap sepsis, and two aspiration pneumonias. Two late complications related to IOERT occurred—one laryngeal necrosis and one laryngeal stenosis, both requiring a laryngectomy. No complications were reported in transporting patients between the surgical suite and radiation suite. No significant deficits in tongue function were reported.

4. OHIO STATE UNIVERSITY IOERT AND HDR-IORT SERIES

4.1. Patient Group and Technical Factors

In 20 patients, the tumor site was accessible to the IOERT applicator. These patients were treated with 6- or 9-MeV electrons. The applicator size ranged in diameter from 5 to

10 cm. A laser-guided, soft docking system was used in a dedicated IOERT suite. A wet gauze bolus 0.5 cm thick was used if required.

In another 20 patients, the treatment areas were poorly accessible to the IOERT applicator and, therefore, they were selected for HDR–IORT. The target area on the tumor bed was measured, and an HDR–IORT applicator that would adequately encompass the target area was selected (*see* Section 2.2) *(72)*.

IORT doses delivered (at 90% isodose line for IOERT and at 0.5 cm depth for HDR–IORT) ranged from 10 to 15 Gy, depending on the amount of residual disease. Two patients received 15 Gy for gross residual disease, and three received 12.4 Gy for microscopically positive margins as determined by frozen section. All others (35 patients with negative margins) received 10 Gy.

External beam irradiation of 50 Gy was planned for all patients. Twelve patients did not receive this planned treatment because of poor medical condition or refusal.

4.2. Results

Table 5 summarizes the treatment results in the initial 40 IORT patients. Median follow-up was 28 months in the HDR–IORT brachytherapy group and 16 months in the IOERT group. Patients who did not complete the prescribed postoperative EBRT had a worse outcome than patients who completed the treatment (2-year local control 50% vs 79%; 2-year survival 33% vs 88%). There was no statistically significant difference in results between patients treated with IOERT or HDR–IORT.

One patient died due to treatment-related complications. No major intraoperative complications were observed. Postoperatively, major treatment-related complications occurred in six patients. These included a subdural hematoma, two cerebrospinal fluid leaks, one nasoethmoid fistula, one case of persistent severe headache, and one fistula outside of the IOERT field.

4.2.1. Results—Intensified Treatment Regimen

An additional 37 patients have been treated on an intensified treatment regimen *(87)*. These patients had previously untreated, resectable squamous cell carcinoma of the oral cavity, oropharynx, or hypopharynx, clinical stage III or IV, before resection. The treatment included a slightly accelerated, hyperfractionated, preoperative EBRT, off-cord dose of 9.1 Gy in seven twice-daily treatments with concurrent continuous infusion cisplatinum (1 mg/m^2/h to a total of 80 mg/m^2) immediately before surgery. After maximal resection, an IOERT (7.5 Gy at 90% isodose with 6-MeV electrons produced by a linear accelerator in the operating room) or HDR–IORT boost (7.5 Gy at 0.5 cm depth) was delivered. In all cases, the frozen-section margins were negative, and the target area for the IORT boost included the closest surgical margins. Beginning on day 29 (21 days after surgery), the patient received a second cycle of cisplatinum (100 mg/m^2 given as a rapid infusion) concomitant with an additional 40 Gy of EBRT delivered in 20 treatments to the primary tumor site and regional draining lymph nodes, and 45 Gy in 20 treatments to the lower neck and bilateral supraclavicular areas. If a histologically positive lymph node larger than 3 cm was present, a postoperative electron boost of 10 Gy in five treatments was delivered. The third and final cycle of cisplatinum was administered on day 50 following completion of the EBRT or during the electron boost.

Of the 37 patients treated, 30 were analyzable; the others were excluded as a result of protocol violations. The preliminary analysis revealed that five oral or pharyngeal fistulas had developed within the first 90 days after initiation of the perioperative concurrent chemo/radiotherapy. Three of these required later surgical corrections. Ten patients, including three with fistulae, had delayed wound healing. In addition, one patient required re-exploration 12 h postoperatively for a hematoma, one had facial and neck edema, two had transient renal insufficiency, and seven had pneumonia. One patient died 40 days after treatment of a lung abscess and multiple infections. Late morbidity included hypothyroidism (six), exposure of mandibular plates (four), bilateral pleural effusion (one), transient Lhermitte's sign (one), and paralysis of the 10th and 12th cranial nerves (one).

The 2-year actuarial overall and disease specific survival was estimated to be 60% and 80%, respectively. Of the 37 patients, 13 died, including 6 with distant metastases. Six of the other seven patients died free of disease. Two patients developed a second primary cancer.

The authors concluded that the use of concurrent surgery, radiotherapy, and chemotherapy showed acceptable morbidity and excellent local, regional, and distant disease control with excellent compliance. However, this was an initial trial designed primarily to assess feasibility, and the encouraging results are the basis for modification of the regimen to add Taxol (taclitaxel) to the postoperative systemic regimen.

5. SUMMARY AND FUTURE DIRECTIONS

The above institutional experiences suggest that IORT, whether administered by electron beam or high-dose-rate brachytherapy, can be added to surgery and EBRT or surgery alone in cases of prior EBRT with no apparent increase in treatment-related morbidity or mortality.

IOERT has been the preferred treatment in easily accessible locations because the duration of treatment in a dedicated IORT suite using an electron beam from a linear accelerator is relatively brief. For less accessible tumors, particularly at the skull base, HDR–IORT is usually possible. Institutions without a dedicated IOERT accelerator can also use HDR–IORT for treatment of the more accessible tumors. The advantage of IOERT, when technically feasible, is a more homogenous and more penetrating dose distribution. HDR–IORT brachytherapy gives a heterogeneous dose that is much higher (200% of prescribed dose) at the surface, has limited penetration, and hence is not suitable for treating bulky gross residual disease.

Preservation of organ function (facial nerve, tongue base, carotid artery, mandible) can be successfully accomplished. When compared to historical controls treated conventionally for incompletely resected cancer (Table 2) and to conventional treatment of recurrent cancer (Table 3), the local–regional control and overall survival following IORT appear superior (Tables 4 and 5). The local–regional control following surgery, IORT, and postoperative EBRT for advanced completely resected head and neck cancer also appears superior to conventional treatment without IORT (Tables 1 and 5). However, randomized clinical trials are needed to assess the efficacy and toxicity of IORT compared to conventional treatment. Such trials for completely resected advanced head and neck cancer are needed because higher doses of conventionally fractionated postoperative radiation therapy have not been shown to improve local–regional control but have been associated with higher complication rates (5). Separate trials could be developed for patients with squamous cell carcinomas, salivary gland malignancies, and soft tissue sarcomas of the head and neck region. Eligible patients would include those with close (<5 mm) or microscopically involved margins, extracapsular lymph node extension, or other high-risk features. Patients with close margins adjacent to facial nerve, tongue base, carotid artery, or other vital structures should be evaluated for organ preservation and quality of life. Surgery and adjuvant IORT could then be combined with conventionally fractionated EBRT or accelerated fractionated EBRT. Accelerated fractionated postoperative EBRT has recently been shown to improve local–regional control rates in a randomized trial (7). Further improvements in local–regional control, freedom from distant metastases, and survival may be obtained by adding concomitant and maintenance cisplatinum-based chemotherapy (88).

In patients with gross residual cancer, particularly in the situation where tumor involves vascular structures, even with the addition of IORT to standard treatment, local–regional tumor control is infrequently obtained, and the rate of distant metastasis and death remains high. The addition of chemotherapy or chemoirradiation (EBRT plus cisplatin-based chemotherapy) preoperatively may increase the rate of complete resection and decrease the incidence of local–regional recurrence and distant metastases for patients who present with local recurrence, involvement of vascular structures or other high-risk factors on imaging studies that would predict for gross residual after standard resection. For previously irradiated patients, the preoperative treatment could consist of chemotherapy alone or low-dose EBRT plus infusion cisplatin (20–40 Gy in 1.8- to 2.0-Gy fractions or 1.2 Gy bid plus daily [5 mg/m^2] or weekly [30 mg/m^2] cisplatin). In previously unirradiated patients, full-dose preoperative irradiation (45–54 Gy in 1.8- to 2.0-Gy fractions) could be combined with simultaneous infusion cisplatin. The addition of a radiosensitizer intraoperatively may also improve local–regional control in patients with gross residual cancer after maximal resection. Local–regional tumor control may also be improved by increasing the IORT field size and treatment depths, as there are many recurrences within and adjacent to the IORT treatment field and in adjacent regional lymph nodes. This is true in both situations of complete and incomplete resection. If preoperative EBRT has not been given, postoperative EBRT should be added (60–63 Gy in 1.8- to 2.0-Gy fractions for previously unirradiated patients, 20–40 Gy for previously irradiated patients) whenever possible, as this is associated with improved local–regional control. Further improvements in local–regional control may be obtained by accelerating the postoperative EBRT (7) and by adding concomitant and maintenance cisplatinum-based chemotherapy (88).

Patients with positive margins have a higher incidence of distant metastases and death (89). Neoadjuvant, concomitant, and maintenance chemotherapy have been shown to decrease the incidence of distant metastases and should be further evaluated (1,8–10). Higher doses of radiation therapy have been associated with improved local–regional control rates for incompletely resected head and neck cancers (20). Similarly, higher doses of radiation therapy have been associated with improved local–regional control in patients with recurrent head and neck cancers (40,41,64). Intraoperative radiation therapy should prove to be a valuable tool to deliver additional radiation therapy without increasing complications, thus improving the therapeutic ratio. Single doses of up to 20 Gy have been shown to be safe even in the patient previously treated with high-dose EBRT.

REFERENCES

1. The Department of Veterans Affairs Laryngeal Cancer Study Group, Induction chemotherapy plus radiation compared with surgery plus radiation in patients with advanced laryngeal cancer, *N. Engl. J. Med.*, **324** (1991) 1675–1690.

2. Lefebrre JL, Chevalier D, Luboinski B, et al. Larynx preservation in piriform sinus cancer: preliminary results of a European Organization for Research and Treatment of Cancer Phase III Trial, *J. Natl. Cancer Inst.,* **88** (1996) 890–899.

3. Al-Sarraf M, LeBlanc M, Giri PGS, et al. Improved overall survival with chemoradiotherapy (CT-RT) vs radiotherapy (RT) in patients (pts) with locally advanced nasopharyngeal Cancer (NPC). Preliminary results of Intergroup (0099) (SWOG 8892, RTOG 8817, ECOG 2388) Randomized Study, Fourth International Conference on Head and Neck Cancer, Toronto, 1996, p. 118.

4. Kramer S, Gelber RD, Snow JB, et al. Combined radiation therapy and surgery in the management of advanced head and neck cancer: final report of study 73-03 of the Radiation Therapy Oncology Group, *Head Neck Surg.,* **10** (1987) 19–30.

5. Peters LJ, Goepfert H, Ang KK, et al. Evaluation of the dose for postoperative radiation therapy of head and neck cancer: first report of a prospective randomized trial, *Int. J. Radiat. Oncol. Biol. Phys.,* **26** (1993) 3–11.

6. Tupchong L, Scott CB, Blitzer PH, et al. Randomized Study of Preoperative Versus Postoperative Radiation Therapy in Advanced Head and Neck Carcinoma: Long-Term Follow-Up of RTOG Study 73-03, *Int. J. Radiat. Oncol. Biol. Phys.,* **20** (1991) 21–28.

7. Ang KK, Trotti A, Garden AS, et al. Importance of Overall Time Factor in Postoperative Radiation Therapy, Proceedings Fourth International Conference on Head and Neck Cancer, Toronto, 1996, pp. 231–235.

8. Laramore GE, Scott CB, Al-Sarraf M, et al. Adjuvant chemotherapy for resectable squamous cell carcinomas of the head and neck: report on Intergroup Study 0034, *Int. J. Radiat. Oncol. Biol. Phys.,* **23** (1992) 705–713.

9. Adjuvant Chemotherapy for Advanced Head and Neck Squamous Carcinoma, Final Report of the Head and Neck Contracts Program. *Cancer,* **60** (1987) 301–311.

10. Schuller DE, Metch B, and Stein DW. Preoperative chemotherapy in advanced resectable head and neck cancer: final report of the Southwest Oncology Group, *Laryngoscope,* **98** (1988) 1205–1211.

11. Holoye PY, Grossman TW, Toohill RJ, et al. Randomized study of adjuvant chemotherapy for head and neck cancer, *Otolarngol. Head Neck Surg.,* **93** (1985) 712–717.

12. Olsen KD, Caruso M, Foote RL, et al. Histopathologic predictors of recurrence after neck dissection in patients with lymph node involvement, *Arch. Otolaryngol. Head Neck Surg.,* **120** (1994) 1370–1374.

13. Chen TY, Emrich LJ, and Driscoll DL. The clinical significance of pathological findings in surgically resected margins of the primary tumor in head and neck carcinoma, *Int. J. Radiat. Oncol. Biol. Phys.,* **13** (1987) 833–837.

14. Scholl P, Byers RM, Batsakis JG, et al. Microscopic cut-through of cancer in the surgical treatment of squamous carcinoma of the tongue. Prognostic and therapeutic implications, *Ann. J. Surg.,* **152** (1986) 354–360.

15. Looser KG, Shah JP, and Strong EW. The significance of "positive" margins in surgically resected epidermoid carcinomas, *Head Neck Surg.,* **1** (1978) 107–111.

16. Zbaeren P and Lehmann W. Frequency and sites of distant metastases in head and neck squamous cell carcinoma, *Arch. Otolaryngol. Head Neck Surg.,* **113** (1987) 762–764.

17. Huang D, Johnson CR, Schmidt-Ullrich RK, et al. Incompletely resected advanced squamous cell carcinoma of the head and neck: the effectiveness of adjuvant vs salvage radiotherapy, *Radiother. Oncol.,* **24** (1992) 87–93.

18. Byers RM, Bland KI, Borlase B, et al. The prognostic and therapeutic value of frozen section determinations in the surgical treatment of squamous carcinoma of the head and neck, *Ann. J. Surg.,* **136** (1978) 525–528.

19. Laramore GE, Scott CB, Schuller DE, et al. Is a surgical resection leaving positive margins of benefit to the patient with locally advanced squamous cell carcinoma of the head and neck: a comparative study using the Intergroup Study 0034 and the Radiation Therapy Oncology Group Head and Neck Database, *Int. J. Radiat. Oncol. Biol. Phys.,* **27** (1993) 1011–1016.

20. Zelefsky MJ, Harrison LB, Fass DE, et al. Postoperative radiation therapy for squamous cell carcinomas of the oral cavity and oropharynx: impact of therapy on patients with positive surgical margins, *Int. J. Radiat. Oncol. Biol. Phys.,* **25** (1992) 17–21.

21. Ahmad K, Cordoba RB, and Fayos JV. Squamous cell carcinoma of the maxillary sinus, *Arch. Otolaryngol.,* **107** (1981) 48–51.

22. Beale FA and Garrett PG. Cancer of the paranasal sinuses with particular reference to maxillary sinus cancer, *J. Otolaryngol.,* **12** (1983) 377–382.

23. Kondo M, Ogawa K, Inuyama Y, et al. Prognostic factors influencing relapse of squamous cell carcinoma of the maxillary sinus, *Cancer,* **55** (1985) 190–196.

24. Korzeniowski S, Reinfuss M, and Skolyszewski J. The evaluation of radiotherapy after incomplete surgery in patients with carcinoma of the maxillary sinus, *Int. J. Radiat. Oncol. Biol. Phys.,* **11** (1985) 505–509.

25. Tsujii H, Kamada T, Arimoto T, et al. The role of radiotherapy in the management of maxillary sinus carcinoma, *Cancer,* **57** (1986) 2261–2266.

26. Gadeberg CC, Hjelm-Hausen M, Sogaard H, et al. Malignant tumors of the paranasal sinuses and nasal cavity. A series of 180 patients, *Acta Radiol. Oncol.,* **23** (1984) 181–187.

27. Rush SE and Bagshaw MA. Carcinoma of the paranasal sinuses, *Cancer,* **50** (1982) 154–158.

28. Hordijk GJ and Brons EN. Carcinomas of the maxillary sinus: a retrospective study, *Clin. Otolaryngol.,* **10** (1985) 285–288.

29. Hu YH, Tu GY, Qi YQ, et al. Comparison of pre- and postoperative radiation in the combined treatment of carcinoma of maxillary sinus, *Int. J. Radiat. Oncol. Biol. Phys.,* **8** (1982) 1045–1049.

30. Knegt PP, de Jong PC, van Andel JG, et al. Carcinoma of the paranasal sinuses. Results of a prospective pilot study, *Cancer,* **56** (1985) 57–62.

31. Lindeman P, Eklund V, and Petruson B. Survival after surgical treatment in maxillary neoplasms of epithelial origin, *J. Laryngol. Otol.,* **101** (1987) 564–568.

32. Sakai S, Hohki A, Fuchihata H, et al. Multidisciplinary treatment of maxillary sinus carcinoma, *Cancer,* **52** (1983) 1360–1364.

33. Schlappack OK, Dobrowsky W, Schratter M, et al. Radiotherapy of carcinoma of the paranasal sinuses, *Strahlenter. Oncol.,* **162** (1986) 291–299.

34. St. Pierre S and Baker SR. Squamous cell carcinoma of the maxillary sinus: analysis of 66 cases, *Head Neck Surg.,* **5** (1983) 508–513.

35. Roa WH, Hazuka MB, Sandler HM, et al. Results of primary and adjuvant CT-based 3-dimensional radiotherapy for malignant tumors of the paranasal sinuses, *Int. J. Radiat. Oncol. Biol. Phys.,* **28** (1994) 857–865.

36. Hong WK, Bromer RH, Amato DA, et al. Patterns of relapse in locally advanced head and neck cancer patients who achieved complete remission after combined modality treatment, *Cancer,* **45** (1985) 1242–1249.

37. Deutsch M, Leen R, Parsons JA, et al. Radiotherapy for postoperative recurrent squamous cell carcinoma in head and neck, *Arch. Otolaryngol.,* **98** (1973) 316–318.

38. Pearlman NW. Treatment outcome in recurrent head and neck cancer, *Arch. Surg.,* **114** (1979) 39–42.

39. Emami B, Bignardi M, Devineni VR, et al. Reirradiation of recurrent head and neck cancers, *Laryngoscope,* **97** (1987) 85–88.

40. Langlois D, Eschwege F, Kramar A, et al. Reirradiation of head and neck cancers, *Radiother. Oncol.,* **3** (1985) 27–33.

41. Pomp J, Levendag PC, and van Putten WLJ. Reirradiation of recurrent tumors in the head and neck, *Am. J. Clin. Oncol.,* **11** (1988) 543–549.

42. Skolyszewski J, Korzeniowski, S, and Reinfuss M. The reirradiation of recurrences of head and neck cancer, *Br. J. Radiol.,* **53** (1980) 462–465.

43. Stevens KR, Britsch A, and Moss WT. High-dose reirradiation of head and neck cancer with curative intent, *Int. J. Radiat. Oncol. Biol. Phys.,* **29** (1994) 687–698.

44. Fu KK, Newman H, and Phillips TL. Treatment of locally recurrent carcinoma of the nasopharynx, *Radiology,* **117** (1975) 425–431.

45. Nisar Syed AM, Feder BH, George FW, et al. Iridium-192 after loaded implant in the retreatment of head and neck cancer, *Br. J. Radiol.,* **51** (1978) 814–820.

46. Thompson RW, Scottie Doggett RL, and Bagshaw MA. Ten year experience with linear accelerator irradiation of cancer of nasopharynx, *Radiology,* **97** (1970) 149–155.

47. Vokes EE, Haraf DJ, Mick R, et al. Intensified concomitant chemoradiotherapy with and without filgrastim for poor prognosis head and neck cancer, *J. Clin. Oncol.,* **12** (1994) 2351–2359.

48. Hartsell WF, Thomas CR, Murthy AK, et al. Pilot study for the evaluation of simultaneous cisplatin/5-fluorouracil infusion and limited radiation therapy in regionally recurrent head and neck cancer (ESTP-C385), *Am. J. Clin. Oncol. (CCT),* **17** (1994) 338–343.

49. Weppelmann B, Wheeler RH, Peters GE, et al. Treatment of recurrent head and neck cancer with 5-fluorouracil, hydroxyurea, and reirradiation, *Int. J. Radiat. Oncol. Biol. Phys.,* **22** (1992) 1051–1056.

50. Spencer S, Wheeler R, Meredith R, et al. Simultaneous hydroxyurea, 5-fluorouracil, and high-dose BID irradiation in previously irradiated patients with recurrent squamous cell cancer of the head and neck, Third International Conference on Head and Neck Cancer, San Francisco, 1992.

51. Emami B and Marks JE. Retreatment of recurrent carcinoma of the head and neck by afterloading interstitial [192]-Ir implant, *Laryngoscope,* **93** (1983) 1345–1347.

52. Mazeron JJ, Langlois D, Glaubiger D, et al. Salvage irradiation of oropharyngeal cancers using iridium 192 wire implants: 5-year results of 70 cases, *Int. J. Radiat. Oncol. Biol. Phys.,* **13** (1987) 957–962.

53. Puthawala AA and Syed AMN. Interstitial reirradiation for recurrent and/or persistent head and neck cancers, *Int. J. Radiat. Oncol. Biol. Phys.,* **13** (1987) 1113–1114.

54. Vikram B and Mishra S. Permanent iodine-125 implants in postoperative radiotherapy for head and neck cancer with positive surgical margins, *Head Neck,* **16** (1994) 155–157.

55. Fee WE Jr, Goffinet DR, Paryani S, et al. Intraoperative iodine-125 implants: their use in large tumors in the neck attached to the carotid artery, *Arch. Otolaryngol. Head Neck Surg.,* **109** (1983) 727–730.

56. Kumar PP, Good RR, Yonkers AJ, et al. High activity iodine-125 endocurie therapy for head and neck tumors, *Laryngoscope,* **99** (1989) 174–178.

57. Chen KY, Mohr RM, and Silverman CL. Interstitial iodine 125 in advanced recurrent squamous cell carcinoma of the head and neck with follow-up evaluation of carotid artery by ultrasound, *Ann. Otol. Rhinol. Laryngol.,* **105** (1996) 955–961.

58. Emami B, Marks JE, Perez CA, et al. Interstitial thermoradiotherapy in the treatment of recurrent/residual malignant tumors, *Am. J. Clin. Oncol.,* **7** (1984) 699–704.

59. Puthawala AA, Syed AMN, Sheiku KMA, et al. Interstitial hyperthermia for recurrent malignancies. *Endocurie Therapy/Hypertherm. Oncol.,* **1** (1985) 125–131.

60. Tupchong L, Waterman FM, and McFarlane JD. Hyperthermia and radiation therapy for advanced regional disease due to recurrent head and neck carcinoma, *Int. J. Radiat. Oncol. Biol. Phys.,* **19** (1990) 1099.

61. Hong WK and Bromer R. Chemotherapy in head and neck cancer, *N. Engl. J. Med.,* **308** (1983) 75–79.

62. Pryzant RM, Wendt CD, Delclos L, Peters LJ, et al. Retreatment of nasopharyngeal carcinoma in 53 patients, *Int. J. Radiat. Oncol. Biol. Phys.,* **22** (1992) 941–947.

63. Benchalal M, Bachaud JM, Francois P, et al. Hyperfractionation in the reirradiation of head and neck cancer, Results of a pilot study, *Radiother. Oncol.,* **36** (1995) 203–210.

64. Wang CC. Reirradiation of recurrent nasopharyngeal carcinoma—treatment techniques and results, *Int. J. Radiat. Oncol. Biol. Phys.,* **13** (1987) 953–956.

65. Lee AWM, Law SCK, Foo W, et al. Retrospective analysis of patients with nasopharyngeal carcinoma treated during 1976–1985: survival after local recurrence, *Int. J. Radiat. Oncol. Biol. Phys.,* **26** (1993) 773–782.

66. Levendag PC, Meeuwis CA, and Visser AG. Reirradiation of recurrent head and neck cancers; external and/or interstitial radiation therapy, *Radiother. Oncol.,* **23** (1992) 6–14.

67. Saroja KR, Hendrickson FR, Cohen L, et al. Reirradiation of locally recurrent tumors with fast neutrons, *Int. J. Radiat. Oncol. Biol. Phys.,* **15** (1988) 115–121.

68. Housset M, Barrett JM, Brunel P, et al. Split-course interstitial brachytherapy with a source shift: the results of a new technique for salvage irradiation in recurrent inoperable cervical adenopathy 4 cm diameter in 23 patients, *Int. J. Radiat. Oncol. Biol. Phys.,* **22** (1992) 1071–1074.

69. Langlois D, Hoffstetter S, Malissard L, et al. Salvage irradiation of oropharynx and mobile tongue about 192 iridium brachytherapy in Centre Alexis Vautrin, *Int. J. Radiat. Oncol. Biol. Phys.,* **14** (1988) 849–853.

70. McCollough KP and Blackwell CR. A dosimetric summary of common bolus materials, (Abstract) *Med. Phys.,* **19** (1992) 835.

71. Chang F, Chang P, Benson K, et al. Study of Elasto-gel pads used as surface bolus material in high energy photon and electron therapy, *Int. J. Radiat. Oncol. Biol. Phys.,* **22** (1991) 191–193.

72. Nag S, Schuller D, Pak V, et al. IORT using electron beam or HDR brachytherapy for previously unirradiated head and neck cancers, *Front. Radiat. Ther. Oncol.,* **31** (1997) 112–116.

73. Nag S, Schuller D, Pak V, Young D, Grecula J, Bauer C, et al. Pilot study of intraoperative high dose rate brachytherapy for head and neck cancer, *Radiother. Oncol.,* **41** (1996) 125–130.

74. Freeman S, Hamaker R, Singer M, et al. Intraoperative radiotherapy of skull base cancer, *Laryngoscope,* **101** (1991) 507–509.

75. Freeman SB, Hamaker RC, Rate WR, et al. Management of advanced cervical metastasis using intraoperative radiotherapy, *Laryngoscope,* **105** (1995) 575–578.

76. Garrett PG, Pugh NO, Ross HR, et al. Intraoperative radiation therapy for advanced recurrent head and neck cancer, *Int. J. Radiat. Oncol. Biol. Phys.,* **13** (1987) 785–788.

77. Garrett PG, Hamaker R, Pugh N, et al. Intraoperative radiation therapy for advanced or recurrent head and neck malignancy. In: *First International Symposium on Intraoperative Radiation Therapy,* Dobelbower, RR and Abe, M, Boca Raton, FL, CRC (1989).

78. Garrett P, Rate W, Hamaker R, et al. Intraoperative radiation therapy for advanced or recurrent head and neck malignancies. In: *Proceedings of the Third International Symposium on Intraoperative Radiation Therapy,* Elmsford, NY, Pergamon (1991).

79. Garrett PG, Rate W, Hamaker R, et al. Surgical resection and intraoperative radiation therapy (IORT) for advanced or recurrent salivary gland malignancies. In: Fourth International Symposium on Intraoperative Radiation Therapy, 1992, pp. 199–202.

80. Rate W, Garrett P, Hamaker R, et al. Intraoperative radiation therapy for recurrent head and neck cancer, *Cancer,* **67** (1991) 2738–2740.

81. Rate W, Garrett P, Hamaker R, et al. Surgical resection and intraoperative radiation (IORT) for advanced neck lymph node metastases. Fourth International Symposium on Intraoperative Radiation Therapy, 1992, pp. 203–206.

82. Foote RL, McCaffrey TV, Olsen KD, et al. Intraoperative electron beam radiation therapy for advanced or recurrent head and neck cancer., Fifth International IORT Symposium, Lyon, France, 1994.

83. Ling SM, Roach M, Fu KK, et al. Local control after the use of adjuvant electron beam intraoperative radiotherapy in patients with high-risk head and neck cancer: the UCSF experience, *Cancer J. Sci. Am.,* **2** (1996) 321–329.

84. Martinez-Monge R, Azinovic I, Alcalde J, et al. IORT in the management of locally advanced or recurrent head and neck cancer, *Front. Radiat. Ther. Oncol.,* **31** (1997) 122–125.

85. Toita T, Nakano M, Takizawa Y, et al. Intraoperative radiation therapy (IORT) for head and neck cancer, *Int. J. Radiat. Oncol. Biol. Phys.,* **30** (1994) 1219–1224.

86. Schmitt TH, Prades JM, Puel G, et al. IORT for locally advanced oropharyngeal carcinomas with major extension into the tongue base, *Front. Radiat. Ther. Oncol.,* **31** (1997) 117–121.

87. Schuller DE, Grecula JC, Gahbauer RA, et al. Intensified regimen for advanced head and neck squamous cell carcinoma, *Arch. Otolaryngol. Head Neck Surg.,* **123** (1997) 139–144.

88. Bachaud JM, Cohen-Jonathan E, Alzieu C, et al. Combined postoperative radiotherapy and weekly cisplatin infusion for locally advanced head and neck carcinoma: final report of a randomized trial, *Int. J. Radiat. Oncol. Biol. Phys.,* **36** (1996) 999–1004.

89. Jacobs JR, Ahmad K, Casiano R, et al. Implications of positive surgical margins, *Laryngoscope,* **103** (1993) 64–68.

27 IORT for CNS Tumors

D. Ortiz de Urbina, N. Willich, R. R. Dobelbower, J. Aristu, J. C. Bustos, D. Carter, S. Palkovic, M. Santos, and F. A. Calvo

1. INTRODUCTION

High-grade malignant gliomas are the most common brain tumors of the adult life and account for about 30–45% of the primary human brain tumors. Of these, nearly 85% are glioblastoma multiforme *(1)*.

Life expectation of patients with malignant brain tumors is still rather short. Even in the most intensive treatment programs, the median survival of glioblastoma patients is very poor. Only a few anecdotal cases are reported as long-term survivors *(2)*.

Glioblastoma multiforme (GBM) and anaplastic astrocytomas (AA) are extraordinarily aggressive tumors. Despite attempts to improve both local and systemic therapy, local persistance or tumor recurrence within 2–3 cm of the primary site is the rule *(3)*. The median survival time and the 5-year survival rate for anaplastic astrocytomas are 36 months and 18%, respectively, and for patients with glioblastoma multiforme, they are only 10 months and less than 5%, respectively *(4)*.

Radiotherapy is the most effective adjuvant therapy modality and is therefore a mandatory treatment after maximal gross surgical resection in the management of high-grade malignant gliomas. The beneficial effect of postoperative irradiation has been documented in randomized clinical trials *(2,5)*.

Brain Tumor Cooperative Group (BTCG) trials have suggested a stepwise relationship between total radiation dose and survival in malignant gliomas *(6)*. Unfortunately, radiation doses greater than 60 Gy are accompanied by unacceptable brain tissue toxicity when conventional external beam radiotherapy is used *(7)*.

From: *Current Clinical Oncology: Intraoperative Irradiation: Techniques and Results*
Edited by: L. L. Gunderson et al. © Humana Press, Inc., Totowa, NJ

In an attempt to improve the outcome of malignant gliomas, multimodality programs including different adjuvant chemotherapy regimens have been the subject of numerous reports over the last decades; prospective randomized clinical trials conducted by the Brain Tumor Study Group (BTSG) (8) and the Radiation Therapy Oncology Group (RTOG)/Eastern Cooperative Oncology Group (ECOG) (2) showed a modest improvement of the median survival time and 18-month survival in patients receiving a 2-chloroethyl-*N*-nitrosourea (BCNU: carmustine) plus radiotherapy. Different prognostic factors including age, performance status, histology, and extent of surgery have been identified in several clinical reports (1).

Intraoperative radiation therapy with high-energy electron beams (IOERT) is an alternative modality as intensification of loco-regional treatment in solid tumors and particularly in high-grade malignant gliomas (9–12). The rationale for IOERT use in malignant brain tumors is based on the usual characteristics of tumor unifocality, pattern of recurrence "in" or very close to the primary site, radiation dose–tumor response correlation, and the possibility to spare normal brain tissue from large doses delivered directly into the tumor bed. In the last decade, several institutions have reported their experience using IOERT in the treatment of intracranial tumors as a feasible and tolerable technique showing encouraging preliminary results when compared with historial controls (13–15).

2. SURGERY WITH AND WITHOUT EXTERNAL BEAM IRRADIATION IN MALIGNANT GLIOMAS

The role of surgical resection in the management of malignant gliomas remains contradictory, as no prospective, randomized clinical trials have been designed to evaluate the impact of the extent of the surgical resection on patient outcome. Extent of resection is generally based on subjective criterion which can lead to either an underestimate or overestimate of the total amount of tumor removed. On the other hand, nobody doubts that cytoreductive surgery is essential in the treatment of patients with high-grade glioma to decrease intracranial pressure and improve focal neurological deficits secondary to mass effect, reduce the steroid dependency, and minimize the tumor burden remaining after surgery. Furthermore, gross tumor removal reduces the number of cells potentially resistant to chemotherapy and/or radiotherapy and, thus, enhances the benefit of the adjuvant therapy.

A BTSG cooperative trial (16) showed that the amount of residual tumor on postoperative computed tomography (CT) scans was inversely correlated with survival time and noted that tumor size after surgery and after radiotherapy was a significant prognostic factor. Ammirati et al. (17) reported that radical tumor removal improved both the functional status and survival of patients when compared with less aggressive surgery. In summary, clinical trials support the strategy of removing as much tumor as possible. Although this strategy is not universally accepted, growing evidence suggests a significant prolongation in the survival time and an improvement in neurological status in such groups of patients, particularly in anaplastic astrocytomas (18).

Technical advances either in neurosurgery (neurosurgical navigation, ultrasonic tissue aspirators, diagnostic ultrasound), imaging diagnosis procedures (enhanced CT/magnetic resonance imaging [MRI] scans, single photon emission computed tomography [SPECT]), or neuroanesthesia techniques provide more aggressive and safer surgical approaches in malignant gliomas. Unfortunately, however, the median survival time in high-grade malignant glioma with surgery alone is stated at 5–6 months (19).

In 1978, the BTCG reported the results concerning the first randomized clinical trial providing evidence that postoperative irradiation significantly improved survival over surgery alone in patients with malignant glioma. The median survival time and the 1-year survival rates were 36 weeks and 24%, respectively, for the irradiated patients versus 14 weeks and 3%, respectively, for the patients managed with surgery alone (8).

Walker et al. (6) retrospectively analyzed the three BTCG studies and showed a direct correlation between radiation dose and survival in patients with malignant gliomas. Median survival times of 13.5, 28, 36, and 42 weeks were seen for patients who received ≤ 45, 50, 55, and 60 Gy, respectively, using daily fractions of 1.7–2 Gy. A statistically significant difference in survival was noted for 50 versus 60 Gy ($p = 0.004$).

Adjuvant chemotherapy has been combined with surgery and conventional radiotherapy as part of the standard approach in the treatment of malignant gliomas. A minimal advantage in terms of survival has been documented with the addition of nitrosoureas (20).

The response of malignant gliomas to standard irradiation techniques is limited both by the extraordinary radioresistance of such tumor cells (21) and by the radiosensitivity of the surrounding normal brain tissue. Many feel that the safe dose that can be delivered to necessary brain volumes is 60 Gy in 1.8- to 2.0-Gy fractions (22), which is below that required to eradicate gross tumor. New radiation technical approaches, such as interstitial brachytherapy (23), stereotactic radiosurgery (24) and intraoperative radiation therapy with high-energy electron beams (IOERT) (9–12) have been introduced in an effort to increase the tumor dose but to spare uninvolved brain tissue from treatment-related injury.

3. INTRAOPERATIVE ELECTRON IRRADIATION

Intraoperative irradiation using high-energy electron beams (IOERT) allows an optimization of the therapeutic ratio of the conventional radiotherapy programs by exploiting the electron beam's uniform-depth dose distribution throughout the target volume with minimal normal brain tissue irradiation. During surgical procedures, IOERT can be used to deliver a high single dose to the tumor volume or the surgical bed that is directly visualized and exposed to the radiation oncologist. This allows a decrease in the possibility of a geographical miss, while sparing normal brain tissue.

In malignant gliomas, because local recurrence is the most frequent cause of treatment failures "within" 2–3 cm around the primary tumor, IOERT is an attractive treatment modality to be explored, in an attempt to improve local tumor control. The published data with IOERT in the treatment of malignant gliomas is made up of a few small series of patients (10,12,14,25–28).

In 1942, Dyke and Davidoff were the first to communicate the use of IORT in the treatment of intracranial tumors in two patients with sarcoma of the brain. After surgical resection both patients received 30 Gy by contact roentgen therapy. Brain edema and inflammatory changes secondary to treatment were found at autopsy in each patient (11).

The first published data noting the use of IOERT in brain tumors was by Abe et al. (9) in 1971 in two patients with recurrent brain tumors. A patient with fibrosarcoma was previously treated by conventional radiotherapy (59.6 cGy). After subtotal removal of recurrent disease, a single dose of 35 Gy was given with 18 MeV through an 8-cm field.

A glioblastoma multiforme patient had been previously treated with 59.4 Gy EBRT, and, after recurrence, was submitted to subtotal surgical resection and 40 Gy single-dose IOERT with 12-MeV electron energy through a 4-cm field. The first patient was free of symptoms for 5 months and died 189 days after IOERT; the second patient developed a radiation-induced necrosis requiring craniotomy on the 63rd day post-IOERT, dying 2 weeks later.

Goldson et al. *(10)* conducted a pilot study at Howard University Hospital, in Washington, and showed the results of using IOERT in a total of 12 patients with different intracranial tumors. A single dose of 15 Gy IOERT was delivered to the tumor in conjunction with 50 Gy EBRT in 25 fractions to the whole brain and an additional 5 Gy cone-down boost to the tumor or tumor bed. They concluded that IOERT as a technique was feasible and clinically applicable in brain tumors.

Several institutions in different countries, mainly in Europe, the United States, and Japan, have included IOERT in phase I–II clinical trials in the treatment of malignant gliomas. A review of that related experience will be discussed.

3.1. Spanish IOERT Experience

The IOERT procedure was introduced in Spain at the University of Navarra in 1984 as a treatment modality of radiation intensification in different locally advanced tumors. Thereafter, the San Francisco de Asís Hospital in Madrid included IOERT as a part of multidisciplinary programs in the treatment of several malignant solid tumors and, particularly, the management of high-grade malignant gliomas. Separate pilot studies at these two major centers reported the preliminary results of using IOERT in intracranial malignant tumors *(12,25)*.

3.1.1. Patient Group and Evaluation

Subsequently, an updated analysis was performed of the joint experience concerning a total of 50 patients with intracranial tumors treated with IOERT at San Francisco de Asís Hospital (30 patients) and at the University of Navarra (20 patients) using nearly identical protocols *(12,25)*. From December 1985 to January 1997, 30 males (60%) and 20 females (40%), with a mean age of 43 years (range 5–73 years) and a Karnofsky performance status ranging from 50% to 100% (median 70%) have been included. A detailed neurological examination and a brain enhanced computed tomography (CT) and/or magnetic resonance imaging (MRI) scans were performed just prior to IOERT, 1 month after the IOERT procedure and every 3 months during subsequent follow-up.

Prior to IOERT, a histological diagnosis, either by stereotactic biopsy or biopsy by open craniotomy was mandatory. Nineteen (38%) primary tumors and 31 (62%) recurrent tumors had pathological reports consisting of astrocytoma grade III (5 patients), anaplastic astrocytoma (16 patients), glioblastoma multiforme (14 patients), anaplastic oligodendroglioma (8 patients), meningeal sarcoma (3 patients), ependymoma grade III (2 patients), anaplastic meningioma (1 patient), and neuroblastoma (1 patient). Lesion location was mainly at the frontal (15 patients), parietal (23 patients), or temporal (9 patients) lobes or retroocular (1 patient), and cerebellum (1 patient).

3.1.2. EBRT Techniques

A total of 42 out of 50 patients (84%) received external beam irradiation (EBRT) with megavoltage equipment (cobalt-60 or 6-MeV photon beam linear accelerator) either as a course of prior treatment before evaluation for IOERT as a component of treatment for recurrence (25 patients: 50%) or as planned adjuvant postoperative treatment after IOERT (17 patients: 34%). A total dose of 45–50 Gy, at 1.8–2.0 Gy/day, 5 days a week, with parallel opposed lateral portals was delivered to the whole brain content. An additional boost of 15 Gy was delivered to a confined volume, including the primary tumor plus 2–3 cm of macroscopic uninvolved brain tissue with 19 patients (38%) receiving adjuvant systemic chemotherapy.

3.1.3. Surgical and IOERT Treatment Procedures

In the operating room, the patient is placed on a mobile table to provide the ability to transport the patient to the radiotherapy unit to subsequently perform an IOERT procedure, if indicated. Based on the enhanced MRI brain scan, a meticulous analysis is performed by the neurosurgeon, radiation oncologist, and anesthesiologist team to select the optimal position of the patient's head before start of the surgical procedure. After the patient's head is immobilized, the neurosurgeon performs a craniotomy to expose the tumor and allow subsequent introduction of the IOERT applicator without any bone structure interfering with the beam.

All the patients underwent maximal surgical resection. The extent of surgery was subtotal in 32 patients (64%) and a total gross tumor removal was performed in 18 patients (36%).

After maximal tumor removal, hemostasis is achieved and the tumor bed is exposed to select the IOERT characteristics related to the applicator size and bevel. The target volume for IOERT is usually the surgical tumor bed plus a 1–2 cm margin of macroscopic normal tissue (Fig. 1). Different factors related to the tumor such as the size, location, and depth are critical in order to achieve success of the IOERT procedure; these factors must be taken into account before surgery and during the surgical exposure.

The most appropriate IOERT applicator size and the angle of the beam incidence into the tumor are then selected by the radiation oncologist (Fig. 1). Five cm (60% of patients) and 6 cm (30%) applicator sizes have been used primarily, but the range has been 3–9 cm. Different beveled angles (0°–45°) were placed at the end of the IOERT applicator to achieve a better geometric adaptation to the anatomic site.

The IOERT energy was chosen according to the required depth of radiation penetration, as related to the thickness of the target tissue. The 90% isodose curve had to encompass the residual tumor or high-risk area. The electron energy was 10 MeV for 4 patients, 12 MeV for 5 patients, 15 MeV for 6 patients, 18 MeV for 23 patients, and 20 MeV for 23 patients. Saline-saturated cotton balls were introduced inside the surgical cavity as tissue-compensating material to homogenize the radiation distribution.

The total single dose of IOERT delivered to the tumor or tumor bed ranged from 10 to 20 Gy. With a primary and/or nonirradiated recurrent tumor, a 15- to 20-Gy dose was used; for a recurrent previously irradiated tumor, 10–15 Gy was given.

3.1.4. Results in Combined Spanish IOERT Series—Primary Tumors

Nineteen patients, 11 males and 8 females, with primary brain tumors have been included in the analysis. The mean age was 45 years and the median Karnofsky performance status was 70% (range 50–80%). This histological diagnosis confirmed an anaplastic astrocytoma (AA—10 patients), anaplastic oligodendroglioma (AO—2 patients), glioblastoma multiforme (GBM—5 patients), meningeal sarcoma (1 patient), and neuroblastoma (1 patient). Complete macroscopic tumor removal at surgery was performed in 8 patients (42%) and subtotal surgical resection in 11 patients (58%).

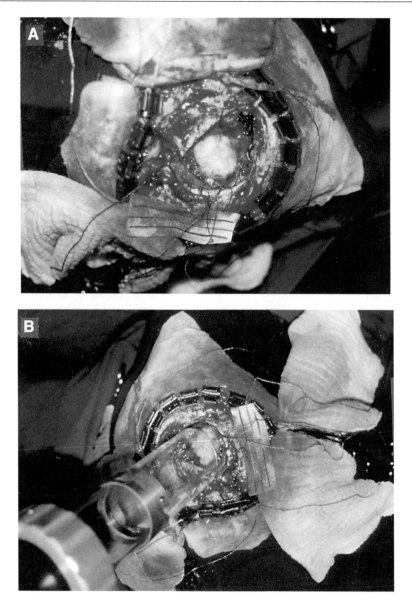

Fig. 1. (A) Craniotomy and tumor bed exposure after surgical resection of glioblastoma multiforme. Saline-soaked cotton is used to fill the tumor cavity to homogenize the dose distribution. **(B)** View of IOERT cone positioning directly on the tumor, avoiding the bone skull.

The most frequent IOERT cone size used was 5 cm (range 5–7 cm), and the energy of IOERT beams ranged from 10 to 20 MeV (median 18 MeV). The median single radiation dose was 15 Gy but ranged from 12.5 to 20 Gy. Thirteen out of 19 patients (68.5%) received fractionated postoperative EBRT (median 50 Gy) to the whole brain.

3.1.4.1. Survival and Disease Control. The 1- and 2-year actuarial survival time, according to Kaplan–Meier method *(29)* have been 70.5% and 36%, respectively, and the median survival time was 21 months (range 1–65 months). Ten out of 19 patients (52.5%) developed tumor progression and the median time to recurrence was 17.5 months (range 3–56 months). Six patients (31.5%) are alive and three have no evidence of tumor relapse.

Twelve patients (63%) died because of tumor progression and 1 patient died without disease because of pulmonary thromboembolism 3 months after IOERT (Table 1).

3.1.4.2. Prognostic Factor Analysis. Patients who underwent complete surgical resection had a median survival time of 22 months and 1- and 2-year survival of 87.5% and 58%, respectively, versus 10.5 months median survival and 53% and 39% 1- and 2-year survival, respectively, in those with subtotal resection. These differences were not statistically significant ($p = 0.18$) by log-rank test. The median time to progression for the group with total resection was 21 months versus 8 months for patients with subtotal resection. Age, Karnofsky index, and tumor size had no significant prognostic value on survival when analyzed by multivariate regression according to the Cox model analysis.

3.1.5. IOERT Results for Recurrent Tumors, Spanish Series

A total of 31 patients had recurrent disease at the time of IOERT, 20 male and 11 females, with a mean age of 40 years and median Karnofsky index of 70% (50–100%). The majority had high-grade gliomas: AA—11 patients; AO—6 patients; GBM—9 patients; meningeal sarcoma—2 patients; atypical meningioma—1 patient; ependymoma—2 patients. In 10 patients (32%), the extent of surgery was a total tumor resection, whereas 21 patients (68%) had a subtotal surgical resection.

Twenty-four patients (77.5%) had previously received EBRT (48–70 Gy) and received no further EBRT at time of relapse. The other seven patients were treated with complementary EBRT (50–54 Gy) after IOERT for their recurrence.

IOERT applicators 5 cm (3–9 cm) in diameter and 18-MeV energy (range 10–20 MeV) were most frequently used for IOERT treatments. The IOERT dose ranged from 12.5 to 20 Gy (median 15 Gy).

3.1.5.1. Survival and Disease Control. One patient was excluded from survival and disease control analyses due to loss at follow-up. The median actuarial survival time for recurrent tumors was 15.5 months (4–80 months); 1-year survival was 58% and 2-year survival was 37%. Seventeen out of 30 patients (56.5%) had a local failure 2–68 months after IOERT (median time to progression: 7 months). At time of analysis, 12 patients were alive (40%)—6 without evidence of disease and the other 6 with disease. Two patients died free of disease at 4 and 16 months (pulmonary thromboembolism, unknown cause) and 16 patients (53%) died because of tumor progression (Table 1).

3.1.5.2. Prognostic Factor Analysis. Considering the extent of surgery versus prognosis in patients with recurrent tumors, those who underwent complete surgical resection had a median survival time and time to progression of 27 months and 6 months, respectively. Patients with subtotal resection had a median survival time of 11 months and median time to progression of 7.5 months.

3.2. Japanese IOERT Experience

In 1989, Yanagawa et al. *(13)* reviewed the results in a total of 27 patients with high-grade malignant glioma treated with 15–50 Gy IOERT plus fractionated EBRT (30–52 Gy, mean dose 50 Gy) and ACNU chemotherapy. Survival rates at 1- and 2-years were 88% and 40%, respectively, and these data compared favorably with patients not treated with IOERT. No adverse effects were noted.

Matsutani et al. *(14)* reviewed the IOERT experience in 170 patients with malignant brain tumors (85 gliomas, 81 metastatic tumors, and 4 other tumors). Thirty patients with GBM (7 primary tumors and 23 recurrent tumors) were included in the analysis. Following total removal macroscopically, the delivered IOERT dose was 10–25 Gy (mean 18.3

Table 1

IOERT for Brain Tumors, Spanish Experience: Local Control and Patient Status

	No. of Patients	Progression Status[a]		Time to Progression Median (Range) (mo)	Survival		Median (Range) (mo)	Patient Status[b]			
		NP	PD		One Year	Two Years		ANED	AWD	DFD	DWD
Primary disease	19	9	10	17.5 (3–56)	70.5%	36%	21 (1–65)	3	3	1	12
Recurrent disease	30	13[a]	17	7 (2–68)	58%	37%	15.5 (4–80)	6	6	2	16

[a] NP = no progression; PD = progression disease.
[b] ANED = alive, no evidence of disease; AWD = alive with disease; DFD = dead, free of disease; DWD = dead, with disease.
[c] One patient not evaluable (lost follow-up).

Gy) and all patients received fractionated EBRT with a dose of 30–80 Gy (mean 58.5 Gy). The median time to tumor progression and the median survival time were 73 weeks and 119 weeks, respectively, and the 1-, 2-, and 3-year survival rates were 97%, 61%, and 33% respectively; 87% of patients were free of tumor for more than 1 year. Four patients (17%) developed a recurrence within the primary site and 19 patients (79%) had a recurrence marginal to the treatment area. Patients receiving a IOERT dose less than 25 Gy showed no acute or subacute side effects.

Nineteen patients with intracranial tumors were treated with IOERT (23–40 Gy) by Shibamoto et al. *(27)* at Kyoto University. Seventeen patients had recurrent tumors and had received prior EBRT (17–65 Gy), 4–112 months before IOERT. The median survival time was 12 months for nine patients with GBM or AA and 51 months for eight patients with anaplastic ependymomas (AE) and AO. Twelve patients had local tumor progression; five recurred outside the IOERT field, two had diffuse regrowth of the tumor in both unirradiated and irradiated areas, and only one patient had an in-field recurrence.

Twenty patients with supratentorial gliomas (11 GBM and 7 AA) were included in a clinical study developed by Fujiwara et al. *(26)* consisting of surgical resection, IOERT (20–25 Gy), and EBRT (40–57.6 Gy). Median survival time was 14 months, which compared favorably with that of the control group (10 months). For GBM, the median survival time and median time to progression were 17 months and 10 months, respectively, whereas for AA, the results were 12 and 7 months, respectively.

Finally, Sakai et al. *(28)* presented their IOERT experience in 44 patients (12 AA and 32 GBM). Surgical resection plus 10–50 Gy IOERT (median 26.7 Gy) and 47–57 Gy EBRT (median, 50.6 Gy) was performed. The overall 2- and 3-year survival were 57% and 38%, respectively, and particularly for GBM, they were 43% and 24%, respectively. The local recurrence of tumor 1 year after IOERT was 63.6%.

3.3. The U.S. IOERT Experience

The reported U.S. clinical experience with intraoperative electron irradiation for tumors involving the central nervous system (CNS) stems from two centers: Howard University and The Medical College of Ohio (MCO) *(30)*. Both institutions conducted pilot studies using IOERT as a supplement to EBRT to boost the radiation dose locally for treatment of primary, recurrent, and metastatic CNS tumors, both above and below the tentorium.

3.3.1. HOWARD UNIVERSITY

In 1984, Goldson and co-workers reported results from 12 patients treated with IOERT for brain tumors *(10)*. Four of the 12 patients were treated for GBM, 5 for AA, 3 for meningiomas, and a solitary patient suffered an oligodendroglioma. The extent of surgical resection ranged from simple biopsy to total removal of the tumor.

3.3.1.1. Radiation Factors. The IOERT dose was 15 Gy in every case, but the EBRT dose ranged from 0 to 55 Gy. The IOERT was administered through 4- to 9-cm applicators using 9- to 12-MeV electron beams. Saline-saturated cotton balls were used in the resection cavity as tissue-compensating material to maintain dose homogeneity. Typically, EBRT commenced 1–2 weeks after IOERT, delivering 50 Gy to the whole brain and 5 Gy to the tumor bed via "cone-down" techniques.

3.3.1.2. Results. Two patients that had biopsies only (without benefit of surgical decompression) developed severe cerebral edema after IOERT. Coma, seizures, and intracranial bleeding were also encountered. Two glioma patients died within 30 days of

IOERT. At the time of a report in 1984, six patients were alive without evidence of tumor 8–42 months after IOERT with 1- and 2-year survival of 60% and 20%, respectively.

3.3.2. MEDICAL COLLEGE OF OHIO

At the MCO, 19 intracranial IOERT procedures were performed on 17 patients with malignant brain tumors. Two patients were treated with IOERT for recurrent disease. There were 12 primary brain tumors and 5 tumors metastatic to the brain. The lesion was supratentorial in 14 cases, infratentorial in 5 cases. Patient age ranged from 13 to 70 years, with a median age of 45 years.

3.3.2.1. Radiation Factors. IOERT doses of 10–20 Gy (median 15 Gy) were administered through 2.5- to 9-cm flat-ended applicators using 6- to 20-MeV electron beams, depending on the depth of the lesion and/or the resection cavity. Saline-soaked cotton balls were used within the resection cavity to help obtain the desired dose distribution. EBRT (up to 77 Gy) was generally administered prior to IORT using 4- to 10-MV X-rays and/or ^{60}Co gamma rays and/or 43-MV neutrons.

3.3.2.2. Results. The average survival time (after initial diagnosis) was 12 months for patients with primary brain tumors (range 2–22 months) and 8.5 months for those with metastatic brain tumors (range 4–13 months). Six of the 12 patients with primary malignant brain tumors survived more than a year after initial diagnosis. The average survival time after IOERT was 6 months for patients with primary malignant brain tumors. Two patients with recurrent glioblastoma expired within 30 days of IOERT. CT scans of these two patients failed to show intracranial hemorrhage or increase in cerebral edema. Delayed bone flap necrosis occurred in three cases.

3.4. University of Münster Experience

3.4.1. PATIENT GROUP

Forty-six patients with malignant brain tumors have been treated with IOERT at the University of Münster *(15)*. The heterogeneous collection consisted of 27 patients with primary brain tumors, 13 patients with recurrent tumors, and 6 patients suffering from brain metastases. Patients age ranged from 32 to 71 years, with a median of 55 years. All tumors were histologically examined after a stereotactic sample excision.

The histological tumor types were distributed as follows: 22 GBM, 14 astrocytoma grade III, 6 metastasis, 3 oligodendroglioma grade III, and 1 ependymoma grade III. According to the intended treatment with surgery and postoperative EBRT, all patients had preoperative CT scans as well as MRI scans. SPECT studies were done using the flowmarker ^{99m}Tc–HMPAO as well as the amino acid analogon ^{123}I-α-methyltyrosine (AMT). Additionally, a CT scan was performed with four markers affixed on the patient's scalp for the calibration of the neuronavigation system.

3.4.2. IOERT AND SURGICAL TREATMENT PROCEDURE

All tumors were resected as completely as possible. For surgery, patients were rested on a mobile table with their head fixed in a Mayfield clamp. The craniotomy hole had to surround the tumor by a margin of at least 2 cm so that no bony structures could obstruct the beam. Until August 1995, the resection hole used to be measured manually in all three dimensions and then filled up with tissue-equivalent wet cotton strips.

An electron applicator, individually modified with lead absorbers, was selected according to the diameter of the resection area. Depending on the measured depth of the tumor bed, electron energies varied from 10 to 18 MeV: 34 patients received 14 MeV, 10 patients received 18 MeV, and 3 patients were treated with 10-MeV electrons for superficially located tumors. All tumors were localized supratentorially and had a size less than 6 cm.

After IOERT, the dose distribution was reconstructed based on 3 d MP rage MRI sequences of the patient's head carried out before and just after surgery. Knowing the exact angle of the incident ray and the exact position of the patient's head during IOERT from verification films, the isodose curves could be superimposed on the corresponding MRI reconstructions from the 3 d MP rage data set. The greatest disadvantage of this system was that dose calculation could only be performed approximately and after therapy. Thus, it could only serve as quality control after treatment but not as a method for treatment planning.

Since August 1995, IOERT of brain tumors is performed with the assistance of a neuronavigation system manufactured by the Radionics Burlington Company. The system uses an articulated sensing arm which transmits back the three-dimensional coordinates of its tip (the operating point) (Fig. 2A).

Before surgery, a CT scan is carried out with four markers affixed to the patients scalp so that these markers appear on the different CT planes. In the operating theater, the neuronavigation arm is mounted on the Mayfield clamp securing the patient's head. The fiducial points, affixed on the patients head during the CT procedure, are touched with the tip of the navigation arm to establish them as reference points for the calibration of the neuronavigation system. This new tomographic stereotactic device is then able to translate the three-dimensional coordinates of the operating point into a corresponding point on the preoperative CT images. For the radiation oncologist, this neuronavigation system is of particularly high value, as it enables him to perform treatment planning in IOERT before therapy.

After surgery, the localization of the arm tip is projected into the corresponding CT slice, showing its position in relation to the former tumor-bearing area. The radiation oncologist is now able to determine the necessary depth and select a suitable dose distribution and electron energy as well as determine the angle of the incident ray. Then, after taping the patients head with sterile plastic foils, a device especially constructed for this purpose, the so-called BDI (beam direction indicator), was fixed on the patient's head. This device can be adjusted so that it indicates the correct angle of the incident ray (Fig. 2B). Now the patient is transferred into the department of radiotherapy, where IOERT can be delivered knowing the exact depth of the target area (i.e., the necessary electron energy) and the angle of the incident ray before irradiation.

For the 37 not previously irradiated patients, the treatment consisted of surgical resection and 20 Gy IOERT, followed by 40–60 Gy cobalt-60 gamma irradiation or megavolt irradiation with photons (10 MV). The seven previously irradiated patients received 25 Gy IOERT without additional EBRT; two patients received only 15 Gy IOERT during the initial phase of the study. The target volume for EBRT (tumor plus 1–2 cm safety margin) had to be completed surrounded by the 90% isodose.

3.4.3. Münster Results

Eight to 10 weeks after IOERT, every patient was subjected to neurological examination, and CT and MRI scans as well as another AMT–SPECT were made. This follow-up program was repeated every 3 months.

The patients with metastases were excluded from survival calculations. At the time of analysis, 10 of 40 treated patients were still alive. Five patients died from other causes,

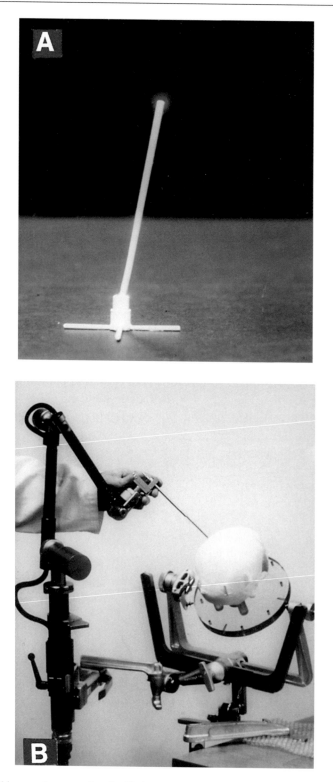

Fig. 2. Technical innovations used at the University of Münster. (**A**) The neuronavigation system with the navigation arm; (**B**) the beam direction indicator (BDI).

19 patients died from local recurrence, and 6 died from relapse outside the treatment area. The median survival time for all patients was 12.5 months. The overall survival probability for all patients 1 year after IORT was 50.5%, and after 2 years, it was 11.2%. The probability for recurrence-free survival for all patients after 1 year was 44.3%, and after 2 years, it was 10.1%.

3.4.3.1. Prognostic Factor Analysis. Stratified by tumor types, the median survival time for the grade III gliomas was 14.9 months, and for the glioblastomas, it was 11.5 months. The 1-year survival probability for the grade III gliomas was 58.8%, and for the glioblastomas, it was 45.5%.

There were differences in survival times and the survival probabilities between primary and recurrent tumors. Whereas primary tumors had a median overall survival time of 11.5 months, the recurrent tumors had a median survival time of 21.1 months. The primary tumors had a 1-year survival probability of 46%, whereas primary tumors had a median overall survival probability of 67.1%.

To estimate the prognostic value of different factors, tumor size, general condition (Karnofsky status), and extent of surgical resection were evaluated by a multivariate analysis (Cox regression). Neither age (younger vs older than 55 years), nor Karnofsky status (below vs above 70%), nor tumor size (larger vs smaller than 55 cm^3) were statistically significant. Only the extent of surgical resection (complete vs incomplete) was found to be statistically significant (Fig. 3A). Twenty-nine out of 40 patients with primary tumors had a total resection. These patients had a median survival time of 14.9 months and a 1-year survival probability of 66.6%. For those patients ($n = 11$) who only underwent subtotal resection, the median survival time was 5 months with a 1-year survival probability of only 18.2%. The log-rank p-value amounted to 0.0009, which is highly significant. When the survival probabilities of glioblastoma patients treated by IOERT with and without EBRT were compared with the historical control treated by postoperative EBRT alone, an improvement was observed (Fig. 3B).

3.4.3.2. Treatment Tolerance. After this combined surgery and intraoperative radiotherapy, most of the patients improved in terms of their neurological symptoms. Twenty-one of 22 patients suffering from intracranial pressure prior to therapy showed an improvement, and other neurological symptoms (e.g., aphasia, paresis, convulsion, psychosyndrome and hemianopsia) also reduced.

Postoperative complications were not encountered more frequently than after surgery and/or conventional radiotherapy. There were two patients with wound infections and healing impairment, one patient with a hemorrhage occurring 2 days after surgery and IOERT (this patient died from this side effect 4 months later), and one patient suffered from postoperative brain edema, this edema being the cause of his death 3.5 months later. No long-term side effects were observed in any patient due to the IOERT, and a brain necrosis could never be shown on MRI or AMT–SPECT.

3.5. Toxicity and Complications

There is a lack of information regarding the tolerance of normal brain tissue to high single doses of electron beam irradiation, such as that used in IOERT, either alone or as a boost after fractionated EBRT. Experimental IOERT studies in dogs confirm that peripheral nerves are the dose-limiting tissue for the clinical use of IOERT *(31,32)*. Peripheral neuropathies in patients usually occurs 6–9 months or longer following IOERT. It has been suggested that IORT doses of < 20 Gy may not result in clinically significant

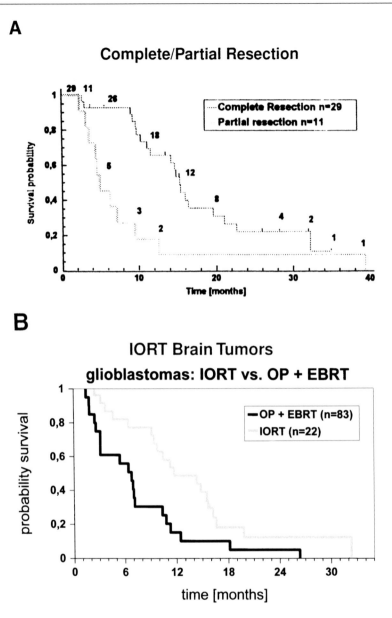

A

Complete/Partial Resection

B

IORT Brain Tumors
glioblastomas: IORT vs. OP + EBRT

Fig. 3. Impact of prognostic factors on survival in the University of Münster series. (**A**) Complete versus partial resection in the total IOERT series of 40 patients; (**B**) survival comparison in glioblastoma patients treated with an operative resection (OP) plus EBRT ($n = 83$) versus IOERT plus EBRT ($n = 22$).

peripheral nerve injury *(31)*. Unfortunately, the data obtained in animal experiments and clinical regarding peripheral nerve tolerance to IOERT cannot be extrapolated to the human brain.

Matsutani et al. *(14)* presented data from high single-dose irradiation in a rat glioma model and from a pilot study using IOERT in malignant gliomas and noted that doses in excess of 26 Gy would induce acute swelling of surrounding brain. According to his experience, delayed necrosis in the treatment area was observed in 33% of patients (10 of 30) receiving a mean IOERT dose of 18.9 Gy (range 15–22 Gy) and an EBRT dose of 61 Gy (range 50–70 Gy). The median time from the IOERT to the diagnosis of necrosis was 14 months (3–40 months) and 6 of 10 patients required surgical decompression. Matsutani suggested that IOERT doses less than 25 Gy combined with EBRT are a safe and tolerable approach.

Fujiwara et al. (26) noted that 6 out of 20 patients had mild IOERT-related complications. One patient who received a 20-Gy IOERT dose developed a radionecrosis 17 months after IOERT and three patients treated with 25 Gy had severe brain edema in the immediate postoperative period, requiring surgical decompression.

Histologically proven brain necrosis in the tissue volume treated by IOERT was shown in 3 of 19 patients treated at Kyoto University (27) and was fatal in one who received a high single dose of 40 Gy. Histological examination of resected specimen from patients with delayed brain necrosis after IOERT for brain tumors have shown widespread coagulation necrosis with scattered heavily damaged tumor cells and blood vessels consisting of fibrinoid necrosis, telangiectasia, and thickened hyalinized vascular wall (33).

Goldson et al. (10) suggest that an IOERT boost of 15 Gy appears to be well tolerated when preceded by some form of surgical decompression. The Spanish experience is in agreement with this consideration, with no long-term sequelae or radionecrosis observed when doses equal or lesser than 15 Gy were used (Fig. 4). Three out of 11 patients in the combined Spanish series (27%) receiving 20 Gy and a high-energy electron beam (18 MeV) with an IOERT cone size of 5 cm, 6 cm, and 6 cm, respectively, developed radiation brain damage consisting of necrosis, 3–4 months after the procedure. All recovered with symptomatic treatment (Fig. 5). Delayed side effects due to the IOERT have not been seen by other groups, such as the University of Münster (15) or The Medical College of Ohio (30).

4. DISCUSSION AND FUTURE POSSIBILITIES

4.1. Local Relapse

Local recurrence is the most frequent cause of treatment failure in high-grade malignant gliomas. Both the extent of surgery and the dose of irradiation in brain tumors are limited, either because of the risk of permanent neurological sequelae with aggressive surgical resections or the risk of unacceptable normal brain injury with irradiation doses high enough to assure tumor control, respectively.

Surgery, conventional EBRT, and a combination of both modalities appear to have reached a therapeutic plateau in local tumor control rates. In an attempt to intensify radiotherapy, IOERT has been incorporated in the management of high-grade malignant gliomas.

A sharp and rapid fall-off is shown by the depth–dose curves for IOERT, allowing delivery of a high single dose to the directly exposed tumor volume or the surgical bed, thereby decreasing the geographical miss rate while sparing surrounding normal brain tissue. Because high-grade gliomas of the brain are generally unifocal lesions and the pattern of recurrence is in or within 2–3 cm of the primary tumor site, IOERT might be an interesting modality treatment to explore further. In addition, IOERT may be appropriate to consider as a rescue treatment in recurrent previously irradiated tumors, because a safe and tolerable single dose can be delivered to small and limited volumes.

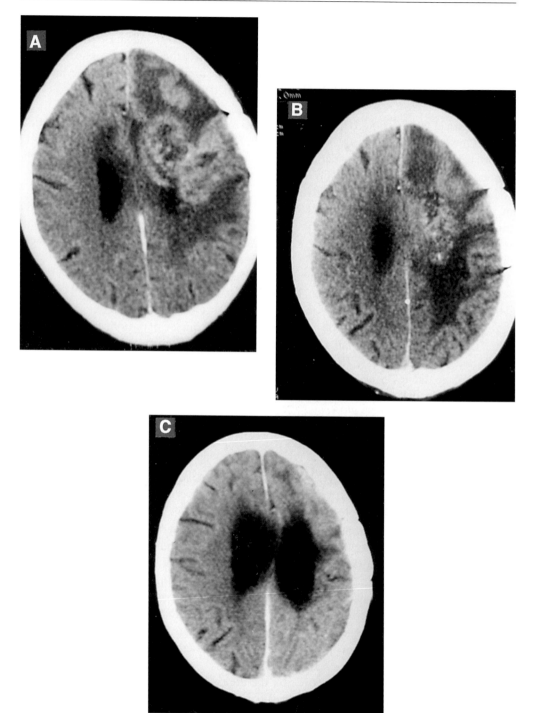

Fig. 4. A 30-year-old man with glioblastoma multiforme treated with 20 Gy IOERT and 70 Gy EBRT. (**A**) Initial preoperative enhanced CT scan; (**B**) a follow-up CT scan at 18 months showing abnormally low density in the white matter with contrast enhancement and mass effect as a result of radionecrosis; (**C**) CT scan at 43 months after IOERT, showing long-term changes on brain tissue after radionecrosis treated with symptomatic treatment.

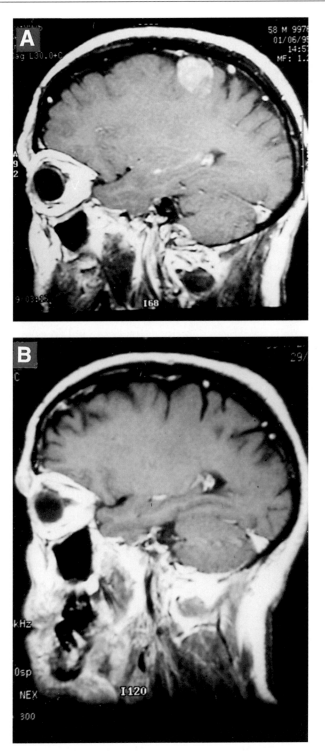

Fig. 5. Magnetic resonance images with gadolinium–diethylenetriaminepentaacetic acid (DPTA) enhancement in a 51-year-old patient with anaplastic astrocytoma: (**A**) prior to IOERT procedure; (**B**) 13 months following 15 Gy IOERT and 50 Gy EBRT.

4.2. IORT Dose and Optimization

Several problems concerning the accuracy and precision in the target volume definition, the optimum dose, and the selection of the electron beam energy are critical aspects
to consider in order to achieve better results by using the IOERT procedure in the treatment of intracranial tumors. In EBRT, CT- and MRI-assisted treatment planning enable
a high precision in target volume definition. In IOERT, on the contrary, accurate pretreatment planning has not been possible so far because the target volume cannot be defined
precisely before an attempt at maximal resection. The margins of the resection area are
defined by the surgeon during the operation. According to these margins, depth–dose
curves and electron energy are chosen and the exact position of the electron cone is
defined by the radiation oncologist and the neurosurgeon in the operation theater. During
this procedure, various difficulties in dose calculation can arise, resulting in the need for
more exact pretreatment planning. In an attempt to overcome this handicap, since August
1995 a method for calculation of posttreatment as well as pretreatment dose distributions
was established at the University of Münster with the neuronavigation system previously
described.

The selection of the electron beam energy depends on the depth of the tissue to be
irradiated, which should include the tumor or tumor bed and the surrounding 2–3 cm,
where viable tumor cells have been described. Because vital areas must be occasionally
irradiated, either a decrease in electron energy or a lower dose may need to be selected.

The optimum dose to be delivered by IOERT remains to be defined. Considering the
known dose-response relationship in malignant gliomas, the largest maximum tolerable
single dose by the normal brain tissue located immediately around the tumor bed should
be used. As previously has been described, it seems that single doses not greater than 20–
25 Gy in addition to 50–60 Gy fractionated external beam irradiation can be safely
delivered (10,14,15,25).

4.3. IOERT Impact on Local Relapse and Survival

It is difficult to draw definitive conclusions about the results obtained from the data
communicated by the different published clinical trials of IOERT in brain tumors. It
seems, however, that several institutions' experiences compare favorably with historical
controls based on conventional treatment (13–15). Multidisciplinary programs, including maximal surgical resection, IOERT, and EBRT, have provided encouraging results,
with 1-year survival rates from 20% to 90% and median survival time from 6 to 27.7
months (Table 2).

The latest data by Matsutani show a median survival time of 29.7 months for IOERT
in malignant brain tumors. Perhaps the excellent 1-, 2-, and 3-year survival probabilities
of 97%, 61%, and 33%, respectively, are partly due to a carefully selected patient group,
characterized by favorable prognostic factors, including astrocytoma grade III or GBM,
peripheral supratentorial lesions, primary therapy, tumor size below 5 cm, total resection,
and preoperative Karnofsky performance status better than 60% (14).

Taking into account this selected group, Willich at the University of Münster noted
that the 1-year survival probability for 17 patients who fulfilled these criteria was 71.5%
(15). The experience at San Francisco de Asís Hospital in Madrid is also in accordance
with these exciting results; a median survival time of 20 months and 1- and 2-year
survival of 52% and 41.5%, respectively, have been observed in a group which included
a majority of patients with GBM. Similar results have been reported by several other
Japanese Institutions (14,26–28).

Table 2
Intraoperative Radiotherapy with IOERT in HighGrade Malignant Gliomas: Anaplastic Astrocytomas and Glioblastoma Multiforme

	Total Patients	IOERT Dose (Median)	EBRT Dose (Median)	Type/No. Pts.	Histology[a]/No. Pts.	Survival %			Recurrence-Free Survival
						Median (Month)	1 Year	2 Years	
European Experience									
Willich et al. (15)	40	20 Gy	40–60 Gy	Primary	AA/GBM	11.5	46	—	1 Year: 44.3%
				Recurrent		21.1	67.1	—	2 Years: 10.1%
Ortiz De Urbina et al. (25)	35	10–20 Gy (15 Gy)	48–80 Gy (50 Gy)	Primary	AA/GBM	20	52.2	41.7	1 Year: 45.6%
				Recurrent		11.5	43.3	28.8	2 Years: 33.3%
U.S. Experience									
Goldson et al. (10)	10	15 Gy	0–55 Gy	Primary	AA/GBM	8	60	20	—
Gouda et al. (30)	11	10–20 Gy	50–70 Gy	Primary	AA/GBM	6	20	—	—
Japanese Experience									
Matsutani et al. (14)	30	10–25 Gy (18.3 Gy)	30–80 Gy (58.5 Gy)	Primary/7 Recurrent/23	GBM	27.7	97	61	87% more than 1 year
Shibamoto et al. (27)	19	23–40 Gy	17–65 Gy	Primary/2 Recurrent/17	AA/GBM/9 AE/AO/8	12 51	45.4 —	9 —	— —
Fujiwara et al. (26)	20	20–25 Gy	40–57.6 Gy	Primary	AA/GBM	12 17	42.8 72	— 9	MTTP[b] = 7 months MTTP = 10 months
Sakai et al. (28)	44	10–50 Gy (26.7 Gy)	47–57 Gy (50.6 Gy)	Primary	AA/GBM	—	—	57	1 Year: 27.4%

[a] AA = anaplastic astrocytoma; GBM = glioblastoma multiforme; IOERT = intraoperative radiation therapy with electron beam; EBRT = external beam radiation therapy; AE = anaplastic ependymoma; AO = anaplastic oligodendrogliomas.

[b] MTTP = median time to progression.

517

Unfortunately, even though the total irradiation dose is increased by incorporating IOERT, relapses continue to occur close to the primary site, either immediately outside the IOERT field or "in" the irradiated volume. Rates of disease-free survival continue to be unsatisfactory. Although Matsutani et al. *(14)* noted that 87% of patients were free of tumor for more than 1 year after completion of protocol treatment, other series note less optimistic results. Willich et al. at the University of Münster *(15)* related a 1- and 2-year recurrence-free survival of 44.3% and 10.1%, respectively, in a group of patients with primary high-grade malignant glioma, whereas Ortiz de Urbina at San Francisco de Asís Hospital (updated data) showed a recurrence-free survival at 1- and 2-years of 45.6% and 33.3%, respectively, in patients with both primary or recurrent malignant glioma. In the Japanese group, Sakai et al. *(28)* shows 63.3% 1-year recurrence-free survival.

4.4. IOERT for Recurrent Disease

Other than chemotherapy programs, there have been few reports concerning local retreatment of recurrent glioma after previous EBRT. The high risk of brain necrosis excludes the possibility of achieving radical doses in a second EBRT course.

IOERT has been explored as an alternative modality treatment in such cases *(25,27)*. Seventeen patients with recurrent glioblastomas were selected for IOERT at the University of Tokyo, receiving a mean dose of 17 Gy (range 10–25 Gy), and the median time from recurrence to death was 36 weeks *(14)*. Shibamoto et al. *(27)* found a median survival time of 12 months for nine patients with recurrent GBM and AA and 51 months for eight patients with less infiltrative tumors (ependymoma or anaplastic oligodendroglioma). In 11 patients with recurrent grade III glioma treated with IOERT at the University of Münster *(15)*, the 1-year survival probability observed was 67.1%.

According to the experience at San Francisco de Asís Hospital, a 1- and 2-year survival time of 58% and 37%, respectively, has been observed in recurrent brain tumors, including different histological diagnosis; 12 out of 30 patients with recurrent intracranial tumors were alive at the time of the analysis, and the median survival time of 15.5 months (range 4–80 months) has ben documented. Particularly considering the group of patients with recurrent GBM or AA, the median survival time was 11.5 months with a 1-year survival of 43.3%.

An additional issue to be considered is that the clinical outcome appears to have improved as a result of both a relief of intracranial pressure by the surgical decompression and debulking and the radiotherapeutic approach. As noted by Willich et al. *(15)*, there was an improvement in Karnofsky performance status from 70% prior to surgery and IOERT to 80% thereafter.

4.5. IOERT Tolerance

The incidence of postoperative complications after IOERT do not increase when compared to that reported for surgery alone *(34,35)*. This observation has been confirmed by the experience of the different groups included in the present chapter. Severe or life-threatening toxicity related to the IOERT is rarely observed when moderate doses not in excess of 20–25 Gy are delivered to small fields. Only anecdotal deaths directly related to the procedure have been described.

5. CONCLUSIONS

It can be concluded that IOERT is an attractive, tolerable, and feasible treatment modality as an antitumoral intensification procedure in intracranial malignant tumors.

The published experiences by several institutions throughout the world suggest that IOERT is an effective complement to surgery and conventional EBRT in the loco-regional management of these kind of tumors. Available data compare favorably with the historical controls, without an increase in side effects.

Further research in IOERT must investigate questions such as the optimum dose, the combination of radiosensitizers, or oxygenomimetic agents to modulate the biological response of the tumor to radiation, the precision intraoperatively to define the target tumor volume, the way to optimize the dose distribution into the tumor by a correct treatment planification, and the accuracy in the delivery of the prescribed dose during the procedure. Prospective cooperative clinical trials would be helpful to investigate the potential benefit of IOERT in an homogeneus group of patients with high-grade malignant glioma in order to draw definitive conclusions. Whether such trials are feasible is an intriguing question.

REFERENCES

1. Leibel SA, Scott CB, and Pajak TF. The management of malignant gliomas with radiation therapy: therapeutic results and research strategies, *Semin. Radiat. Oncol.,* **1** (1991) 32–49.
2. Nelson DF, Diener-West M, Horton J, Chang Ch, Shoenfeld D, and Nelson JS. Combined modality approach to treatment of malignant gliomas. Re-evaluation of RTOG 7401/ECOG 1347 with long-term follow-up: a joint Radiation Therapy Oncology Group and eastern Cooperative Oncology Group study, *Natl. Cancer. Inst. Monogr.,* **6** (1988) 279–284.
3. Wallner KE, Galicich JH, Krol G, Arbit E, and Malkin MG. Patterns of failure following treatment for glioblastoma multiforme and anaplastic astrocytoma, *Int. J. Radiat. Oncol. Biol. Phys.,* **16** (1989) 1405–1409.
4. Leibel SA, Scott CB, and Loeffler JS. Contemporary approaches to the treatment of malignant gliomas with radiation therapy, *Semin. Oncol.,* **21** (1994) 198–219.
5. Medical Research Council Brain Tumor Working Party, A medical research council trial of two radiotherapy doses in the treatment of grades 3 and 4 astrocytoma, *Br. J. Cancer,* **64** (1991) 769–774.
6. Walker MD, Strike TA, and Sheline GE. An analysis of dose-effective relationship in the radiotherapy of malignant gliomas, *Int. J. Radiat. Oncol. Biol. Phys.,* **5** (1979) 1725–1731.
7. Marks JE, Baglan RJ, Prassad SC, and Blank WF. Cerebral radionecrosis: Incidence and risk in relation to dose, time, fractionation and volume, *Int. J. Radiat. Oncol. Biol. Phys.,* **7** (1981) 243–252.
8. Walker MD, Alexander E, Hunt WE, MacCarty CS, et al. Evaluation of BCNU and/or radiotherapy in the treatment of anaplastic gliomas. A cooperative clinical trial, *J. Neurosurg.,* **49** (1978) 333–343.
9. Abe M, Fukuda M, Yamano K, Matsuda S, and Handa H. Intraoperative irradiation in abdominal and cerebral tumours, *Acta Radiol.,* **10** (1971) 408–416.
10. Goldson AL, Streeter OE, Ashayeri E, Collier-Manning J, Barber JB, Fan and K-J. Intraoperative Radiotherapy for Intracranial Malignancies, *Cancer,* **54** (1984) 2807–2813.
11. Dyke CG and Davidoff KM. *Roentgen Treatment of Disease of the Nervous System.* Philadelphia: Lea and Febiger; pp. 111–12, 1942.
12. Calvo FA, Abuchaibe O, Vanaclocha V, and Aguilera F. *Intracranial Tumors in Intraoperative Radiotherapy: Clinical Experiences and Results* (Felipe A. Calvo, Manuel Santos, and Luther W. Brady, eds.), Springer-Verlag, Berlín Heidelberg, Germany, pp. 31–6, 1992.
13. Yanagawa S, Doi H, Sakai N, and Yamada H. (1989), Intraoperative radiation therapy (IORT) of malignant gliomas, *Strahlenther. Onkol.,* **165** (1981) 781.
14. Matsutani M, Nakamura O, Nagashima T, Asai A, et al. Intraoperative radiation therapy for malignant brain tumors: rationale, method, and treatment results of cerebral glioblastomas, *Acta. Neurochir. (Wien),* **131** (1994) 80–90.
15. Willich N, Palkovic S, Prott FJ, Morgenroth C, Heidgert S, and Wassmann H. IORT for malignant brain tumors. In Intraoperative Radiation Therapy in the Treatment of Cancer (Vaeth JM, ed.), *Front. Radiat. Ther. Oncol.,* **31** (1997) 93–96.
16. Wood JR, Green SB, and Shapiro WR. The prognostic importance of tumor size in malignant gliomas: a computed tomographic scan study by the Brain Tumor Cooperative Group, *J. Clin. Oncol.,* **6** (1988) 338–343.

17. Ammirati M, Vick N, Liao Y, Ciric Y, and Mickhael M. Effect of the extent of surgical resection on survival and quality of life in patients with supratentorial glioblastomas and anaplastic astrocytomas, *Neurosurgery,* **21** (1987) 201–206.

18. Quigley MR and Maroon JC. The relationship between survival and the extent of the resection in patients with supratentorial malignant gliomas, *Neurosurgery,* **29** (1991) 385–389.

19. Berger MS. Malignant astrocytomas: surgical aspects, *Semin. Oncol.,* **21** (1994) 172–185.

20. Lesser GJ and Grossman S. The Chemotherapy of High-Grade Astrocytomas, *Semin. Oncol.,* **21** (1994) 220–235.

21. Suit HD, Baumann M, and Skates S. Clinical interest in determinations of cellular radiation sensitivity, *Int. J. Radiat. Biol.,* **56** (1989) 725–737.

22. Leibel SA and Sheline GE. Tolerance of the brain and spinal cord to conventional therapeutic irradiation: radiation injury to the nervous system, (Gutin PH, Leibel SA, and Sheline GE, eds.), New York, NY, Raven, pp. 239–56, 1991.

23. Scharfen CO, Snee PK, Wara WM, Larson DA, et al. High activity iodine-125 interstitial implant for gliomas, *Int. J. Radiat. Oncol. Biol. Phys.,* **24** (1992) 583–591.

24. Loeffler JS, Alexander III E, Shea M, Wen PY, et al. Radiosurgery as part of the initial management of patients with malignant gliomas, *J. Clin. Oncol.,* **10** (1992) 1379–1385.

25. Ortiz de Urbina D, Santos M, García Berrocal I, Bustos JC, et al. Intraoperative radiation therapy in malignant glioma: early clinical results, *Neurol. Res.,* **17** (1995) 289–294.

26. Fujiwara T, Homna Y, Ogawa T, Irie K, et al. Intraoperative radiotherapy for gliomas, *Neurooncol,* **23** (1995) 81–86.

27. Shibamoto Y, Yamashita J, Takahashi M, and Abe M. Intraoperative radiation therapy for brain tumors with emphasis on retreatment for recurrence following full-dose external beam irradiation, *Am. J. Clin. Oncol. (CCT),* **17** (1994) 396–399.

28. Sakai N, Yamada H, Andoh T, Nishimura Y, and Yanagawa S. Brain Tumors, in Intraoperative Radiation Therapy (Schildberg FW, Willich N, and Krämling HJ, eds.). Fourth International Symposium IORT. Verlag, Munich, pp. 172–7, 1992.

29. Kaplan EL and Meier P. Non-parametric estimation from incomplete observation, *J. Am. Stat. Assoc.,* **53** (1958) 457–481.

30. Gouda JJ, Brown JA, Carter D, and Dobelbower RR. Malignant brain tumors treated with IORT, in Intraoperative Radiation Therapy in the Treatment of Cancer (Vaeth J, ed.), *Front. Radiat. Ther. Oncol.,* **31** (1997) 87–91.

31. Kinsela TJ, DeLuca AM, Barnes M, Anderson W, Terrill R, and Sindelar WF. Threshold dose for peripheral neuropathy following intraoperative radiotherapy (IORT) in a large animal model, *Int. J. Radiat. Oncol. Biol. Phys.,* **20** (1991) 697–701.

32. Vujaskovic Z, Gillette SM, Powers BE, Larue SM, et al. Intraoperative radiation (IORT) injury to sciatic nerve in a large animal model, *Radiother. Oncol.,* **30** (1994) 133–139.

33. Funata N, Tanaka Y, and Matsutani M. Histopathology of radiation injury of the brain with special reference to intraoperative radiotherapy-induced changes: Intraoperative radiation therapy (Abe M, eds.), Pergamon, New York, pp. 401–2, 1991.

34. Blomstedt GC. Infections in neurosurgery: a retrospective study of 1143 patients and 1517 operations, *Acta. Neurochir.,* **78** (1985) 81–90.

35. Gaillard T and Gilsbach JM. Intra-operative antibiotic prophylaxis in neurosurgery: a prospective, randomized, controlled study on cefotiam, *Acta. Neurochir.,* **113** (1991) 101–109.

28 IORT for Breast Cancer

Joyce A. Battle, Jean-Bernard DuBois,
Hollis W. Merrick, and Ralph R. Dobelbower, Jr.

CONTENTS

1. INTRODUCTION

Over the past 50 years, there has been a steady increase in the reported incidence of female breast cancer. This has been due partly to causative factors such as environmental chemicals and diet, and partly to the more widespread use of mammography, which, since the 1980s, has proven particularly useful in the detection of early breast cancers.

Breast cancer is the most common neoplasm in women worldwide; in the United States, it accounts for approximately 30% of new cancer cases among women (1–3). The U.S. breast cancer death rates have declined over the past 10 years, which again may be a result of early detection as well as improved treatment methods (2,4). Despite this, breast cancer remains the second leading cause of cancer deaths in females in the United States, and projected figures indicate that approximately 44,190 deaths and 181,600 new cases of breast cancer will occur in 1997 (2).

2. RATIONALE FOR IORT IN BREAST CANCER TREATMENT

Early detection of breast cancer often allows the patient and her physicians to consider therapeutic options that are not available in the later stages of the disease. One of these options is breast-conserving treatment, which consists of limited excision of breast tissue (i.e., lumpectomy, segmental mastectomy, quadrantectomy), axillary lymph node resection, and a follow-up course of external beam radiation therapy (EBRT). When compared with total mastectomy, breast-conserving therapy has been demonstrated to provide the physical and psychological benefits of good cosmesis without compromising tumor control or survival (5–7).

From: *Current Clinical Oncology: Intraoperative Irradiation: Techniques and Results*
Edited by: L. L. Gunderson et al. © Humana Press, Inc., Totowa, NJ

Table 1
Histology

Tumor Type	No. of Patients
Infiltrating ductal	60
Infiltrating lobular	7
Mucinous	3
Medullary	1
Ductal carcinoma *in situ*	1
Total	72

The advent of intraoperative radiation therapy (IORT) brought an additional weapon to the battle against cancer. Since its introduction in the 1960s in Japan and in the 1970s in the United States, IORT has been employed in the treatment of deep-seated tumors of the pelvis, abdomen, and brain. The theory behind IORT is easily understood: Higher radiation doses can be given directly to the tumor bed, providing a tumoricidal dose while sparing adjacent radiosensitive organs, nerves, and other normal tissues such as the skin.

However, although multiple centers began to report their results of using IORT for treatment of cancers of the pancreas, stomach, colon, rectum, and central nervous system, this promising modality was virtually ignored as an option in breast cancer treatment. As recently as 1990, there were no papers on IORT for breast cancer presented at the biennial International Symposium on Intraoperative Radiation Therapy. During the 1990s, however, several centers began to demonstrate that IORT, in combination with breast-conserving surgery and conventional EBRT, could be a formidable addition to the anticancer arsenal. The rationale behind these pilot studies was that smaller boost volumes, with skin and subcutaneous tissues excluded, could result in better cosmesis and less fibrotic change without compromising treatment efficacy.

3. THE MEDICAL COLLEGE OF OHIO AND MONTPELLIER IORT SERIES

The Medical College of Ohio (MCO) (Toledo, OH, U.S.A.) and the Centre Regional de Lutte Contre le Cancer (CRLC) (Montpellier, France) each have reported their retrospective analyses of breast cancer patients treated with conservative surgery and IORT followed by EBRT *(6,8)*. In this combined series, 72 patients between the ages of 33 and 81 were followed for a period of up to 12 years (minimum follow-up period: 2 years). Each patient had biopsy-proven carcinoma (Table 1) which had been discovered at an early stage (Table 2).

3.1. Treatment Methods

3.1.1. SURGERY

At the time of surgery, lumpectomy was performed to remove the tumor, utilizing frozen sections to ensure that there was a satisfactory tumor-free margin. Axillary lymph node dissection was performed during the procedure on all patients.

3.1.2. IORT

Intraoperative irradiation (IORT) was delivered to the tumor bed. In order to ensure that the entire tumor bed was encompassed by the IORT field, the mammary parenchyma

Table 2
Staging

Tumor Stage[a]	No. of Patients
Stage I (T_1N_0)	31
Stage IIA (T_1N_1 or T_2N_0)	32
Stage IIB (T_2N_1)	9
Total	72

[a]According to criteria established by the American Joint Committee on Cancer (AJCC).

was loosely sutured so that the lateral margins were brought into apposition, as illustrated in Figs. 1 and 2. The applicator was then positioned to encompass the entire tumor bed, preferably with a 1-cm margin.

The MCO and CRLC IORT devices have been described elsewhere (9,10). Both are hard-docking devices that provide excellent dose localization.

The tumor beds were completely encompassed by 1- to 3-in. circular fields using flat-ended applicators, generally at a 100-cm focus-surface distance. Doses of 10 Gy (69 patients) or 15 Gy (3 patients) were delivered using 6- to 20-MeV electron beams. At the CRLC, the electron beam energy was 6 MeV in every case. At the MCO, the electron beam energy was varied in accordance with the measured thickness of the breast tissue at the site of the lumpectomy wound. The radiation dose was specified at the depth of maximum dose in the MCO series and at the half-thickness of the 90% isodose in the CRLC series.

Following IORT, the retaining sutures were removed. The incision was then closed in the conventional fashion.

3.1.3. EBRT

All 72 patients received a course of conventional postoperative EBRT, beginning when primary healing was satisfactorily established. Treatment was delivered over 5–6 weeks for a total of 45–50 Gy in fractionated doses of 1.8 or 2.0 Gy. Most patients were treated with opposing (often noncoplanar) fields of 6-MV photons modified with wedge filters (15°–45°, as appropriate). When indicated, the regional lymphatics were also irradiated to similar doses.

3.2. Results of IORT Series

At both centers, patients were assessed for perioperative and postoperative complications, cosmesis, and local tumor control.

3.2.1. Tolerance

No significant complications associated with IORT were observed at either institution. The use of IORT added only 30–35 min to the total operating time, and none of the patients experienced any difficulties due to the additional exposure or anesthesia. Postoperative drainage, length of hospital stay, and interval until the onset of postoperative radiation therapy were not significantly different from patients who underwent lumpectomy without IORT. At CRLC, three patients, who were excluded from the study because they had received larger IORT doses, did experience lymphocele formation at

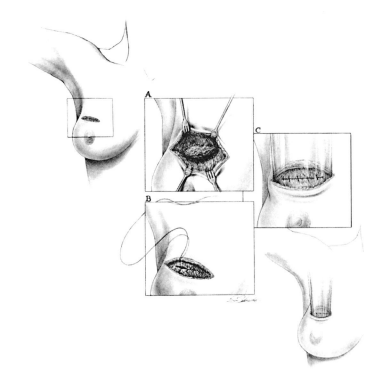

Fig. 1. The procedure of IORT for resected breast cancer is depicted. After an excisional biopsy has been performed, the margins of the breast tissue are loosely approximated by sutures to include them in the IORT field. The applicator is placed deep to the skin and the radiation is administered directly to the base and margins of the excision site.

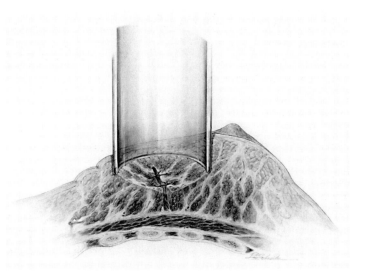

Fig. 2. Close-up view of the proper placement of the applicator in the breast biopsy site. The margins are shown approximated so that the IORT field can encompass the entire circumference of the tumor bed. This enables the margins and the base of the excision site to be treated simultaneously.

the drainage site of the lumpectomy; it was felt that this problem was due to the higher radiation dose, as no such complications were seen with doses of 10 Gy.

3.2.2. COSMESIS

Patients at both centers enjoyed excellent cosmetic results. The majority experienced no visible untoward sequelae of radiation therapy, such as cutaneous telangiectasia, cutaneous or subcutaneous sclerosis, visible tissue deformation or asymmetry, or pain. Eight of the 72 patients developed minor fibrosis at the lumpectomy site, which was palpable but not painful. In five of these eight patients, the induration disappeared within a few months; in the other three, cosmesis was affected but only mildly so. The patients themselves were uniformly pleased with the cosmetic results.

3.2.3. LOCAL CONTROL

Most importantly, none of the 72 patients in this combined series have experienced local tumor recurrence. This is especially significant when compared to studies of lumpectomy with postoperative external beam radiation therapy but without IORT, in which local recurrence rates of 10–15% have been reported (11–14). Because patients in these two IORT series had a minimum follow-up of 2 years, the lack of any local relapse to date is very encouraging.

These results may be partially due to patient selection, as only patients with stage I or stage II disease were deemed eligible for treatment by this method. However, 41 of the 72 patients in this series (57%) presented with stage II disease, with 9 of 72 (12.5%) at stage IIB; yet these patients achieved the same excellent local control as their stage I counterparts.

4. THE POTENTIAL ADVANTAGES OF IORT

Intraoperative radiation therapy in conjunction with breast-conserving surgery and postoperative external beam radiation therapy has demonstrated, to date, an impressive ability to prevent local recurrence in early breast cancer. The authors believe that much of the success of this modality is the result of the surgical and radiotherapeutic techniques employed at MCO and CRLC. As described earlier, the adaptations that were made to the standard lumpectomy procedure—in particular, the use of retaining sutures to draw the lateral aspects of the breast wound into the radiation field—facilitate accurate positioning of the applicator, thus ensuring that the entire tumor bed will receive a uniform radiation dose while greatly decreasing the possibility that some areas of the margins will be missed.

Delivery of the initial radiation dose through the surgical incision allows for a higher single dose than can be achieved with EBRT. Because the radiation may be aimed precisely at the tumor bed, there is less danger of radiation exposure to surrounding normal tissue. In addition, because this precise high dose is given at the time of surgery, the patient requires fewer postoperative EBRT treatments. This reduces radiation exposure to the skin, the lung, and normal subcutaneous tissues, which contributes to the low incidence of radiation-related sequelae and to the generally excellent cosmetic results. In addition, dosimetric studies have demonstrated that IORT provides a remarkably homogeneous dose distribution, rendering it superior to implanted radioisotopes (15,16).

5. CONCLUSIONS

The results obtained in the MCO/CRLC series are significant not only for their implications in the treatment of early breast cancer but for the future of IORT itself. As Hanks and Lanciano stated in their editorial in the *International Journal of Radiation Oncology,*

Biology and Physics (17), IORT has proven to be quite effective in controlling local disease in areas such as the gastrointestinal tract. However, when used for patients with a high risk of distant metastases and a lack of effective systemic therapy, such as pancreatic cancer, IORT does not significantly improve survival despite the improved local control. For IORT to achieve its greatest impact in patients with high systemic as well as local risks, effective systemic therapy must be added as a component of treatment. For a variety of reasons, large randomized clinical trials have been difficult to conduct, and most studies now underway involve retrospective or prospective case reviews by single institutions.

The effectiveness of IORT when combined with breast-conserving surgery and postoperative EBRT should therefore be regarded as encouraging, not only from the perspective of the treatment of breast cancer but as an indication of the next direction of IORT. When combined with carefully constructed surgical procedures and followed, where appropriate, with EBRT and effective chemotherapy, IORT has now been shown to have the ability to enhance survival and improve the quality of life for some patients with cancer.

Intraoperative irradiation as a single treatment modality is not "the cure." However, when used in conjunction with other modalities of treatment, IORT has the potential to be a valuable component in the fight against cancer.

REFERENCES

1. Azzena A, Zen T, Ferrara A, Brunetti V, Vasile C, and Marchetti M. Risk factors for breast cancer. Case-control study results, *Eur. J. Gynaecol. Oncol.*, **15** (1994) 386–392.
2. Parker SL, Tong T, Bolden S, and Wingo PA. Cancer statistics, 1997, *CA*, **47** (1997) 5–27.
3. Rozenberg S, Liebens F, Kroll M, and Vandromme J. Principal cancers among women: breast, lung and colorectal, *Int. J. Fertil. Menop. Stud.*, **41** (1996) 166–171.
4. Sondik EJ. Breast cancer trends: incidence, mortality, and survival, *Cancer*, **74(3 Suppl)** (1994) 995–999.
5. Fisher B and Anderson S. Conservative surgery for the management of invasive and noninvasive carcinoma of the breast: NSABP trials. National Surgical Adjuvant Breast and Bowel Project, *World J. Surg.*, **18** (1994) 63–69.
6. Hiraoka M and Abe M. Breast conservation treatment for breast cancer, *Jpn. J. Cancer Chemother.*, **20** (1993) 2126–2132.
7. Morrow M, Harris JR, and Schnitt SJ. Local control following breast-conserving surgery for invasive cancer: results of clinical trials, *J. Natl. Cancer Inst.*, **87** (1995) 1669–1673.
8. Merrick HW, Battle JA, Padgett BJ, and Dobelbower RR. IORT for early breast cancer: a report on long-term results, *Front. Radiat. Ther. Oncol.*, **31** (1997) 126–130.
9. Bagne FR. Physical aspects and dosimetric considerations for intraoperative radiation therapy with electron beams. In Dobelbower RR Jr. and Abe M (eds.), *Intraoperative Radiation Therapy*, CRC, Boca Raton, FL, 1987 pp. 35–58.
10. DuBois J-B, Hay M, Gely S, Saint-Aubert B, Rouanet P, and Pujol H. IORT in breast carcinomas, *Front. Radiat. Ther. Oncol.*, **31** (1997) 131–137.
11. DiPaola RS, Orel SG, and Fowble BL. Ipsilateral breast tumor recurrence following conservative surgery and radiation therapy, *Oncology*, **8** (1994) 59–68.
12. Fisher B and Redmond C. Lumpectomy for breast cancer: an update of the NSABP experience, *Monogr. Natl. Cancer Inst.*, **11** (1992) 7–13.
13. Mansfield CM, Komarnicky LT, Schwartz GF, et al. Ten-year results in 1070 patients with stages I and II breast cancer treated by conservative surgery and radiation therapy, *Cancer*, **75** (1995) 2328–2336.
14. Margolese RG. Recent trends in the management of breast cancer. 4. Diagnosis and management of local recurrence after breast-conservation surgery, *Can. J. Surg.*, **35** (1992) 378–381.
15. Beteille D, Vignolo C, Muraro S, et al. Laser heating of thermoluminescent plates: application to intraoperative irradiation measurements, *Radiother. Oncol.*, **37** (1995) 250.
16. Mansfield CM. Intraoperative Ir 192 implantation for early breast cancer, *Cancer*, **66** (1990) 1–5.
17. Hanks GE and Lanciano RM. Intraoperative radiation therapy: cut bait or keep on fishing?, *Int. J. Radiat. Oncol. Biol. Phys.*, **34** (1996) 515–517.

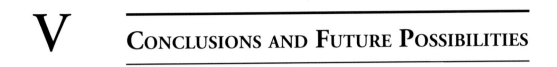

V CONCLUSIONS AND FUTURE POSSIBILITIES

29 Conclusions and Future Possibilities—IORT

Leonard L. Gunderson, Christopher G. Willett, Felipe A. Calvo, and Louis B. Harrison

CONTENTS

PATIENT SELECTION, MULTISPECIALTY TREATMENT APPROACHES
NEW TECHNOLOGY AND DEDICATED FACILITIES
LOCAL CONTROL VERSUS PERIPHERAL NEUROPATHY ISSUES
DISTANT CONTROL
TREATMENT TOLERANCE
REFERENCES

Experience thus far has demonstrated that variable combinations of external beam irradiation (EBRT), intraoperative irradiation (IORT) with electrons (IOERT) or high dose rate brachytherapy (HDR-IORT) and surgical resection are feasible and practical in settings where close interdisciplinary cooperation exists, and that these aggressive approaches appear to impact local control with and without survival. With primary colorectal cancers that are unresectable for cure or for locally recurrent colorectal cancers, both local control and long-term survival appear to be improved with the aggressive combinations including IORT when compared with results achieved with conventional treatments. These findings are consistent from various institutions and countries (MGH, Mayo, Pamplona, Japan; *see* Chapters 14–16). When residual disease exists after resection of gastric cancers, IOERT with or without external radiation has achieved encouraging survival results (Chapter 11). Excellent local control and long-term survival have been achieved with abdominal and pelvic soft tissue sarcomas with IORT-containing treatment approaches for both primary and recurrent lesions (Chapters 18 and 19). In the randomized National Cancer Institute trial, improved local control was achieved with lower small-bowel morbidity with IOERT plus EBRT versus EBRT alone in patients with marginally resected primary retroperitoneal sarcomas. Mayo Clinic investigators have reported excellent results for locally recurrent as well as locally advanced primary abdominal and pelvic sarcomas. Long-term salvage of approximately 30% has also been achieved with IORT-containing treatment approaches for locally recurrent gynecologic and renal malignancies (Chapters 22 and 23, respectively). With locally unresectable pancreatic cancer, an apparent improvement in local control has been noted with IOERT

From: *Current Clinical Oncology: Intraoperative Irradiation: Techniques and Results*
Edited by: L. L. Gunderson et al. © Humana Press, Inc., Totowa, NJ

plus EBRT, but survival has not been altered because of a high incidence of abdominal failure, both liver and peritoneal (Chapter 12). In the treatment of pediatric malignancies with IOERT or HDR–IORT, single-institution reports reveal excellent local control and survival (Chapter 26). In lung cancer management, IOERT has reported promising local control rates when integrated in the multidisciplinary treatment of Pancoast tumors (boosting a tumor bed chest wall region after preoperative chemoradiation plus resection), or in parenchymal lesions with or without mediastinal involvement (Chapter 24). Extremity soft tissue sarcomas are technically simple to treat with IORT (either IOERT or HDR–IORT) with attractive results in terms of cosmesis, function, and limb preservation rates (Chapter 20). IORT in the context of multimodal treatment for bladder cancer has proven to be able to sterilize transitional cell carcinoma and should be evaluated more extensively as an addition to chemo-EBRT for bladder preservation (Chapter 23). IORT is also being evaluated in other sites, including bone sarcomas, marginally resected or locally recurrent head and neck cancers, and selected CNS and breast cancers (Chapters 21, 25, 27, and 28, respectively).

1. PATIENT SELECTION, MULTISPECIALTY TREATMENT APPROACHES

Optimization of results with IORT treatment approaches will continue to be dependent on proper patients selection as well as appropriate multispecialty treatment (facilities and equipment; aggressive skilled team of multispecialty physicians—surgeon(s), radiation oncologist, and medical oncologist). Previously untreated patients remain the best overall candidates for the aggressive IORT-containing treatment approaches discussed in this book, as optimal combinations of EBRT (with and without sensitizers), resection, IORT (with and without dose modifiers), and systemic therapy can be used as planned sequential treatment to optimize both local and distant control of disease.

The best long-term results will be achieved in patients without evidence of distant metastases at time of treatment and in whom good systemic treatment options can be given to high-risk patients in planned sequential fashion. Use of adequate pretreatment staging evaluations is necessary before subjecting patients to the potential risks of the locally aggressive techniques discussed in this book. More frequent use of laparoscopy, chest and abdominal computed tomographies (CTs), and newer imaging techniques including positron emission tomography (PET)-scanning and tumor-specific antibody studies would be desirable after preoperative EBRT (with and without chemo) and prior to exploration, resection, and IORT.

In the future, an area of conceptual interest is the systematic evaluation of IORT for the management of tumor sites and stages in which adjuvant or neoadjuvant EBRT has proven to be a mandatory treatment component. This means the evaluation of "adjuvant IORT," in the strict understanding of the concept (treatment of an anatomical region at high risk for local recurrence following resection with negative but narrow margins). In some of these settings, the use of IORT may allow a decrease in the dose of EBRT with an improvement in the overall therapeutic ratio. This may optimize further the benefits in terms of improvements in the therapeutic index seen when using IORT plus EBRT with and without chemo for known residual disease after maximal resection. Several European groups have already activated clinical trials, including IORT as a component of the adjuvant loco-regional irradiation segment of treatment (1–3). Preliminary results are excellent in every parameter analyzed, and locally advanced primary rectal cancer is the disease model most frequently selected to date for such pilot studies.

2. NEW TECHNOLOGY AND DEDICATED FACILITIES

Some of the technical problems and nuisance aspects of IORT, encountered in the 1980s and early 1990s, can be overcome with dedicated or semidedicated IOERT or HDR-IORT facilities. This can be built as an operating room (OR) in the Radiation Oncology Department as done for IOERT at the National Cancer Institute (NCI), Medical College of Ohio, Thomas Jefferson University, Howard University, and others, and as done at Memorial Sloan-Kettering Cancer Center (MSKCC), Georgetown, and Beth Israel–New York for HDR-IORT. The most ideal situation is to place an IORT facility within or near the OR suite, which has been done at the Mayo Clinic, Massachusetts General Hospital (MGH), M. D. Anderson Cancer Center (MDACC), Ohio State, Beth Israel—New York, and some European institutions. Either approach simplifies the treatment of patients, necessitates fewer reoperations (refused by some patients and physicians), and avoids transportation and sterility problems. It also prevents the need to shut down the outpatient treatment machine for a "potential" case. However, the dedicated IOERT option in an OR setting is quite expensive if an existing OR has to be retrofitted for proper shielding and a new linear accelerator has to be purchased as the electron source.

New technologies should improve the availability of IORT from the perspective of cost-effective alternatives. These technologies include mobile HDR units, as being used at MSKCC and other institutions for HDR–IORT, and mobile IOERT machines [Mobetron (4) and NOVAC-7 (5)]. For the mobile HDR machine, a shielded facility is necessary in either the OR area or in the Radiation Oncology Department. Instead of shielding an entire OR room, however, technology now exists to create a shielded box (room within a room) into which the patient can be placed for the HDR–IORT component of treatment after surgical resection, and placement of the Harrison-Anderson-Mick (HAM) applicator has been accomplished. However, many existing ORs are small and may not be able to accommodate the increasing complexity of such procedures. The Mobetron IOERT unit has built-in shielding in a C-arm design (Fig. 1) and could theoretically be moved from one operating room to another, if indicated. The Mobetron is a magnetron-driven X-band accelerator with electron energies of 4–12 MeV and 90% depth doses of 1.0–4.0 cm. If large IOERT fields are necessary, as for retroperitoneal sarcomas, such cases may need to be performed in an operating room with limited shielding in the floor to allow use of larger IOERT applicators. An alternative mobile IOERT option recently described is the NOVAC-7, which is a prototype device made of a miniature linear accelerator initially installed in a fixed robotic arm (2). The electron energy capability is more limited than the Mobetron unit, with the highest energy in the range of 7–10 MeV. The most recent version of NOVAC-7 is fully transportable. The potential technical limitations of the mobile IOERT machines are uncertain in view of their recent development.

The existence of both dedicated facilities and new technologies increases the likelihood of evaluating IORT in combination with "curative resection" and reduced dose EBRT with and without chemotherapy in adjuvant disease settings where adjuvant EBRT doses necessary to achieve local control approach or exceed an acceptable level of normal tissue tolerance. An excellent example of this philosophy was the randomized NCI

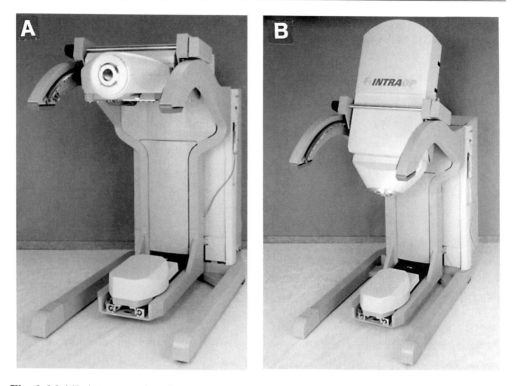

Fig. 1. Mobile intraoperative electron treatment system (Mobetron) with compact beam stopper allows use in an existing operating room with little or no additional shielding required: (**A**) Mobetron in transportation configuration; (**B**) Mobetron in treatment configuration. (With permission from Gunderson LL et al., Seminars in Oncology, **24** [1997] 715–731.)

abdominal sarcoma trial in which adjuvant-type doses of EBRT resulted in excessive small-bowel morbidity in addition to poor local control, but the combination of IOERT with lower-dose EBRT resulted in excellent local control and a low incidence of small-bowel morbidity. For lesions of various histologies in which marginal resection with narrow or microscopically positive margins has been accomplished, the use of moderate-dose EBRT (45 Gy in 25 fractions of 1.8 Gy over 5 weeks) plus IORT of 10–12.5 Gy may be preferable to high-dose EBRT of 60–65 Gy with regard to both local control and normal tissue morbidity.

3. LOCAL CONTROL VERSUS PERIPHERAL NEUROPATHY ISSUES

Acute and late morbidity and local disease control are thus far acceptable in patients who can be treated with curative intent utilizing a full component of adjuvant EBRT (with or without chemo), gross total resection, and IORT. That good local control results are being realized is not unexpected, as a substantially higher radiation dose can be delivered to the target tissue with combined EBRT–IORT approaches while the dose to the adjacent normal tissues is markedly less. Accordingly, there is a large "therapeutic gain." The history of radiation therapy shows that whenever higher radiation doses can be delivered with safety to the target volume, there is an improvement in local control with and without survival *(6)*.

Skilled surgeons must attempt to accomplish a gross total resection whenever that is safely feasible. This both improves the chance of long-term local control and decreases the risk of peripheral neuropathy in previously irradiated and unirradiated patients, as lower doses of IORT can be utilized in combination with EBRT for microscopic residual (or less) versus gross residual disease.

When a full component of EBRT (45–55 Gy in 1.8- to 2.0-Gy fractions with and without chemotherapy) can be given to *previously unirradiated patients,* the IORT dose can be limited to 10–12.5 Gy (prescription minimum dose) in patients with a gross total resection but marginally negative or microscopically positive margins. The chance for local control will be 85–90%, and the risk of grade 2 or 3 neuropathy is ≤5%.

In a *previously irradiated patient,* the EBRT dose usually has to be limited to 20–30 Gy in 10–15 fractions. If the surgeon can accomplish a gross total resection, an IORT dose of 15–17.5 Gy (prescription minimum dose) has a reasonable chance of achieving local control (≥50%) when combined with preoperative EBRT of 20–30 Gy plus infusion 5-FU or cisplatin, and the risk of grade 3 neuropathy may be as low as 5% *(7,8).* The risk of grade 3 neuropathy appears higher with IORT doses ≥20 Gy *(7–13)* but may be necessary with gross residual disease after maximal resection or in retreatment situations. When tumor-related risks are higher, as in the latter circumstances, the degree of treatment-related risk that both the patient and physician may be willing to undertake will clearly be higher, especially if a reasonable chance of tumor control exists.

3.1. Radiation Sensitizers and Dose Modifiers

When gross total resection cannot be accomplished, in-field disease control is not optimal. Evaluation of dose modifiers during both IORT (intraoperative hyperthermia, sensitizers) and EBRT dose delivery is warranted.

Intraoperative hyperthermia (IOHT) would be of interest to evaluate in close approximation to IORT in view of its known ability to sensitize hypoxic tumors to irradiation. However, animal studies at Colorado State University (CSU) have demonstrated that IOHT has an additive effect on peripheral nerve intolerance when combined with IOERT *(14),* and data suggest that the IORT dose should be ≤15 Gy when combined with IOHT. Feasibility pilot studies have been conducted at Mayo Clinic to evaluate ultrasound technology to deliver IOHT via the IOERT Lucite applicator using a water-filled insert (Fig. 2) *(15).* Clinical phase I/II studies are in the development phase in which previously irradiated patients who develop subsequent local recurrence will be treated with limited-dose EBRT with and without chemotherapy, maximal resection, and IOERT plus IOHT.

Patients with locally advanced cancers in whom local regional failure is a common pattern of relapse represent an excellent setting for testing *hypoxic cell sensitizers* in combination with the best currently available modalities (surgery, EBRT plus concomitant chemo, IORT, possible maintenance chemotherapy). IORT is an ideal model for addressing hypoxic cell radioresistance, as using a large single dose of radiation does not allow reoxygenation to occur. At least part of the local failure rate in large or recurrent tumors at any site may be due to hypoxia. The 2-nitroimidazoles, such as etanidazole, have been studied in conjunction with radiation therapy to sensitive hypoxic cells to irradiation, because up to several logs more cells are killed for the same dose of radiation in the presence of normal oxygen levels as compared to hypoxic conditions. The degree of radiosensitization depends on the concentration of sensitizer in the tumor at the time of irradiation *(16).*

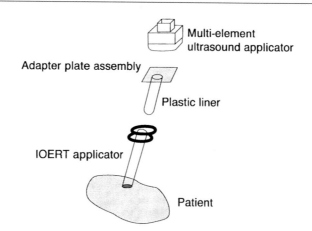

Fig. 2. Ultrasound-directed IOHT. An adaptor plate assembly positions the multielement ultrasound applicator above the IOERT Lucite applicator. The adaptor plate contains a plastic liner filled with sterile degassed water that is inserted into the IOERT applicator to transport ultrasound to induce therapeutic heating. (Reproduced from ref. *12.*)

In Radiation Therapy Oncology Group (RTOG) 89-06, 42 patients with locally advanced malignancies were entered in an escalating dose scheme for Etanidazole of 5.5, 7.5, 9, 10.5, and 12.0 g/m^2 *(17).* Etanidazole was given via intravenous infusion over 15 min, followed within 20–30 min by IOERT. Multiple tissue samples from tumor, tumor bed, and/or normal tissue were obtained with simultaneous plasma samples. Etanidazole concentrations in tissue and serum were determined in 33 of the 42 patients. The median time to maximum serum concentration was 25 min. Median time to maximum tissue concentration was 40 min. Tissue concentrations began falling approximately 1 h after infusion. Acute drug toxicities were minimal up to the maximum chosen target dose of 12 g/m^2. Toxicities reported during follow-up appeared to be related to surgery and/or irradiation, not to drug. The concentration of sensitizer in tumor/tumor bed tissues with the 12-g/m^2 dose level (988 μg/mL mean tissue concentration and 430 μg/mL median) was 10-fold greater than in a previous trial at the dose level of 2 g/m^2 of Etanidazole. A sensitizer enhancement ratio for the hypoxic cell of 2 to 2.5 was projected. On the basis of tissue biopsy information, IORT should be given ~40 min after the start of a 15-min infusion, allowing time for maximum intracellular uptake into tumor cells. The tolerable single-dose level of 12 g/m^2 has potential with other high-dose radiation settings such as brachytherapy or stereotactic radiosurgery.

RTOG attempted to test the addition of Etanidazole to standard treatment for locally advanced recurrent colorectal cancers in randomized phase III trials. The number of IORT institutions within RTOG was insufficient to successfully meet accrual objectives and the study was closed. For such trials to be successfully accomplished, international cooperation will be necessary. The International Society of IORT (ISIORT) has interest in ultimately conducting phase II and randomized phase III trials testing issues of importance to IORT institutions (IOERT and HDR-IORT).

4. DISTANT CONTROL

With most locally advanced primary or recurrent malignancies, distant metastases continue to be a major issue, especially in patients with high-grade lesions. Incorporation

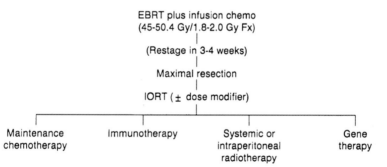

A: Multimodality IORT schema – chemosensitive tumors; low-risk distant metastases

EBRT plus infusion chemo
(45-50.4 Gy/1.8-2.0 Gy Fx)
|
(Restage in 3-4 weeks)
|
Maximal resection
|
IORT ± dose modifier
|
Maintenance chemo (multidrug)

B: Multimodality IORT schema – chemosensitive tumors; high-risk distant metastases

2-3 cycles multidrug chemotherapy
|
(2-5 week rest)
|
EBRT plus infusion chemotherapy
(45-50.4 Gy/1.8-2.0 Gy Fx)
|
(Restage in 3-4 weeks)
|
Maximal resection
|
IORT ± dose modifier
|
Maintenance chemo (multidrug)

C: Multimodality IORT regimen – chemosensitivity uncertain

EBRT plus infusion chemo
(45-50.4 Gy/1.8-2.0 Gy Fx)
|
(Restage in 3-4 weeks)
|
Maximal resection
|
IORT (± dose modifier)

| Maintenance chemotherapy | Immunotherapy | Systemic or intraperitoneal radiotherapy | Gene therapy |

Fig. 3. Potential investigational IORT schemas based on chemosensitivity of disease site and risk of distant metastasis (IORT = intraoperative irradiation, EBRT = external beam irradiation, chemo = chemotherapy). (**A**) Chemosensitive tumor—low-risk distant metastasis (DM); (**B**) chemosensitive tumor—high-risk DM; (**C**) chemosensitivity uncertain. (With permission from Gunderson LL et al., Seminars in Oncology, **24** [1997] 715–731.)

of systemic therapy into locally aggressive treatment regimens will be necessary in order to maximize disease control and survival. Such strategies will differ for chemosensitive versus chemo-uncertain malignancies (Fig. 3). Systemic strategies by disease site were discussed within the chapters on disease site results and future possibilities. These may need to be tested in randomized phase III international studies. Although distant disease control improvement is an important issue, we should not lose sight of the importance of local control, even for tumor systems in which better local control does not necessarily result in improved survival.

5. TREATMENT TOLERANCE

In situations where IORT doses of 15–20 Gy need to be utilized in proximity to a peripheral nerve, randomized studies are indicated to evaluate radioprotectors with and without fractionated IORT. In in vivo studies, pretreatment with the radioprotector amifostine (WR 2721) has demonstrated protection of a variety of normal tissues, including bone marrow stem cells, dorsal root ganglion and intestinal cells, and renal, lung, and liver tissue *(18,19)*. In both phase II *(20,21)* and phase III clinical studies *(22)*, amifostine has also demonstrated the ability to reduce cisplatin-induced neurotoxicity with no evidence of simultaneous tumor protection. In view of the IOERT dose limitations of peripheral nerve and an increase in neuropathy as a function of IORT dose, an evaluation of IOERT with and without amifostine is indicated. Although the amifostine daily dose in fractionated EBRT pilot studies has been 300–400 mg/m^2/day, chemotherapy studies have shown that single doses of 740–900 mg/m^2 can be given. Because a dose of 900 mg/m^2 produces more risk of hypotension, a dose of 740 mg/m^2 has been suggested as an IORT pretreatment dose (on the day of IORT ± the prior day) to be followed by several doses of 300–400 mg/m^2 in the early postop period. Phase II limited institution studies will be conducted under the aegis of the ISIORT group before proceeding with a randomized phase III study. In the phase II study, tissue and serum levels will be obtained to determine the ideal timing of amifostine prior to IORT.

Other strategies to be tested in clinical situations in which the planned IORT boost dose for gross residual is known to be related with increased severe toxicity include the following:

1. Design of presurgical treatment components (fractionated EBRT, chemoirradiation, induction chemotherapy followed by preoperative EBRT, etc.) to induce tumor downstaging and improved resectability. This increases the likelihood of a gross total resection and the ability to use IORT doses of 10–12.5 Gy instead of 15–20 Gy.
2. Incorporation of modern EBRT technology in IORT trials that allows safe escalation of total EBRT doses to limited target volumes. Such technology includes three-dimensional planning systems, high precision conformal therapy (multileaf collimation), and beam-intensity-modulated radiotherapy. These types of trials may permit a reduction in the IORT boost dose by increasing the dose within reduced EBRT fields beyond the normal adjuvant level of 45–50 Gy.
3. Interstitial permanent seed implant of gross residual disease in conjunction with an IORT dose of <20 Gy in an attempt to improve local control, by virtue of substantial dose escalation, with less risk of nerve intolerance.

An exceptional method of IORT dose escalation in recurrent-residual, unresectable, or previously treated EBRT patients that may need a single IORT dose of ≥15 Gy for a reasonable chance of local tumor control would be fractionated IORT doses of 7.5–10 Gy. Potential methods of accomplishing fractionated IORT would include the following: (1) Deliver the first IORT fraction before attempted resection and the second fraction after resection but just before surgical reconstruction (4- to 10-h interval) and (2) deliver first IORT fraction after resection and the second fraction at time of re-exposure of the target volume 24 h later and/or 1–4 weeks later (surgical use of a zipper system for initial closure of a wound when planned reoperation is indicated may facilitate the integration of fractionated IORT—*see* Fig. 4).

Results with fractionated IORT have never been reported, and the clinical feasibility is questionable. The described strategies may become acceptable options with progress

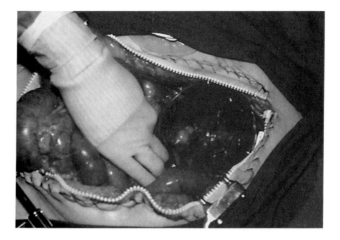

Fig. 4. Recurrent pelvic sarcoma surgically resected and incision temporarily closed with a zipper system for delayed IOERT treatment. Note the final position of the IOERT applicator in the pelvis and the small bowel being removed from the target volume.

in the surgical–anesthetic arena. Although Gillette et al. initiated animal studies to test fractionated IORT, grant funding was not sufficient to allow the animals to be followed to adequate intervals after treatment (E. Gillette, personal communication).

It should be remembered that these areas of investigation will require integrated teams of surgeons, radiation oncologists, medical oncologists, and physicists who are willing to push the therapeutic envelope. The teams will have to be skilled in all aspects of their craft and be willing to accept potentially higher treatment-related risks in the pursuit of improved outcomes. There will only be a handful of institutions in each country that have both the physician expertise and the facilities to explore these horizons. Increasing cooperation among these institutions is an important step in the direction of progress. To a large extent, this spirit of collaboration was the seed that both started the production of this text and encouraged the organization of the ISIORT.

REFERENCES

1. Azinovic I, Calvo FA, Santos M, et al. Intense local therapy in primary rectal cancer: multi-institutional results with preoperative chemoradiation plus IORT, *Front. Radiat. Ther. Oncol.,* **31** (1997) 196–199.
2. Eble MJ, Lehert TH, Herfarth CH, et al. IORT as adjuvant treatment in primary rectal carcinomas: multimodality treatment, *Front. Radiat. Ther. Oncol.,* **31** (1997) 200–203.
3. Valentini V, Cellini N, De Santis M, et al. Chemoradiation therapy and IORT in locally advanced rectal cancer: preliminary results in 36 patients, *Front. Radiat. Ther. Oncol.,* **31** (1997) 213–215.
4. Meurk ML, Goer DA, Spalek G, and Cock T. The Mobetron: a new concept for intraoperative radiotherapy. In Vaeth J and Meyer J (eds.), *The role of Intraoperative Radiation Therapy in the Treatment of Cancer,* S. Karger: Basel. *Front. Radiat. Ther. Oncol.,* **31** (1997) 65–70.
5. Fantini M, Santori F, Soriani A, Creton G, Banassi M, and Begnozzi L. IORT Novac 7 a linear accelerator for electron beam therapy (Abstract). 6th International Symposium of IORT. San Francisco, September 1996.
6. Suit H. Local control and patient survival, *Int. J. Radiat. Oncol. Biol. Phys.,* **23** (1992) 653–660.
7. Gunderson LL, Nelson H, Martenson JA, et al. Locally advanced primary colorectal cancer: intraoperative electron and external beam irradiation +/– 5-FU, *Int. J. Radiat. Oncol. Biol. Phys.,* **37** (1997) 601–614.
8. Gunderson LL, Nelson H, Martenson JA, et al. Intraoperative electron and external beam irradiation with or without 5-fluorouracil and maximum surgical resection for previously unirradiated, locally recurrent colorectal cancer, *Dis. Colon Rectum,* **39** (1996) 1379–1395.

9. Shaw EG, Gunderson LL, Martin JK, et al. Peripheral nerve and ureteral tolerance to intraoperative radiation therapy: clinical and dose-response analysis, *Radiother. Oncol.,* **18** (1990) 247–255.

10. Kinsella TJ, DeLuca AM, Barnes M, et al. Threshold dose for peripheral neuropathy following intraoperative radiotherapy (IORT) in a large animal model, *Int. J. Radiat. Oncol. Biol. Phys.,* **20** (1991) 697–701.

11. LeCouteur RA, Gillette EL, Powers EL, et al. Peripheral neuropathies following experimental intraoperative radiation therapy (IORT), *Int. J. Radiat. Oncol. Biol. Phys.,* **17** (1989) 583–590.

12. Gillette EL, Gillette SM, Vujaskovic Z, et al. Influence of volume on canine ureters and peripheral nerves irradiated intraoperatively. In Schildberg FW, Willich N, and Krämling H (eds.), *Intraoperative Radiation Therapy—Proceedings 4th International Iort Symposium,* Munich, 1992, Essen. Verlag Die Blaue Eule, pp. 61–63, 1993.

13. Kinsella TJ, Sindelar WF, DeLuca AM, et al. Tolerance of the canine bladder to intraoperative radiation therapy: an experimental study, *Int. J. Radiat. Oncol. Biol. Phys.,* **14** (1988) 939–946.

14. Vujaskovic Z, Gillette SM, Powers BE, et al. Effects of intraoperative irradiation (IORT) and intraoperative hyperthermia (IOHT) on peripheral nerve, *Int. J. Radiat. Oncol. Biol. Phys.,* **34** (1996) 125–131.

15. Bourland JD, Gunderson LL, Peterson IA, et al. Intraoperative hyperthermia via IORT electron applicator cones. In Schildberg FW, Willich N, and Kramling H (eds.), *Intraoperative Radiation Therapy,* Essen. Verlag Die Blaue Eule, (1993), pp. 411–414.

16. McNally NJ, Denekamp J, Sheldon P, et al. The importance of timing and tumor concentration of sensitizer, *Radiat. Res.,* **73** (1979) S68–80.

17. Halberg FE, Cosmatis D, Gunderson LL, et al. RTOG 89-06: a phase 1 study to evaluate intraoperative radiation therapy and the hypoxic cell sensitizer etanidazole in locally advanced malignancies, *Int. J. Radiat. Oncol. Biol. Phys.,* **28** (1993) 201–206.

18. Peters GJ and van der Vijgh WJF. Protection of normal tissue from the cytotoxic effects of chemotherapy and radiation by amifostine (WR-2721): preclinical aspects, *Eur. J. Cancer,* **31A (Suppl 1)** (1995) S1–S7.

19. Capizzi RL. The preclinical basis for broad-spectrum selective cytoprotection of normal tissues from cytotoxic therapies by amifostine (ethyol®), *Eur. J. Cancer,* **32A (Suppl 4)** (1996) S5–S16.

20. Glover DJ, Glick JH, Wecter C, et al. Phase I/II trials of WR-2721 and cisplatin, *Int. J. Radiat. Oncol. Biol. Phys.,* **12** (1986) 1509–1512.

21. Mollman JE, Glover DJ, Hogan WM, and Furman RE. Cisplatin neuropathy: risk factors, prognosis and protection by WR-2721, *Cancer,* **61** (1988) 2192–2195.

22. Kemp G, Rose P, Lurain J, et al. Amifostine pretreatment for protection against cyclophosphamide-induced and cisplatin-induced toxicities: results of a randomized control trial in patients with advanced ovarian cancer, *J. Clin. Oncol.,* **4** (1996) 2101–2112.

INDEX